CLINICAL INTEGRATION:

SURGERY

Student reviewers

Our medical textbooks are assessed and reviewed by the following medical students:

University of Aberdeen School of Medicine and Dentistry: Dylan McClurg
Barts and The London School of Medicine and Dentistry: Jay Singh
University of Birmingham College of Medical and Dental Sciences: Hannah Morgan
Cardiff University School of Medicine: Chloe Chia
The University of Edinburgh Medical School: Tanith Bain
University of Exeter Medical School: Zoe Foster
Hull York Medical School: Maalik Imtiaz
King's College London GKT School of Medical Education: Karan Sagoo
University of Liverpool School of Medicine: Sophie Gunter
University of Manchester Medical School: Holly Egan
Newcastle University School of Medical Education: Jenita Jona James
Norwich Medical School: Aneesa Khan
University of Nottingham School of Medicine: Tom Charles
University of Sheffield Medical School: Rebecca Nutt
St George's, University of London: Nawshin Basit
Swansea University Medical School: Jack Bartlett
University of Central Lancashire School of Medicine: Katie Chi Kei Cheung
University College London Medical School: Camila Nicklewicz

We are grateful for their essential feedback.

Additional student reviewers wanted

We are keen to recruit more student reviewers, particularly at UK medical schools where we don't currently have anyone in post. If you would like to apply for the position, please contact Simon Watkins (simon.watkins@scionpublishing.com) and explain why you would be suitable for the role.

Feedback, errors and omissions

We are always pleased to receive feedback (good and bad) about our books – if you would like to comment on any of our books, please email info@scionpublishing.com.

We've worked really hard with the authors to ensure that everything in the book is correct. However, errors and ambiguities can still slip through in books as complex as this. If you spot anything you think might be wrong, please email us and we will look into it straight away. If an error has occurred, we will correct it for future printings and post a note about it on our website so that other readers of the book are alerted to this.

Thank you for your help.

Hx Ex Ix Rx

CLINICAL INTEGRATION:
SURGERY

Edited by

Samuel Chee (MBBS (Hons))

Manda Raz (MBBS (Hons))

Asiri Arachchi (MBBS Dip Surg Anatomy FRACS (General Surgery))

Scion

© **Scion Publishing Ltd, 2021**

First published 2021

A CIP catalogue record for this book is available from the British Library.

ISBN 9781911510772

Scion Publishing Limited

The Old Hayloft, Vantage Business Park, Bloxham Road, Banbury OX16 9UX, UK

www.scionpublishing.com

Important Note from the Publisher

The information contained within this book was obtained by Scion Publishing Ltd from sources believed by us to be reliable. However, while every effort has been made to ensure its accuracy, no responsibility for loss or injury whatsoever occasioned to any person acting or refraining from action as a result of information contained herein can be accepted by the authors or publishers.

Readers are reminded that medicine is a constantly evolving science and while the authors and publishers have ensured that all dosages, applications and practices are based on current indications, there may be specific practices which differ between communities. You should always follow the guidelines laid down by the manufacturers of specific products and the relevant authorities in the country in which you are practising.

Although every effort has been made to ensure that all owners of copyright material have been acknowledged in this publication, we would be pleased to acknowledge in subsequent reprints or editions any omissions brought to our attention.

Registered names, trademarks, etc. used in this book, even when not marked as such, are not to be considered unprotected by law.

Typeset by Evolution Design & Digital Ltd, Kent, UK

Printed in the UK

Last digit is the print number: 10 9 8 7 6 5 4 3 2

CONTENTS

ABOUT THE EDITORS

Dr Samuel Chee
MBBS (Hons)
Samuel Chee is an Australian junior doctor with a keen interest in orthopaedic surgery, trauma and teaching. He completed his MBBS from Monash University, Australia in 2018, and is currently studying for his MTrauma (Orth) at the University of Newcastle, Australia. He is also an adjunct lecturer for Monash University, providing teaching to medical students at The Alfred Hospital.

Dr Manda Raz
MBBS (Hons)
Manda Raz is an Australian doctor affiliated with Peninsula Health in Melbourne, with a broad interest in academia, research and acute care medicine. He completed his MBBS from Monash University, Australia. Dr Raz is the recipient of several scholarships, awards and medals for his academic achievements and contribution to empirical research and clinical governance. He is also the author and editor of multiple books and reference works spanning a number of clinical, legal and administrative specialties, and is currently studying for his MBioethics.

Dr Asiri Arachchi
MBBS Dip Surg Anatomy FRACS (General Surgery)
Asiri Arachchi is a general surgeon, researcher and academician, and is currently pursuing subspecialty fellowship training in colorectal surgery. He has an interest in teaching and mentoring doctors and students.

LIST OF CONTRIBUTORS

Marjorie Burgess MBBS (Hons) GradDipSurgAnat
Cases 25, 27–29

George He MD BMedSc
Cases 81–82, 84–8; reviewed Cases 21, 83, 88–90

Mohit Jain MBBS MS
Case 4

Emily Mogridge MBBS (Hons) GradDipSurgAnat
Cases 51–60

Carolyn Neil MD BSc (Biomed) and **Christopher Hancock** MD
Cases 41–50

Marie Nguyen MD BMedSc
Cases 21, 83, 88–90; reviewed Cases 81–82 and 84–88

Dion Paul MD
Cases 31, 34, 37

Ashray Rajagopalan MBBS (Hons)
Cases 22–24, 26, 30

Emma-Leigh Rudduck MD BBiomedSci
Cases 61–70

Nicholas E. Savage BMedSc MD
Cases 1–3, 5–10; contributed to Case 4

Abhishekh Srinivas BMedSc (Hons) MD
Cases 35, 38–40

Eren Tan MBBS (Hons)
Cases 11–20

Luke Wang MBBS BMedSc
Cases 71–80

Qing Xue MD
Cases 32–33, 36

Silvana F. Marasco MBBS, PhD, FRACS and **Sylvio C. Provenzano Jr.** MD, MSc, FRACS
supervised the writing of Cases 1–10.

PREFACE

Following on from the success of *Clinical Integration: Medicine*, we, the editors, felt there was a gap in resources when it came to clinically applicable surgical cases for medical students. From my experiences going through medical school, studying for the clinical exams (or OSCEs) was certainly more difficult when the topic was surgical, especially in the more niche specialties such as ENT, Plastics and Paediatric Surgery. We aim for *Clinical Integration: Surgery* to be used as a tool to prepare for medical school clinical exams, especially in the final years where information synthesis and the management of certain conditions become important.

The book is a compilation of case studies that have been written by doctors who are either training or have an interest in that specialty. A history, examination, investigations and management section are provided, with certain key words being highlighted for further discussion. These points of discussion are intended to prompt readers to understand why the case was written in such a way and deepen their knowledge of the case diagnosis.

Clinical Integration: Surgery can be used in many ways. It can be read from front to back as a study tool to learn about different surgical topics and their work-up and management. It can also be used as a testing tool, where the reader could review the case history and examination to formulate a list of differential diagnoses, and then review the investigations to identify the true diagnosis and propose a management plan to compare to what is provided.

We hope that this book is a pleasure to read as much as it was to write.

Samuel Chee
Manda Raz
Asiri Arachchi

ABBREVIATIONS

AAA	abdominal aortic aneurysm
AAD	acute aortic dissection
ABCDE	airway, breathing, circulation, disability and exposure
ABG	arterial blood gas
ABI	ankle–brachial index
AC	alternating current
ACDF	anterior cervical discectomy and fusion
ACE	angiotensin-converting enzyme
ACL	anterior cruciate ligament
ACS	acute coronary syndrome
ACTH	adrenocorticotrophic hormone
ADLs	activities of daily living
ADPKD	autosomal dominant polycystic kidney disease
AFP	alpha-fetoprotein
AJCC	American Joint Committee on Cancer
AKI	acute kidney injury
ALP	alkaline phosphatase
ALT	alanine aminotransferase
AMP	adenosine monophosphate
AOM	acute otitis media
AP	anteroposterior
aPTT	activated partial thromboplastin time
ARDS	acute respiratory distress syndrome
ASIA	American Spinal Injury Association
ASOT	antistreptolysin O titre
AVM	arteriovenous malformation
AVPU	Alert; responds to Voice, responds to Pain, Unresponsive
BAL	blood alcohol level
BAV	bicuspid aortic valve
BCC	basal cell carcinoma
BGL	blood glucose level
BMD	bone mineral density
BMI	body mass index
BP	blood pressure
BPH	benign prostatic hyperplasia
bpm	beats per minute

BTM	biodegradable temporising matrix
CABG	coronary artery bypass graft
CAP	community-acquired pneumonia
CCB	calcium channel blocker
CCP	cyclic citrullinated peptide
CEA	carcinoembryonic antigen
CES	cauda equina syndrome
CK	creatine kinase
CKD	chronic kidney disease
CMP	calcium, magnesium and phosphate
CMV	cytomegalovirus
CN	cranial nerve
CNS	central nervous system
COPD	chronic obstructive pulmonary disease
CPA	cerebellopontine angle
CPB	cardiopulmonary bypass
CPR	cardiopulmonary resuscitation
CRP	C-reactive protein
CSF	cerebrospinal fluid
CSL	compound sodium lactate
CSM	cervical spondylotic myelopathy
CT	computed tomography
CTA	CT angiography
CTB	CT brain
CUS	compression ultrasonography
CVS	cerebral vasospasm
CXR	chest X-ray
dADLs	domestic activities of daily living
DC	direct current
DCM	degenerative cervical myelopathy
DHCA	deep hypothermic circulatory arrest
DIC	disseminated intravascular coagulation
DOAC	direct oral anticoagulant
DRE	digital rectal examination
DVT	deep vein thrombosis
EBUS	endobronchial ultrasound
EBV	Epstein–Barr virus
ECG	electrocardiography

ED	Emergency Department
EDH	extradural haemorrhage
eGFR	estimated glomerular filtration rate
EMG	electromyography
ENT	ear, nose and throat
ERCP	endoscopic retrograde cholangiopancreatography
ESR	erythrocyte sedimentation rate
ETT	endotracheal tube
EUA	examination under anaesthesia
EVAR	endovascular aneurysm repair
EVD	external ventricular drain
EVLT	endovenous laser therapy
FAST	focused assessment with sonography in trauma
FBC	full blood count
FBE	full blood examination
FDG	fluorodeoxyglucose
FDP	flexor digitorum profundus
FDS	flexor digitorum superficialis
FESS	functional endoscopic sinus surgery
FISH	fluorescence *in situ* hybridisation
FNA	fine needle aspirate/aspiration
GABHS	group A beta-haemolytic streptococcus
GBM	glioblastoma multiforme
GCS	Glasgow Coma Scale
GGT	gamma-glutamyl transpeptidase
GI	gastrointestinal
GORD	gastro-oesophageal reflux disease
GP	general practitioner
GTN	glyceryl trinitrate
HAP	hospital-acquired pneumonia
Hb	haemoglobin
hCG	human chorionic gonadotrophin
Hct	haematocrit
HDL	high density lipoprotein
HHT	hereditary haemorrhagic telangiectasia
HIT	heparin-induced thrombocytopenia
HIV	human immunodeficiency virus
HLM	heart-lung machine
HOCM	hypertrophic obstructive cardiomyopathy
HPOA	hypertrophic pulmonary osteoarthropathy
HPV	human papillomavirus
HR	heart rate
HTM	heart team meeting
HTN	hypertension
ICC	intercostal catheter
ICH	intracranial haemorrhage
ICP	intracranial pressure
ICU	intensive care unit
IDC	indwelling urinary catheter
IDH	isocitrate dehydrogenase
IE	infective endocarditis
Ig	immunoglobulin
IHD	ischaemic heart disease
IM	intramuscular
INR	international normalised ratio
IPJ	interphalangeal joint
IV	intravenous
IVC	inferior vena cava
IVDU	intravenous drug use(r)
IVP	intravenous pyelogram
JVP	jugular venous pressure
KUB	kidneys, ureter, bladder
LAD	left anterior descending
LCL	lateral collateral ligament
LDH	lactate dehydrogenase
LDL	low density lipoprotein
LFT	liver function test
LITA	left internal thoracic artery
LL	lower limb
LMCA	left main coronary artery
LMN	lower motor neurone
LMWH	low molecular weight heparin
LOC	loss of consciousness
LV	left ventricular
LVH	left ventricular hypertrophy
MCL	medial collateral ligament
MCPJ	metacarpophalangeal joint
MC&S	microscopy, culture and sensitivities
MDT	multidisciplinary team
MEN	multiple endocrine neoplasia

MGMT	methyl guanine methyl transferase	PNET	primitive neuroectodermal tumour
MI	myocardial infarction	PR	per rectum
mJOA	modified Japanese Orthopaedic Association	PSA	prostate-specific antigen
		PT	prothrombin time
MMA	middle meningeal artery	PTH	parathyroid hormone
MMSE	mini mental state examination	PTS	post-thrombotic syndrome
MOCA	Montreal Cognitive Assessment	PTX	pneumothorax
MR	mitral regurgitation	PVD	peripheral vascular disease
MRA	magnetic resonance angiography	RA	rheumatoid arthritis
MRI	magnetic resonance imaging	RadA	radial arteries
MRSA	methicillin-resistant *Staphylococcus aureus*	RCA	right coronary artery
		RCC	renal cell carcinoma
MS	multiple sclerosis	RHD	rheumatic heart disease
MUA	manipulation under anaesthesia	ROM	range of motion
MVA	motor vehicle accident	RR	respiratory rate
NAI	non-accidental injury	RSI	rapid sequence induction
NEC	necrotising enterocolitis	RTx	radiotherapy
NF	neurofibromatosis	RUQ	right upper quadrant
NGT	nasogastric tube	RVA	radiofrequency vein ablation
NIHSS	National Institutes of Health Stroke Scale	SABR	stereotactic ablative body radiotherapy
NOF	neck of femur fracture	SAH	subarachnoid haemorrhage
NSAID	non-steroidal anti-inflammatory drug	SAM	systolic anterior motion
NSCLC	non-small cell lung cancer	SBP	systolic blood pressure
OA	osteoarthritis	SCC	squamous cell carcinoma
OME	otitis media with effusion	SCLC	small cell lung cancer
OP-CAB	off-pump CABG	SCM	sternocleidomastoid
OPG	orthopantomogram	SGLT2	sodium-glucose co-transporter-2
ORIF	open reduction, internal fixation	SIADH	syndrome of inappropriate antidiuretic hormone secretion
PAD	peripheral arterial disease		
pADLs	personal activities of daily living	SIRS	systemic inflammatory response syndrome
PCA	patient-controlled analgesia		
PCI	percutaneous coronary intervention	SLE	systemic lupus erythematosus
PCKD	polycystic kidney disease	SLNB	sentinel lymph node biopsy
PCL	posterior cruciate ligament	SLT	straight leg test
PCR	polymerase chain reaction	SOB	shortness of breath
PDA	patent ductus arteriosus	SPECT	single-photon emission CT
PE	pulmonary embolism	SPF	sun protection factor
PET	positron emission tomography	STI	sexually transmitted infection
PFT	pulmonary function test	SVC	superior vena cava
PICC	peripherally inserted central catheter	SVG	great saphenous vein
PIPJ	proximal interphalangeal joint	T2DM	type 2 diabetes mellitus
PND	paroxysmal nocturnal dyspnoea	TAI	traumatic aortic injury

TAVR	transcatheter aortic valve replacement	UFH	unfractionated heparin
TB	tuberculosis	UL	upper limbs
TBI	traumatic brain injury	UMN	upper motor neurone
TBSA	total body surface area	URTI	upper respiratory tract infection
TEVAR	thoracic endovascular aortic repair	UTI	urinary tract infection
TFT	thyroid function test	UV	ultraviolet
TIA	transient ischaemic attack	VA	visual acuity
TNM	tumour, node, metastasis	VATS	video-assisted thoracoscopic surgery
TOE	transoesophageal echocardiogram	VBG	venous blood gas
TSH	thyroid-stimulating hormone	VSD	ventricular septal defect
TTE	transthoracic echocardiography	VTE	venous thromboembolism
TTF	thyroid transcription factor	WBC	white blood cell
TURP	transurethral resection of the prostate	WCC	white cell count
UEC	urea, electrolytes and creatinine		

CASE 1: Aortic stenosis

History

- A patient attends the cardiothoracic surgery outpatient clinic for a work-up of **aortic stenosis** [1] [2] [3]. She was referred by her primary care physician when echocardiography suggested aortic stenosis.
- The patient, a **76-year-old** [4] **woman** [5], explains that she has been suffering **chest pain** [6] for the last 2 months. She notes that it is particularly noticeable on exertion and that she has also been more short of breath recently. Her husband, who has attended the clinic with her, states that she has also been feeling faint when performing activities lately.
- She has a past medical history of **hyperlipidaemia, hypertension** [7] and gout. She was recently told by her GP that she falls into the pre-diabetes category.

1 Aortic stenosis is defined as blood flow across the aortic valve becoming impaired due to a pathological narrowing. The aortic valve is composed of three leaflets (or cusps) suspended within the sinuses of Valsalva in the proximal aorta. The coronary vessels arise from two of the three sinuses of Valsalva and fill during diastole. The leaflets are named the left coronary leaflet, the right coronary leaflet and the non-coronary leaflet. The point where each leaflet meets the next leaflet on the aortic wall is termed the commissure. In terms of surgical anatomy, two landmarks are important to understand. Firstly, the anterior leaflet of the mitral valve is below the commissure between the left coronary leaflet and non-coronary leaflet. Secondly, the bundle of His is below the commissure between the right coronary leaflet and non-coronary leaflet. Aortic stenosis is the most common valvular disease in developed countries and occurs in approximately 3% of those aged ≥75 years.

2 Broadly, there are three forms of aortic valve stenosis: degenerative calcific aortic stenosis, bicuspid aortic valve (BAV), and rheumatic aortic stenosis. Degenerative aortic stenosis makes up approximately 80% of cases of aortic stenosis. Given that it is a degenerative disease, its prevalence increases with age. This condition occurs in a morphologically normal valve (i.e. a trileaflet valve). BAV occurs in approximately 1 in 200 people. It is the most common congenital heart abnormality. Bicuspid aortic valves typically have a smaller cusp and a larger cusp (which is made of the second and third normal cusps fused together). Although it is a structural defect, it is associated with other congenital and acquired cardiovascular diseases. BAV stenosis is the reason for most of the cases which are not degenerative aortic stenosis. It usually presents 20 years earlier than degenerative aortic stenosis. Rheumatic aortic stenosis is becoming less common and is now rare in developed countries. It typically causes mild aortic stenosis.

3 Aortic stenosis causes a disturbance in normal physiology. The left ventricle's normal response to compensate for aortic stenosis is to hypertrophy. Hypertrophy results in greater muscle mass, lower compliance, diastolic dysfunction, higher systolic ventricular pressure, longer systolic time and less coronary perfusion, resulting in chronic ischaemia.

4 Advanced age is associated with degenerative aortic stenosis. As mentioned previously, BAV stenosis tends to present earlier. Most cases of aortic stenosis presenting before age 50 are related to a BAV. In those over 70, degenerative aortic stenosis is the most common underlying aetiology.

5 Males are approximately 20% more likely to have some form of aortic stenosis. Women are more likely to have advanced disease and be of advanced age at presentation.

6 Most patients have some symptoms at presentation of aortic stenosis. However, they may present without symptoms with the investigation of a cardiac murmur or on echocardiography for another reason. Syncope, angina and dyspnoea have been described as the classic symptoms of aortic stenosis. Most commonly patients complain of fatigue and then dyspnoea. Angina is the next most common presenting symptom. The underlying cause for angina in aortic stenosis is due to the fact that it can reduce coronary blood flow while increasing myocardial demand, resulting in subendocardial ischaemia. This can also present as exertional angina. Furthermore, aortic stenosis leads to ventricular hypertrophy which then increases myocardial oxygen demand. Accordingly, angina is more common in patients with both aortic stenosis and ischaemic heart disease. Currently, it is understood that increasing aortic stenosis severity is associated with angina. Syncope is a worrying symptom which indicates end-stage disease or conduction disturbance. Approximately 35% of patients with significant aortic stenosis experience symptoms of pulmonary vein hypertension. These include dyspnoea, orthopnoea, paroxysmal nocturnal dyspnoea (PND) and peripheral oedema.

7 There are several possible past medical history findings relevant to aortic stenosis. As mentioned, a congenital BAV can be the underlying cause of aortic stenosis, particularly in younger patients. Rheumatic heart disease may also be the underlying aetiology for aortic stenosis. Patients with chronic

kidney disease (CKD) on dialysis have a significantly increased risk of developing aortic stenosis. High levels of low density lipoprotein (LDL) cholesterol have also been found to be associated with the development of aortic stenosis. There are risk factors that are shared with aortic stenosis. These include hypertension, diabetes and hyperlipidaemia. Lastly, a history of radiation therapy to the chest is also a risk factor for the development of aortic stenosis.

Examination

- The patient was **short of breath** [1] upon entering the room. However, her dyspnoea settles while talking. She is conscious and alert.
- Her blood pressure is **140/110mmHg** [2].
- Her radial pulse is **weak and delayed** [3].
- Her **chest is free of scars and deformity** [4].
- Her **apex beat is forceful** [5] but not displaced and a **thrill** [6] is felt in the aortic region.

- On auscultation, there is a **grade 4/6 systolic murmur radiating to the carotids** [7].
- There is also an **S4 sound** [8].
- The abdomen is soft and non-tender. There are **no peripheral signs** [9]. The patient is instructed to undergo several investigations before being seen next.

1 General inspection may give more information regarding the patient's symptoms as well as overall state. Dyspnoea at rest indicates a significant reduction in function. The patient may be in pain or clutching their chest. Conscious state should be assessed.

2 Narrow pulse pressure is a feature of aortic stenosis. This is defined as <25% of the systolic value. This is due to a drop in stroke volume caused by the stenosis itself.

3 Classically, the pulse in aortic stenosis is slow-rising and weak. The pulse can also be delayed. However, systemic hypertension or inelastic arteries in older patients can prevent this finding from being clear. Palpating the brachial artery may allow the pulse findings in aortic stenosis to be felt, despite these factors. Overall, these signs are uncommon.

4 As always, it is important to inspect the chest. This may give rise to signs of pulmonary disease. Scars from previous surgery may also be seen including from sternotomy, thoracotomy or pacemaker insertion.

5 The apex beat may be forceful in patients with left ventricular hypertrophy (LVH).

6 A palpable murmur is known as a thrill and can be felt with grade 4 or higher murmurs.

7 In terms of auscultation, the classic murmur of aortic stenosis is a systolic murmur greater than grade 3/6. It is heard as a crescendo-decrescendo murmur that peaks in mid-systole. This is due to pressure within the left ventricle

building and the velocity of blood flow across the aortic valve increasing. This causes turbulent flow resulting in a murmur. Classically, the murmur also radiates to the carotid. However, it can be difficult to differentiate this from a carotid bruit. In severe aortic stenosis, the murmur may be quiet and high pitched due to reduced flow.

8 In terms of the heart sounds themselves, the S2 may be diminished and single. This is due to the aortic component of the S2 (comprising the pulmonary and aortic sounds) becoming soft due to the aortic leaflets having less mobility. In normal physiology, the aortic valve closes before the pulmonary valve, allowing the two components of S2 to be heard. However, in aortic stenosis, aortic valve closure is delayed so that it can occur at the same time as pulmonary valve closure. This can also contribute to the single S2 sound heard. In very severe aortic stenosis, aortic valve closure may become so delayed that it occurs after pulmonary valve closure. This produces the sound of a normal split S2. However, it is termed a paradoxically split S2 because the aortic component is occurring after the pulmonary component instead of before. Additionally, due to hypertrophy of the left ventricle, there may be an S4 sound. An S4 sound is caused by blood entering a stiff ventricle.

9 Aortic stenosis can cause an acquired von Willebrand deficiency. This may result in epistaxis or bruising as well gastrointestinal (GI) bleeding associated with angiodysplasia. This is most common in severe aortic stenosis.

Investigations

- The patient returns to clinic having undergone several investigations for her **presumed aortic stenosis** [1].
- **Full blood examination, kidney and liver function tests and coagulation studies** [2] are all normal.
- **Electrocardiography (ECG)** [3] shows evidence of left ventricular hypertrophy and left atrial enlargement.
- Her **chest X-ray** [4] is clear but shows calcification of the aortic valve.
- **Transthoracic Doppler echocardiography** [5] shows a mean gradient across the aortic valve of 45mmHg and $0.8cm^2$ valve area.
- The patient also undergoes **coronary angiography** [6] using cardiac catheterisation, which finds no evidence of ischaemic heart disease.
- She does not undergo **cardiac stress testing** [7].
- **Other investigations** [8] are considered but not performed.

[1] There are several differential diagnoses to consider in a patient presenting with aortic stenosis without echocardiography findings. Aortic sclerosis can produce a murmur similar to that of aortic stenosis. As mentioned, hypertrophy of the ventricle can lead to ischaemia of the muscle. Additionally, ischaemic heart disease and aortic stenosis can often exist at the same time within one patient. Another differential diagnosis for aortic stenosis is hypertrophic cardiomyopathy. It produces stenosis not involving the aortic valve itself and can produce a similar murmur to aortic stenosis. Manoeuvres increasing afterload, such as hand gripping or squatting, typically make a murmur of hypertrophic cardiomyopathy softer. Hypertrophic cardiomyopathy can be diagnosed using echocardiography.

[2] Blood tests to be considered include full blood examination (FBE), kidney function, liver function and coagulation studies. These allow assessment of comorbidities that may complicate the surgical process. Additionally, von Willebrand levels and platelet function tests may be considered to investigate for haematologic abnormalities associated with aortic stenosis.

[3] Electrocardiography (ECG) is useful for indicating left ventricular hypertrophy (LVH) and evidence of left atrial enlargement. LVH is seen on ECG as increased R wave amplitude in left-sided leads and increased S wave depth in right-sided leads. It is commonly diagnosed as S wave depth in V1 and tallest R wave height in V5 or V6 added together being >35mm. There may also be T wave inversion in V6. Left atrial enlargement produces a bifid P wave in lead II (also known as P mitrale) and enlarges the negative portion of P wave in V1. Patients with aortic stenosis can also have pathology of the conduction system. These include atrioventricular block, hemiblock or bundle branch block.

[4] Chest X-ray (CXR) may be used in the diagnosis of aortic stenosis. It allows assessment of pulmonary oedema, which indicates heart failure. Additionally, it allows assessment of cardiac size as well as dilatation of the ascending aorta or valve calcification. There may also be evidence of LVH. It is also used in the immediate preoperative setting to ensure there is no pneumonia or other pathology.

[5] Transthoracic Doppler echocardiography allows definitive assessment of aortic stenosis. It uses the reflection of sound waves to examine the heart as it functions. Doppler ultrasound works by recognising sound waves that are specifically reflected by moving particles (including red blood cells). This test is both sensitive and specific for diagnosis of aortic stenosis. It is indicated for any unexplained systolic murmur, a single second heart sound, BAV or symptoms of aortic stenosis. The gradient of pressure across the aortic valve can be calculated from the blood velocity through the valve. Overall, the mean gradient is more useful than the peak gradient. Aortic stenosis is considered moderate when the mean gradient is >25mmHg and severe when the gradient is >40mmHg. However, it is possible for severe aortic stenosis to exist with a low gradient if left ventricular function is reduced. This may be seen in a very late presentation or a patient with a cardiomyopathy. The valve area can also be determined. The normal aortic valve area is approximately $3-4cm^2$. Symptoms usually develop in patients with an aortic valve area $<1cm^2$. Currently, aortic stenosis is considered mild when the valve area is $>1.5cm^2$, moderate when $1-1.5cm^2$ and severe when $<1cm^2$.

[6] Cardiac catheterisation allows actual measurement of the pressure gradient across the aortic valve with a pressure transducer. Pressure can be measured in the ventricle then the aorta, or simultaneously. However, as it is an invasive test, it is usually reserved for those with inconclusive echocardiography. In patients over 40 years of age being considered for operation, coronary angiography is also performed. This is due to the fact that aortic stenosis frequently coexists with coronary artery disease. Additionally, a coronary artery bypass graft (CABG) can be performed at the same time as the surgery for aortic stenosis.

[7] Stress testing through exercise with ECG monitoring is generally not advisable in patients with severe aortic stenosis. Dobutamine stress echocardiogram may be used

in those patients in whom the diagnosis has been difficult to determine. Abnormal findings at stress echocardiogram include onset of symptoms, inadequate blood pressure increase or drop, bradycardia, arrhythmia or ST segment depression, increased gradient across the valve with exercise or reduction in ejection fraction.

[8] Other tests that may be considered included dobutamine stress echocardiogram and cardiac magnetic resonance imaging (MRI).

Management

Immediate

Discuss the **likely prognosis with no management** [1] with the patient, as well as the possible **management modalities and indications for each** [2] [3] [4] [5]. Given that the patient is symptomatic but not prohibitively high risk, book her in for an elective surgical aortic valve replacement. Discuss the **risks** [6] of the procedure beforehand. Ensure the patient receives a **dental review and consider antibiotic prophylaxis** [7] for bacterial endocarditis.

Short-term

Perform an aortic valve replacement with cardiopulmonary bypass. Excise the diseased aortic valve and replace it with a **bioprosthetic valve** [8] [9]. **Close the chest** [10] and extubate the patient in theatre. Monitor the patient for **24 hours in the cardiac care unit** [11] before moving to the cardiothoracic surgery ward.

Long-term

Consider **anticoagulation** [12] while in hospital and for the first 3 months. Follow the patient up in the **cardiothoracic outpatient clinic** [13] after her operation.

[1] The natural history of aortic stenosis, as with many other treatable diseases, is not fully understood. Aortic valve replacement is favoured when the gradient is severe, due to the poor prognosis associated with untreated disease. This is true whether the stenosis produces symptoms or not.

[2] Broadly, there are three presentations for aortic stenosis: clinically unstable, clinically stable but symptomatic, and clinically stable but asymptomatic. In the first category, medical therapy or balloon valvuloplasty is appropriate. For those in the second category, patients are managed according to surgical risk. Those in the low risk categories are more likely to undergo surgery and those in the high risk category are more likely to undergo transcatheter aortic valve replacement (TAVR) or balloon valvuloplasty. Those in the third category may be considered for surgery based on their echocardiography findings.

[3] No medical therapy has been shown to improve survival in those with aortic stenosis. However, it can be used to treat frequently occurring comorbid conditions including ischaemic heart disease, hyperlipidaemia, hypertension and heart failure. Additionally, it can be used to manage heart failure symptoms. These typically include angiotensin-converting enzyme (ACE) inhibitors and diuretics.

[4] TAVR is an emerging alternative to surgery. It avoids the need for surgery, cardiopulmonary bypass or cardiac arrest. A stent-mounted bioprosthetic valve is placed within the aorta. Patients classed as high risk may undergo TAVR. TAVR has similar mortality and symptom reduction as surgery. However, it has a different complication profile. TAVR has been found to be non-inferior to surgery in both high and low risk patients although valve durability remains questionable and pacemaker rates remain higher in TAVR.

[5] Balloon aortic valvuloplasty is another procedure performed using cardiac catheterisation. It uses a balloon to dilate the stenosed aortic valve and is reserved for patients who have prohibitively high risk for other interventions. This is used as a bridging procedure to TAVR or surgery in acute situations as the re-stenosis rate is very high.

[6] The 30-day mortality for aortic valve replacement is approximately 3% in developed countries. The risk is higher for women than men. Mortality rises when concurrent CABG is performed. Long-term survival is similar for mechanical and bioprosthetic valves. In terms of early mortality, acute cardiac failure, myocardial infarction (MI), neurologic complications, bleeding and infection predominate. Another significant complication is replacement valve endocarditis (discussed within *Case 2*). Lastly, peri-valvular leak or structural compromise of tissue valve can occur. If this is severe it may require re-operation.

7 Dental review before cardiac surgery is important as dental procedures can cause a transient bacteraemia, resulting in an increased risk of infective endocarditis. Therefore, any required dental procedures should occur before the aortic valve is replaced. Local guidelines should be reviewed regarding the need for antibiotic prophylaxis for patients with structural heart defects in general, as well as for peri-operative administration.

8 This Case will discuss isolated surgical aortic valve replacement. This procedure may also be used in the management of aortic regurgitation. General anaesthesia is established and the patient is prepped and draped. Median sternotomy or a right anterior thoracotomy is performed, and cardiopulmonary bypass is established. A cross clamp is applied across the aorta. Transverse aortotomy is performed approximately 15mm above the right coronary artery (RCA) and 30mm above the aortic valve itself. The pulmonary trunk may need to be dissected off the aorta. The valve is excised. Neat excision of the valve is a technically challenging but critical aspect of the procedure. All calcium is removed from the annulus.

9 Prosthetic valves are the most common option used for aortic valve replacement. The annulus must be sized to allow appropriate fit. The replacement valve can be attached using an interrupted or continuous suture technique. An allograft aortic valve may be used instead of a mechanical replacement valve. These are often termed bioprosthetic valves. Bioprosthetic valves may sit on a stent to allow appropriate attachment. Lastly, the aortic valve can be replaced with the patient's own pulmonary valve (autograft). The pulmonary valve is then replaced with a pulmonary allograft. This double valve procedure is known as the Ross procedure and is typically reserved for young patients. Overall, mechanical valves have the advantage of lasting longer but patients require lifelong warfarin. Bioprosthetic valves carry the advantages of decreased risk of thromboembolism (long-term anticoagulation is not required) and overall decreased risk of haemorrhage. New sutureless bioprosthetic surgical aortic valves are available which reduce cross clamp and cardiopulmonary bypass times.

10 Once the replacement valve is placed, the aortotomy is closed and air is evacuated from the heart. Carbon dioxide is used to reduce the likelihood of air embolism. This is due to the fact that carbon dioxide is more soluble than air in blood, so bubbles become dissolved without causing an embolism. Closure of the pericardium protects the heart from damage in the case of future resternotomy. Total operative time is approximately 3 hours.

11 Rigorous postoperative care is essential in all cardiac surgery. Care for patients after valve surgery is similar to other cardiac surgery procedures. Patients with mechanical prostheses require warfarin anticoagulation with target international normalised ratio (INR) 2.0–3.0 usually commencing the day after surgery. Some atrial pathologies raise the INR requirement. Currently, there is no consensus regarding anticoagulation protocol for bioprostheses. Patients with atrial fibrillation for >48 hours after surgery should be anticoagulated with warfarin or more commonly a NOAC (non-vitamin K antagonist oral anticoagulants) until the restoration of sinus rhythm. Left atrial pressure is usually maintained at a higher pressure than normal to account for the higher required filling pressure of the left ventricle. Sinus tachycardia may need to be managed with beta blockers.

12 After the short-term postoperative period, patients may stay in a hospital ward with lower level care for several days before discharge. They may require anticoagulation, as previously discussed. They will also require antibiotic prophylaxis before dental procedures and any medical procedure involving infected tissue (such as the drainage of an abscess). These patients should be followed up in outpatient clinic.

13 Most patients who undergo aortic valve replacement enjoy significant symptom and functional status improvement and achieve improved survival. More than 90% have been found to achieve New York Heart Association (NYHA) functional class I or II at 3 years.

CASE 2: Infective endocarditis

History

- A patient presents to the Emergency Department (ED) with **suspected infective endocarditis** [1] .
- He is a **62-year-old male** [2] who has been feeling unwell for the last three weeks [3] .
- He states he has been feeling feverish and experiencing **shaking and shivering** [4] . He has also been fatigued with decreased exercise tolerance.
- He has **no history of rheumatic fever** [5] .

- He has risk factors for **infective endocarditis** [6] including a heart murmur which was identified by his general practitioner (GP) **many years ago** [7] , and generally poor dentition. He states he had several teeth extracted about a year ago.
- He has no relevant family or past medical history. He does not drink, smoke or use recreational drugs.

[1] Infective endocarditis (IE) is an infection causing inflammation of the endocardial surface of the heart, associated valvular structures, chordae tendineae, ventricular septal defects (VSDs), patent ductus arteriosus (PDA) or intracardiac devices such as prosthetic valves or pacemakers. It is characterised by vegetations on the surface of the endocardium or within it (as an abscess). Two conditions are necessary to cause IE: bacteraemia and endothelial injury. IE most commonly affects the valves of the heart as defective valves produce turbulence and consequently injury to the endothelium. Microorganisms within the bloodstream attach to this area, leading to the formation of a vegetation by processes of clotting, inflammation and proliferation. Inside the vegetation, microorganisms are protected from phagocytosis and antibiotics. Predisposing conditions to IE are valve defects (stenosis or regurgitation), rheumatic heart disease (RHD), congenital heart disease, BAV and prosthetic material. The left-sided valves are affected in the vast majority of IE not related to drug use. The aortic valve is affected more commonly than the mitral valve. In IE related to drug use, about half of IE affects the tricuspid valve and the other half affects the aortic valve. In developed countries, the incidence of IE is approximately 2–10 per 100 000 people per year.

[2] Men are more affected by IE than women in a ratio of approximately 3:1, although the proportion might differ amongst populations.

[3] IE can be acute or subacute (chronic). Acute IE is a severe form of the disease. It is caused by virulent microorganisms and can be a threat to life within days. Subacute IE is an indolent form of the disease that can develop over a period of weeks or months.

[4] The most common presenting symptoms of IE are related to the infective process, rather than its effects on haemodynamics or other sequelae from immunological or vascular phenomena. Fever, chills and rigors are the most

common complaints and are present in almost all patients with IE. However, as with other infective conditions, elderly patients or those who are immunocompromised may present without fever. This can make the diagnosis more difficult in those populations. Other general symptoms related to infection and systemic disease can occur and include night sweats, fatigue, weight loss, anorexia and muscle pain. IE can also present with weakness, arthralgia, headache and dyspnoea. These symptoms can be constitutional or caused by septic emboli. IE can also present with chest pain. This can be due to heart failure from compromised valve function or an embolus to a coronary artery. Back pain can also be present in IE due to discitis from septic emboli. Symptoms of progressing heart failure, including progressive dyspnoea, oedema, cough and orthopnoea, may also indicate IE. Haematuria can arise from renal emboli. Symptoms of stroke can occur with intracranial haemorrhage or stroke due to septic embolism. Lastly, anaemia can be from chronic disease and usually worsened by iron deficiency.

[5] The differential diagnoses for IE reflect the fact that it can present with general symptoms. History of rheumatic fever is a hint for possible valvular disease, although active carditis occurs in younger individuals. RHD can cause mainly constitutional symptoms. These symptoms include polyarthritis, symptoms of carditis, subcutaneous nodules, Sydenham's chorea, erythema marginatum and a preceding streptococcal infection. Atrial myxoma is also a differential for IE. Patients can have systemic features due to inflammatory reaction as well as emboli from impaired haemodynamics. The disease progression of atrial myxoma is often undulating, whereas IE is usually progressive. There are other forms of endocarditis with sterile vegetations including Libman–Sacks endocarditis and non-bacterial thrombotic endocarditis which should also be considered.

6 There are several risk factors for IE. The most significant risk factors include past history of IE, the presence of prosthetic valves, congenital heart disease and recipients of heart transplant. A past history of IE is associated with a higher incidence of recurrence and worse outcomes overall. Prosthetic valves carry a greater risk of IE than native valves, particularly if implant happened within one year prior. In terms of congenital heart disease, PDA, VSDs and aortic stenosis are associated with a higher incidence of IE. This is likely due to the changes in haemodynamics and subsequent areas of turbulence and low pressure allowing bacterial accumulation on the endocardium.

7 Other risk factors include the presence of intravascular devices (electronic cardiac devices or intravascular catheters), acquired degenerative valve disease, mitral valve prolapse, hypertrophic obstructive cardiomyopathy (HOCM), intravenous (IV) drug use, dental procedures and diabetes mellitus. Implanted devices and catheters can cause endovascular injury; in addition a catheter can be a direct port of entry of microorganisms into the bloodstream. Acquired degenerative valve disease and HOCM cause endocardial injury and allow bacterial adherence. RHD was, in the past, a leading risk factor for IE. However, RHD is becoming significantly uncommon in more economically developed countries. In both adult and paediatric populations, mitral valve prolapse is associated with an increased risk of IE. IV drug users are at an increased risk of developing acute endocarditis. The most common offending pathogen is *Staphylococcus aureus*. The tricuspid and aortic valves are most commonly affected in IV drug users. However, this patient group is also more likely to develop left-sided IE than the general population. Dental procedures can cause transient bacteraemia of the normal commensal flora of the mouth, especially in individuals with poor dental hygiene.

Examination

- On general inspection, the patient **appears relatively well** [1].
- His **temperature is 38.5°C but otherwise his vital signs are stable** [2].
- His **fingertips do not appear ischaemic, but Janeway lesions and Osler nodes are present** [3].
- On auscultation of the chest, the heart sounds are dual and there is a **grade 3 out of 6 systolic murmur** [4]. It is loudest in the mitral area and radiates to the axilla.
- The abdomen is soft and non-tender but the **spleen** [5] can be palpated.
- **Neurological examination is normal** [6]. Fundoscopic examination shows no retinal changes.
- There are no **other abnormal examination findings** [7].

1 General inspection is likely to be unremarkable. It may be clear that the patient is fatigued, in pain, feverish or has had a stroke due to embolism. It is also important to inspect the patient's dentition, as this is one of the most common sources of infection. Anaemia is common in patients with subacute endocarditis. Individuals with acute IE appear generally or severely ill.

2 Fever is usual in IE. Patients with acute IE often have a high fever and more severe constitutional symptoms. However, low grade or no fever and less severe symptoms is a common presentation in subacute IE.

3 The peripheral signs of IE are broadly related to two phenomena. The first group are the vascular phenomena, due to parts of a vegetation breaking off creating septic emboli. These emboli can travel to any part of the body to produce both clinical signs and complications of the disease. Septic emboli, depending on size and final destination, can cause stroke, gangrene (fingers or limbs), abdominal pain (spleen or gut), haematuria/bacteriuria (kidneys) and even MI. Janeway lesions are painless haemorrhagic papules or macules of the soles and palms and are related to microabscesses caused by microorganisms, particularly *Staphylococcus aureus*. The second group are the immunologic phenomena. In terms of clinical signs, these include Osler nodes, which are painful, nodular lesions mainly on the tips of the fingers and toes. Roth spots can be seen on fundoscopy as a red spot with pale centre. Petechiae and clubbing can also occur in patients with IE. Splinter haemorrhages and conjunctival haemorrhages can be caused by either embolic or immunologic phenomena. The classical peripheral signs of IE occur late in the disease and therefore are not commonly seen.

4 IE can be associated with a new heart murmur or change to a pre-existing murmur. However, while a heart murmur is commonly found in patients with IE, the classically described 'changing murmur' is rare. IE without valve regurgitation or stenosis does not cause a cardiac murmur. For IE involving the aortic valve, a short diastolic murmur is often heard. However, it can be difficult to appreciate this due to tachycardia. IE involving the mitral valve often causes mitral regurgitation and a pansystolic murmur radiating to the axilla. Large vegetations on the mitral valve can obstruct the flow of blood, causing an effective mitral stenosis. The murmur of mitral stenosis is a low-pitched rumbling diastolic murmur. Particularly in drug users, the tricuspid valve can be affected. This typically causes tricuspid regurgitation and is heard as a pansystolic murmur heard loudest at the left lower sternal border.

5 Examination of the abdomen may reveal spleen enlargement.

6 A full neurological exam, including fundoscopy, should always be performed to identify neurological complications.

7 Signs of heart failure, including basal crackles, effusions, oedema and skin rash, particularly of the shins, and tachypnoea can also indicate IE.

Investigations

- The **modified Duke criteria** [1] [2] are considered for diagnosis of IE and guide subsequent investigations. Blood cultures have been taken before commencing antibiotics in the ED.
- **Transthoracic echocardiography has already been performed** [3] before referral to the cardiothoracic surgery team. It shows moderate mitral regurgitation with an oscillating vegetation of about 30mm attached to the anterior leaflet. A transoesophageal echocardiogram is then performed to better characterise the valve/heart compromise.

- The patient fulfils both the **vascular** [4] and **immunologic** [5] phenomena criteria with the peripheral stigmata of IE found on examination.
- **MRI brain is unremarkable** [6].
- Full blood examination demonstrates **microcytic anaemia and a raised white cell count** [7]. C-reactive protein is also elevated.
- Routine blood tests are ordered daily for the rest of the patient's admission. **Other investigations are considered** [8].
- The blood cultures return positive showing growth of *Staphylococcus aureus*, susceptible to flucloxacillin.

1 There are several diagnostic criteria guidelines for IE. One that is used commonly is the modified Duke criteria, divided into major and minor diagnostic criteria. The first major criterion is blood cultures positive for typical IE organisms with specific collection requirements and multiple samples, and the second criterion is specific echocardiographic findings of IE. The minor criteria are the presence of a predisposing heart condition or IV drug use, fever >38°C, vascular phenomena suggestive of embolisation, immunologic phenomena specific to IE, positive blood culture not meeting the major criterion and echocardiographic findings not meeting the major criterion. The criteria requirements for the diagnosis of IE are 2 major, 1 major and 3 minor, or 5 minor. A detailed description of the Duke criteria should be used for clinical purposes for those with positive blood cultures and native valves. These criteria cannot be applied to those with a prosthetic valve or pacing system, when blood cultures are negative or when the right heart is affected. Although knowledge of the clinical aspects of IE is important, most diagnoses are made through the use of blood cultures and echocardiography.

2 For the modified Duke criteria, the first major criterion is two separate blood cultures positive for typical IE organisms, persistently positive blood cultures for microorganisms consistent with IE, single positive blood culture for *Coxiella burnetii* or antiphase I IgG antibody titre >1800. These typical organisms include viridans streptococci,

Staphylococcus aureus, *Streptococcus bovis*, community-acquired enterococci or the HACEK group (*Haemophilus* spp., *Aggregatibacter* spp., *Cardiobacterium hominis*, *Eikenella* spp. and *Kingella*). The majority of IE is caused by Gram-positive bacteria. *Staphylococcus aureus* is the most common, then *Streptococcus viridans*, which is an oral streptococci. Both coagulase-negative and coagulase-positive *Staphylococci* are found in prosthetic valve IE. Gram-positive organisms, such as *Streptococcus bovis*, can cross the bowel wall in conditions like bowel malignancy or ulcerative colitis and result in IE. The HACEK group are Gram-negative organisms which are slow growing. Although they are a well-known cause of IE, they are only found in approximately 2% of cases. *Coxiella burnetii* is the organism responsible for Q fever and should be considered in those in contact with animals and negative blood cultures. Fungal microorganisms, most commonly *Candida* spp. *and Aspergillus* spp., cause IE in approximately 2% of cases. IV drug users, those with prosthetic valves and patients with long-term intravascular catheters are at highest risk of IE due to fungal microorganisms. Fungal IE causes larger vegetations, widespread and metastatic infection and valvular invasion with negative blood cultures. Blood cultures should be obtained urgently before empiric antibiotic treatment is commenced. To meet the minor criteria, a patient must have positive blood culture, which does not meet the major criteria or serologic evidence of an infection that is consistent with organisms known to cause IE.

Modified Duke criteria	
Requires 2 major, or 1 major and 3 minor, or 5 minor criteria	
Major criteria	Minor criteria
• Blood cultures positive with typical IE organisms • Echocardiography findings including: oscillating intracardiac mass on valve, abscess or new partial dehiscence of prosthetic valve or new valvular regurgitation	• Predisposing heart condition or IV drug use • Fever >38°C • Vascular phenomena suggestive of embolisation • Immunologic phenomena specific to IE • Positive blood culture not meeting the major criterion • Echocardiographic findings not meeting the major criterion

3 Transthoracic echocardiography (TTE) is always requested in cases of bacteraemia and even with a low suspicion of IE; however, its sensitivity is only about 50%. On the other hand, a transoesophageal echocardiogram (TOE) has sensitivity of >90%. Therefore, when TTE cannot rule out IE and IE is suspected, a TOE should be obtained. The echocardiogram findings that meet the Duke's criteria are: oscillating intracardiac mass on valve, abscess or new partial dehiscence of prosthetic valve or new valvular regurgitation. An oscillating intracardiac mass in the context of IE is a vegetation. Differential diagnoses for intracardiac masses include thrombus, primary tumour such as myxoma or metastasis. Abscesses can occur on the valves as well as within the myocardium. They are associated with worse outcomes in IE. Dehiscence of prosthetic valve refers to a breakdown of sutures leading to detachment of the prosthesis from the annulus. Its presence is considered a major criterion for the modified Duke criteria.

4 Evidence of vascular phenomena forms one of the minor criteria for IE. This includes evidence of major arterial emboli, septic pulmonary infarct in right-sided disease, mycotic aneurysm, intracranial haemorrhage, conjunctival haemorrhages and Janeway lesions. Computed tomography (CT) can be used to detect splenic and renal infarction. Intracranial haemorrhage or stroke can be investigated through CT or MRI. Septic pulmonary infarcts can occasionally be seen on CXR but the definitive imaging modality is CT. They can cause lung abscesses. A mycotic aneurysm is defined as dilation of an artery due to infection. Mycotic

aneurysms commonly occur in the aorta or intracranial vessels. Embolisation causes the presenting manifestation of left-sided IE in approximately 10% of cases. However, approximately 50% of patients with left-sided IE have some evidence of vascular phenomena on physical exam or imaging. The brain is commonly compromised.

5 Evidence of immunologic phenomena forms the other minor criterion for IE. This includes positive rheumatoid factor. Complement levels can be low in those with glomerulonephritis as complement is consumed as part of the immunologic process. Positive antineutrophil cytoplasmic antibodies also suggests glomerulonephritis. Biopsy of the kidney may show crescentic glomerulonephritis or endocapillary proliferative glomerulonephritis. Roth spots and Osler nodes fulfil this criterion.

6 Neurologic investigation is vital for patients with suspected or confirmed IE. Neurologic abnormalities occur in approximately 25% of patients with IE at presentation. These abnormalities can include stroke, transient ischaemic attack, meningitis, abscess and symptoms such as seizure, headache and focal neurologic deficit. Cerebrospinal fluid (CSF) examination may be used to investigate meningitis. As mentioned, intracranial manifestations of IE can be investigated with MRI or CT. This may affect timing of surgery and detect lesions not producing symptoms.

7 There are several other tests that should be performed in these patients. FBE may show leucocytosis and anaemia. Kidney function tests can show evidence of acute kidney injury from immunologic or antibiotic-induced glomerulonephritis, sepsis or heart failure. Liver function tests (LFTs) and coagulation studies should be ordered as baseline. Erythrocyte sedimentation rate (ESR) and C-reactive protein (CRP) are often raised. Urinalysis may show microscopic haematuria, proteinuria or pyuria due to glomerulonephritis or embolic event in the kidney. Electrocardiography should be performed, especially if the patient is for surgical management. ECG is also useful to assess for formation or extension of abscess close to the conduction system. If abnormalities of conduction are found, another TOE should be performed.

8 Positron emission tomography (PET) scan can be used when there is difficult identifying the source of infection or for confirming endocarditis, when there is a high suspicion. PET can identify a high fluorodeoxyglucose (FDG)-avidity spot on a valve and an abscess elsewhere in the body, which may be a source or an embolic complication.

Management

Immediate

Assess the need for **urgent resuscitation** [1]. Consult the **infectious diseases team** [2].

Short-term

Commence the patient on **IV antibiotics** [3]. Discuss the patient at the IE team meeting, and consider **surgery** [4] [5]. Perform a **coronary angiogram** [6] to exclude ischaemic heart disease. Discuss the benefits and risks of surgery with the patient and his family. A couple of days later, perform **surgery for infective endocarditis** [7] through median sternotomy.

Establish cardiopulmonary bypass and open the left atrium. Excise the mitral valve and replace it with a bioprosthetic valve. Wean the patient from bypass into sinus rhythm. Send the excised mitral leaflets for microscopy, culture and sensitivities (MC&S). Insert a peripherally inserted central catheter (PICC) and administer antibiotics for 6 weeks.

Long-term

Monitor the patient in ICU [8] following the surgery. Ensure an **uneventful postoperative recovery** [9] and **follow the patient up in clinic** [10]. Discuss appropriate **preventive strategies for IE** [11] with the patient.

[1] Patients with IE, especially in its acute form, can have compromised cardiac function as well as septic shock. These may require urgent resuscitation.

[2] Patients with IE should be reviewed by a multidisciplinary team (MDT). This team should include infectious diseases specialists, cardiologists and cardiothoracic surgery specialists.

[3] IV antibiotics successfully treat IE without the need for surgery in approximately 65% of cases. While the risk of an embolic event is high in IE in general (>20%), the commencement of antibiotic therapy is associated with a lower rate of new embolic events. Blood cultures (ideally several) should be obtained before commencing antibiotics, to allow targeted therapy. Because it can be difficult for antibiotics to penetrate the vegetation, long courses of antibiotic therapy are necessary. Once antibiotic therapy is commenced, blood cultures should be obtained in a serial fashion every 2 days until they are negative. The duration of antibiotics is counted from the first day of negative blood cultures and will generally last at least 6 weeks. Broadly, aminoglycosides are often used in conjunction with an antibiotic affecting the cell wall such as beta-lactam or vancomycin. This allows increased entry of the aminoglycoside through the cell wall. Patients with multi-resistant organisms frequently do not recover with antibiotic therapy alone. Even in subacute disease, this constant bacteraemia can lead to valvular abnormalities. For antibiotic therapy alone, repeat echocardiograms should be obtained if new complications are suspected.

[4] In general, patients deteriorate significantly before improving, following such operations with severe systemic inflammatory response. This has to be taken into account when selecting the operative candidate and indicating surgery. The surgeon's experience plays a major role in the surgical management of infective endocarditis. Nevertheless, there are some well-defined indications for surgery in the context of IE: cardiac failure, uncontrolled sepsis, perivalvular abscess, intracardiac fistula and large vegetations (10mm is considered large, and mobile vegetations on the anterior leaflet of mitral valve have a higher risk of embolisation despite antibiotics). Infection with *Staphylococcus aureus*, multi-resistant organisms or fungi often require early surgical intervention. Advanced patient age is not an absolute contraindication to surgery, as it lowers mortality in all age groups – it should be assessed on a case-by-case basis.

[5] The timing of surgery for IE takes is a matter of wide variability, hence management within an endocarditis team is ideal. Some factors that influence decision-making are haemodynamic instability, size and location of vegetation, increasing vegetation, presence of abscess or prosthetic valve, recent haemorrhagic or large embolic stroke. Early surgery, when possible, has been shown to have long-term mortality benefits.

[6] Pre-operative coronary angiogram is indicated for those with history of ischaemic heart disease (IHD) and aged over 40 years. Unfortunately, it is not always possible, especially in aortic valve endocarditis due to high risk of septic emboli.

[7] Surgery for IE has several goals. First, infected tissue must be completely removed. Secondly, repair of the affected/resected parts of the heart and restoration of function. Given that these are open-heart operations, cardiopulmonary bypass is necessary. Intraoperative TOE is used to identify other affected areas/valves, fistulae and abscesses, and assess surgical repair. Surgeons should consider whether to repair or replace the affected valve. Prosthetic valves carry a significantly increased risk of recurrence of IE in the setting of active infection (when microorganisms from surgical specimen still grow in culture). If cultures of resected valve

are positive, an entire 6-week postoperative antibiotic course is recommended. In patients operated on with culture-negative IE, polymerase chain reaction (PCR) from the surgical specimen is an important tool to precisely identify the aetiologic agent.

8 Patients who have had operations for IE should undergo the same postoperative monitoring as those who have had other valve operations. Immediate postoperative care in the intensive care unit (ICU) includes invasive arterial monitoring, central venous line continuous ECG, temperature and urine output. Alpha and beta agonists are used commonly. A Swan–Ganz catheter can be inserted in selected cases for assessment of cardiac output and intravascular volume status with right atrial and pulmonary artery pressures. Antibiotic levels should be assessed as these patients often have compromised renal function. For the same reason, renal function should be assessed in the postoperative period. Full blood count and reactants can be used to monitor the resolution of infection. If the patient remains septic, other possible sites should be considered – comparing the pre-operative CT with a recent one can aid in identification of other sources of infection.

9 Mortality is directly affected by the pre-operative status of the patient, the degree of cardiac injury and complexity of procedure. For prosthetic valve IE, the mortality is higher.

This is likely due to difficulties associated with re-operation, the increased frequency of abscess and insidious disease progression. For those with healed IE (outpatient setting), mortality is much lower. The 10-year survival for IE with valve replacement is approximately 60%. There are several factors associated with poorer outcomes for patients with IE treated through surgery. Haemodynamic disturbance, staphylococcal infection, older age, renal dysfunction, length of cardiopulmonary bypass time, non-healed IE, prosthetic valve IE and emergency procedures are all associated with higher in-hospital mortality.

10 Patients are usually monitored with serial full blood examinations and CRP to assess for recurrence. Echocardiography should be performed to establish a new baseline for valvular function. These patients usually undergo follow-up in cardiology and infectious diseases clinics.

11 Patients with risk factors for IE including previous IE history, prosthetic heart valves, congenital heart disease, acquired valvular disease, hypertrophic cardiomyopathy and mitral valve prolapse are at increased risk of IE during transient bacteraemia. Antibiotic prophylaxis should be considered in these patients when undergoing dental procedures, and all surgical procedures including colonoscopy and gastroscopy, especially if they are having polyp removal or other instrumentation.

CASE 3: Ischaemic heart disease

History

- A **58-year-old** [1] **man** [2] presents to his GP with a **history** [3] of **indigestion** [4] mainly on weekends, which has been getting worse in the last 2 months.
- When questioned about these **episodes** [5], he says that he normally has breakfast and then **works hard in the garden** [6].
- He **becomes sweaty and has to stop** [7] for a drink to relieve the heartburn.
- Last weekend, he felt a strong pain that lasted for 5 minutes.
- The patient denies any other medical background such as **hypertension** [8], **dyslipidaemia** [9], **diabetes** [10], major surgery or allergies. He has no other relevant past medical history. He only takes over-the-counter medication for indigestion.
- His **father** [11] died of a heart attack aged 60 and his **brother** [11] had coronary artery bypass graft (CABG) surgery at the age of 48.
- He smokes **10 cigarettes** [12] per day, has a **poor diet** [12], does **not exercise regularly** [12] and drinks a **moderate amount of alcohol** [12]. He has been counselled on these risk factors previously.
- He works as a travel agent and is **stressed** [13] about the current financial aspects of his job.

[1] Advancing age is the single most important risk factor for ischaemic heart disease (IHD). Postmenopausal women are also at greater risk of developing IHD.

[2] IHD is more common in males. However, due to the high prevalence of this disease overall, it is still an important disease to consider in females.

[3] IHD presentations occur in three broad categories: angina pectoris, acute coronary syndrome (ACS) or silent ischaemia.

[4] Angina pectoris is a pain, discomfort or feeling of heaviness, squeezing or tightening of the chest. It is often felt behind the sternum or over the left precordium. It may radiate from the chest to the jaw, shoulder, back or arm. Some patients find that it is a feeling similar to heartburn.

[5] When investigating pain, it is important to identify the location and radiation, character (pain, heaviness, tightness or discomfort) and severity, duration, relieving and precipitating factors.

[6] Angina pectoris is often brought on by exertion, when myocardial oxygen consumption is increased. Any activity that raises the double product (systolic blood pressure multiplied by the heart rate), such as exercise or emotional distress, can trigger angina in patients with coronary artery obstructions. Chronic angina is caused by a gradual and fixed obstruction of the coronary arteries by plaque of atheroma, which eventually calcifies. If a plaque ruptures (becomes unstable), platelet adhesion and clot formation cause an ACS.

[7] Angina pectoris can be associated with shortness of breath, palpitation, diaphoresis, nausea, vomiting and anxiety. It can also present with epigastric discomfort and fatigue. Although angina pectoris is a common manifestation of IHD, it is not always present. Some 15% of patients with IHD do not present with angina. Silent ischaemia occurs most often in patients with diabetes mellitus. This is due to cardiac autonomic neuropathy as well as the possibility of increased pain threshold. An increased proportion of elderly females also have silent ischaemia, including ACS.

[8] Hypertension has been consistently demonstrated to be associated with an increased risk of IHD. Both systolic and diastolic hypertension contribute to the development of the disease. The pathogenesis relates to the formation of atherosclerosis, increased endothelial dysfunction and changes in the microcirculation.

[9] Dyslipidaemia is also associated with the development of IHD. Elevated LDL cholesterol and low levels of high density lipoprotein (HDL) cholesterol are associated with IHD. This is likely due to the fact that HDL cholesterol is related to the process of removing LDL cholesterol from the vessel wall.

[10] Patients with diabetes mellitus have a significantly higher rate of IHD, because chronic hyperglycaemia affects the vascular wall.

[11] Family history of ACS and premature IHD are both associated with increased rates of IHD.

12 There are several lifestyle factors associated with IHD. These include cigarette smoking, obesity, poor diet, sedentary lifestyle and heavy alcohol intake. Smoking is the second most important risk factor for IHD following age. The association between smoking and the development of the disease is dose-dependent. The overall mechanism is likely due to the acceleration of atherosclerosis as well as platelet activation, coronary artery vasospasm and increasing blood pressure.

13 Psychosocial stress and depression have been found to be associated with IHD.

Examination

- General inspection reveals an **overweight man with significant central adiposity** [1].
- He enters the room **independently, not obviously in pain** [2] and is comfortable at rest.
- There is no obvious **shortness of breath (SOB), cyanosis, pallor or oedema** [3].
- His **vital signs are unremarkable** [4].
- His hands are normal apart from some **tar staining and xanthomata and capillary refill is <2 seconds** [5].
- His **radial pulse is strong and regular** [6] and there is no **radio-radial or radio-femoral delay** [7].
- His **carotid examination** [8] is normal, his **JVP** [8] is not elevated and there is no **hepatojugular reflux** [8].
- There is **xanthelasma** [9] but his mouth is normal.
- Inspection of the chest reveals **no scars, deformities or visible pulsations** [10].
- Palpation of the chest reveals **no thrills or heave, and the apex beat is not displaced** [11].
- The **heart sounds are dual and there are no murmurs** [12].
- The **lungs are clear** [13] and **abdominal examination is normal** [14].
- There are **no scars on the legs or arms** [14] and no missing limbs or toes.

1 Central adiposity and overweight are significant risk factors for ischaemic heart disease. The metabolic syndrome is made up of dyslipidaemia, hypertriglyceridaemia, hypertension, obesity and insulin resistance causing hyperglycaemia. The components of the metabolic syndrome are significant risk factors for vascular disease, including IHD.

2 General inspection should guide several parts of the assessment of the patient. This includes assessment of conscious state, pain and hydration status. It is good practice to include ABC (airway, breathing, circulation) assessment to identify a patient with a potentially life-threatening condition.

3 In patients with IHD, shortness of breath (SOB) is a common symptom of left main coronary artery obstruction or an ACS. The combination of SOB and oedema is associated with heart failure/valvular heart disease. Cyanosis suggests underlying respiratory failure, heart failure or both. Congenital heart disease is another cause of cyanosis but rare in adults. Pallor suggests anaemia or other non-cardiac chronic disease.

4 Assessment of vital signs is crucial for adequate evaluation of any patient. This patient's vital signs present an overall stable picture, despite mild hypertension. It is not uncommon to see completely normal vital signs in patients with chronic IHD. Patients with ACS, though, can present with single or multiple signs of physiological struggle: tachycardia, SOB, hypo- or hypertension, diaphoresis, anxiety; even altered mental status and shock.

5 The hands may exhibit signs of tar staining due to smoking and xanthomata due to hypercholesterolaemia. These are risk factors for IHD.

6 Pulse is important to assess for arrhythmias. A weak and thready pulse indicates that cardiac output is compromised.

7 Radio-radial and radio-femoral delay indicate aortic dissection or, rarely, coarctation of the aorta.

8 A carotid bruit may be present, suggesting extensive atherosclerosis. A raised jugular venous pressure (JVP) and hepatojugular reflux suggest hypervolaemia which may be due to heart failure. A raised JVP may also be due to tricuspid valve pathology or heart block.

9 Xanthelasma suggests chronically raised cholesterol. Other important considerations around the eyes include conjunctival pallor, corneal arcus indicating hypercholesterolaemia and hypertensive or diabetic retinopathy on fundoscopic examination. The mouth may show anaemia or cyanosis.

10 The presence of scars and their location can be a clue for other medical conditions.

11 In heart failure, palpation of the precordium may reveal a displaced apex beat and the apex beat may also be heard over a wider area.

12 In most cases of chronic stable IHD, the heart examination is essentially normal. Auscultation should assess the first and second heart sounds, any extra heart sounds and any murmurs. A third heart sound, although normal in athletes, may be heard in IHD and myocardial hypertrophy due to diastolic dysfunction. A fourth heart sound may also be heard in decompensated heart failure. The heart sounds are often best heard between the left lower and left upper sternal border.

13 In general, patients with IHD are or were smokers and might also have associated lung disease. Basilar rales or crepitations indicate fluid overload. Common cardiac causes of pulmonary oedema are heart failure or valvular

heart disease; common lung causes are chronic obstructive pulmonary disease (COPD), bronchiectasis or pneumonia; always think of other non-cardiac causes of pulmonary oedema, such as renal or endocrine diseases.

14 Peripheral vascular disease is associated with coronary artery disease. Palpation of the abdomen can reveal an abdominal aortic aneurysm. Scars on the arms or legs, or missing limbs or toes may suggest previous bypass surgery, or amputation secondary to peripheral vascular disease.

Investigations

- The patient undergoes **several tests** [1] [2] [3] to exclude a cardiac cause for his indigestion.
- **FBE** [4], **fasting lipid profile** [5], **HbA1c** [6], and **thyroid function tests** [7] are all within normal limits.
- **Functional tests** [8] are considered.
- A **resting ECG** [9] was normal.
- An exercise ECG (stress test) performed days later was considered positive: it was interrupted within 4 minutes due to symptoms of the usual 'indigestion' associated with **upsloping ST depression on**

antero-septal leads and frequent premature ventricular contractions [10].
- His **CXR** [11] and **echocardiography are normal** [12].
- Although **other imaging** [13] is considered, ultimately coronary angiography shows **90% stenosis on the proximal segment of the left anterior descending (LAD), 70% of the circumflex coronary and 70% of the right coronary artery (RCA)** [14].

1 It was difficult to establish from the patient's history whether his symptoms of 'indigestion' were associated with exertion (gardening) or feeding (after breakfast). The GP thought of two main differential diagnoses in this case: coronary artery obstruction and dyspepsia. As the patient has risk factors for IHD (hypertension, overweight, sedentary lifestyle and current smoker – at least) and IHD carries higher risk to life than GI diseases, the GP decided to assess/exclude IHD first.

2 It is important to note the differences in diagnosis/ management between chronic stable IHD and acute coronary syndrome. ACS is a medical emergency, so the patient should be transferred to a hospital, whereas in stable IHD the diagnosis and treatment are mostly done as outpatient.

3 The strategy to balance low risk/simple/cheap to high risk/more complex/expensive diagnostic modalities applies in any case. Blood tests and CXR and more specific cardiac tests (ECG and echocardiogram) will give a snapshot of the patient's general health condition and aid in diagnosing cardiac disorders.

4 FBE can assess for anaemia. Anaemia results in reduced oxygen delivery and is associated with GI causes for blood loss. In patients with IHD, anaemia can exacerbate angina.

5 A fasting lipid profile should be used to diagnose dyslipidaemia, a component of the metabolic syndrome and risk factor for IHD.

6 Fasting blood glucose or HbA1c diagnose/exclude diabetes. Diabetes is a significant risk factor for IHD.

7 Thyroid function should be assessed in hypertension and IHD. Hyperthyroidism results in an increased cardiac output and systolic hypertension; hypothyroidism is associated with IHD.

8 The choice of functional tests (exercise ECG, exercise echocardiogram, dobutamine stress echocardiogram, myocardial perfusion test) should respect the low- to high-risk scale and will depend on contraindication/accuracy of the simpler test (e.g. inability to run on a treadmill or non-diagnostic exercise ECG, prompting a dobutamine echocardiogram or myocardial perfusion scan).

9 ECG is often normal in patients with stable angina. Left ventricular (LV) hypertrophy is common in untreated chronic hypertension. Other ECG abnormalities that can be caused by IHD are Q waves (in silent ischaemia), left bundle branch block and active arrhythmias.

10 An exercise stress ECG adds further information to a resting ECG. The ECG is performed before, during and after exercise and allows assessment of overall exercise capacity, achieved maximum heart rate and symptoms during exercise. The patient follows exercise protocols on a treadmill or bicycle. The ECG may show the ST segment becoming flat or depressed. Some factors indicate particularly poor prognosis. These include exercise limited by symptoms to be less than 6 metabolic equivalents, an inability to mount a systolic blood pressure >120mmHg or the development of ventricular arrhythmias. A stress ECG is not appropriate for patients who have poor conditioning, significant obesity, physical impairments or significant coexisting illness.

11 CXR is a non-invasive test that is helpful in determining other causes of chest pain. It is also useful in assessing the complications of advanced IHD including cardiomegaly, pulmonary oedema and pleural effusions. Calcification of the arteries may also be seen, indicating atherosclerosis. Also, lung disease can be appreciated in CXRs.

12 Echocardiography is indicated in known or suspected heart disease including valvulopathy and heart failure, including assessment of LV function (global or segmental). Echocardiographic signs that are indicative of IHD are wall motion abnormalities or wall thinning. Transoesophageal echocardiography is performed intraoperatively to assess cardiac function by the anaesthesia team.

13 Information regarding coronary artery morphology in the chronic setting of IHD will be required in cases when there is suspicion of myocardial ischaemia. CT coronary angiography is used to screen for coronary artery obstruction. However, functional testing (i.e. coronary angiography) is the gold standard to define coronary artery anatomy and degree of obstruction. This information is used when considering interventional treatment.

14 Coronary angiography is an invasive procedure performed by direct injection of contrast (radio-opaque dye) into the coronary arteries via catheterisation of either the right radial artery or femoral arteries. X-ray is used to capture the image. Angiography often underestimates the degree of stenosis overall. An obstruction causing a diameter loss of 50% is equivalent to a loss of 75% in the area. An obstruction of ≥50% causes significant obstruction to flow.

Management

Immediate

Initial measures to deal with chronic stable IHD include:

- encouragement to improve lifestyle with **healthy eating** [1] and habit management (**weight loss** [2], **regular exercise** [3] and **smoking cessation** [4])
- **blood pressure control** [5]
- **antiplatelets** [6]
- **symptomatic medication** [7]
- **cholesterol level control** [8]
- **diabetes education/management (for diabetic patients)** [9].

Short-term

Discuss the patient at the **h**eart **t**eam **m**eeting **(HTM)** [10]. Choose management based on the risks and benefits of myocardial revascularisation by either **PCI** [11] or **CABG** [12] [13]. **Review all previous information** [14], including **medication** [15], in clinic. Offer the patient **CABG** [16] on **pump** [17] [18]. Discuss risks and benefits of the procedure and alternatives with the patient and obtain consent for surgery.

The proposed operation is CABG **using the LITA to the LAD; and two SVG grafts, to obtuse marginal and RCA** [19]. Monitor the patient postoperatively **in the ICU** [20] and consider **discharge** [21] when the patient feels well.

Long-term

Optimise the patient's **medications** [22] before discharge and ensure he is followed up in the **cardiothoracic outpatient clinic** [23].

1 There are several dietary approaches for IHD. Reducing saturated fats and trans fatty acids are appropriate.

2 Maintaining or achieving a body mass index (BMI) of <25.0 and reducing waist circumference is recommended.

3 Current recommendations are at least 150 minutes of moderate intensity exercise over at least 3 days each week with resistance training for healthy individuals. Exercise prescription will vary with a patient's condition and this regimen might not be applicable to all patients before definitive treatment (either PCI or CABG).

4 All patients should be advised to quit smoking. Counselling and other cessation therapies are appropriate for this.

5 Current blood pressure (BP) treatment should aim for <140/90mmHg. For those with diabetes, BP goal should be <130/80mmHg. Beta blockers reduce heart rate and contractility. This subsequently reduces oxygen demand in the myocardium and has been shown to reduce risk. A combination of ACE inhibitor and calcium channel blocker (CCB) are appropriate for those with diabetes. However, effective drug combinations each have their own benefits and drawbacks.

6 Antiplatelet therapy reduces the risk of acute MI and sudden death. Low dose aspirin is appropriate for this purpose. In those who have received percutaneous intervention, combining aspirin with another antiplatelet such as clopidogrel or ticagrelor is indicated.

7 Nitrates can be used to reduce anginal symptoms.

8 All patients with clinically significant IHD should receive intensive therapy to manage dyslipidaemia – statins are the first line if no contraindications.

9 Adequate glycaemic control is vital in reducing cardiovascular risk. Current recommendations suggest maintaining HbA1c below 7.5%. However, intensive control of HbA1c <6.0% is associated with lower cardiovascular risk.

10 A heart team is composed of cardiologists and cardiac surgeons to discuss patient management, who meet regularly.

11 In percutaneous coronary intervention (PCI), a stent is placed within the stenotic vessel, allowing the vessel diameter to increase and slowing the progression of further stenosis. PCI is associated with lower mortality benefit and increased need for revascularisation procedures.

12 The patient's coronary anatomy (proximal LAD obstruction and two other major arteries with severe disease) indicates surgery on prognostic (quantity of life) and symptomatic (quality of life) grounds. Although PCI can be done in many cases, it may not be beneficial in the long term. Hence, discussion in the HTM is sometimes indicated. Guidelines are established regarding indication for PCI and CABG; however, these are constantly evolving.

13 Current indications include >50% stenosis of the left main coronary artery (LMCA), or LMCA-equivalent disease which involves >70% stenosis of the proximal LAD and left circumflex arteries. Other indications include >70% stenosis in more than three vessels, survivors of ST elevation MI (STEMI) with failed medical or PCI therapy, non-ST elevation MI (NSTEMI) patients with ongoing ischaemia, multivessel disease in patients with diabetes and left ventricular systolic dysfunction with proximal LAD stenosis or significant multivessel disease.

14 History should identify comorbidities and possible risk factors. Physical examination should include identification of viable grafts: differential BP in both arms to identify possible subclavian artery stenosis, which can affect LITA flow; Allen test for radial arteries; presence of long saphenous vein. Other preoperative investigation, according to patient's morbidity, are at the surgeon's discretion: lung function tests, duplex scan of carotid and vertebral arteries, CT scan, MRI, etc.

15 The decision to cease aspirin should be individualised and there is no current consensus. Clopidogrel is associated with increased bleeding risk and should be ceased for at least 5 days in elective cases. Beta blockers and CCBs can be continued up to the time of operation; ACE inhibitors are usually ceased the night before the operation.

16 The surgical myocardial revascularisation, or CABG, involves utilising a source of oxygenated blood (e.g. from the aorta) and employing an autologous conduit (e.g. an artery or vein) to bypass a stenotic segment of coronary artery.

17 CABG can be performed with or without the aid of the heart-lung machine (HLM). When the HLM is used, high dose heparin is administered and big cannulae are used to draw venous blood from the patient and return it to the arterial system. The HLM does the work of the heart and lungs as it exchanges O_2 and CO_2 in the oxygenator and pumps the oxygenated blood back to the body. When the HLM takes control of the whole circulation, both the heart and lungs will be depleted of blood, what surgeons call cardiopulmonary bypass (CPB). During CPB, the heart is isolated from the circulation completely by clamping the ascending aorta and cardioplegia (a solution to arrest and preserve the heart) is injected intermittently into the coronary arteries or coronary sinus. This allows for the heart to be operated on without motion or blood. In other words, the operation itself involves anaesthesia, sternotomy, harvest of grafts, establishment of CPB, anastomoses (revascularisation), termination of CPB, haemostasis and closure of sternotomy.

18 When CPB is not used for revascularisation (off-pump CABG or OP-CAB), the heart will be beating and supporting the circulation throughout that time. Special equipment is used to expose the coronary arteries and stabilise them whilst the anastomosis is performed. Results of both on-pump and off-pump strategies are comparable, coming down to a surgical preference. There is a tendency for OP-CAB to use fewer grafts than CABG.

19 The most common conduits are the left and right internal thoracic arteries (LITA and RITA respectively), the great saphenous vein (SVG) and the radial arteries (RadA). The LITA is normally used as pedicled (it draws blood from its source, the left subclavian artery). SVG and RadA are free grafts as they can be connected from the aorta or even the LITA as source of blood supply. The SVG can be harvested skeletonised or with its vasa vasorum; open incision or endoscopically. Access to the heart is done via sternotomy. Other incisions are necessary if a radial artery or SVG are required.

20 The key to excellent outcomes in cardiac surgery is multidisciplinary/collaborative teamwork. ICU plays a vital role in patient recovery.

21 Major complications of cardiac surgery happen in part by the procedure and in part by the patient's comorbidities, and include death, MI, stroke, bleeding/transfusion and mediastinitis. Temporary atrial fibrillation is very common.

22 Aspirin or other antiplatelet agent is introduced on the day of the operation if there is no bleeding. Antihypertensives are resumed according to need, but beta blockers (as they help in preventing atrial fibrillation) should be the first choice if no contraindications. Ideally the patient is discharged with antiplatelet, beta blocker and statin.

23 Follow-up for patients undergoing CABG involves an MDT including the GP, cardiologist and allied health. Secondary prevention for IHD will need to be continually monitored with GP and cardiologist. Cardiac rehabilitation programmes are a great and safe way to improve patient recovery.

CASE 4: Lung cancer

History

- A patient has been referred to the cardiothoracic surgery clinic for work-up of **possible lung cancer** [1] [2]. He is a 64-year-old man who presented to the ED following a fall at home. He complained of chest pain on the right side.
- A CXR could not determine any rib fractures or lung abnormality. The emergency physician decided to exclude rib fractures by performing a CT scan; this showed a nodule in the right upper lobe and no rib fractures. The patient's pain was managed, and he was referred to the cardiothoracic surgery outpatient clinic.

- On **history** [3] he reports a daily morning **cough** [4] but denies any **haemoptysis** [5], **chest pain** [6], **dyspnoea** [7] or **voice changes** [8].
- He has **no other complaints** [9] [10] [11] of note.
- He has a medical history of hypertension, hyperlipidaemia and anxiety but **no lung conditions** [12].
- He reports a 50 pack year **smoking history** [13] over 40 years. He denies any family history of lung or oesophageal cancer.
- He is a retired **builder** [14] and is not sure if he has had any **asbestos exposure** [15].

[1] The lungs are paired organs that sit within the chest cavity and connect to the trachea through the bronchi. They are the major respiratory organ system. Respiration involves ventilation, gas diffusion (mainly of oxygen and carbon dioxide) and circulation. When abnormal cells proliferate in an uncontrolled manner, it is termed cancer. These abnormal cells do not contribute to the function of the organ and can inhibit the functioning of adjacent healthy tissue. Lung cancer occurs when the abnormal cells have developed from lung tissue. Primary lung cancer begins in the lungs and may spread to lymph nodes or other organs in the body, such as the brain. When cancer cells spread from one organ to another, they are called metastases.

[2] Lung cancer is the most common cancer and is still responsible for the most cancer-related deaths worldwide. It is becoming more common overall, and more common relative to other cancers. However, survival is improving. This is likely due to both a decline in smoking as well as improved diagnosis and treatment. Lung cancer affects more men than women, mainly due to respective lifestyle choices.

[3] Lung cancer symptoms may be caused by the tumour itself, regional or distant spread or from systemic effects (paraneoplastic syndromes). Symptoms can be categorised as thoracic (generally from local effects) and extrathoracic (generally from metastases). Thoracic symptoms include cough, haemoptysis, dyspnoea, chest pain and hoarseness of voice.

[4] Cough is present in the majority of those presenting with lung cancer. It is common in subtypes involving the central airways, including squamous cell and small cell

carcinomas. In keeping with this, in a patient who smokes or has formerly smoked, a new cough should trigger further work-up.

[5] Haemoptysis is common in patients diagnosed with advanced lung cancer. Its presence largely depends on the type and stage of cancer.

[6] Chest pain is another common symptom for those with advanced lung cancer. It is caused by extension of the tumour into the mediastinum, pleura, chest wall or spine. It usually occurs on the same side as the tumour and may be described as dull or aching.

[7] Dyspnoea may also occur in lung cancer. It may be caused by obstruction of the airway either by compression, a mass within the wall extending into the lumen of the airway or through an intraluminal obstruction. Additionally, lung cancer can cause pneumothorax and pleural effusion. These conditions themselves may cause dyspnoea.

[8] Hoarseness of voice may occur if the recurrent laryngeal nerve is affected by the mass.

[9] There are several syndromes associated with lung cancer. Superior vena cava (SVC) syndrome occurs when the SVC is obstructed and interrupts venous return from the head, causing a feeling of congestion in the head as well as dyspnoea. Pancoast syndrome occurs where a superior tumour invades the brachial plexus and sympathetic chain.

[10] Effects of lung cancer not related to local or metastatic causes are considered to be paraneoplastic. Hypercalcaemia can arise from bony metastasis or tumour secretion of

a parathyroid hormone-related protein. The syndrome of inappropriate antidiuretic hormone secretion (SIADH) is frequently caused by small cell lung cancer (SCLC) and results in hyponatraemia. Ectopic production of adrenocorticotrophic hormone (ACTH) can cause Cushing syndrome.

11 Extrathoracic symptoms can manifest from any organ affected and therefore can have numerous symptoms. Hypertrophic pulmonary osteoarthropathy (HPOA) is considered present when clubbing or periosteal proliferation is associated with lung disease. It causes a painful and symmetrical arthropathy.

12 Patients with a history of lung disease such as pulmonary fibrosis or COPD have an increased risk of developing lung cancer. The risk for lung cancer is increased approximately 7-fold in patients with pulmonary fibrosis and is independent of the contributory risk of smoking. COPD is the most common independent risk factor, other than smoking, for lung cancer, increasing the risk of lung cancer by 6 to 13-fold.

13 Cigarette smoking accounts for the majority of lung cancer. The risk of developing lung cancer for a current smoker compared to a non-smoker is approximately 20-fold.

Second-hand smoke exposure is associated with an increased risk of lung cancer, even though the carcinogen dose is much lower than with active smoking. Smoking appears to produce a relationship between intensity of exposure and relative risk, with spouses, children and workplace contacts at increased risk.

14 Exposure to second-hand smoke, asbestos, radon and metals such as arsenic, chromium and nickel have all been associated with an increased risk for developing lung cancer. Radiation therapy can increase the risk of lung cancer in those treated for other malignancies. Air pollution and diesel exhaust exposure have also been linked to the incidence of lung cancer. This risk is proportional to the extent of exposure.

15 There are several occupational and environmental exposures associated with the development of lung cancer. The best-known factors are asbestos and radon. Patients with asbestos exposure complicated by interstitial fibrosis, known as asbestosis, are much more likely to develop lung cancer than patients with asbestos exposure alone. The risk of lung cancer is dose-dependent but varies according to the type of asbestos fibre. In the UK asbestos was used in construction up until 1999.

Examination

- The patient has a **normal appearance** [1] and is distinctly overweight.
- Examination of the **vital signs** [2] reveals the patient to have a mild tachypnoea (resting rate 25) and a low grade temperature of 37.1°C. He is saturating at 94% on air with an audible dry cough.
- Examination of the hands reveals **bilateral clubbing** [3].
- Examination of the **face and neck is normal** [4].

- Notably, there is no **miosis, ptosis or anhidrosis** [5].
- His **haemodynamic examination is unremarkable** [6].
- **Respiratory examination is normal** [7], except for tenderness at the site injured by the fall.
- His abdomen is **soft and non-tender** [8].
- **Peak flow measurement** [9] is performed and found to be lower than normal and a **sputum sample** [9] is taken.

[1] On general appearance, patients with lung cancer can occasionally appear cachectic as a consequence of advanced disease. Confusion or neurologic signs/symptoms can indicate brain metastasis.

[2] Vital signs are a pertinent adjunct to all examinations. The majority of early stage lung cancer patients have normal vital signs. Patients can present with tachycardia, tachypnoea, low saturations and a low grade fever. These abnormal vital signs can be attributed to poor gas exchange and poor ventilation. Fevers can result from a malignant process generally driven by a cytokine response.

[3] Any thorough examination starts at the hands and moves up and then down the body in that order, to ensure a systematic approach. Clubbing (spoon-shaped nails or drumstick fingers) is seen in patients with chronic hypoxia

or paraneoplastic syndrome (it can also rarely occur in the absence of disease). Cyanosis can be seen in the extremities (fingernail beds), mucous membranes (lips and conjunctiva) and skin. HPOA is characterised by periostitis, digital clubbing and painful arthropathy – it generally presents as painful finger or wrist joints but can also occur in the knees and ankles.

[4] Cyanosis can be assessed by inspecting the patient's lips. Pallor can be assessed by assessing their conjunctiva. Lung cancer does not contribute directly to any other head signs; however, metastasis can. While assessing the neck, the trachea should be observed for deviation or tugging. While the majority of the patients have normal tracheal anatomy, mass effect from the tumour can be associated with deviation. Pemberton's sign is performed by asking the patient to lift both their arms above their shoulders; a

positive sign is indicated by facial congestion, cyanosis and respiratory distress. This is generally indicative of mass effect causing compression of the SVC. Lymph node metastasis can present as palpable lymphadenopathy and the cervical chain, supraclavicular and axillary nodes must be assessed.

5 It is important to perform a neurological examination when there is a complaint of pain in shoulders or hands, weakness in the affected limb and atrophy of muscles of the upper limb. This is due to brachial plexus involvement. The ulnar nerve (roots C8–T1) is the first to be affected from tumours originating from lung apex and invading the chest wall, also known as Pancoast tumours or superior sulcus tumours. Pancoast tumours are not common, accounting for <5% of lung cancers. Pancoast syndrome is a possible clinical presentation of these tumours, when there is ipsilateral upper limb (hand, arm or shoulder) pain, weakness or paraesthesia and Horner's syndrome (miosis – constricted pupil; ptosis – drooping of eyelid; and anhidrosis – hemifacial sweating). Horner's syndrome occurs with invasion of the stellate ganglion or ansa subclavia, both part of the sympathetic chain.

6 The cardiovascular examination is usually normal, but associated ischaemic heart disease is frequent, as smoking is a common risk factor.

7 The respiratory examination starts with inspection of the chest wall and assessing for any asymmetrical movements or posture. Assess for the use of accessory muscles in respiration. Perform percussion on the back and the anterior chest wall. Following that, auscultate the back and the anterior chest wall. Patients with lung cancer can have unilateral percussion dullness secondary to the mass or an associated pleural effusion. Decreased breath sounds can be heard over the mass or due to a pleural effusion.

8 Abdominal examination is usually normal; however, the patient can have metastasis which can present as ascites, hepatomegaly or discomfort. Common sites for metastasis from lung cancer are adrenals, liver, brain, bone and lymph nodes (supraclavicular).

9 A complete examination also includes peak flow measurement and a sputum sample as an adjunct to the respiratory examination.

Investigations

- The patient undergoes several investigations to identify the nodule found on CT. He has a panel of **blood tests** [1].
- There were no previous **chest X-rays** [2] nor **chest CTs** [3] to compare so a **PET scan** [4] was ordered.
- The scans, blood tests and history allow for consideration of **differential diagnoses** [5].
- Following the investigations and diagnosis the patient is found to have a 2.5cm nodule in his right upper lobe with high FDG avidity. Mediastinal lymph

nodes are small (<10mm) and do not show FDG avidity on the PET scan. This allows for the patient to be staged based on the **TNM criteria** [6] [7] [8] [9].
- The definitive diagnosis is, however, made only by **tissue sampling** [9], in this case with a **CT-guided core biopsy** [10] [11].
- The biopsy returns as a **non-small cell lung cancer (NSCLC)** [12] [13] [14] with **immunohistochemistry** [15] being positive for TTF1 and CK7.

1 When a CT is suspicious of a lung malignancy, an assortment of blood tests is performed to predict the likelihood of metastasis. Abnormal tests can direct further imaging. These tests include a full blood count (FBC), electrolytes including calcium, LFTs and lactate dehydrogenase (LDH). Deranged LFTs could indicate liver metastasis. Hypercalcaemia should trigger additional imaging for bone metastasis and consideration of paraneoplastic syndrome. Elevated alkaline phosphatase (ALP) in conjunction with gamma-glutamyl transpeptidase (GGT) can suggest liver metastasis; however, an isolated raised ALP can suggest bony metastasis. Hyponatraemia can suggest a paraneoplastic effect (found normally in SCLC) and further tests should be performed at the time of initial evaluation to prevent delays in treatment.

2 Early stage lung cancer often appears as a solitary pulmonary nodule. Where possible, CXR should be compared

with previous chest imaging to determine age of the lesion and to attempt to quantify a growth pattern. CXR indicating new or enlarging focal lesion, pleural effusion, pleural nodularity, enlarged chest nodes, post-obstructive pneumonia or segmental atelectasis can be suggestive of malignancy.

3 While CXR is the first radiographic modality for lung cancer, further characterisation should be performed by a contrast CT scan. Malignant non-solid or part solid nodules often grow slower and can appear stable for longer. CT is useful for characterising the lesion anatomically, allowing guidance for tissue biopsy procedures. CT findings suggestive of malignancy include large lesion size >15mm, irregular or spiculated borders, upper lobe lesion or development of solid component within a ground glass region. Multiple nodules in a patient with known extrathoracic malignancy is suggestive of metastasis. CT can aid in staging of the tumour by contributing to knowledge regarding the local extent of the tumour, nodal involvement and metastasis presence. However, confirmation by tissue biopsy is mandatory. At times, it is difficult to differentiate cancer from inflammatory nodules.

4 Positron emission tomography (PET) has become a great aid in the diagnosis, staging and follow-up of patients with cancer. During PET, a small amount of radioactive glucose (fluorodeoxyglucose-18 or FDG) is administered. Areas with high metabolic activity (brain, heart, diaphragm, inflammatory and cancer cells) will take up larger amounts and this is shown on the PET scan. In early stages of disease, it defines the metabolic activity of the nodule. Malignant and infective ones tend to be very active, whereas benign tumours show no or minimal FDG avidity (the one exception to this rule is well differentiated carcinoid (neuroendocrine) neoplasia). It is also helpful in identifying possible lymph node involvement – in other words, staging the cancer. In advanced stages, it is used to monitor response to chemo- or radiotherapy. In addition, distant metastasis can be easily identified.

5 The differential diagnosis for lung cancer can include metastatic nodules, benign lung tumours, non-specific granuloma, tuberculous granuloma, pneumonia (empyema/ abscess), tracheal tumour, thyroid mass, hamartoma, bronchogenic cyst, lymphoma and granulomatosis with polyangiitis.

6 Once diagnosis is confirmed and appropriate imaging has been performed, the patient can be staged for their lung cancer. Staging is based on tumour size (T), nodal involvement (N) and whether or not metastasis (M) is present. The TNM staging system is a universally accepted system to illustrate the extent of disease burden and is regularly reviewed by international societies. The TNM stage and the patient's functional status (ECOG - Eastern Cooperative Oncology Group scoring system) allows for clinicians to determine the most appropriate treatment pathway.

7 The primary tumour is graded based on size, invasion of local structures and associated features (*see Table*). 'T' stands for tumour size, 'N' for presence of cancer in lymph node stations (regional spread), and 'M' for presence of metastasis (distant spread). The lower case prefix means it is based on clinical (cTNM) or pathological (pTNM) staging.

American Joint Commission on Cancer TNM staging for non-small cell lung cancer – 8th edition	
Tumour size	
Tx	Size of tumours cannot be measured
T1	Subdivided into T1a (<1cm), T1b (>1cm but <2cm) and T1c (>2cm but <3cm)
T2	3–5cm, involving the main bronchus or those that have associated atelectasis
T3	>5cm but <7cm or invading chest wall, pericardium or phrenic nerve
T4	>7cm or if the tumour is invading the diaphragm
Node (regional spread)	Node stations: 1–4 (superior mediastinal nodes), 5–6 (aortic nodes), 7–9 (inferior mediastinal nodes), 10–14 (N1 nodes)
N0	No nodes affected
N1	Ipsilateral hilar or pulmonary nodes
N2	Ipsilateral mediastinal or subcarinal lymph nodes
N3	Contralateral mediastinal, hilar nodes and ipsilateral or contralateral scalene nodes or supraclavicular nodes
Metastasis (distant spread)	
M1a	Limited to chest
M1b	Single extrathoracic metastasis
M1c	Multiple extrathoracic metastases

8 Metastatic disease is subdivided into three classifications: M1a if it is limited to the chest, M1b if there is a single extrathoracic metastasis and M1c if there are multiple extrathoracic metastases.

9 As mentioned previously, the stages are based on the TNM and are broken down into four stages, where stage 0 is for carcinoma *in situ* and stage I disease is deemed curable with localised disease. Stage IV is where there is widespread disease and metastasis. The staging system allows for algorithmic approach to the management of patients and allows for prognosis of the diagnosis.

10 Lung cancer diagnosis relies on histopathological examination. Tissue samples can be obtained through several tests, always favouring the less invasive over a more invasive modality. The choice of test and the likelihood of diagnosis will depend on tumour location (for instance, a central tumour might be diagnosed on sputum, whereas a peripheral one might need fine needle aspirate (FNA or core biopsy). Sputum cytology is a non-invasive modality commonly used. While collection is simple, it does not provide ideal samples for immunohistochemistry or molecular studies and is therefore generally used in practice when the patient is unable to undergo any invasive or minimally invasive procedure in the context of overwhelming metastatic disease.

Minimally invasive procedures include imaging guided biopsy, bronchoscopy and pleural aspiration. Image-guided biopsy may be used for the lesion itself as well as lymph nodes and suspected metastatic spread. Bronchoscopy allows for analysis of the bronchial tree and also allows for a variety of other sampling techniques such as bronchial washing, brushing or endobronchial ultrasound (EBUS) guided biopsy. A new modality is navigational bronchoscopy, which can reach small peripheral nodules. Bronchoscopy may also stage the disease, especially EBUS, as it can biopsy mediastinal nodes. Pleural aspirates in patients who present with pleural effusions can also be sent for analysis to confirm metastatic disease. Invasive procedures include cervical mediastinoscopy, anterior mediastinotomy and video-assisted thoracoscopic surgery (VATS). These surgical procedures are used to obtain diagnosis or staging, when a less invasive means is not possible.

11 The major objective of the biopsy is to differentiate between malignant or benign disease, and primary lung or metastasis, so treatment can be implemented accordingly. This will also determine the best surgical approach. For instance, if a nodule is from lung origin, the best outcome is achieved with anatomical resection (lobectomy), whereas if metastasis, a wedge resection or stereotactic ablative body radiotherapy (SABR) could be options (provided that the primary source of cancer is controlled).

12 Lung carcinomas are classified based on histopathologic subtype. Lung cancer is divided into two broad categories: non-small cell lung cancer (NSCLC) and small cell lung cancer (SCLC).

13 Neuroendocrine tumours are classified as small cell carcinoma (also known as oat cell carcinoma or SCLC), large cell neuroendocrine carcinoma, typical and atypical carcinoid. They usually arise in the central airways and continue to grow and infiltrate from this point. SCLC are very aggressive and metastasis occurs early in the process. SCLC accounts

for approximately 15% of all bronchogenic carcinomas. SCLC shows a strong correlation with cigarette smoking and is extremely rare in those who have never smoked.

14 About 80–85% of lung cancers are NSCLC. The main subtypes of NSCLC are adenocarcinoma, squamous cell carcinoma (SCC), large cell carcinoma, sarcomatoid carcinoma and adenosquamous carcinoma. Adenocarcinoma is the most common, accounting for approximately 50% of NSCLC cases, followed closely by SCC. It begins in mucus-producing cells found in the lining of the airways. Histologic diagnosis requires evidence of either neoplastic gland formation, pneumocyte marker expression or intracytoplasmic mucin. SCC occurs in the cells lining the surface of major airways; hence they tend to have a central location (close to pulmonary hilum).
Large cell carcinoma is a malignant epithelial neoplasm lacking both glandular and squamous or neuroendocrine differentiation by light microscopy, immunohistochemistry, and lacking cytologic features of small cell carcinoma. It is usually present as a large peripheral mass with prominent necrosis.
Sarcomatoid carcinoma is a broad term that represents a heterogeneous group of NSCLC. These include pleomorphic carcinoma, spindle cell carcinoma, giant cell carcinoma, carcinosarcoma and pulmonary blastoma. A histologic diagnosis of sarcomatoid carcinoma is associated with overall worse survival. These represent less than 1% of all lung cancers.

15 Immunohistochemistry stains allow classification and differentiation of lung cancers. Adenocarcinoma are generally positive for thyroid transcription factor (TTF-1), mucin, CK7, napsin-A, surf-A, surf-B and PAS-D. TTF-1 defines the adenocarcinoma as primary lung origin. SCC is classically positive for p63, p40, and cytokeratin 5 and 6 (CK5 and 6), and generally negative for CK7 (it is difficult to precisely identify its origin in patients with history of other SCCs such as skin, head-and-neck or colorectal).

Management

Immediate

The patient is stable.

Short-term

Discuss the patient at the thoracic MDT **meeting** [1]. His lung cancer is classified as a clinical Stage IIB NSCLC. Using a multimodal approach considering the disease pathology and patient factors, offer the patient **surgery** [2], with lobectomy being the **procedure of choice** [3] [4] [5]. Consider the **management of higher stage NSCLC and SCLC** [6] [7] [8] [9]. In the outpatient clinic, ideally with a support person, give that diagnosis to the patient. Explain the **management course** [10]:

it will include a surgical resection (lobectomy) and with the potential for adjuvant chemotherapy and radiotherapy. Following the procedure, monitor the patient and ensure an **uncomplicated recovery** [11].

Long-term

Discuss the histology results at the Thoracic MDT. It confirms that the lesion was completely excised with adequate margins and he had two positive lymph nodes. His staging is pT1cN0M0, finalised at Stage IA3 NSCLC – it is considered cured and he will be regularly followed up (consult and CT) for up to 5 years, unless recurrence is identified. Follow the patient up in the cardiothoracic surgery clinic **in 5 years** [12].

1 All lung cancer cases, once diagnosed and appropriately investigated, should be discussed at a Thoracic MDT with specialists from thoracic surgery, medical oncology, radiation oncology, pulmonology, palliative care and allied health. This is to ensure the patient is seen from different angles and the best care pathway is chosen for that individual. Appropriate staging and characterisation of the cancer allows for a suitable management plan to be formulated. Management varies between NSCLC and SCLC. NSCLC is predominantly managed surgically from Stages I–II with a curative intent. Stages IIIB–IV are managed with a symptom control intent. Stage III is highly debatable as surgically curative and depends on local team indication/research protocols. SCLC is predominantly managed with systemic therapy and radiotherapy, and surgical resection is only beneficial in T1–T2 disease with no nodal involvement.

2 The major roles of surgery in intrathoracic cancer are:
- curative – with intent to cure by resection of the organ, or part of it, and/or adjacent structures (e.g. lobectomy or pneumonectomy with lymph node dissection)
- diagnostic or staging – to diagnose the disease and/or determine its extent (e.g. mediastinoscopy with node biopsy or VATS with wedge resection)
- palliative – to control symptoms (e.g. pleurodesis to treat large symptomatic neoplastic pleural effusions, pericardial drainage for tamponade or airway stents for tracheal obstruction)
- debulking – there is no intention to cure, but to remove mass to control symptoms (e.g. resection of large anterior mediastinal mass after chemotherapy)
- supportive – to assist in other therapeutic modalities (e.g. insertion of a portacath for administration of chemotherapy)
- reconstructive – for cosmetic or functional intentions (e.g. harvesting of muscle flap for chest wall reconstruction).

3 Preoperative assessment is a essential process prior to any discussion at the MDT. A patient's past medical history, in particular cardiac and respiratory issues, is reviewed prior to any decision-making. A preoperative pulmonary function test assesses the patient's preoperative pulmonary reserve and diffusion capacity (DLCO) are important predictors of postoperative complications and mortality. Patients with FEV_1 and DLCO >80% are generally considered low risk and can in the main tolerate even a pneumonectomy without any significant lung dysfunction. Patients with <80% in these values should undergo further testing prior to considering any operative intervention. Other tests that can be considered according to patient needs are exercise ECG or echocardiogram, myocardial perfusion scan and ventilation-perfusion scan (V/Q scan).

4 Thoracic surgeries can be performed via open thoracotomy (a rib spreader provides visualisation) or VATS (video-assisted, that can be achieved with a camera and instruments via one or more ports – currently the most common way to perform thoracic surgery). The most common procedures are:
- wedge resection or atypical segmentectomy – a piece of lung (not respecting anatomic landmarks) is resected. Used for diagnosis or cure (in case of metastatic disease in the lung).
- lobectomy – a pulmonary lobe is resected (anatomic resection), often associated with mediastinal lymph node dissection. Used for cure.
- pneumonectomy – the whole lung is resected, often associated with mediastinal lymph node dissection. Used for cure.
- mediastinoscopy – an instrument is placed within the pre-tracheal fascia and this gives access to high mediastinal lymph nodes anterior and to the right of the trachea. Used for staging or diagnosis.
- anterior mediastinotomy – an incision over the second rib cartilage gives access to lymph nodes on the left side of the mediastinum. Used for diagnosis or staging.

5 In pleurodesis, adhesions between the visceral and parietal pleura are created with either talc or resection of parietal pleura. This procedure is used for palliation.

6 In early stage (Stage I–II) NSCLC, anatomical resection (lobectomy or pneumonectomy as opposed to wedge resection) offers best long-term survival. Lobectomy, when possible, is the gold standard treatment for early stage NSCLC. Lobectomies are mostly performed as VATS. The 5-year disease-free survival from surgery alone for Stage I, II and III disease is approximately 60–70%, 35–45% and 15–20%, respectively. Depending on staging and cancer pathology, adjuvant chemotherapy can increase the 5-year disease-free survival by approximately 10%. Patients who cannot undergo surgery (those who refuse or are not operative candidates) are offered radiotherapy either by the means of SABR or conventional fractionated radiotherapy. SABR allows for high dose radiation delivered using image guidance and high-precision targeting. Currently, SABR and wedge resections show similar local control and 5-year survival.

7 Stage III NSCLC management is often complex and at times controversial. This is because the tumour size, local extension and nodal involvement widely vary in this stage. Stage III is subclassified into IIIA, IIIB and IIIC. The treatment is generally a combination of local and systemic therapy. Operative intervention is offered generally in Stage IIIA if the surgical resection is deemed technically feasible with either a lobectomy or pneumonectomy (removing the entire lung) along with concurrent chemoradiotherapy and ideally within a research protocol. Stage IIIB and C generally involve contralateral lymph nodes and therefore are deemed unresectable and treated similarly to Stage IV disease. The prognosis of Stage III cancer is generally poor.

8 Stage IV NSCLC has a palliative approach to treatment. Patients are often referred to medical oncology, radiation oncology and palliative care for symptom management. Goals of care are determined with the patient and clinician and a combination of systemic and/or symptom control medication regime is given to provide comfort during end of life care.

9 SCLC at presentation is often a disseminated disease. Rarely, these patients present with a solitary nodule without regional nodal involvement or distant metastasis, in which case surgical management can be offered similar to that described for NSCLC. However, SCLC is known to be very chemosensitive and therefore systemic chemotherapy and adjuvant radiotherapy are an essential part of management. Patients with both limited stage and extensive stage SCLC have shown benefit in undergoing prophylactic cranial irradiation to decrease the risk of brain metastasis. As previously described, SCLC is an aggressive disease process where even patients with limited disease have a 5-year survival rate of 10%, in contrast to those with extensive disease, with studies quoting 5-year survival rates of 1–2%.

10 Any operative procedure carries risks from the general anaesthesia or surgery itself. Surgical risks can be subdivided into general and specific. General risks include; infection (pneumonia/empyema), bleeding, deep vein thrombosis or pulmonary embolism. Specific risks include prolonged air leak (bronchopleural fistula), atrial fibrillation, middle lobe torsion (right-sided surgery), chylothorax and nerve injury (phrenic or recurrent laryngeal nerves).

11 Postoperative recovery can occur either on the ward or ICU, depending on the surgical procedure, the patient's functional status and local logistics. Chest drain(s) are inserted after the procedure to evacuate any effusion/blood or air. They are removed when there is no air leak and a drainage of less than 150ml/24h (according to surgical preference). Loco-regional administration of local anaesthetic via extra-pleural or epidural catheter is a great way to decrease use of opioids, control pain and encourage early mobilisation. Hospital stay is around 3–5 days, according to patient's pre-op conditions and surgery. The MDT is key to early recovery, relying heavily on allied health involvement, such as physiotherapy, pain team, pharmacist, occupational therapy and social work.

12 Following curative treatment patients are generally followed up for a total of 5 years. Most guidelines suggest 3-monthly follow-up for the first 2 years followed by 6-monthly follow-up for the next 3 years. Clinical follow-up is accompanied by radiological imaging, generally a CXR and a CT scan, and on occasion PET scan. Studies have suggested that most recurrences occur within 2 years of treatment and therefore intensive follow-up for the first 2 years is vital. Patients are urged to stop smoking and reduce any environmental carcinogenic exposure such as second-hand smoke or asbestos exposure.

CASE 5: Mediastinal mass

History

- A patient has been referred to the general thoracic clinic for an incidental **mediastinal mass** [1] [2] discovered on CXR.
- The patient is a **63-year-old female** [3] with **no current symptoms** [4] [5].
- She has a **past history of mild myasthenia gravis** [6] which is adequately managed with an oral acetylcholinesterase inhibitor. She has no other past medical history and no relevant family history.
- She **does not smoke but enjoys alcohol infrequently** [7]. She is a retired gym teacher who lives alone.

[1] The mediastinum is the space between the two pleural cavities. It is surrounded by the chest wall anteriorly and spine posteriorly. The superior boundary is the thoracic inlet, which comprises the spine, first ribs and manubrium, and the diaphragm inferiorly. It can be divided into sections: anterior, middle and posterior. The anterior mediastinum contains the thymus gland, internal thoracic vessels, lymph nodes and fat. The thymus gland is made of left and right lobes and lies anterior to the fibrous pericardium. It is most prominent in children. The middle mediastinum contains the pericardium, heart, great vessels, trachea, oesophagus and phrenic and vagus nerves. The posterior mediastinum contains the thoracic duct, descending aorta and autonomic ganglia and nerves. Lymph nodes within the mediastinum are divided into lower mediastinal lymph nodes, subcarinal lymph nodes and upper mediastinal lymph nodes.

[2] There are several differential diagnoses to consider for a mediastinal mass. Masses can be divided into two categories: primary and secondary. Primary disease location is related to the anatomy of the mediastinum and native tissue types within each section. However, it is important to remember that migration can occur from one compartment to another. Primary mediastinal masses can be benign or malignant, with approximately 30% being malignant. Diseases likely to arise in the anterior compartment include germ cell tumours, thymomas, retrosternal goitres, aortic arch aneurysms and lymphadenopathy. Half of all mediastinal masses occur in the anterior mediastinum. However, lymphadenopathy can also occur in the middle compartment along with mediastinal cysts and ascending aorta aneurysms. Lastly, posterior mediastinal masses can be due to neurogenic tumours, which can be benign or malignant, oesophageal disease including duplication, tumours and diverticula, hiatus hernias or bronchogenic cysts. Secondary masses typically result from lymphatic spread via mediastinal lymph nodes. Primary neoplasms that spread to the mediastinum commonly include lung, oesophagus, larynx, thyroid and stomach. The 'terrible Ts', which are differential diagnoses for anterior mediastinal mass, include thymic tumours, teratoma, thyroid mass and terrible lymphadenopathy.

[3] Age and gender of the patient make some diseases more likely than others. A bimodal age distribution has been described, with peak incidences occurring in those aged <10 years and those aged 60–70 years. Overall there is equivalent incidence between genders, although males are more likely to present as children and females are more likely to present later in life. Among those aged <10 years the most common diagnoses include neurogenic tumours, mesenchymal tumours, cysts, lymphoid tissue disease and germ cell tumours. In those >60 years, the most common diagnoses include thymic lesions, cysts, metastatic carcinomas and mesenchymal tumours.

[4] Mediastinal masses are usually asymptomatic, with most being discovered incidentally through chest imaging. They are more commonly symptomatic in children than adults. Malignant masses are more likely to cause symptoms. Symptoms can be divided into thoracic symptoms and systemic symptoms. Within the thoracic categorisation, symptoms can be considered based on structure affected. Airway compression can cause dyspnoea, stridor, haemoptysis and cough. Oesophageal compression can cause dysphagia. Recurrent laryngeal nerve disruption can cause a hoarse voice. Superior vena cava obstruction can cause facial swelling. Sympathetic ganglion involvement may cause a Horner's syndrome. Chest wall invasion may cause pain or a palpable mass. Systemic symptoms include those typically described in cancer, such as fever, weight loss, fatigue and night sweats. These are usually related to the release of hormones, antibodies or cytokines.

[5] The time course regarding development of symptoms is also important for the delineation of likely diagnoses. For example, thymoma or other slow growing tumours may have an insidious progression of symptoms. On the other hand, lymphoma may have a relatively rapid onset. There are some presentations related to mediastinal mass that require

urgent action. These include tracheal obstruction, bronchial obstruction, thoracic aortic aneurysm rupture and aortic dissection. These conditions may all be further investigated with imaging if required. Although most mediastinal masses are identified through imaging, some may present through the symptoms mentioned above. Common differential diagnoses to consider for those presentations include masses arising in the lungs, oesophagus, trachea, larynx or neck.

6 There are risk factors associated with the differential diagnoses for a mediastinal mass. Family history of any of the differential diagnoses for mediastinal mass is likely to be significant. Conditions associated with thymomas

include myasthenia gravis, pure red cell aplasia and hypogammaglobulinaemia. Conditions associated with lymphoma include radiation exposure, immunodeficiency or -suppression, and autoimmune diseases. Lack of dietary iodine and female gender are associated with retrosternal goitre.

7 Smoking status and alcohol intake should also be determined as well as any current medications. General fitness should be assessed, given that surgery may be considered. A social history is an important part of any initial work-up.

Examination

- **General inspection** [1] shows a comfortable woman in the clinic room, who appears well. She is not short of breath and is showing no signs of myasthenia gravis.
- Her **vital signs** [2] are stable and she is afebrile.

- There is **no stridor, hoarseness of voice, facial swelling, sign of Horner's syndrome or haematologic malignancy** [3].
- Her **chest is clear on auscultation** [4].

1 General inspection should first identify whether the patient appears well, sick or critical. As mentioned previously, patients are most likely to appear critical from airway obstruction or significant circulatory compromise, most likely due to aortic pathology. However, other facets of general inspection may also yield important findings. Patients with thymoma, which is associated with myasthenia gravis, may appear to have reduced facial expression, fatigue and weakness. Those with metastatic cancer or severe systemic illness may appear cachectic. Dyspnoea or oxygen requirement may indicate poor candidacy for surgery.

2 Assessment of vital signs is also important for those with a mediastinal mass. Those with airway obstruction or underlying respiratory pathology may be hypoxic. Patients with lymphoma may exhibit B symptoms, one of which is fever. The presence of B symptoms is associated with more

advanced lymphoma. Secondary infection of mediastinal cysts or the mediastinum itself can cause fever and subsequent sepsis.

3 Symptoms are often related to adjacent structures affected by the mass. This is the same for signs produced. Additionally, myasthenia gravis can produce ptosis, diplopia and slow or slurred speech. Haematologic malignancy may produce pallor, petechiae, hepatosplenomegaly or an abdominal mass. A testicular mass may be found in germ cell tumours.

4 Malignant mediastinal masses may produce pleural effusion. This may be seen as 'stony' dullness on percussion and decreased chest expansion. Clinical signs are most likely in moderate effusions (>300ml).

Investigations

- The patient's initial **CXR is reviewed** [1]. It shows a mass with regular margins and bulging in the right upper mediastinal contour.
- The appropriate **next steps for investigation are considered** [2].
- **Blood tests** [3] including FBC, thyroid function tests, kidney function tests and other investigations are normal. In keeping with her known myasthenia gravis, acetylcholine receptor antibody is positive.
- She undergoes a CT scan which shows a **solid,**

enhancing mass in the anterior mediastinum [4]. It appears to not involve any other structures and there are no abnormal lymph nodes.
- **Other non-invasive diagnostic techniques** [5] [6] are considered.
- She is then considered for **several invasive diagnostic techniques** [7] [8] [9] [10] [11]. However, ultimately the lesion is thought to be almost certainly a thymoma on imaging and potential management is discussed with the patient.

1 A large proportion of mediastinal masses are discovered incidentally, most commonly through chest radiography. If a mass is suspected clinically, chest radiography is indicated, although in modern practice CT is usually the first-line imaging modality. Posteroanterior and lateral views should be obtained, allowing localisation of the mass as well as estimation of size and composition.

2 Although definitive diagnosis of mediastinal mass will eventually require some form of tissue diagnosis, possibilities can be narrowed based on patient demographics, location of the mass and signs or symptoms produced. While the mass may appear to arise from the mediastinum (particularly on chest radiography), it is important to confirm that the mass is not arising from adjacent structures like the lungs, pleura or chest wall.

3 There are several laboratory tests that can aid in the diagnosis of mediastinal mass. For suspected thymoma, full blood count and acetylcholine receptor antibody are useful tests. FBC allows assessment of general fitness for surgery as well as assessing whether pure red cell aplasia is present. Acetylcholine receptor antibody is positive in myasthenia gravis, although it may be subclinical. Approximately 30% of patients with thymoma have myasthenia gravis. For a mass suspected to be a retrosternal goitre, thyroid function tests (TFTs) should be ordered. However, most retrosternal goitres are non-functioning. For suspected germ-cell tumours, alpha-fetoprotein (AFP) and beta-human chorionic gonadotrophin (beta-hCG) should be ordered. All young men with anterior mediastinal mass should trigger high suspicion of germ-cell tumour. Children with a paravertebral mass (and therefore suspected neurogenic tumour) should be evaluated for increased noradrenaline and adrenaline production, which is raised in neuroblastoma and ganglioneuroblastoma. Lastly, for suspected haematological malignancy, LDH, full blood count and smear, flow cytometry, HIV serology and hepatitis B and C serology should be ordered.

4 Ultimately, CT is the most useful imaging modality for the evaluation of a mediastinal mass and is the next progression of investigation following chest radiography. Some patients may benefit from IV contrast which will provide better characterisation of the mass. CT is useful in differentiating between different types of masses. Typical descriptions include fatty masses (low radiodensity), cystic masses (smooth appearance and homogeneous attenuation) and solid masses. Although there may be features to suggest a benign or malignant mass, CT cannot definitively distinguish between these. CT has been found to be the most accurate imaging modality for most types of mediastinal mass, with MRI being slightly superior in some diseases. Thyroid goitres have a characteristic appearance on CT and do not typically require more invasive investigation.

5 MRI is similarly able to distinguish between different tissue types. It can be particularly useful in assessing vascular involvement or thyroid masses when the use of IV contrast is contraindicated. MRI is also particularly useful in assessing neurogenic tumours, particularly in children. Other imaging modalities may also be used, although not as widely as CT. PET scanning, which is used for pre-operative staging of thoracic malignancy, has been used for mediastinal mass evaluation but is not routine. It does have value in differentiating benign from malignant tumours and in monitoring disease response to treatment.

6 For testicular masses, testicular ultrasound can be used. This imaging modality is highly sensitive for the detection of testicular masses. Barium swallow may be used to assess oesophageal cysts, as the cyst may communicate with the oesophagus itself. Radioactive iodine thyroid scan can be used to evaluate the extent of the thyroid gland.

7 The decision to pursue more invasive diagnostic techniques is based on several factors including symptoms, location and size of mass and the likelihood of malignancy. However, definitive tissue diagnosis is usually required prior to initiating therapy (particularly if the management is invasive). Pre-treatment diagnosis has the potential to inform requirement for neoadjuvant therapy as well as avoid surgery in cases where it is unlikely to provide benefit, such as lymphoma.

8 Image-guided percutaneous needle biopsy can be performed with either CT or ultrasound. Needles can either be a fine needle or a core needle. Fine needle biopsies usually suffice for solid masses, while core needle biopsies may be required for suspected lymphoma and thymoma. The advantages of these techniques are that they are low risk and can be performed without the need for admission. There are several approaches that can be utilised, but common ones include parasternal, paravertebral, suprasternal and subxiphoid approaches. The approach is chosen based on the size and location of the target lesion. Most centres avoid needle biopsy of suspected thymoma due to the potential for tumour seeding in the needle tract.

9 An alternative percutaneous needle biopsy is endoscopic biopsy with ultrasonography. This can be performed bronchoscopically (EBUS) or via the oesophagus (EUS). These techniques use a fine needle. A disadvantage of these techniques is that they can only biopsy tissue adjacent to the oesophagus or bronchi. These techniques are used commonly for lymph node sampling – most commonly for lung cancer. However, they are also useful for mediastinal mass assessment – particularly those in the middle compartment.

10 Other invasive tests may be useful for the assessment of mediastinal mass. A bone marrow biopsy has the potential to diagnose lymphoma or leukaemia. Haematological or metastatic malignancies may affect lymph nodes peripherally. A lymph node biopsy may be useful in this case.

11 Surgical diagnostic procedures are typically performed with a minimally invasive approach but may require conversion to an open procedure. They are typically utilised when the target lesion is not amenable to percutaneous or endoscopic biopsy techniques or when needle biopsy techniques do not yield a diagnosis. Mediastinoscopy is a commonly used procedure with high diagnostic value. It involves an incision being made above the manubrium, allowing a mediastinoscope to be passed into the mediastinum. Another minimally invasive procedure is an anterior mediastinotomy (Chamberlain procedure). This involves a small transverse parasternal incision. These are most commonly used for lymph node biopsy for lung cancer staging but have value in mediastinal mass assessment. VATS may also be employed for the diagnosis and treatment of mediastinal mass. It has the advantage of exposure to all compartments of the mediastinum and the potential to be curative, although it is an invasive procedure and usually requires hospitalisation. Lastly, there is the uncommon potential for the requirement of sternotomy or thoracotomy for diagnosis of mediastinal mass.

Management

Immediate

The patient is otherwise well and does not require immediate intervention.

Short-term

Discuss **potential management plans** [1] with the patient. Refer the patient for a **preoperative anaesthesia work-up** [2]. **Consider different surgical approaches** [3] [4] [5] [6]. Perform a thoracoscopy and remove the entire thymus. Extubate the patient on the operating table and take her to the recovery bay [7] where her vital signs are monitored. **Monitor for complications** [8]. **Discharge the patient** [9] [10] when safe to do so.

Long-term

Follow up the patient in the thoracic oncology clinic [11].

---

[1] Mediastinal masses do not typically present in an acute fashion. Urgent management is thus rarely required.

[2] From an anaesthesia perspective, there are two structures which may be affected by a mediastinal mass. Superior vena cava involvement may impair the delivery of drugs. If the function of the superior vena cava is significantly affected, alternative intravenous access can be obtained through a lower extremity peripheral IV line or femoral line. Superior vena cava compression can also cause venous congestion of the head when the patient is laid supine for surgery. Airway compromise can also be dangerous, particularly around the time of induction. Fibreoptic intubation is often required, as mediastinal masses can change the shape of the trachea.

[3] The most appropriate surgical approach is determined based on the location and size of the lesion, likely or confirmed diagnosis and surgeon preference.

[4] For anterior masses, surgical resection approaches include minimally invasive options such as VATS (chest, subxiphoid or cervical approaches) or open approaches (through thoracotomy or median sternotomy).

[5] For middle and posterior compartment masses, thoracotomy or VATS approach is usually employed, with similar guiding principles to those detailed previously.

[6] Thoracotomy is a commonly employed approach in thoracic surgery. Thoracotomy through the left and right sides allows exposure of different structures. The left exposes the aorta and lower oesophagus while the right exposes the upper oesophagus, superior vena cava, trachea and carina. Most mediastinal masses require the use of a right-sided thoracotomy. The surgery itself first requires induction of anaesthesia and securing the airway. This must be performed with the use of a double-lumen endotracheal tube to allow deflation of one lung. The patient is positioned in a lateral decubitus position with the upper arm extended above their head. An incision is made just below the tip of the scapula and dissection continues down to the latissimus dorsi fascia. In a muscle-sparing approach, the anterior aspect of latissimus dorsi is dissected off the chest wall. The muscle is then retracted posteriorly. In a posterolateral approach, the latissimus dorsi muscle is transected. The serratus anterior can be spared in a similar manner by dividing its fascia inferiorly and retracting the muscle anteriorly and superiorly. An appropriate intercostal space should be identified (usually 4th or 5th intercostal space) which often requires the use of a scapular retractor. Intercostal muscles are then dissected from a small portion of the superior aspect of the rib. A small part of the rib posteriorly can be removed to aid rib spreading, although this is not commonly done in modern thoracotomy techniques. The reason for the rib resection was to enhance exposure and avoid inadvertent rib fractures. The pleural space is then entered, taking care not to injure the underlying lung. Once the operation itself is complete, closure is required. The inferior and superior ribs are fixed to each other with a large absorbable suture. The subcutaneous tissue and skin should then be closed. A chest drain is invariably required.

7 For thymectomy specifically, it is important to ensure that the entire thymus is resected by making sure that the cervical limbs of the thymus that extend superiorly are also removed. All fatty tissue is incorporated in the specimen from the diaphragm up to above the innominate vein and from phrenic to phrenic laterally.

8 Immediately following the operation, monitoring of cardiopulmonary function should occur frequently. Haemodynamic stabilisation, early extubation and adequate pain relief are priorities. Encouragement of specific manoeuvres used to increase lung volume and function should also occur. Pleural drains are typically placed on suction of 20cm of water.

9 The most common complication of thoracotomy in the setting of mediastinal resection is bleeding, usually from the area of resection itself or a disturbed intercostal artery.

High chest drain output is usually the guide for the need for re-exploration. Pain is another significant complication of thoracotomy and a large reason behind the increasing use of VATS. Infection is not common in thoracotomies for mediastinal resection.

10 Venous thromboembolism prophylaxis should be implemented based on individual patient factors. The chest drain(s) should be removed when there is no air leak, drain output is little or nothing, there is reasonable respiratory function and imaging shows lung re-expansion.

11 Follow-up for patients with a mediastinal mass is heterogeneous due to the fact that it is primarily based on the underlying aetiology. Some benign-appearing masses may never undergo definitive investigation or resection but remain monitored through imaging.

CASE 6: Mitral regurgitation

History

- A **62-year-old** [1] **female** [2] presents to the cardiac surgery outpatient clinic after being referred from her cardiologist for **mitral regurgitation** [3] [4] [5] [6].
- She presents with **shortness of breath on exertion, fatigue and orthopnoea** [7]. These symptoms have been developing for the last year.
- She has experienced no chills, sweats or cough. She has **no past medical history** [8].
- She is on **no medications** [9].

- Her **family history** [10] includes ischaemic heart disease and upon further questioning her mother had a "valve problem".
- She **exercises regularly, has a good diet and does not smoke or drink alcohol excessively** [11].
- She is a retired painter who **lives with her partner at home** [12].
- **Complications of mitral regurgitation are considered** [13].

[1] Mitral regurgitation (MR) caused by rheumatic heart disease (RHD) is more common in elderly populations as the incidence of RHD and rheumatic fever has been decreasing significantly in developing countries. Rheumatic fever and RHD remain common in indigenous populations in Australia. Mitral prolapse typically presents in middle-aged individuals as it is slowly developed, particularly in late adolescence.

[2] MR due to RHD is more common in men. Mitral prolapse incidence is similar among sexes, although males are more likely to undergo surgery and at an earlier age than females. Mitral annular calcification is more common in females.

[3] MR is defined as the leakage of blood through the mitral valve during systole. The mitral valve is between the left atrium and left ventricle. It has two leaflets; one anterior and one posterior. The property of leaflets meeting together with a pressure-tight seal is known as coaptation. The commissures (edge of leaflet intersection on each side) are called the anterolateral and posteromedial commissures. Papillary muscles (which arise within the ventricle) attach to the ventricular surface of the mitral valve leaflets through chordae tendineae. These cords prevent prolapse of the leaflets during systole. The factors that allow the mitral valve to prevent regurgitation include the integrity and length of the chordae tendineae, integrity and position of the papillary muscles to which they attach, the surface of the valves themselves and maintenance of normal annular diameter.

[4] MR is classified as either acute or chronic. It can also be stratified into primary and secondary disease. Primary disease is caused by abnormalities of the valve apparatus. Secondary disease occurs when another condition causes changes that compromise the mitral valve's normal function, resulting in regurgitation. In the acute phase of RHD, myocarditis can result in annular dilatation, preventing a complete leaflet seal. This causes acute MR which can improve over time. Following remission of the acute phase, progressive posterior leaflet thickening and restriction may occur with associated chordae shortening, resulting in chronic MR. Annular dilatation usually occurs over time, exacerbating the regurgitation further.

[5] Degenerative mitral valve disease includes mitral valve prolapse and leaflet flail. Prolapse itself is relatively common (approximately 2% incidence) and in the majority of cases does not result in regurgitation. However, overall it is the most common cause of MR managed with surgery in developed countries. The underlying pathophysiology is due to leaflet redundancy and thickening related to myxomatous degeneration. The prolapsing leaflet then places more strain on the chordae, resulting in elongation and potential rupture. In some patients the leaflet thickening may be more predominant, while in others chordal rupture contributes more to regurgitation. Annular calcification is a degenerative cause of MR and thus more common in elderly populations. It is often seen in patients with left ventricular hypertrophy.

[6] Myocardial infarction can cause papillary muscle dysfunction or even rupture which can subsequently produce acute MR. Chronic ischaemic MR occurs as a result of posterior leaflet tethering due to development of a more globular left ventricular shape, pulling the posteromedial papillary muscle away from the posterior mitral annulus. Other rare causes of MR include infective endocarditis and left ventricular aneurysms. It is important to note that chronic MR can be exacerbated by other conditions, resulting in an acute presentation.

[7] The spectrum of presentations of MR is wide. Those with mild chronic MR may never develop symptoms, while those with acute MR may present in acute pulmonary oedema with significant haemodynamic instability. Acute MR, which can be caused by chordal rupture or infective endocarditis, manifests as sudden onset symptoms of pulmonary hypertension.

These include dyspnoea, fatigue, orthopnoea, PND, syncope and chest pain. Chronic MR is often asymptomatic for a significant period of time. The first symptom is usually exercise intolerance and dyspnoea on exertion, with the symptoms of pulmonary hypertension slowly presenting thereafter. Severe MR leads to back pressure of blood into the lungs, leading to congestion and raised pulmonary pressures. Over time the right ventricle develops strain due to the higher afterload (higher pulmonary artery pressures) and tricuspid regurgitation due to right ventricular failure and tricuspid annular dilatation occurs. Right ventricular failure can manifest as leg swelling and chronic fluid retention. There are several presenting symptoms that are less commonly associated with MR including palpitations, diaphoresis, presyncope and cough. Palpitations may be due to atrial fibrillation, which may be caused by MR and is often related to left atrial dilatation.

8 There are several conditions associated with causes of MR. A history of RHD or a likely-sounding story of rheumatic fever is significant. This may include an illness with fevers, joint pain, sore throat, skin changes or signs of heart failure. Marfan syndrome and some other connective tissue diseases are associated with mitral prolapse. History of IE, IHD, left ventricular systolic dysfunction and hypertrophic cardiomyopathy are also significant. Left ventricular systolic

dysfunction can create MR through dilatation. As the ventricle itself becomes larger, with the chordae tendineae remaining the same length, the leaflets can become dragged down to the point that they do not meet during systole. This results in a classically central regurgitation. Ischaemic heart disease usually causes MR through the same mechanism.

9 Medications may suggest the aforementioned conditions. Some anorectic and dopaminergic drugs are associated with MR.

10 Mitral prolapse can be familial or more commonly sporadic. Family history of MR or any of the underlying conditions associated with it may be significant.

11 Cessation of smoking and of excessive alcohol consumption is always advised. Diet and exercise advice is also particularly important in cardiovascular disease.

12 Assessment of social background is an important part of the work-up of any patient and allows management goals to be better considered.

13 There are several complications associated with the natural history of mitral regurgitation. These include atrial fibrillation, pulmonary hypertension, left ventricular dysfunction and congestive heart failure.

Examination

- The patient appears comfortable at rest in the clinic room. However, she was **breathless when she walked in from the waiting room** [1] .
- Her **vital signs** [2] are stable and she is afebrile.
- Her **pulse is irregular** [3] and her **JVP is not elevated** [3] .

- **Inspection and palpation of her chest are normal** [4] .
- Auscultation reveals dual heart sounds and a **pansystolic murmur radiating to the axilla** [5] [6] .
- She also has **coarse bibasal crepitations and pitting oedema** [7] to the mid-shin.

1 Although there are several examination findings associated with MR, mild or moderate MR may not have any findings. Most patients present with symptoms on exercise only. The patient should be generally inspected for signs of pain or distress. Their body habitus and general exercise tolerance should be assessed as they may have bearing on fitness for surgery. Dyspnoea is another important sign relevant to MR as it indicates more advanced disease. It carries a poor prognosis as it indicates exhaustion of cardiac compensation. Lastly, aids which the patient brings should also be considered. Oxygen requirement is relevant in the context of MR as well as surgical candidacy. Orthopnoea may be demonstrated by the requirement for several pillows while supine.

2 Fever may suggest endocarditis or another cause of SOB – for example pneumonia. Acute MR may cause acute pulmonary oedema resulting in low oxygen saturations. It may also result in cardiogenic shock manifesting as

tachycardia, tachypnoea, hypotension and inadequate tissue perfusion. Chronic MR may also show signs of right heart failure including low oxygen saturation, but rarely manifests as shock.

3 Severe MR may result in a small volume pulse (in keeping with a narrow pulse pressure). MR can be associated with atrial fibrillation, due to left atrial enlargement. It is therefore important to assess pulse rate and rhythm. Atrial fibrillation will be palpated as an irregularly irregular pulse. It is useful to auscultate and then palpate the carotid pulse. The JVP should also be assessed, given that mitral regurgitation can be associated with right ventricular failure in late stages.

4 The chest should be inspected for signs of underlying respiratory disease which may be relevant for fitness for surgery. Scars indicating previous thoracic surgery are important to assess. MR can cause left ventricular dilatation which may be palpated as a displaced apex beat.

5 MR is heard as a soft systolic murmur. In acute MR, the regurgitation may be so severe that it does not cause a murmur, especially in combination with poor ventricular function or hypotension.

6 Chronic MR may have more signs associated with it. The classic description of this murmur is a holosystolic or pansystolic (occurs over the entire course of systole) murmur that sounds high-pitched or blowing. It may radiate to the left axilla and is best heard at the apex. Accentuating manoeuvres include increasing preload (raising the legs) or afterload

(Valsalva). A quiet S1 may be heard, which is due to the mitral valve not closing forcefully. An S3 heart sound indicates left ventricular dilatation.

7 The posterior chest wall should be inspected for scars and auscultated for lung sounds. Coarse crackles are heard in pulmonary oedema whereas poor air entry is heard in pleural effusion. These conditions can be associated with left ventricular failure and pulmonary hypertension. Sacral and peripheral oedema should also be assessed.

Investigations

- **Differential diagnoses** [1] for this woman's presentation are considered.
- **Routine blood tests** [2] are normal.
- Electrocardiography shows **atrial fibrillation and signs of left ventricular hypertrophy** [3].
- Her **CXR is normal** [4].
- Her cardiologist sent forward a transthoracic echocardiogram showing MR. To further assess the problem, a **transoesophageal echocardiogram**

is performed [5]. The left ventricular ejection fraction is 45%, there is severe left atrial dilation and severe mitral regurgitation. The posterior leaflet is myxomatous and prolapsing.
- **Other tests are considered** [6] [7] [8] [9].
- **Coronary angiogram is normal** [10].
- Her MR is classified as **grade D which is symptomatic and severe** [11].

1 The differentials for acute presentation of MR include acute coronary syndrome, IE, pneumonia, acute pulmonary oedema or arrhythmias. However, acute MR may occur in response to one of these conditions or cause them as a complication. The differentials for chronic MR presentation include IHD, subacute infective endocarditis, mitral stenosis, aortic or pulmonary valve disease or atrial myxoma. These conditions can also cause or exacerbate chronic MR.

2 Blood tests to be considered include full blood examination, kidney function, liver function and coagulation studies. These allow assessment of comorbidities that may complicate the patient's ability to tolerate an operation.

3 ECG may show left ventricular hypertrophy if significant and chronic MR is present. It may also show signs of prior infarction or underlying rhythm disturbance such as atrial fibrillation. Left atrial enlargement may cause a broad P wave.

4 CXR in those with chronic MR may have several characteristic features including left atrial enlargement, prominent left atrial appendage and left ventricular hypertrophy. Signs of pulmonary venous hypertension may also occur.

5 Echocardiography is typically the best modality for diagnosing MR and assessing severity. Both transthoracic and transoesophageal echocardiography are used. Echocardiography allows assessment of valve anatomy and haemodynamics as well as complications. The assessments made during echocardiography can be considered as

qualitative (visual assessment) and quantitative (based on measurements). Severity is determined based on several variables. Severe lesions are usually easily recognised but it can be more difficult to determine severity when regurgitation is intermediate or mild. As such, a few parameters are used to assess severity. The first are structural parameters which include left atrial size, LV size and changes to the mitral apparatus. The second is colour flow Doppler which can visualise the 'jet' of flow from the LV back into the left atrium during systole. The pulmonary veins are also analysed to determine if regurgitation is causing backward flow in the pulmonary veins. Pulmonary artery pressure can be estimated with echocardiography, although it is known to not be very reliable. Mitral prolapse and flail as well as endocarditis can be assessed. The ejection fraction in MR does not represent true cardiac output, as part of the ejection volume is regurgitating into the left atrium.

6 Exercise stress testing may be useful for patients with severe mitral regurgitation who are asymptomatic. It can be used to uncover LV dysfunction that is not obvious on resting echocardiography. This is important as it predicts LV function following surgery.

7 Cardiac MRI may be used in conjunction with echocardiography.

8 Right heart catheterisation may be used to determine pulmonary artery pressures, as well as estimating left atrial pressure through a wedge pressure. Pulmonary hypertension indicates significant changes to normal haemodynamics.

9 Brain natriuretic peptide (BNP) levels are associated with MR consequences including LV dysfunction and increased left atrial volume. It can be used to monitor patients with MR.

10 As with other non-urgent cardiac conditions potentially involving surgery, coronary angiogram is often performed preoperatively to assess for the need for concurrent CABGs.

11 The severity of primary and secondary MR is typically graded by considering echocardiographic features and the presence of symptoms. One such grading system is the American Heart Association/American College of Cardiology Mitral Regurgitation guidelines. MR is graded as either 'at risk', 'progressive', 'asymptomatic severe' or 'symptomatic severe' (grades A–D). Severity categories are mostly used to inform large-scale research; each patient's disease is considered individually and within the context of other factors.

Management

Immediate

The patient is otherwise well and does not require emergency intervention.

Short-term

Given this patient's severe and symptomatic MR, **she will benefit from mitral valve surgery** [1] with concurrent **surgical therapy for her atrial fibrillation** [2]. Discuss the **alternatives to surgery** [3] [4] [5] with the patient, and obtain consent to have the procedures performed. Consider the **acuity of her disease** [6]. Perform a preoperative transoesophageal echocardiogram. It shows disease localised to the posterior leaflet and it is decided that a **repair, rather than replacement, is suitable for**

this patient [7] [8] [9]. Refer the patient to a cardiac surgeon specialising in mitral valve surgery and perform a minimally invasive operation. This involves peripheral cannulation of the femoral vessels to attach the patient to cardiopulmonary bypass. A right mini-thoracotomy is performed and thoracoscopic surgery is performed to repair the valve. Following the procedure, **monitor her closely in the critical care unit** [10]. Discharge the patient from hospital, ensuring the **postoperative course is stable** [11].

Long-term

Follow the patient up in the **outpatient clinic** [12] and review her postoperative echocardiogram to ensure an adequately functioning valve.

1 The indications for surgery vary between primary and secondary MR. For primary MR, surgery is indicated for symptomatic and severe MR. For asymptomatic and severe MR, additional echocardiographic parameters, the presence of AF and risk are considered. Typically, surgery is recommended as soon as signs of LV dilatation are identified on echocardiography. If referring to a specialist centre with a high repair rate (rather than replacement) then referral even before LV dilatation is warranted. For secondary MR, surgery is indicated for symptomatic and severe MR. If surgery is not indicated, periodic monitoring is suggested. Overall, the threshold for surgery is lowering over time as outcomes improve.

2 Atrial fibrillation is commonly associated with chronic MR. These two conditions have a bidirectional relationship. Chronic MR can cause dilatation of the left atrium, resulting in atrial fibrillation. Atrial fibrillation can also cause enlargement of the left atrium, resulting in loss of coaptation of mitral valve leaflets and regurgitation. Atrial fibrillation may persist even after definitive treatment for MR. There are some surgical procedures which are considered in patients with AF undergoing mitral valve surgery, to prevent recurrence

of atrial fibrillation postoperatively. These include left atrial appendage removal and the maze procedure. The atrial appendage allows turbulent flow and therefore its presence increases the risk of thromboembolism formation. The maze procedure involves creating a 'maze' of scar tissue on the atria, isolating abnormal electrical circuits, and reverting the patient back to sinus rhythm. Typically, the maze is now performed with radiofrequency or cryotherapy.

3 MR can be managed within four broad categories: periodic monitoring, medical, transcatheter and surgical. Periodic monitoring is employed in all patients with MR who do not require intervention, as it is usually a progressive disease.

4 Medical management is considered as an adjunct or alternative to definitive surgical management. Those with symptomatic MR with preserved ventricular function require no specific therapy. Hypertension should be treated appropriately to reduce LV afterload. Those with impaired ventricular function (both primary and secondary MR) are treated in the same way as heart failure with reduced ejection fraction. Drug classes used include ACE inhibitors, beta blockers and diuretics for fluid overload. Cardiac resynchronisation therapy may also be required. Overall, there is a larger place for medical management in secondary MR – severe primary MR is a surgical condition if the patient can tolerate an operation. Concurrent conditions should also be managed appropriately in all patients with MR. Common conditions include IHD, atrial fibrillation and tricuspid regurgitation.

5 Transcatheter management of MR is currently limited to mitral valve repair. Although transcatheter mitral valve replacement is possible, it is still being developed. Transcatheter mitral valve repair involves 'clipping' of the mitral valve leaflets. Access is obtained through the femoral vein and the catheter is advanced to the right atrium, by which the left atrium is accessed by piercing through the interatrial septum. The procedure is performed with echocardiography guidance. This procedure is typically used in patients who cannot tolerate surgery, as the results are suboptimal compared to surgery. In-hospital and long-term mortality is similar between transcatheter and surgical therapy. However, transcatheter repair is much more likely to leave residual MR.

6 Acute MR causing haemodynamic instability is an emergency and requires urgent correction of valve function. Diuretics may be used to decrease afterload (allowing more blood to preferentially eject through the aortic valve) and reduce intravascular volume (thereby reducing annular dilatation and reducing regurgitation).

7 Surgery for MR can involve repair or replacement of the mitral valve. Repair is preferred when feasible and currently the use of mitral valve repair is increasing. This is due to the fact that anticoagulation is required for mechanical valves and bioprosthetic valves have a short life expectancy. Large studies have validated the durability of mitral valve repair.

8 Mitral valve repair can be performed as open (via sternotomy) or as minimal access (via right thoracotomy, using thoracoscopic techniques or robotic and femoral vessels cannulation).

9 Mitral valve replacement can also be performed minimally invasively or via median sternotomy. Mechanical or bioprosthetic valves may be used to replace the excised valve. Mechanical valves carry the disadvantage of requiring lifelong anticoagulation but are more durable.

10 Patients should be monitored postoperatively in a critical care unit, as for other cardiac operations. Decreasing afterload is a priority following mitral valve repair or replacement, as it allows better cardiac performance. This can be accomplished with glyceryl trinitrate (GTN) or nitroprusside. Anticoagulation is commenced with warfarin soon after the operation (usually the evening of postoperative day 1 or 2). For patients with mitral valve replacement, the optimal INR is 2.5–3.5. As mentioned previously, this is continued for life for mechanical replacements. Patients who received a bioprosthetic valve receive anticoagulation for a variable amount of time, depending on surgeon preference.

11 Complications of surgery include postoperative stroke, stenosis of the valve prosthesis, recurrent regurgitation, peri-prosthesis leak and endocarditis of native or prosthetic valves. Systolic anterior motion (SAM) results in left ventricular outflow obstruction. SAM usually occurs in patients with hypertrophic cardiomyopathy but can also occur in patients who have undergone mitral repair.

12 Follow-up is important to assess for late complications of treatment and monitor for recurrence of regurgitation. However, surgical management of MR has been shown to be durable and allow excellent long-term survival with freedom from re-operation. Antibiotic prophylaxis should be considered for prevention of infective endocarditis for dental and other procedures.

CASE 7:   Pleural empyema

History

- A **62-year-old female** [1] [2] presents to the ED with **suspected empyema** [3] [4]. The surgical team is called to review her.
- She was admitted in the same hospital for **pneumonia five weeks ago** [5]. This had resolved, and she returned home.
- However, she has presented again with one week of decline. She has been unwell for the last week with **fevers, shortness of breath and pain** [6]

on the right side of her chest. Additionally, she feels fatigued and has lost 2kg of weight with no intention to do so.
- She has rheumatoid arthritis which is managed with **infliximab** [7] but has been otherwise well.
- She has **no history or recent surgical interventions or trauma** [8]. She denies alcohol or illicit drug use. She is retired and currently lives with her husband in a safe environment at home.

[1] Empyema is more common in men. It occurs in males compared to females in approximately a 2:1 ratio.

[2] Empyema is more common at the extremes of age (<18 years old and >65 years old). The most frequent age of presentation for adults is approximately 60–70 years old.

[3] Empyema, which is also known as pleural empyema, empyema thoracis and pyothorax, is the presence of frank pus caused by microorganisms within the pleural space. The extreme case is empyema necessitatis, when pus drains spontaneously through the chest wall (rare currently due to antibiotics). Empyema can be caused by invasion of the pleural space from pyogenic bacteria, fungi, parasites or mycobacteria. This can occur from an adjacent pneumonia or from another source (haematogenic or lymphatic spread), known as primary and secondary empyema, respectively. Empyema develops in up to three stages known as the exudative stage, fibrinopurulent stage and organisational stage. The exudative stage involves the accumulation of sterile pleural fluid secondary to inflammation. In the absence of progression from this stage, the disease is known as a simple parapneumonic effusion. The fibrinopurulent stage, which can begin after 48 hours, occurs when bacteria invade the pleural space and fibrin is deposited on the pleural membranes. Loculations and adhesions then form. A loculation is an isolated pocket of fluid that has been separated from other fluid by fibrous septi. This stage includes both complicated parapneumonic effusion and empyema. The organisational stage, which occurs after 1–2 weeks, involves the development of a thick pleural peel and septations due to growth of fibroblasts and capillaries. These can inhibit lung expansion, which is known as trapped lung.

[4] The incidence of empyema has been slowly rising after its initial drop following the development of antibiotics. The

incidence is approximately 10 in 100 000 person years in developed countries.

[5] Approximately 70% of cases with empyema involve a history of recent pneumonia. Pneumonia can cause effusion through increased vascular and pleural permeability, release of inflammatory cytokines and neutrophil chemotaxis. This effusion can subsequently become infected. Therefore, risk factors for pneumonia are also risk factors for empyema. Risk factors for community-acquired pneumonia (CAP) include residence in a nursing home, contact with children, chronic respiratory diseases, chronic comorbidities including chronic heart disease and diabetes, alcohol misuse, smoking and poor oral hygiene. Risk factors for hospital-acquired pneumonia (HAP) include poor infection control, intubation and mechanical ventilation, low head of bed height, H2 antagonist use, reintubation and persistent sedation. Most cases of empyema are related to CAP. If a pneumonia fails to respond to antibiotic therapy, it should be investigated for the presence of an effusion.

[6] The presentation for someone with empyema depends on their stage of disease development. The usual scenario is a patient with risk factors, history of recent pneumonia and symptoms suggesting infection. Fever and rigors are common. Constitutional symptoms such as fatigue, weight loss and anorexia are also common. Patients can also have a productive cough. This is likely due to the preceding pneumonia if present. Pleuritic chest pain may be present and is due to inflammation and subsequent irritation of the parietal pleura. A large pleural effusion can cause SOB. However, SOB can also be due to underlying pneumonia. Compared to pneumonia, patients with empyema usually have a subacute presentation rather than acute disease progression. They usually report a progression of symptoms from a few days to up to two weeks. Presentation may be delayed in patients with anaerobic infections.

7 There are several factors that increase the risk of developing empyema from pneumonia. These include IV drug use, alcohol abuse, aspiration, poor dental hygiene, malnutrition, extremes of age, partially treated pneumonia, pneumonia requiring hospital admission and gastro-oesophageal reflux. Comorbid lung disease is also a risk factor. This is likely due to reduced lung clearance from diseases such as bronchiectasis, COPD, asthma and lung cancer. Immunosuppression is another risk factor for empyema development. This immunosuppression may be caused by blood disease, chemotherapy, HIV/AIDS or malnutrition. Like many other diseases, immunosuppression can conceal symptoms, resulting in delayed presentation and diagnosis. Past history of empyema is also a risk factor for developing empyema again.

8 However, there are other potential causes for empyema. It can result from direct contamination of the chest from trauma or surgery, rupture of lung abscess or by extension from the mediastinum (oesophageal perforation) or abdomen. Thoracic trauma is related to an increased risk of empyema. Approximately 5% of patients with significant thoracic trauma develop empyema. Additionally, a haemothorax left without treatment can lead to empyema without a primary effusion. Surgical interventions in the thorax can also result in empyema. These interventions include thoracic surgery, chest drain insertion or thoracentesis. A significant proportion, as high as 20%, of all cases of empyema are related to non-pneumonic processes.

Examination

- The patient is sitting in her bed in the ED. She looks **unwell** [1] and is **complaining of pain** [1] in her right chest.
- Her **temperature is 39.1°C** [2] and her oxygen saturations are 95%.
- Her **respiratory rate is 27 breaths/minute** [2]. Her BP is 100/65mmHg and heart rate is 104 beats per minute (bpm).
- Her chest shows **normal expansion and work of breathing** [3].
- Her **chest wall is not tender** [4].
- The base of her right chest is **dull to percussion** [5] and there are **decreased breath sounds** [6].
- There are **no peripheral signs** [7].

1 General inspection can vary significantly in patients with empyema. Approximately 30% of patients do not have clinical signs. Some patients may appear relatively comfortable with normal posture. Some may show obvious distress and pain with altered posture or breathing. They may be overtly short of breath or tachypnoeic. Some patients, particularly older patients, can present with confusion. They may show signs of associated diseases. Supplemental oxygen may also be seen. Walking aids may indicate frailty or underlying musculoskeletal condition requiring immunosuppressive medication.

2 The vital signs are important to examine in any patient, particularly in one with a suspected infective process. As with any infection, the patient may be pyrexic. Patients with empyema can have a particularly high temperature. Patients with sepsis may be hypotensive and tachycardic with an increased respiratory rate. Approximately 35% of patients with empyema present with a septic picture.

3 Clinical signs of effusion are generally absent if the volume of effusion is <200ml. Examination of the chest itself should begin with inspection. Assessment of breathing pattern involves measuring rate, time of inspiration to expiration ratio. Assessment of effort of breathing involves inspecting for accessory muscle use and tracheal tug. Patients with empyema may be tachypnoeic with increased work of breathing. Empyema may show signs of reduced chest expansion due to pleuritic pain and inflammation causing decreased lung expansion on the side of the effusion. There may be signs of recent surgical intervention or trauma in the form of scars, dressings or obvious chest wall deformity.

4 Palpating the chest and asking the patient to speak allows assessment of voice transmission, also known as tactile fremitus. This is decreased in effusion but increased in diseases causing consolidation, such as pneumonia. In empyema, there may be appreciable chest wall oedema or warmth.

5 Percussion of the chest wall in empyema may yield a classically 'stony dull' sound. In a patient in erect position, the lowest part of the pleural cavity is the posterior base. In a free-flowing effusion, fluid will accumulate here. However, empyema in the organising phase may not demonstrate this attribute. In left-sided effusions, Traube's space will be dull to percussion. The superior aspect of the effusion may be appreciable on percussion with a return of normal resonance.

6 Auscultation will likely demonstrate decreased breath sounds since the lung on the side of the empyema is experiencing reduced ventilation. Conversely, areas of consolidation may have easily heard breath sounds with bronchial breathing.

7 There are not many peripheral signs of empyema. Patients with underlying respiratory disease or lung cancer may show clubbing of the fingernails.

Investigations

- The patient's blood tests during her admission for pneumonia approximately 5 weeks ago are reviewed and show that she had a **CRP of 121mg/L** [1].
- The patient undergoes **new blood tests** [2] while she waits for a CXR in the ED. They show leucocytosis, a CRP of 300mg/L with normal kidney and liver function. Blood cultures are also taken.
- After some time, supine CXR shows a **large lenticular-shaped mass in the right chest with loculations** [3].

- Thoracic ultrasound [4] is considered but **CT of the chest** [5] is ultimately ordered. CT shows large retained fluid collection with loculations and internal septa, suspicious of empyema.
- Ultrasound-guided thoracentesis is subsequently performed, and **frank pus was aspirated** [6].
- **Culture of pleural fluid is ordered** [7].
- **Differential diagnoses** [8] for this case are considered.

[1] A person with pneumonia who has albumin <30g/L, sodium <130mmol/L, platelet count >400 x 10⁹/L or CRP >100mg/L is at increased risk of developing empyema.

[2] There are several blood tests useful for diagnosis of empyema. An FBE, specifically the white blood cell count and CRP level, can give information regarding the systemic response to infection expected from empyema. However, a lack of CRP rise or leucocytosis does not necessarily rule out the possibility of empyema. Blood cultures may be used to ascertain the offending organism. Even when a pleural fluid culture is negative, blood cultures can be positive. As with blood cultures for other diseases, when patient condition permits, the culture should ideally be taken before the commencement of antibiotic therapy. Blood cultures may have been performed recently due to pneumonia. The infecting organism of the pneumonia may not be the same organism causing the empyema. Kidney function can be affected by metabolic response, antibiotics and contrast for CT imaging. LFTs are also frequently performed due to the association between liver dysfunction and effusion.

[3] In general, a CXR should be ordered for all patients with significant respiratory complaint and a septic picture. Chest X-ray in empyema can show an effusion as well as features suggesting the organising phase of the disease. Approximately 300–500ml (depending on the size of the patient) is required to show blunting of the costophrenic angle. However, loculated effusions usually make an obtuse angle with the chest wall and form a 'lenticular' shape. Conversely, pleural effusion is usually concave towards the lung. Loculations and diffuse consolidation of the lung also suggest empyema. Lastly, it is possible to identify pleural thickening, which is also associated with empyema. There are some findings that suggest the need for surgical drainage over medical management. These include loculations, hydro-aerial levels, signs of pleural thickening and effusion occupying >50% of the hemithorax. One particular sign is the posterior inverted 'D' shape on the lateral view. Overall, plain radiography of the chest in empyema varies significantly based on the viscosity of the fluid as well as the presence of loculations and the patient's position.

[4] Ultrasonography of the chest can be used for the diagnosis and assessment of empyema and as triage for patients who might need further radiological imaging. It is frequently used when further assessment is required regarding loculations or pleural thickening found on plain chest radiography. It is also useful in critically ill patients who are limited to a supine position. It is more sensitive than CXR in detecting pleural effusions. It has limited use in patients with thick chest walls. Empyema on ultrasound can show the presence of fluid that is echogenic, loculations and septations. Ultrasonography findings can fall in the spectrum from homogeneous anechoic (transudative effusion) to complex septated findings (fibrinopurulent stage). Ultrasound is very useful to guide both thoracentesis and chest drain insertion.

[5] Chest CT is the most important radiological modality used in empyema. It takes images of adjacent 1–3mm slices through the chest during a single breath hold. IV contrast allows differentiation between pleural membranes and empyema, characterising the complexity of the infectious process. It is more sensitive than CXR for determining smaller effusions. Empyema is usually seen on CT as loculated effusions along the lower posterior pleural surface. Visceral and parietal pleural thickening with contrast enhancement is the hallmark of empyema, as inflammatory tissue (perfused by systemic circulation) receives contrast on the arterial phase of the CT. The 'split pleura' sign is caused by contrast enhancement of both parietal and visceral pleura, forming a 'halo' around the whole or part of the effusion. The presence of air/gas within the pleural space (without recent chest surgery or drains) indicates infection. In advanced empyema, entrapment of lung is commonly associated with collapse/consolidation and loss of lung volume. CT has the advantage of assessing other lung diseases (e.g. cancer, COPD) and underlying causes of empyema such as oesophageal perforation or lung cancer. When one or more hydro-aerial cavities are seen on CXR, CT is critical to differentiate between lung abscess and empyema, although at times this can be difficult. It is also used to guide drainage of pockets of pus.

MRI and PET scan play a very limited role in the diagnosis of empyema.

6 Pleural fluid is collected through thoracentesis. This procedure can also be curative in some conditions as it drains fluid from the pleural space. Fluid is usually drained from the posterolateral aspect of the back, over the diaphragm. The needle should be inserted at the superior rib margin to avoid the intercostal neurovascular bundle. Once fluid is aspirated, it can be analysed in several ways. In empyema, the fluid may be frank pus and may have a putrid odour. Frank pus is essentially diagnostic for empyema. In complicated parapneumonic effusion the fluid may appear cloudy. Pleural fluid pH <7.2 suggests empyema. Other markers of pleural fluid indicating empyema include total protein concentration >30g/dl, LDH >2 times upper limit of normal for serum, glucose <3.3mmol/L and white cell differential showing >90% leucocytes.

7 Positive Gram stain or culture occurs in approximately 60% of cases and allows targeted antibiotic therapy. Empyema is often caused by more than one microorganism. Typical causative organisms vary between preceding CAP and HAP. In CAP, the most common organisms are Gram-positive aerobic bacteria such as *Streptococcus milleri*, *S. pneumoniae* and staphylococci. Cases following HAP are almost all staphylococci, including methicillin-resistant *Staphylococcus aureus* (MRSA).

8 There are several differential diagnoses to consider in a patient with suspected empyema. These include a pneumonia itself without effusion. Although there are no obvious differentiating history or exam findings, a pneumonia will be seen on CXR as lung consolidation without associated effusion. Another diagnosis to consider is an uncomplicated parapneumonic effusion. Patients with uncomplicated parapneumonic effusion may be less likely to have a fever. Additionally, the pleural fluid will be sterile with a pH >7.2. Lung abscess presents with a productive cough and sputum with an offensive odour. Effusions can be associated with several inflammatory conditions including rheumatoid arthritis and systemic lupus erythematosus. Lung abscess will show a cavitating lung lesion with air-fluid level. A significant proportion of pleural effusions are due to malignant causes and this may be a differential diagnosis for empyema. However, malignant pleural effusion is likely to present with a longer history of symptoms. Thoracentesis, CXR and CT are able to differentiate between malignant pleural effusion and empyema. It is also possible for a malignant pleural effusion to become infected, causing empyema. Haemothorax, due to anticoagulation or haemophilia, trauma or surgical intervention, can present with a similar syndrome to empyema. Additionally, it can become infected. However, the pleural fluid will be overtly bloody with a high haematocrit. Chylothorax can also present in a similar manner to empyema. However, it does not cause infective symptoms such as fever. Additionally, analysis of pleural fluid can provide further differentiation.

Management

Immediate

Provide **fluid resuscitation** [1] and admit in the thoracic surgery unit. Commence the patient on **antibiotic therapy** [2] [3] and insert a **chest drain** [4].

Short-term

Monitor the patient with repeat chest X-rays. Several loculations persist. Given her immunocompromised status, consider **fibrinolytic therapy** [5] and **surgery** [6]. Perform a **VATS procedure** [7], and prepare for potential conversion to **open procedure** [8] if lung entrapment is too severe and decortication is not possible with VATS. Monitor the patient in **ICU postoperatively** [9]. **Discharge** [10] the patient when safe to do so.

Long-term

Follow the patient up in the **outpatient clinic** [11] [12].

1 Patients with empyema may be septic, which requires management. This may require urgent IV antibiotics, fluid resuscitation and the use of vasopressors or inotropes. This may need to occur before a diagnosis of empyema is made. Broadly, the goal of treatment of empyema is to evacuate infective material from the pleural space. This is accomplished initially through pleural fluid drainage supported by antibiotic therapy. However, chest tube drainage does not resolve the issue in complex multiloculated effusions. For those who are not fit for surgery, intrapleural fibrinolytics may be used. For those fit enough, surgery is performed to clear the pleural space and allow lung re-expansion.

2 There are two stages to antibiotic therapy for empyema. Firstly, there is the empiric therapy used before positive pleural aspirate cultures return. Empiric antibiotics should be chosen based on local hospital/area guidelines and are usually administrated intravenously until clear clinical improvement. They should cover likely organisms causing empyema, including aerobic and anaerobic types. Broadly, antibiotics that penetrate the pleural space should be used.

These include penicillins (with or without beta-lactamase), cephalosporins and metronidazole. Aminoglycosides do not penetrate the pleural space well and should be avoided. Anaerobes can be difficult to culture and can also secondarily infect empyemas. Therefore, even if anaerobe culture is negative, empiric antibiotic therapy should be continued. Antibiotic therapy administration should not be delayed by pleural fluid sampling or drainage. Empiric antibiotic therapy does not need to cover atypical organisms including *Legionella*, *Chlamydia* and *Mycoplasma* spp. as they do not usually infect effusions.

3 In the second stage, antibiotic therapy for empyema is directed based on culture results of infecting organisms. Some pathogens are more likely to be the sole organism responsible for infection. These include *Streptococcus pneumoniae* and *Staphylococcus aureus*. When they are the sole organism cultured, antibiotic therapy can be directed specifically at them. However, most cases involve a polymicrobial infection. In this case, it is likely that the infection will include several anaerobic pathogens. Subsequently, antibiotic therapy is directed based on the likely source of infection (HAP, CAP or aspiration). There is no current consensus regarding duration of antibiotics for empyema and complicated parapneumonic effusions. Generally, therapy lasts 1–3 weeks.

4 Tube thoracostomy allows drainage of infected material within the pleural space. Some suggest that thoracentesis should occur in patients with pleural fluid thickness of >2cm on imaging. This is due to the fact that smaller effusions are expected to resolve with antibiotics alone. Tube thoracostomy is recommended for patients with pH <7.2, LDH >1000IU/L, glucose <40mg/dl and loculated effusions. There is no current consensus on ideal drain size – it is a balance between smaller drain size being less invasive and larger drain size allowing frank pus to drain. Extensive septation is associated with poor outcomes, especially in small bore tubes. Drains usually fail due to blockage. Tube thoracostomy should be followed up with chest X-ray to ensure position and confirm drainage. Isolated loculations can be managed with observation, CT/ultrasound-guided drainage or more invasive treatment which includes fibrinolytics and surgery, depending on size, location and symptoms. Complications of chest drain insertion include damage to surrounding structures, bleeding, subcutaneous emphysema and even death.

5 The pathophysiology of empyema involves deposition of fibrin around the lung and chest wall. Thus fibrinolytic therapy can be used to break down loculations and adhesions before the establishment of a pleural rind. Examples of fibrinolytics include tissue plasminogen activator (tPA), DNase and streptokinase. Although it has been shown to have some benefit in patients with empyema, it is not recommended as part of routine treatment. It is especially useful in patients who are not resolving with tube thoracostomy alone but are not surgical candidates.

6 The surgery for empyema is known as pulmonary decortication. It involves debriding granulation tissue and fibrous rind that lies on both the visceral and parietal pleura (although the rind typically only forms on the visceral pleura). The goals of therapy are to evacuate infected tissue and promote lung expansion to eliminate space within the pleural cavity. There are two broad ways of performing the surgery: through VATS or open. VATS has been shown to be effective in relatively loose adhesions. However, when a thick rind is present, open thoracotomy is used. Surgery is indicated for those who do not respond to antibiotics and tube thoracostomy. Approximately 30% of patients with empyema require surgery.

7 The procedure starts with establishment of single lung ventilation with a double-lumen endotracheal tube or normal tube with a bronchial blocker (this allows deflation of the operated lung). The patient is placed in lateral decubitus with the affected side up. In cases of fluid level on imaging (possible broncho-pleural fistula), single lung ventilation is mandatory to protect the non-operated lung, as effusion can soil it. Access to the chest is gained through VATS or an open approach. The location of incision is chosen based on the location of the empyema itself. The pleural space is assessed. Loculations and adhesions are broken down and the pleura is decorticated. Decortication of the lung should allow re-expansion, although this is not always possible. The intercostal nerves around the area of incision are blocked with local anaesthetic. The chest is then closed, which involves placing pericostal sutures, repairing muscles divided on approach and closing the skin. One or more chest drains should be placed. Some recommend an anterior drain (for air), a posterior and high, and a posterior and low for fluid/effusion/blood. The patient should be extubated as soon as possible as this is associated with better outcomes. The patient will likely require ICU admission.

8 Complications of surgery for empyema include haemorrhage, especially in the setting of coagulopathy, anticoagulants or antiplatelets, arrhythmias, particularly atrial fibrillation, cardiac ischaemia and myocardial infarction and pulmonary oedema.

9 Postoperatively, pain management is vital for these patients. Pain following thoracic surgery can usually be managed with regional anaesthesia: intercostal blocks and/or paravertebral catheter with continuous infusion of local anaesthetic. Epidural block in empyema carries a risk of paravertebral abscess so is not generally accepted. Standard assessment of vital signs should occur. Care should be taken not to overhydrate patients with empyema postoperatively. Nutritional support is critical as empyema is a highly catabolic state. The chest tube should be observed for output. Early physiotherapy is essential to recruit lung and eliminate pleural space – the ultimate goal of surgery. Patients require deep vein thrombosis (DVT) prophylaxis (mechanical, pharmacological or both) while admitted.

10 There are several possible complications of empyema. Acutely, patients with empyema can suffer from septic shock, pulmonary oedema following fluid drainage and respiratory failure. In the long term, patients with empyema can suffer respiratory failure due to pleural thickening restricting lung expansion and bronchopleural fistula. Lastly, there is the possibility of chronic empyema. Chronic empyema requires surgery due to the fact that tube thoracostomy cannot drain the pleural rind.

11 Mortality of empyema is approximately 5% but is higher for patients with comorbidities or those who are immunocompromised. Morbidity increases with the stage of empyema. Mortality is highest in those requiring open surgery. Both mortality and morbidity increase if treatment is inadequate or delayed.

12 Most patients are discharged from hospital with oral antibiotics. FBE and CRP levels should be assessed within a few weeks to ensure adequate response. A CXR should be performed within a few weeks to assess lung re-expansion and any leftover effusions. However, CXR findings can take several months to become normal. Some patients can experience poor pulmonary function due to restriction of lung expansion from pleural thickening. This usually resolves within 6 months, although if symptoms persist it may be an indication for repeat decortication.

CASE 8: Spontaneous pneumothorax

History

- The cardiothoracic surgery team is asked to see a patient with **suspected pneumothorax** [1] [2] [3] [4] (PTX) in the ED.
- The patient is a **23-year-old male** [5] who was at a concert last night when he developed **severe left-sided chest pain and shortness of breath** [6] [7]. He presented to hospital the day after the pain occurred.
- The patient has experienced **two previous episodes of PTX** [8] : the first managed with observation and the second with needle aspiration.
- He takes no medication and has no significant medical or family history of PTX. He has had **no recent surgical interventions** [9] .
- He has been **smoking casually since the age of 17 years** [10] .
- He is a **university student who lives with his family** [11] .

1 PTX is defined as the presence of air within the pleural space. Usually, the source of this air is the lung itself, but it can also arise from the outside (as in penetrating trauma) or from the oesophagus following perforation. The pleural space is bound by the visceral pleura on the surface of the lungs and the parietal pleura on the surface of the chest wall. Normally the pleural space is held in slight negative pressure (the relatively rigid chest wall maintains structure while the elastic recoil of the lungs is constantly pulling them inwards). However, if an abnormal communication forms between the pleural space and the alveoli, gas will flow into the pleural space. The pressure in the pleural space increases and subsequently prevents the lung from expanding normally. When only one episode of air leaking into the pleural space occurs, it develops a PTX. However, if air continues to leak, it is defined as a broncho-pleural fistula.

2 PTX may be classified according to the mechanism as spontaneous or traumatic. Traumatic pneumothorax may be due to penetrating or blunt mechanisms as well as iatrogenic. Spontaneous PTX can be further categorised, depending on the presence or absence of underlying lung disease, as primary or secondary. Primary spontaneous PTX is caused by rupture of small blebs ('lung blisters' containing air) at the apical segments of upper or lower lobes without associated lung disease. It recurs in approximately 20% of the cases. Current theories for bleb formation include genetic (mutations to the folliculin gene), congenital (air sacs growing faster than vessel in upper lobes) and mechanical (more negative intrapleural pressure in tall individuals). These blebs may eventually rupture, causing a PTX.

3 Secondary spontaneous PTX occurs in the presence of lung disease when the underlying lesion is close to the pleural surface. The most common causes are COPD, bullous/cystic disease or lung abscess. At some point in the disease, a PTX can happen.

4 Tension PTX occurs when the air leak itself acts as a one-way valve, permitting increasing pressure in the pleural space. It causes impaired ventilation and can also prevent venous return to the heart, resulting in obstructive shock. Tension PTX is a clinical diagnosis.

5 Primary spontaneous PTX is more common in young males (aged 20–30 years), whereas secondary spontaneous PTX is more common in individuals >50 years old. This reflects the increasing incidence of chronic lung disease with age. However, it is still possible for secondary spontaneous PTX to occur in young patients.

6 Spontaneous PTX usually presents with acute pleuritic pain (associated with breathing). The pain is typically on the same side as the PTX although it can also be central. PTX may also cause dyspnoea, although this can vary significantly between patients. The severity of dyspnoea depends on the degree of impairment to ventilation as well as reserve respiratory function. As such, patients with secondary spontaneous PTX are more likely to be dyspnoeic. Patients with spontaneous PTX may less commonly develop cough or orthopnoea. A spontaneous PTX can be associated with haemothorax, as small collateral vessels (systemic vessels from the chest wall supplying the area of inflammation or bulla on the lung surface) are torn when the bleb bursts.

7 The differential diagnoses for acute onset chest pain and dyspnoea include acute coronary syndrome, pulmonary oedema or exacerbation of heart failure, pulmonary embolus, acute asthma (although this is less likely to cause chest pain), acute exacerbation of COPD, pneumonia, acute aortic dissection and anxiety. An appropriate history should further investigate the likelihood of these differentials.

8 Obtaining a past medical history from the patient is important in spontaneous PTX. Patients may have had this condition before (recurrent spontaneous PTX) or have underlying pulmonary disease likely to cause a secondary spontaneous PTX. Important medical conditions include COPD, severe asthma, tuberculosis (TB), cystic fibrosis and lung malignancy (primary or metastatic). PTX in the young patient may be associated with Langerhans cell histiocytosis or thoracic endometriosis. Other lung conditions are likely to be relevant. Diseases such as Marfan syndrome, Ehlers–Danlos syndrome and homocystinuria are associated with primary spontaneous PTX.

9 Iatrogenic causes of PTX include central line access, mechanical ventilation, thoracentesis, insertion of permanent pacemaker, removal of a previously inserted chest drain and

other intrathoracic procedures. Mechanical ventilation is most likely to produce a PTX in patients with previous lung disease, severe pneumonia or respiratory distress syndrome.

10 Cigarette smoking is a significant risk factor for the development of spontaneous PTX (it increases the risk 10-fold in women and 20-fold in men). The development of blebs is thought to be related to smoking, although blebs also occur in non-smokers. Family history of PTX in general increases the risk of PTX.

11 Social history is an important part of the work-up for all patients.

Examination

- The patient has **stable vital signs** [1]. He appears to be in modest pain and mildly distressed.
- He is on **5L per minute of oxygen through a Hudson mask** [2].
- He has **no signs of trauma or underlying lung disease** [3].
- He has a **tall and slender body habitus** [4].
- The nurse responsible for the patient explains that he was tachypnoeic on presentation but has settled with oxygen administration. His **blood oxygen saturation was 91% but has now risen to 99%** [5].
- Otherwise, his vital signs are stable, and he is afebrile.

His hands are inspected and show no signs of underlying lung disease. His **capillary refill time is normal** [6].
- Examination of his **neck and JVP are also normal** [7].
- His chest has **no scars or obvious deformity** [8]. His chest is hyper-resonant on percussion on the left side, with decreased tactile fremitus felt on the left.
- Additionally, **reduced breath sounds are heard on the left side** [9].
- Consideration is given as to how this patient would present with **tension pneumothorax** [10] or if **intubated** [11].

1 Examination following the trauma primary survey acronym of ABC (airway, breathing and circulation – please refer to *Case 9*) is an excellent tool to identify life-threatening situations and act accordingly. In the case of PTX, there is a spectrum from the almost asymptomatic patient to the severely haemodynamically compromised with a tension PTX.

2 On general inspection, it should be noted whether the patient appears well, unwell or critical. Critical appearance may be due to tension PTX or another underlying cause for their presentation – there are several life-threatening causes for sudden onset chest pain or SOB. The patient may appear to be in pain or distress. Cough and stridor may also be heard. They may be on oxygen through nasal prongs or Hudson mask to increase their blood oxygen saturation. This may be a sign of long-standing pulmonary disease (such as COPD requiring the use of home oxygen) or more likely an acutely administered intervention in the ED.

3 General inspection may also yield signs of underlying pulmonary disease. This includes changes in posture and overall colour. Patients with severe emphysema may appear pink, cachectic and breathe with pursed lips. Patients with severe chronic bronchitis may appear cyanotic (due to

hypoxaemia) and obese. It is also important to consider whether the patient may have been involved with any trauma or surgery.

4 Tall and slender body habitus is also associated with primary spontaneous PTX. This is thought to be due to the fact that the pleural pressure is more negative at the apex of the lung, making subpleural blebs more likely to form and subsequently rupture.

5 The vital signs in patients with a potential PTX are used to stratify risk and guide management. The patient may be tachypnoeic, due to either pain or decreased ventilatory capacity. They may also have reduced oxygen saturations. However, this represents significantly reduced ventilatory capacity and is not always present. Patients with underlying lung disease may have reduced oxygen saturations at baseline.

6 Inspection of the hands can alert to acute or chronic lung disease. Peripheral capillary refill time is abnormally long with haemodynamic instability caused by tension PTX. Peripheral cyanosis may be present in those with underlying lung disease. Clubbing represents chronic lung disease or paraneoplastic syndrome. Asterixis may be present in those with carbon dioxide retention, as seen in type 2 respiratory failure.

7 The JVP may be raised in tension PTX or in pulmonary hypertension. Pulmonary hypertension has several possible causes, including COPD or other lung disease.

8 The chest should be inspected for scars. These may indicate previous surgery or chest tube insertion. This may suggest underlying lung disease or recurrence of primary spontaneous PTX. Radiotherapy used in lung cancer can cause the overlying skin to be dry and scaly. Chest wall deformities should also be considered. Hyperexpansion (barrel chest) is associated with chronic lung conditions – most commonly asthma and COPD. Other chest wall deformities such as pectus excavatum may be associated with development of spontaneous PTX.

9 The chest should then be palpated. This may reveal displacement of the apex beat, which may be seen in tension PTX. Chest expansion should be assessed. Chest hyperexpansion may be seen in tension PTX. Reduced chest expansion may be seen in simple PTX. The chest should be generally percussed, including the supraclavicular region and axilla. PTX causes hyper-resonance, as the underlying tissue below the site of percussion is much less dense. PTX may be felt as decreased vibration when assessing tactile vocal fremitus. Auscultation of the chest is vital in the assessment of PTX. Reduced breath sounds are heard over the affected area. They may be reduced or totally absent.

10 Tension PTX is an uncommon presentation that carries high mortality. It is mostly seen in trauma in the pre-hospital setting or emergency rooms and in ICU. Tension PTX commonly presents with respiratory distress, tachypnoea and chest pain. Hypoxia also occurs but less commonly. Jugular vein distension and tracheal deviation are uncommon signs. Overall, the most common signs are decreased breath sounds and hypertympanic percussion on the affected side. Cardiovascular compromise and obstructive shock associated with tension PTX is caused by decreased venous return (due to either increased intrathoracic pressure or dynamic obstruction of IVC/SVC with mediastinal shift). As a consequence, hypotension and tachycardia, including pulsus paradoxus (a fall in blood pressure during inspiration >10mmHg) can be seen. Please refer to *Case 9* for more details on tension PTX.

11 PTX presentation in ventilated patients in ICU or during anaesthesia, besides its usual physical examination, can be associated with decreased oxygen saturation, subcutaneous emphysema, sudden increase in both peak and plateau airway pressures, pulsus paradoxus (seen as oscillation of the arterial trace during respiratory cycle) and even haemodynamic instability with tension PTX.

Investigations

- The **need for urgent management is considered** [1].
- As the patient is deemed stable, IV access is obtained, and **routine blood tests are taken** [2]. They later return as normal.
- An arterial blood gas sample is taken on arrival, before the administration of oxygen. The patient was found to be **hypoxaemic with a mild respiratory alkalosis** [3].
- Electrocardiography shows **no change** [4].
- Mobile erect CXR occurs in the ED [5].
- It shows a **large left-sided PTX** [6].
- Ultrasound also occurs, showing the absence of **lung sliding** [7].
- CT [8] is used preoperatively to ensure that all disease is resected.
- **Other tests are considered** [9].

1 The diagnostic pathway with imaging for PTX is based on the stability of the patient. For unstable patients with suspected tension PTX, investigations should not delay management. Increasingly, bedside ultrasound is utilised in urgent situations. This usually occurs concurrently with resuscitation measures.

2 Routine blood tests are likely to have been performed in the ED. Full blood examination may show mild leucocytosis. Given that PTX can present with symptoms that have several possibilities, troponin levels and D-dimer levels may also be ordered. For secondary spontaneous PTX, blood tests may be useful for detecting the underlying lung disease. Coagulation studies are useful for patients who are to undergo an invasive procedure (either chest tube or surgery).

3 Arterial blood gas (ABG) may augment the assessment of decrease in respiratory function due to PTX. It is indicated for patients with significant decrease in peripheral oxygen saturation (<92%), those with ostensible respiratory distress involving tachypnoea or accessory muscle use, or those with a history of respiratory failure. Patients with significant PTX may be hypoxaemic (PaO_2 <60mmHg) – type 1 respiratory failure. Tachypnoea produces hypocapnoea. Hypercapnoea ($PaCO_2$ >50mmHg) is a sign that the patient is becoming tired (respiratory pump failure) – type 2 respiratory failure – and is frequently associated with hypoxaemia. It is most common in patients with underlying lung disease.

4 ECG is part of triage for chest pain in the ED, even in young patients.

5 For haemodynamically stable patients, erect CXR is the primary diagnostic imaging modality – inspiratory/ expiratory views help in diagnosing small PTX. X-ray is also used to assess the evolution of PTX. Patients may not require CXR if they are going to have a chest CT scan for another reason. PTX is seen on CXR as a clear margin between the line representing the edge of the lung and the chest wall. This distance correlates with the size of the PTX. CXR may also show a deep, lucent costophrenic angle on the same side as the PTX. Large PTX can show diaphragmatic flattening as the pressure pushes the diaphragm downwards. PTX may be confused with large bullae. Occasionally, skin folds and ribs may also give the appearance of PTX. For secondary spontaneous PTX, the underlying cause may be seen on CXR.

6 The size of the PTX may be estimated – when there is <2cm between the parietal and visceral pleura at the level of the hilum, it is deemed a small PTX. When there is >2cm, it is deemed large. However, lung collapse does not always occur in a uniform manner, so this categorisation system does not always accurately reflect the volume of air within the pleural space or loss of ventilatory capacity. Note that American and European guidelines define size of PTX differently.

7 Ultrasound may be used for the diagnosis of PTX. It is particularly useful in urgent situations and has been shown to be more sensitive than CXR. It is also commonly used

for the diagnosis of PTX in ventilated patients. PTX is seen on ultrasound as the presence of a lung point. The parietal pleura creates a broad reflective surface for the ultrasound and is seen as a white line. When lung is present immediately below the parietal pleura, lung sliding is seen. However, in PTX, where there is no lung immediately below the parietal pleura, no lung sliding will be present. Lung point, which is diagnostic of PTX, is seen as the meeting of lung sliding on one side of the screen and the absence of lung sliding on the other. This indicates the border of the PTX. However, in large PTX, when the lung is almost completed deflated and not touching the chest wall, there will be no lung point. Horizontal lines along the interior surface of the pleura may also be seen. They are caused by the presence of air.

8 CT can be used to investigate the underlying cause of spontaneous PTX – it is used when secondary spontaneous PTX is suspected or as a pre-op work-up in any patient with PTX. It is very accurate for defining underlying lung disease and determining the size and location of the PTX. PTX is seen as a clear space between the visceral and parietal pleura. Blebs and bullae are well defined even on a non-contrast low dose protocol chest CT.

9 More sophisticated or invasive tests can be used electively (away from ED setting) to investigate the causes of a secondary spontaneous PTX. This may include genetic testing for specific syndromes, flexible bronchoscopy with microbiology or cytology sampling, or lung biopsy for interstitial lung disease. PET, CT-guided FNA or EBUS are complementary tools to diagnose nodules or masses identified during the investigation of a PTX.

Management

Immediate

As mentioned, the patient was **administered oxygen on arrival** [1] . He **otherwise appears stable** [2] . The PTX is moderate but there is **no evidence of respiratory compromise** [3] [4] . Given the patient has had two previous episodes, an urgent **pigtail catheter is not indicated** [5] [6] .

Short-term

Contact the cardiothoracic surgery team for admission and monitoring. Perform a **VATS with resection of blebs** [7] [8] [9] and subsequently **pleurodesis the next day** [10] [11] .

Long-term

Discharge [12] the patient once clinically improving. Follow up the patient with repeat CXR to assess for recurrence. Discuss **potential prevention measures** [13] .

1 The primary goal of management of a PTX is to keep the patient oxygenated and haemodynamically stable. To achieve that, the next steps will depend on the vital signs (respiratory and pulse rates, BP, oxygen saturation), severity of symptoms and the size of the PTX. The measures to be taken can escalate accordingly from observation to oxygen therapy, to needle aspiration, to insertion of a thin or large bore intercostal catheter (ICC), to VATS. Upright positioning (raising the head of the bed) can improve respiratory function. For patients with oxygen saturations <96%, oxygen may be administered. However, caution must be used when administering oxygen to patients with CO_2 retention (as is commonly seen in COPD), as it may exacerbate type 2 respiratory failure. In these patients, oxygen saturation of 88–92% should be adequate. Some believe that oxygen administration will increase the partial pressure of oxygen within the pleural space, and as oxygen is better absorbed than nitrogen, the PTX would resolve quicker.

2 For patients with PTX and respiratory distress requiring mechanical ventilation, immediate chest tube insertion should always follow intubation, because positive pressure ventilation can create a tension PTX. Needle decompression might have to be performed concomitantly to intubation or soon thereafter, even before ICC insertion.

3 Small pneumothoraces typically resolve within 10 days. A CXR may be repeated several hours later to monitor progression and another one performed at discharge – invasive management is usually not required. Outpatient follow-up is important – they should be seen within a few days of discharge. Larger pneumothoraces can be managed with observation or chest tube placement. Broadly, the more evidence of altered respiratory function, the more likely that a chest tube is required. Patients with any size PTX who are unstable or show signs of tension should have a chest tube placed. Secondary spontaneous PTX follows these management principles but consideration should also be given to improving the patient's primary disease.

4 There are several procedures used in the acute management of PTX. A needle thoracostomy is used for decompressing the chest when features of tension PTX are evident. It is inserted in the second intercostal space, midclavicular line. Following this, a chest tube is typically placed.

5 A pigtail catheter (catheter thoracostomy) is a less invasive way to allow air to escape from the chest than a chest tube. It is inserted percutaneously using Seldinger technique (needle puncture, insertion of a wire, followed by dilation of the track and placement of the pigtail catheter). Thoracic drains with air leak should not be clamped (air will accumulate within the chest and cause, at least symptoms; at worst tension PTX. Indeed, some units do not clamp any drain ever to maintain a unified protocol and avoid this situation). The drainage system is 'part of the patient' and should be examined to assure the drain is secured and inside the chest, the water seal is functional and to ensure no kinks,

obstruction or disconnection. Patients with chest drains should be monitored for symptoms (pain, SOB, subcutaneous emphysema) and haemodynamic/respiratory instability. Documentation about the presence of air leak and the amount of fluid drainage is critical for decision-making and management.

6 A large-bore chest tube (tube thoracostomy) may be used to drain fluid and air. Insertion technique is described in *Case 9*. This is not typically required for spontaneous PTX unless tension is present or there is a complicating factor, such as the presence of an effusion or blood.

7 The decision to offer/perform primary VATS (even before insertion of an ICC) depends on the patient's stability, available logistics and consent. The goal of surgery in spontaneous PTX is to control the source of air leak (by resecting the blebs or bullae – currently done with surgical staples, but previously by cutting and oversewing) and prevent recurrence (by creating adhesion between the visceral and parietal pleura). Indications for surgery include recurrent episodes of PTX on one side, bilateral PTX, haemopneumothorax, persistent air leak for several days despite chest tube placement, for high risk occupations (such as pilot or scuba diver), if pregnancy is contemplated or for patients who developed life-threatening PTX requiring a chest tube. Secondary PTX has a high recurrence rate due to underlying lung disease. Patients on their first presentation of spontaneous PTX, who are stable and have indication for surgery (as above for primary PTX and any patient with secondary PTX) can have corrective surgery even before chest drainage – depending on availability of a surgical team and local logistics. Whilst surgery is discussed in detail, non-operative techniques for pleurodesis do exist. However, they are reserved for patients who are not candidates for surgery (usually seen in secondary spontaneous PTX). This may involve the intrapleural administration of talc (the most common), tetracycline derivative (rare due to availability) or seldom autologous blood (risk of infection).

8 VATS is by far the most commonly used surgical approach to spontaneous PTX. The objective of surgery is to resect the probable cause of air leak (the bleb or bulla) and prevent recurrence (with pleurodesis). Before the advent of VATS, a small muscle-sparing axillary thoracotomy was used to manage it. For convenience and improved operative visualisation, single lung ventilation (the operated lung is deflated whilst the contralateral lung provides ventilation) is achieved with a double lumen endotracheal tube. Alternatively, a bronchial blocker can be inserted via a normal endotracheal tube to exclude the one lung. This deflates the operated lung and creates a large operative field within the chest. Shafted instruments are then inserted into the pleural cavity via ports (openings through the chest wall – either direct or via trocars). Depending on the surgical preference, there could be one (uniportal), two or more ports. Uniportal VATS has been accepted recently with great enthusiasm as it requires a single entry of about 2–3cm and potentially less postoperative pain. As opposed to laparoscopic surgery, CO_2 insufflation is not mandatory in the chest (although it might improve visualisation in some cases), as the chest wall is a rigid non-collapsible cavity.

9 General anaesthesia is established with a double lumen endotracheal tube and the patient is positioned in a lateral decubitus with the affected side up. IV antibiotics are given and the chest tube (if *in situ*) is removed once single lung ventilation is commenced – otherwise a tension PTX can occur under positive pressure ventilation (communication with the anaesthetist is critical). One or more ports (according to surgeon preference) are established. The camera is inserted and the interior of the chest wall visualised (it can also assist in placement of other ports). The pleura is inspected and location of the blebs identified. Blebs at the apex of the upper lobes are the most common source of air leak in primary spontaneous PTX, although they can also occur at the apex of the lower lobes – hence usefulness of pre-op CT.

10 Pleurodesis is adhesion between visceral and parietal pleura. The purpose of these adhesions is to obliterate the pleural space and avoid lung collapse by a future PTX or effusion. Pleurodesis is classified as mechanical or chemical, according to the way it creates adhesions. Chemical pleurodesis is the most used form of pleurodesis and is performed by spraying talc or tetracycline, as powder or slurry, inside the thoracic cavity. Advantages of chemical pleurodesis are that it is readily available, quick and gives thorough distribution within the chest during VATS with low recurrence rates. It can be done on the ward through a chest tube (reserved for high risk patients) and is cheap. Disadvantages are pain, fever and absorption of talc by the body when small particle talc (<5 microns) is used. Mechanical pleurodesis involves pleurectomy (the parietal pleura is actually dissected and resected or is removed by abrasion with rough material – sandpaper-like or gauze). Its advantages include low recurrence (for resection only) but disadvantages are more bleeding and potential to damage nerves at the thoracic inlet, including ansa subclavia (causing Horner's syndrome), vagus (vocal cord palsy) and phrenic nerves. Blebs and/or bullae are resected with surgical staples

(the stapler provides 2 or 3 lines of staples and cuts the tissue simultaneously). A wedge resection (surgical biopsy) at the apex of the upper lobe is recommended, even if no obvious disease is identified. This is particularly useful to obtain tissue for histopathology and diagnosis of lung disease (for example, in lymphoangiomyomatosis, where patients may quickly progress to transplant). Lung volume reduction surgery can be performed in very selected patients with severe COPD and PTX, when emphysema is limited to upper lobes.

11 Pain control is critical to expedite mobility and respiratory physiotherapy, and hence prevent DVT and lung collapse. A combination of agents is required, with the goal to avoid opioids as they depress respiratory centre and cough. Local anaesthetic is liberally used around the port and drain sites and as intercostal nerve blocks. A paravertebral catheter can be inserted under video assistance for post-op continuous infusion. Liposomal bupivacaine (effects last 48–72 hours), where available, can be used.

12 Most patients who have undergone VATS can be returned to the ward. They should be assessed with regular post-anaesthetic observations. Venous thromboembolism prophylaxis is required. Typically, the chest drains are placed on suction for a period of time before being transitioned to a simple underwater valve device, then removed once there is no air leak and drainage is <100ml/24h (this amount is a guide only as there is variability between patients and surgeon's preference).

13 Following resolution of the PTX, whether that be through observation, thoracostomy or surgery, patients should be re-evaluated around 3 weeks after their procedure. The patient should be assessed for signs of recurrence or pain from pleurodesis. A CXR is commonly performed to confirm re-expansion. Additionally, patients should be counselled on reducing behaviour that puts them at risk of recurrence. This includes the cessation of smoking and of the use of illicit drugs. Air travel should be avoided for at least 2 weeks. Scuba diving should be avoided for life if possible. The patient should avoid exercise for 2 weeks, although more vigorous exercise may require a longer period.

CASE 9: Thoracic trauma

History

- A patient arrives by ambulance to the trauma bay. He has experienced significant **thoracic trauma** [1] [2].
- The team leader **assigns roles** [3] and obtains a **handover from the paramedics** [4] [5].
- A **25-year-old man** [6] was involved in a **high speed motor vehicle accident** [7].
- He was restrained by a seatbelt when slippery road conditions caused him to veer, resulting in the car hitting the guardrail and **rolling over several times** [8].
- He **was confused** [9] at the scene and brought by road ambulance to the closest **Major Trauma Centre** [10].
- His wife was following him in another car and told the paramedics that he has no **allergies, does not take medications nor has significant past medical history** [11]. Their **last meal** [11] before the crash was 5 hours earlier.

[1] Understanding chest trauma relies on anatomical knowledge of the thorax and surrounding structures. The contents of the chest include the mediastinum and lungs. Within the mediastinum is the heart, aorta, trachea and oesophagus. The floor of the chest is the diaphragm. However, several organs are partially covered by the lower ribs and may be injured in what appears to be isolated thoracic trauma. These include the liver, spleen and kidneys.

[2] The cardiac box is the area of chest overlying the heart. It is bound by the clavicles superiorly, xiphoid inferiorly and the midclavicular line laterally. Penetrating trauma to this area is very likely to result in cardiac trauma.

[3] As with many aspects of emergency care, consideration should be given to record-keeping, consent for treatment and obtaining forensic evidence. Team structure is vital in the assessment and management of trauma. There should be a team leader responsible for supervising and checking decisions as well as directing assessment and assigning tasks.

[4] Given that trauma can be unpredictable and high pressure, a common pathway has been developed to aid clinical thinking and communication. Patients who have undergone trauma experience a pre-hospital phase (retrieval and delivery to hospital). During this time, clinicians at the receiving hospital should prepare themselves for the arriving case. Within the hospital phase, triage must first occur. This is particularly important in resource-limited environments or where there are multiple or mass casualties. Trauma patients are often assessed and initially managed in non-tertiary centres before being transported to metropolitan centres for definitive care.

[5] There is a classically described trimodal distribution of death in trauma. The first peak occurs in minutes after the event when injuries are not compatible with life. These injuries include high spinal cord injury, damage to the heart or great vessels or catastrophic damage to the airways. The second peak occurs within hours following the event. Injuries causing death in this time frame relevant to thoracic trauma include haemopneumothorax, tension PTX, ruptured spleen, liver lacerations and injuries causing significant blood loss. The 'golden hour' after the event requires fast assessment and resuscitation to prevent mortality. The third peak occurs days to weeks after the injury and usually involves sepsis or multi-organ dysfunction due to the significant physiologic disturbances related to major trauma.

[6] Trauma is a leading cause of death in those under the age of 40 in developed countries. Trauma is more common in males aged 10–30 years. Alcohol and drugs are often involved.

[7] There are several mechanisms of trauma. Blunt trauma frequently results from motor vehicle accidents (including motorbike collisions and cyclists), falls and interpersonal violence. Penetrating trauma can be caused by bullets or knives and other objects used to stab. It can also result from situations where the patient collides with something sharp such as in a motor vehicle accident or fall. Thermal injury can complicate thoracic trauma or be the sole mechanism.

[8] Specific mechanisms of injury can predict injury patterns. Mechanisms likely to cause significant thoracic trauma include frontal or side impacts in motor vehicle accidents, ejection from vehicle, pedestrian impact with motor vehicle, penetrating trauma to anterior chest and thoracoabdominal region.

9 Confusion in trauma is a sign of concussion, low cardiac output or both. Body physiology is altered in severe trauma. Decreased blood volume due to fractures or bleeding leads to decreased end-organ tissue perfusion and cellular ischaemia with subsequent oedema and inflammation. The central nervous system (CNS) response to trauma is targeted to protect the CNS and cardiovascular system: keep blood pressure and retain fluid. This is achieved by increasing heart rate and systemic vascular resistance.

10 Obtaining a history of the events from retrieval personnel is vital. However, this handover should not delay the primary survey. It should include information on the entire course of the patient's journey from traumatic event to delivery to hospital. The patient's initial status, eyewitness accounts, initial assessment and management and events during transport are crucial. Patients who have experienced significant trauma are often placed in a cervical collar and on a spinal board for transport.

11 More detailed history, whoever it is obtained from, should not delay the primary survey. Important aspects of the history are represented with the acronym 'AMPLE'. This includes allergies, current medications, past medical history, last meal and events surrounding the injury. This information may be gleaned from the patient themselves, retrieval personnel, family or eyewitnesses. Past medical history may yield conditions requiring medical input later in the patient's recovery.

Examination

- The **primary survey begins immediately** [1].
- The **airway** [2] [3] is assessed and found to have no injury.
- His **breathing** [4] is assessed next.
- He can barely speak, is taking shallow breaths and is tachypnoeic; his **left hemithorax is hyperinflated and hypertympanic** [5] [6] in relation to the right and his **trachea is deviated to the right** [5] [6].
- There is decreased **air entry on the left and he is hypoxic** [7].
- The **circulation** [8] [9] is assessed; he is **tachycardic in shock** [10] [11].
- His **neurological state** [11] deteriorates rapidly and he is found to have a Glasgow Coma Scale (GCS) score of 5.
- This initial assessment triggers **immediate intubation with rapid sequence induction (RSI)** [12] by one team and left hemithorax needle decompression followed by an intercostal drain by another team.
- The patient's temperature is maintained to **prevent hypothermia** [13]. The patient's haemodynamics responded to the procedures above and liberal fluid resuscitation.
- A **secondary survey** [14] can now be completed. The chest is examined in more detail with the use of adjunctive investigation modalities.
- Injuries to the **chest wall and nearby bony structures** [15], the **lungs** [16], the **heart and great vessels** [17] [18] and **other structures within the chest** [19] [20] are considered.
- Other than significant chest trauma, he appears to have **no other major injuries** [21]. The cardiothoracic surgery team is contacted to make them aware of this patient.

1 As the patient arrives at hospital, a primary survey occurs with resuscitation administered concurrently. The primary survey follows the acronym ABCDE: Airway with restriction of cervical spine movement, Breathing, Circulation, Disability (neurologic status) and Exposure and environmental control. Note that thoracic trauma can affect A, B and C simultaneously, hence mortality is high. The objective of the primary survey is to identify and correct life-threatening injuries.

2 The 'A' part of the primary survey is for Airway. The upper airway can be obstructed by direct trauma, foreign body (teeth fragments, dental prosthesis, soil) or fluid (blood and vomit). Fracture of laryngeal bones and cartilages can make it difficult to establish airway control, so urgent tracheostomy might be required. Swelling and haematoma originating from nearby vessel injuries can also obstruct the airway.

Signs of upper airway obstruction include stridor and hoarse voice, and intercostal muscle use. Bleeding or vomit within the airway may be suctioned. Ultimately, a secure airway is required if there is obstruction.

3 Lower airway obstruction occurs due to tracheobronchial tree injury. Although this type of injury is not very common, it usually causes death. Signs of lower airway obstruction include haemoptysis, large subcutaneous emphysema or cyanosis. CXR typically shows huge subcutaneous emphysema and a collapsed lung with PTX. Most injuries occur close to the carina. Potential complications include tension PTX or pneumopericardium. Intubation and ventilation have the potential to worsen the injury. If a chest tube is inserted, oxygenation and symptoms can get worse as air can leak preferentially through the drain as opposed to entering the lungs. CT can raise a high index of suspicion, but bronchoscopy confirms the injury. Management involves intubation with advanced techniques (bronchoscopic guidance) where the endotracheal tube is placed beyond the disruption, in the case of tracheal injury, or in the contralateral bronchus, in case of bronchial injury.

4 'B' is for 'Breathing'. Assessing breathing requires complete exposure of the patient (including the neck, which may involve briefly opening the cervical collar). The chest should be inspected, palpated and auscultated in search of tracheal deviation, rib fractures/crepitation, flail segments or open cavity.

5 These are the signs of a tension PTX. In severe chest trauma, the association of hypotension, hypoxia and tachycardia should call attention for a possible tension PTX, hence inspection of the chest must be done quickly to exclude or confirm it.

6 Tension PTX occurs when pressure builds in the pleural space. Injury to either lung or chest wall can cause a one-way valve, allowing air to enter the pleural space but not exit. This means that during the negative pressure of inspiration in the pleural space, more air is brought in. The affected hemithorax keeps filling with air up to the point that lung expansion is hampered and the intrathoracic pressure prevents venous return into the chest (intrathoracic pressure is higher than venous pressure in the inferior vena cava (IVC) and SVC). Distended jugular veins is another sign of tension PTX, but not always present on the severely hypovolaemic patient. Tension PTX can be rapidly diagnosed by physical examination and confirmed with ultrasound. However, ultimately it is a clinical diagnosis and additional diagnostic modalities should not delay treatment.

7 Open PTX occurs when there is free passage of air through the chest wall; in other words, when an open thoracic wound can be seen, moving air in and out of the chest. It is sometimes termed a 'sucking chest wound'. Air will enter the pleural space preferentially instead of the trachea, resulting in inadequate ventilation. This leads to hypoxia and hypercapnoea. These wounds are often managed in the pre-hospital setting with an occlusive dressing taped on three sides, producing a one-way valve, or simply, a closed dressing if the patient tolerates it. Massive haemothorax not only affects breathing but circulation as well. It is defined as collection of >1500ml of blood within one side of the chest. It commonly results from injury to the large blood vessels within the thorax. This collection can prevent normal lung expansion and therefore hamper normal ventilation. Signs of massive haemothorax include shock, signs of hypovolaemia, absent breath sounds and dullness to percussion on one side.

8 'C' is for Circulation. Thoracic trauma can affect A, B and C on the primary survey. Assessment includes determining whether there are cool peripheries and/or skin mottling. The pulse should be assessed for quality as well as rate and rhythm. Blood pressure (and pulse pressure) and blood oxygen saturation should be monitored along with

electrocardiography assessment. Massive haemothorax (mentioned above) affects B and C.

9 Cardiac tamponade can also occur in chest trauma. It is defined as accumulation of fluid within the pericardial space resulting in reduced cardiac output. The pericardium is not very compliant and so only a small amount of fluid is needed to start restricting cardiac function. It most commonly occurs due to penetrating injuries. Beck's triad of clinical signs for cardiac tamponade include hypotension, muffled heart sound and jugular venous distension. However, in the hypovolaemic patient the jugular vein may not distend, and muffled heart sounds will almost invariably be present in obese patients and even difficult to hear in a noisy resuscitation room, making it hard to identify the Beck's triad. Nevertheless, pulsus paradoxus (an exaggerated drop in systemic BP during inspiration) is present with mechanical or spontaneous ventilation. It is very difficult to synchronise pulse and ventilation when the patient is tachycardic. So, in practice, the pulse tends to disappear during inspiration if there is tamponade and especially when the patient is already hypotensive/hypovolaemic. Pulsus paradoxus can also occur in severe acute asthma. Tension PTX and cardiac tamponade can present in similar ways, but inspection of the chest will give clues to a PTX. Cardiac tamponade is diagnosed by ultrasound.

10 Trauma can also result in circulatory arrest. This is defined as the state of being unconscious with the absence of a pulse. The potential underlying cardiac rhythms include pulseless electrical activity, ventricular fibrillation and asystole. Potential causes include (from airway to circulation) profound hypoxia, tension PTX, hypovolaemia, tamponade and severe myocardial contusion. Significantly, the cardiac event may have occurred before the injury. Cardiopulmonary resuscitation (CPR) following traumatic circulatory arrest can be either closed (following advanced life support guidelines) or open – ED thoracotomy. The latter is used in select patients, mostly with penetrating injury when deterioration was witnessed by health staff. ED thoracotomy carries severe complications, so it is only performed by trained teams.

11 Neurologic status can be determined using the Glasgow Coma Scale (GCS). The motor score of the GCS best correlates with overall outcomes. Decreased level of consciousness may be due to decreased cerebral oxygen delivery, direct cerebral injury or other causes including hypoglycaemia and drugs.

12 Definitive airway control is employed in those with reduced conscious state, to improve oxygenation and prevent aspiration of gastric content.

13 The primary survey requires complete exposure of the patient for assessment. However, after the survey is complete, it is important to maintain the patient's body temperature to prevent or correct hypothermia. This can be accomplished through the use of forced air warming blankets, maintaining an appropriate temperature of the room and infusing warmed fluids/blood.

14 The secondary survey is a more rigorous assessment of the patient once they are more stable. It is a head-to-toe evaluation of the patient including history and exam. The goal is to identify life-threatening injuries not found on primary survey. The secondary survey can be augmented with the use of diagnostic tests. It is important because many injuries can only be appreciated after adequate resuscitation. For instance, when a patient is in shock, bleeding from minor vessels cannot be noted as blood volume is low and systemic vascular resistance is very high (the patient is 'shut down'). Once the cardiac output and BP increase, those vessels start to bleed, and the patient can even become unstable again. This typically happens with injury to the intercostal and visceral arteries. Another example is a simple PTX, that develops after intubation and positive pressure ventilation.

15 Bony injuries that may occur in thoracic trauma include rib fracture, sternal fracture, sternoclavicular dislocation and scapular fracture. All of these injuries usually occur in high energy/deceleration trauma and intrathoracic structures are likely affected. Aortic rupture should be suspected when first rib or scapular fractures occur. Thoracic trauma may also cause flail chest. This occurs when three (or more) ribs are broken in two (or more) places, producing a segment of chest wall that moves independently with ventilation. This produces a paradoxical chest wall movement where the segment becomes depressed during inspiration (it is sucked in by the negative pressure of the pleural space) and pushed out during expiration. This prevents the underlying lung from ventilating effectively.

16 Pulmonary contusion (bruising of the lung) often occurs in thoracic trauma and is more common in young patients – their non-ossified bones are more likely to bruise the underlying lung than break. Pulmonary contusion is often, but not always, associated with rib fractures. Hypoxaemia can result from impaired ventilation and diffusion from either of these pathologies. However, it can also result from pain impairing normal chest wall movement. Haemothorax may be caused by damage to the lung, great vessels or intercostal vessels in trauma. When the collection becomes >1500ml, it is termed 'massive' (discussed within *Examination Note 7*).

17 Blunt cardiac injury may also result from thoracic trauma, particularly within the cardiac box. It is usually caused by high energy blunt trauma mechanisms. It can result in myocardial contusion as well as rupture. Cardiac rupture often causes cardiac tamponade (as blood from the ruptured chamber is ejected into the pericardial space). As such, it presents in a similar manner to tamponade. Blunt cardiac injury can also disrupt the coronary vessels and cardiac valves.

18 Traumatic aortic injury (TAI) can occur in high energy trauma. It usually causes immediate death. Those who survive do so because the adventitia contains the rupture, usually at the aortic isthmus. Speculation about the mechanisms of TAI associated with rapid deceleration include a combination of shear forces, hydrostatic tension inside aorta, squeezing by bony structures (manubrium, first rib, clavicle and vertebrae) and developmental structure of different parts of the descending aorta. There are usually no specific physical examination findings for TAI.

19 The diaphragm may also be injured in thoracic trauma. This may be through blunt trauma (produce large tears) or penetrating trauma (producing small perforations). Examination findings are usually absent.

20 Oesophageal injury may also occur in thoracic trauma, mostly with penetrating mechanisms. Ruptured oesophagus usually causes a pneumo- or haemothorax with severe haemodynamic instability. There may be ingesta (food matter) within the chest tube.

21 The secondary survey may also discover other pathology, as thoracic trauma is commonly associated with injuries to other body areas.

Investigations

- Investigations are performed as adjuncts to the primary and secondary survey. **Bloods** [1] are taken from the patient's IV access sites.
- ECG leads are attached, and the patient is monitored with **constant telemetry** [2]. His vital signs are used to partially guide resuscitation.
- Ultrasound is used to assess the patient. There is **no free fluid in the peritoneum or in the pericardial space** [3].
- CXR performed within the resuscitation bay shows **rib fractures, scapular fracture, small bilateral haemothorax and a haematoma on the left at the apex (apical cap sign)** [4].
- Once the patient is stabilised and preliminary management is done, a full body CT scan is performed. CT finds **bilateral multiple rib fractures, left scapular fracture, pulmonary contusions, bilateral pneumo-haemothorax, small left apical extrapleural haematoma and a small haematoma at the aorto-pulmonary window** [5].
- **Other investigation modalities are considered** [6] [7].
- The radiologist reviews the imaging and a gated CT angiogram is performed and an **aortic flap identified** [8].

1 Once IV access is obtained, blood samples are taken for analysis. Initial full blood examination may reveal anaemia, although this will depend on resuscitation performed so far. For example, some helicopter transport units carry blood transfusion products. Anaemia due to acute haemorrhage is likely to be normocytic. Assessment of renal and liver function is also important as it has bearing for the patient's ongoing resuscitation and recovery. Liver failure can produce coagulopathy, which is relevant for management in general. Coagulation studies themselves are important for the same reason. Many people in the community are anticoagulated; it is important to be able to recognise this and consider the underlying reason even if a history is not obtainable. Serum amylase and lipase levels are also important as blunt abdominal injury can cause pancreatitis. Cardiac troponin can be used for the diagnosis of myocardial injury, although this may not necessarily be due to cardiac contusion. Lastly, a valid group and hold should be sent to the laboratory. This facilitates the administration of cross-matched blood products.

2 ECG is essential for monitoring in all trauma patients. However, those who have experienced thoracic trauma particularly require an ECG. This is due to the fact that blunt cardiac injury can cause arrhythmias.

3 A focused assessment with sonography in trauma (FAST) scan is a rapid and non-invasive test that can be performed at the bedside and is considered as an adjunct to primary and secondary survey. It is a very useful tool but does rely on operator knowledge. It is used in a screening manner for pericardial effusion and haemoperitoneum. An extended protocol (eFAST) has been developed to also assess for PTX by placing the probe on the anterior chest. Ultrasonography can be used more generally to evaluate the structure and function of the heart and ascending aorta.

4 CXR is a vital tool in the diagnosis of injuries caused by thoracic trauma. This should be accomplished through a mobile device rather than the patient being transported to radiology. Supine images may be necessary but may make it difficult to observe a PTX. Mediastinal injury (including aortic, oesophageal and tracheobronchial) may be appreciable

through this modality. Additionally, pulmonary contusion and haemothorax can be diagnosed through CXR. CXR should also be utilised for checking positioning of various devices following insertion (endotracheal tube, chest drain, nasogastric tube).

5 The decision to obtain further imaging – CT in most cases – or take the patient for operative management in trauma is complex and invariably depends on individual factors. The actual environment within a CT scanner room does not lend itself well to resuscitation or life-saving interventions. Therefore, patients should be adequately resuscitated and stabilised before being scanned. CT can be used to identify injury to the upper and lower airway, pneumothorax, haemothorax, chest wall injuries, pericardial effusion, cardiac contusion, diaphragmatic injury, oesophageal injury and aortic disruption. The CT is typically done without the use of contrast first, followed by IV contrast administration. The actual scan is performed during the arterial phase.

6 MRI is not commonly used in thoracic injuries. However, it may be used to evaluate the spinal cord and associated structures as well as assisting with the prognostication of traumatic brain injuries.

7 Other useful modalities in the assessment/management of thoracic trauma are:
- laryngoscopy – diagnosis of upper airway injury
- flexible bronchoscopy – diagnosis of tracheobronchial injury and advanced airway management
- endoscopy – investigation of oesophageal injury.

8 Currently, the diagnosis of TAI relies on the usual emergency CT scan. In cases where injury is not clear, an ECG gated CT angiogram with thinner slices can be used to better define the aorta. Angiographic study of the aorta is rarely used in modern practice and is reserved for cases where a gated CT cannot rule out TAI. A CT scan can show important signs of direct aortic injury (intimal flap, pseudoaneurysm and intramural haematoma) and indirect aortic injury (aorto-pulmonary window and periaortic haematoma, irregular lining of the intima, and major change in the aortic diameter).

Management

Immediate

As the patient is assessed and bedside investigations occur, **problems are managed concurrently [1] [2]**. Given the mechanism of injury and examination findings, **needle decompression of the left side and bilateral chest tubes insertion [3] [4]** occurred earlier.

Short-term

There are **several conditions [5] [6]** sometimes found in thoracic trauma that are not present in this patient. Note the **drain output [7]** upon placement of the chest tube. Monitor the patient closely, given the potential need for **surgery [8]**. Consider the **role of rib fixation for rib fractures [9]**. Treat the **scapular fracture conservatively [10]**. **Admit the patient to**

ICU for ventilation [11] [12]. Perform a tertiary survey 24 hours following the injury. Manage the TAI subacutely with a **thoracic endovascular aortic repair** [13]. Treat any **postoperative and post-traumatic sequelae** [14]. Extubate the patient when safe and transfer him to the trauma ward to continue recovery.

Long-term

Follow up the patient in the outpatient clinic with repeat CXR to assess for any reoccurrence of haemothorax.

1 The majority of thoracic trauma does not require operative intervention. Most can be treated with smaller procedures and resuscitation.

2 Resuscitation occurs as the patient is assessed. Obvious haemorrhage is stemmed if possible. If the patient is not intubated but haemodynamically unstable, oxygen is administered. The patient may then require intubation with ventilation. Fluid resuscitation occurs with possibility of activation of the massive transfusion protocol. Advanced life support and CPR may also be required. Pain management should be a priority and, if the patient is conscious, is likely to facilitate ventilation and lung recruitment.

3 Needle decompression is performed when tension PTX is suspected. The needle is placed in the 2nd intercostal space, midclavicular line. A sudden rush of air both confirms and solves the tension PTX. Finger thoracostomy is an alternative to this and occurs in the 5th intercostal space, midaxillary line. The advantage of this procedure is the ability to confirm that the lung re-expands through palpation. Following either of these procedures, an ICC should be placed.

4 Intercostal catheters may be small (<20Fr) or large (>20Fr) bore and are used to manage both pneumo- and haemothoraces. Large bore (usually about 30Fr in size) ICCs are almost universally used in the management of trauma as the drainage of blood and clot may be needed. ICCs may be placed in trauma before definitive imaging is obtained – in obvious significant thoracic trauma they would likely be placed essentially on patient arrival. ICCs are placed in the 5th intercostal space, midaxillary line in the 'triangle of safety'. The triangle of safety is made up of the lateral edge of pectoralis major, the lateral edge of latissimus dorsi; and the base of the triangle is the mid-humeral point. A small incision is made at the superior border of the rib to avoid the neurovascular bundle. Blunt dissection is performed down to the pleura. Once the pleural cavity is entered, a finger sweep is performed. The chest tube is inserted with forceps. The tube is connected to an underwater seal drainage system and respiratory swing is confirmed. The tube is sutured, and a sterile dressing is placed. A CXR confirms correct ICC positioning.

5 Tracheobronchial injury is usually treated with surgery although conservative management may be used in selected patients (small laceration and endotracheal tube cuff able to be inflated distal to the injury to allow ventilation).

6 Acute cardiac tamponade is an emergency. It can be managed percutaneously or surgically. However, in the setting of traumatic cardiac tamponade, surgical drainage is preferred. This can be performed through sternotomy, thoracotomy or laparotomy. As with most procedures involving opening of the pericardium, a drain should be left in the pericardial space to prevent recurrence of tamponade.

7 Haemothorax is usually caused by lung lacerations, bleeding intercostal vessel or internal mammary artery. Most haemothoraces can be managed with chest drainage. Indications for urgent thoracotomy (as opposed to thoracotomy in the emergency department) include haemothorax with volume >1500ml, hourly drain output >200ml/hour for 4 hours or 100ml/hour for 8 hours, large unevacuated haemothorax, cardiac tamponade, chest wall defect resulting in impaired ventilation, massive air leak impairing lung expansion or great vessel injury affecting haemodynamic function. VATS may be used in less critical patients for thoracic exploration and management.

8 Most common sources of bleeding in blunt chest trauma are intercostal arteries, internal thoracic arteries and lung.

9 The treatment of rib fractures is mostly supportive, with heavy involvement of chest physiotherapy and pain control. Oral or IV narcotics may be inadequate, necessitating loco-regional block with epidural, paravertebral or intercostal local anaesthetic administration. Operative rib fixation has the capacity to provide significant benefit to patients. However, the indications for it are very patient-specific. Flail chest, where the structural abnormality is directly affecting respiratory physiology, is agreed upon as a definite indication for fixation. Other indications where rib fixation is considered include severe chest wall deformity, sustained requirement for mechanical ventilation, chronic pain, lung herniation, fracture non-union and in instances where thoracotomy has occurred for another reason.

10 Fractures of the scapula and sternum may occasionally be fixated operatively, usually in the context of significantly displaced or unstable fractures. Adequate pain management is an essential part of management for these patients.

11 Patients with cardiac contusion should receive at least 24 hours of cardiac monitoring.

12 Pulmonary contusions do not typically require operative management. They are most likely to impair lung function, necessitating mechanical ventilation for longer periods. Major parenchymal lung injuries requiring some type of operative management are rare. Air leak and haemorrhage are usually solved with chest drainage although they may require surgery.

13 Thoracic endovascular aortic repair (TEVAR) is a minimally invasive procedure carried out by cardiothoracic surgeons, vascular surgeons and interventional radiologists. Depending on local preferences, they may work alone or in teams. The procedure involves cannulating the femoral artery and placing a stent (endograft) across the area of disruption. It is not usually used in the acute setting and is usually performed once the patient is stable. The goal of TEVAR in TAI is to prevent free rupture of the aorta.

14 Although a patient may survive initial resuscitation and operative management, they are still at risk of dying. As mentioned earlier, this is usually from sepsis or multi-organ dysfunction and failure. Acute kidney injury, acute respiratory distress syndrome (ARDS), cardiac arrest, cerebrovascular accident, DVT, pneumonia and urinary tract infection (UTI) are all common sequelae of trauma. ARDS and pneumonia are particularly common following chest trauma.

CASE 10: Type A aortic dissection

History

- There is a patient in the ED who has suspected **aortic dissection** [1] [2].
- He is a **55-year-old** [3] **male** [4] with sudden onset **sharp chest pain radiating through to his back** [5] and **syncope** [6].
- He has **hypertension and ischaemic heart disease** [7], but both are managed adequately with medical therapy.
- He has no features of connective tissue disorders. He has **no family history** [8] of aortic dissection.
- He does not **smoke or use illicit drugs** [9].
- His diet and exercise habits are poor. He is unemployed and does not engage in any **heavy lifting** [10].

[1] Acute aortic dissection (AAD) is a medical emergency, as mortality for non-operated cases reaches 50% in the first 48 hours. AAD is defined as blood leaving the normal aortic lumen and dissecting the inner and outer layers of the media to form a false lumen. This is usually precipitated by a tear in the intimal layer. The initial tear may arise in an ulcerated area of atheromatous disease in the aorta or arise *de novo*. The dissection can progress distally (anterograde) or proximally (retrograde). Usually the intimal tear is within 10cm of the aortic valve. Aortic dissection is considered acute if it is less than 14 days old, after which it is termed chronic. Pathologically, cystic medial necrosis or degeneration is commonly seen. The incidence of aortic dissection is approximately 1–3 per 100 000 people annually.

[2] Aortic dissection is a difficult diagnosis to make clinically, as several other serious diseases can present in a similar manner. Acute coronary syndrome shares several symptoms with aortic dissection. Additionally, ECG changes and reduced renal function can occur in both diseases. Pulmonary embolism is another potential cause of chest pain and haemodynamic compromise. Other serious causes of acute chest pain include myocarditis, pericarditis, tension PTX and oesophageal perforation. One needs to think about AAD to diagnose it, as clinical presentation can mimic many diseases, from stroke to kidney stones (related to dissection/obstruction of the arterial supply to that organ).

[3] Increasing age is associated with development of aortic dissection. The peak incidence is between 55 and 65 years of age. However, patients with dissections involving the ascending aorta are usually younger than those with descending aorta. In patients with risk factors such as genetic or structural abnormalities or drug use, age of onset tends to be lower. Most patients presenting with type A AAD will have pre-existing ascending aortic dilatation or aneurysm.

[4] Male gender is a significant risk factor for development of AAD.

[5] The most common presenting complaint of aortic dissection is sudden onset and severe chest or back pain. It can often be described by patients as 'sharp', 'tearing' or 'ripping'. The pain may change character and location as the false lumen becomes larger through further dissection. The pain can also radiate to the back or neck and arms due to involvement of aorta distal to the arch. A small proportion of patients present without chest pain. The pain is not likely to change in intensity over time. This is in contrast to the chest pain of an ACS which can increase over time as ischaemia progresses. However, pain can migrate as the dissection progresses.

[6] Other symptoms are non-specific and include diaphoresis, nausea and vomiting, syncope and dyspnoea. Many associated symptoms are due to ischaemic syndromes from occlusion of branches of the aorta. Occlusion of the coronary vessels can result in infarction or angina. Occlusion of the arch vessels can result in stroke. Around 10% of patients with ascending aortic dissection will have a stroke. Mental status changes can be caused by cerebral hypoperfusion due to either cardiogenic shock, hypovolaemic shock or occlusion of the arch vessels. Abdominal pain can occur from visceral ischaemia due to occlusion of the coeliac trunk and mesenteric arteries. Low urine output can occur due to kidney hypoperfusion with renal involvement or tamponade. Pain or paralysis in the lower limbs are due to interruption of arterial supply or spinal cord ischaemia (descending aorta dissection involving intercostal branches). The dissection can rupture into several spaces including the pleura, resulting in haemoptysis and dyspnoea; retroperitoneum, causing shock; or pericardium, causing tamponade. Dissection around the aortic root typically results in acute aortic incompetence. This

can lead to heart failure; however, haemodynamic instability is mostly due to tamponade or free rupture.

7 Several diseases are associated with aortic dissection and can be categorised as degenerative, structural, connective tissue, trauma and other. Aortic dilatation and hypertension are significantly associated with aortic dissection and the most common aetiology. Several structural abnormalities including bicuspid aortic valve, annulo-aortic ectasia and coarctation are risk factors. Aortic degeneration and cystic changes resulting in damage to the aortic media are associated with type A AAD. Genetic disorders include Marfan syndrome, Turner, Noonan and vascular Ehlers–Danlos. Past history of giant cell arteritis and other connective tissue disorders are also weakly associated with dissection. Cannulation of the aorta during cardiac surgery or coronary

artery catheterisation can also lead to an intimal tear and subsequent dissection. Other associations include pregnancy and infection.

8 Family history of aortic aneurysm or dissection raises the likelihood of a patient developing the disease. The term familial thoracic aortic aneurysm and dissection (familial TAAD) is used for significant family history but in the absence of any known connective tissue syndromes.

9 Use of tobacco, cocaine and amphetamines may also be associated with dissection.

10 Heavy lifting is associated with aortic dissection, particularly in young people, and is thought to be due to the significant increase in BP during this activity.

Examination

- On general inspection, the patient appears to be in pain and has clearly altered consciousness. He has no physical features of **connective tissue disorders** [1].
- Examination of the vital signs reveals the patient to be **tachycardic, tachypnoeic** [2] and **hypotensive** [3].
- His **pulse is absent in the right arm** [4] and there is a **significant blood pressure difference** [5]

(25mmHg) between the left and right arms.
- The **JVP** [6] is raised but there are no other changes in the **neck or face** [7].
- **Inspection of the chest** [8] is normal.
- However, a **diastolic murmur** [9] is heard in the aortic area on **auscultation** [10].
- The abdomen is **soft with no masses** [11].
- There are **no focal neurological deficits** [12].

1 Marfan syndrome, a defect in fibrillin synthesis, is significantly associated with aortic dissection and represents around 10% of dissections presenting under the age of 40. Around 30% of patients with Marfan syndrome develop aortic dissection. Features of Marfan syndrome include tall stature, long and thin fingers, pectus excavatum, hyper-flexible joints, high arched palate and a narrow face. Features of Ehlers–Danlos syndrome include changes to skin such as translucency, bruising and early ageing as well as changes to joints resulting in hyper-flexibility. In patients with the vascular type of Ehlers–Danlos syndrome, there is an increased risk of developing aneurysms, arterial dissections and pseudoaneurysms.

2 The patient may be tachycardic in an attempt to compensate for decreased end-organ tissue perfusion. However, a late sign may be bradycardia. Other signs of shock should be assessed, including cool and clammy peripheries as well as prolonged capillary refill. The respiratory rate may increase due to pain, distress or due to ischaemic tissue and subsequent metabolic acidosis with respiratory compensation. Oxygen saturation may be reduced due to general haemodynamic compromise. Temperature is unlikely to be increased.

3 Hypertension is commonly seen in type B dissections and type A AAD. Hypotension in these cases is associated with mechanical complications such as free rupture or tamponade. Cardiac tamponade is caused by blood/plasma leaking through the dissected adventitia.

4 A weak, delayed or absent pulse suggests blocked blood flow to peripheral vessels. This can result from a flap of intima blocking a vessel or compression from haematoma. The location of the pulse affected (carotid, brachial or femoral) can suggest location of the malperfusion syndrome. Malperfusion syndrome is associated with poor outcomes in general, including increased mortality.

5 A BP difference of >20mmHg is also associated with dissection. This is caused by the same mechanism as a weak or absent pulse.

6 The JVP may be raised. This could indicate cardiac tamponade or coronary dissection.

7 Expansion of the aorta can cause compression of the superior vena cava. This can cause dyspnoea, headache, facial swelling and cyanosis, distended neck veins and upper limb and neck oedema.

8 The chest should be inspected for signs of trauma, scars indicating previous chest surgery and central capillary refill. Asymmetrical chest expansion may indicate haemothorax. Palpation may reveal areas of tenderness in chest trauma. Percussion may be dull in haemothorax.

9 Aortic dissections, particularly of the ascending aorta, can spread proximally towards the heart to involve the aortic valve itself. This can cause acute aortic regurgitation caused by unseating of the aortic valve cusps, or dilation of the aorta resulting in an incomplete seal between the leaflets. Aortic regurgitation is heard as an early diastolic decrescendo murmur best heard at the upper right sternal border. It is also associated with hypotension and wide pulse pressure. It occurs in approximately half of dissections involving the ascending aorta. Aortic regurgitation can cause dyspnoea. Peripheral signs of aortic chronic regurgitation are not usually seen. These include Quincke's sign (pulsations seen after compression of the nail bed), de Musset's sign (bobbing of the head synchronised with each heartbeat) and Corrigan's pulse (a pulse that is bounding and forceful).

10 Auscultation can also allow assessment of tamponade. Cardiac tamponade will cause muffled heart sounds.

11 The abdomen should be assessed to determine signs of descending aorta involvement, particularly below the diaphragm. This may be felt as a large, pulsating and expanding mass in the abdomen. Signs of peritonism may indicate peritoneal bleeding.

12 Focal neurologic deficit results from involvement of branch arteries or extensive dissection where the aorta expands and compresses local structures. Stroke and altered consciousness can occur from either extension of the dissection into the carotids or low cardiac output. Horner's syndrome (ipsilateral ptosis, miosis and anhidrosis) is rare in AAD and is caused by stretching of the ansa subclavia. Hoarseness of the voice can occur from involvement of the left recurrent laryngeal nerve, as it runs around the aortic arch. Acute paraplegia is due to spinal cord ischaemia and more commonly occurs in dissections involving the descending aorta, due to the fact that it supplies the intercostal vessels.

Investigations

- The patient undergoes several investigations to determine the presence and **type of aortic dissection** [1]. These are conducted urgently from the ED.
- **ECG is normal** [2].
- **Laboratory studies** [3] show normal FBE, tests of kidney function show raised creatinine, D-dimer is positive, troponins are negative, and toxicology is negative.
- **Chest X-ray** [4] shows widening of the mediastinum.
- Aortic dissection is **strongly suspected** [5].
- **CT with contrast** [6] shows that the dissection is confined to the ascending aorta and also involves the brachiocephalic artery.
- **Other investigations are considered** [7].
- It is determined that he has an acute DeBakey type II (type A) dissection.
- **Transoesophageal echocardiogram** [8] in the operating theatre shows an ascending aortic dissection.
- There is associated **acute aortic regurgitation and dilation of the aortic root** [9].

1 There are two classification systems used to categorise aortic dissection. The DeBakey classification divides dissection into three types: type I involves ascending and descending, II involves only ascending and III involves only descending aorta. The Stanford classification, which is more commonly used, describes type A dissections as any involving the ascending aorta and arch (including descending aorta or not), whilst type B dissections involve only the descending aorta.

2 The ECG is usually normal in aortic dissection. If the ECG is normal, it suggests that the chest pain is not caused by an ACS. However, ECG can also show inferior ST elevation indicating right coronary dissection as well as any other type of ST segment elevation MI or when the dissection leads to myocardial ischaemia. This makes the test less helpful as it does not allow an ACS to be excluded. ECG may also show signs of pericarditis, evidenced by widespread ST segment elevation, or pericardial tamponade which is seen as low voltage and electrical alternans.

3 Laboratory tests may show a leucocytosis consistent with acute inflammatory processes of the aortic wall. Tests of kidney function may show creatinine elevation, indicating that the renal arteries are involved or that there is an acute kidney injury due to hypoperfusion. D-dimer is a test with very high sensitivity but low specificity. If it is negative, dissection is unlikely. Troponins may be elevated if the dissection causes ischaemia of the myocardium. Toxicology should be performed in those with acute aortic syndromes. Cross-match should be performed in anticipation for the need for whole blood transfusion.

4 CXR has the potential to show abnormalities associated with the aorta. These include mediastinal widening or changes in the aortic contour or knuckle. Widening of the mediastinum occurs most commonly in dissections involving the descending aorta. Other possible findings include pleural effusion and tracheal shift. CXR is least useful as a diagnostic test for ascending aorta dissections.

5 Although not specific, the triad most commonly associated with aortic dissection are sudden onset chest pain, variation in pulse (lack of proximal extremity or carotid) or blood pressure differential between the left and right arms, and mediastinal widening on chest radiograph.

6 CT is the most common modality used for diagnosing aortic dissection, as it is readily available in any ED. It has the advantage of producing images in a short time period. It has the ability to identify the aortic tear, re-entry points, affected branches and pericardial effusion. By doing so, it helps the surgeon to choose the best site for arterial cannulation and operative planning. CT can also differentiate other forms of acute aortic syndromes, such as intramural haematoma or penetrating atherosclerotic ulcers. Overall the sensitivity and specificity of CT in aortic dissection approach 100%. The use of contrast limits its use in patients with allergies or renal insufficiency. If timed appropriately, CT with contrast can also rule out PE. This makes it a useful test for acute chest pain with features of haemodynamic compromise.

7 MRI is increasing in use as an imaging technique for diseases of the thoracic vessels. Although MRI is not commonly used in the diagnosis of AAD, it is a good tool for long-term follow-up, as it does not use radiation. Contrast medium is not required although gadolinium can be used. The disadvantages of MRI include high cost, lack of availability and long time to complete. Additionally, MRI is not appropriate for patients in critical condition.

8 Transoesophageal echocardiography (TOE) is a useful and accurate diagnostic test for aortic dissection. TOE is not as readily available as CT, but it can be performed relatively quickly, even if the patient is in critical condition with low procedure-associated morbidity. TOE has sensitivity and specificity of >90% and approaching 100% for both ascending and descending aortic dissections. It can also be used to identify complications including pericardial effusion, tamponade, aortic regurgitation, coronary artery involvement, dilation of aortic root and ascending aorta as well as changes in ventricular function. In theatres it assists in identifying tamponade, positioning arterial cannulae (when a guidewire is used), assessing the aortic valve and weaning off cardiopulmonary bypass.

9 Echocardiography is also used to diagnose aortic regurgitation. Acute aortic regurgitation can be caused by aortic dissection or aortic valve endocarditis. Chronic aortic regurgitation is most often due to chronic aortic root dilation or bicuspid aortic valve. Echocardiography with colour Doppler shows the regurgitation of blood from the aorta back into the left ventricle. Echocardiography also allows assessment of left ventricular size as well as function during systole. However, these are typically normal in acute aortic regurgitation. Transoesophageal imaging is more accurate than transthoracic for diagnosis of aortic regurgitation.

Management

Immediate

Contact the **cardiothoracic surgery team** [1] immediately. Obtain **IV access** [2] and commence **medical therapy** [3]. Insert an **arterial line** [4], **intubate** [4] the patient and insert a **urinary catheter** [4]. Contact the blood bank for urgent blood grouping and cross-match. Take the patient urgently to the operating theatre and then discuss the **operation with family** [5].

Short-term

Perform urgent surgery [6] which includes

replacement of the diseased segment of aorta [7] with a Dacron graft and aortic valve repair or aortic root replacement, using cardiopulmonary bypass. Take the patient to the **ICU** [8] after the operation. Monitor closely for **acute renal failure** [9] and repeat **echocardiography and CT imaging** [10]. Discharge the patient when it is safe to do so.

Long-term

Discuss prevention measures of aortic dissection [11] and follow the patient up in the cardiothoracic outpatient clinic.

1 Given that management differs between ascending and descending dissections, early determination of dissection location is important. Type A aortic dissection is a cardiac surgical emergency due to the potential for rupture. It requires urgent consultation with a cardiothoracic surgery team. Type B dissections can often be treated with medical care rather than invasive intervention. However, in complicated type B dissections which include those with rupture, visceral or peripheral ischaemia, rapid expansion or persistent pain, urgent surgery can be also required. Type B dissections are most commonly managed by vascular surgeons through an endovascular approach. The natural history of acute type A dissections is approximately 50% mortality at 48 hours and 90% mortality at 1 year. In practical terms, currently type A AAD is approached via sternotomy and type B is for medical treatment or TEVAR.

2 Two large-bore IV cannulae should be placed if this has not already been done. Medical management is used acutely to control pain, decrease the likelihood of disease progression and optimise the patient as much as possible during surgery. Pain control may include IV opioids or PCA.

3 Management to reduce propagation of the dissection is termed 'anti-impulse therapy'. Anti-impulse therapy involves lowering the BP and decreasing LV contraction. Antihypertensive therapy is usually accomplished with IV beta blockers (if no contraindications). Blood pressure should be reduced without affecting mental status or urine output. The aim is a systolic BP around 100–120mmHg. Heart rate should be reduced to <60bpm. Once the heart rate is reduced, vasodilator therapy should be given. An IV infusion of vasodilator such as nitroprusside, which can be tightly titrated, is used.

4 Patients with AADs require blood pressure monitoring through an arterial line to allow frequent monitoring. Those who are haemodynamically unstable require intubation, particularly if imaging is required. A urinary catheter allows precise measurement of urinary output.

5 Consent should be obtained for urgent surgery, although it is not necessary if it is an emergency and the patient is unconscious. Most patients with dissection of the ascending aorta undergo emergency surgery. Reasons they may not include significant comorbidities, advanced age and patient refusal. Mortality of surgery for dissection of the ascending aorta is approximately 10–35%. The mortality of patients undergoing only medical management is approximately 50% in the first 48 hours, with only 20% surviving 2 weeks.

6 The goal of surgery is to exclude the entry and re-entry tears located in aortic root, ascending aorta and arch, re-establish flow into true lumen, and repair or replace the aortic valve. If required, coronary artery bypass is also performed. The technique itself involves establishing cardiopulmonary bypass, inspection of the aorta, managing disease associated with the aortic root or valve, replacing the diseased aorta with graft (typically Dacron) and then weaning cardiopulmonary bypass. Endovascular grafting can be used in selected patients with dissections involving the descending thoracic aorta as an attempt to avoid the need for future TEVAR.

7 This surgery is very complex with different surgical and circulatory support techniques, including cerebral and myocardial protection as its main points. As such,

the simplest technique will be described here. A median sternotomy is performed. Once cardiopulmonary bypass is established with femoral artery and right atrium cannulation, the body temperature is decreased to about 20°C for deep hypothermic circulatory arrest (DHCA). Then, the circulation is ceased for 10–20 minutes, the patient's blood is drained into the oxygenator and the ascending aorta is resected from the aortic valve to just proximal to the brachiocephalic trunk. A Dacron graft is anastomosed at this level with care to join both layers of the dissected aorta. The Dacron graft is then cannulated, de-aired and clamped proximal to the cannula. Circulation is resumed and the patient is rewarmed. During rewarming, the aortic valve is repaired (sometimes the aortic root is replaced – a graft with a valve is used and the coronary arteries are re-implanted to this graft) and the graft is anastomosed to the ascending aorta, just above the aortic valve. Once the temperature reaches 36–37°C, the patient is weaned off cardiopulmonary bypass. If the aortic arch is involved, the arch vessels may be anastomosed to the graft separately or together as a cuff. This typically involves a longer period of DHCA.

8 Postoperatively, hypertension must be controlled as it is associated with an increased risk of bleeding, re-dissection and rupture. Since the dissection may have affected branch vessel and organ perfusion, pulses and tests of organ function should be performed regularly. Any sign of malperfusion should be followed by immediate imaging and appropriate treatment. Control of hypertension can be achieved through beta blockers, CCBs and ACE inhibitors. Beta blockers have also been shown to reduce the rate of aortic dilatation, as well as being protective of aortic complications for those with Marfan syndrome.

9 There are several factors associated with impaired recovery from surgery. These include age over 70 years, haemodynamic compromise, renal failure, pulse changes, ischaemic ECG changes, prior acute MI, previous aortic valve replacement and neurologic impairment.

10 Patients who have had an aortic dissection also need monitoring for the development of aortic aneurysms. This is typically done through CT with contrast and allows assessment of the diameter of the aorta. Echocardiography should be performed in those who have had valve reconstruction. Periodic use of echocardiography and CT imaging is required after dissection repair. Lastly, patients should be counselled on avoiding heavy lifting as well as heart rates >100bpm. Cardiovascular risk factors should be assessed and managed.

11 Prevention for aortic dissection includes management of hypertension as well as other cardiovascular risk factors including smoking. Patients with either Marfan or Ehlers–Danlos syndrome should be monitored using echocardiography for aneurysm of the aortic root. This condition is associated with dissection.

CASE 11: Acoustic neuroma

History

- A **48-year-old** [1] **Asian** [2] female presents to the **ED** [3] with a 12-hour history of **sudden right-sided hearing loss** [4], **sensation of fullness** [5] in the right ear and **tinnitus** [6].
- She complains of **difficulty understanding speech** [7] and some mild **unsteadiness of gait** [8], but denies **vertigo** [9].
- She also denies **fever** [10], **otalgia** [11], **otorrhoea** [12], **trauma** [13], **facial numbness** [14], **facial weakness** [15], **morning headaches** [16], **nausea** [17], **vomiting** [17], **neck pain** [18], **photophobia** [18] or **recent URTI** [19].
- She has a past history of **recurrent otitis media** [20] requiring grommets in childhood; however, she denies past history of **ischaemic heart disease** [21], **neurofibromatosis** [22] or **multiple sclerosis** [23].

[1] The median age at diagnosis of acoustic neuroma is 50 years.

[2] Acoustic neuromas are more common in Asians, with an incidence of approximately 2.6 per 100 000 person years.

[3] Acoustic neuromas can present acutely to the ED or subacutely to the outpatient department. It is important to consider this diagnosis in any patient with sensorineural hearing loss.

[4] If hearing loss is present, most acoustic neuromas will present with gradual onset of hearing loss, with a median duration of up to 2 years. However, up to 20% of patients presenting with hearing loss will experience this suddenly, occurring instantly or over the course of several hours. This hearing loss may also occasionally resolve spontaneously; however, it is still important to conduct a full investigation despite the recovery of hearing. Overall, approximately 5% of patients presenting with an acoustic neuroma will describe sudden sensorineural hearing loss. Sudden sensorineural hearing loss as a condition is poorly understood and is mostly idiopathic in nature. There are multiple theories attempting to explain the phenomenon.

[5] Sensation of fullness is a common symptom that is associated with hearing loss. This may be due to conductive hearing loss (e.g. middle ear effusion) or sensorineural hearing loss (e.g. retrocochlear pathology).

[6] Tinnitus (ringing in the ear) is a very common symptom of many ear conditions. It is usually associated with hearing loss; however, it can occasionally be present without hearing loss. The presence of tinnitus may be indicative of an underlying pathology, but is commonly a diagnosis in itself (subjective idiopathic tinnitus).

[7] Difficulty understanding speech (poor speech discrimination) is a symptom indicating dysfunction of the cochlear nerve (retrocochlear dysfunction). In the setting of poor speech discrimination, the possibility of a retrocochlear pathology (e.g. acoustic neuroma, cerebellopontine angle meningioma) needs to be excluded.

[8] Often patients with acoustic neuroma may present with a mild balance disturbance (disequilibrium). This can be very minor, and often patients will not mention it, and thus it will only be elicited on careful, directed questioning.

[9] Vertigo (the hallucination of movement) is a much less common symptom of acoustic neuroma.

[10] Fever in the setting of hearing loss may be associated with an infective condition (e.g. acute otitis media, labyrinthitis, meningitis).

[11] Otalgia may indicate an infective or inflammatory process in the ear, such as acute otitis media.

[12] Otorrhoea may indicate an infective or inflammatory process in the ear, such as acute otitis externa, or acute otitis media with tympanic membrane perforation.

[13] Recent trauma (especially trauma to the temporal bone) may cause hearing loss due to a fracture of the temporal bone. If a fracture is suspected, this should be assessed with a temporal bone CT. Given the course of the facial nerve through the temporal bone, assessment of the facial nerve in a patient with temporal bone fracture is crucial.

[14] Facial numbness may indicate pathology in the peripheral cutaneous nerves; however, the possibility of trigeminal nerve pathology (e.g. trigeminal nerve compression, herpes zoster ophthalmicus) needs to be considered.

15 The facial muscles (except those of mastication – the pterygoids, masseter and temporalis) are controlled by the facial nerve (cranial nerve VII). Unilateral weakness of the face may indicate a lower motor neurone (facial nerve) pathology or an upper motor neurone (central) pathology (e.g. stroke). Presence of forehead sparing (i.e. intact occipitofrontalis movement) favours an upper motor neurone cause due to the bilateral neural supply of the temporal branch of the facial nerve.

16 Headaches (especially morning headaches) are a symptom of increased intracranial pressure (ICP). In this cause, a large acoustic neuroma causing mass effect and compression of the 4th ventricle may result in hydrocephalus, causing morning headaches.

17 Nausea and vomiting are also symptoms of increased ICP, along with morning headaches.

18 Neck pain and photophobia are signs of meningism, and are concerning for meningitis. Hearing loss can occur secondary to meningitis due to infection and ischaemia of the cochlear nerve fibres and hair cells. Alternatively, some causes of hearing loss (e.g. cholesteatoma, acute otitis media) may develop meningitis as a complication.

19 The most common theory of sudden sensorineural hearing loss (i.e. sensorineural hearing loss over <12 hours) is viral infection of the cochlea. Many patients presenting with sudden sensorineural hearing loss report a recent viral upper respiratory tract infection (URTI) within the past 30 days; however, a viral URTI as a cause is usually extremely difficult to prove, if not impossible.

20 Recurrent otitis media (especially with perforation or requiring grommets) is a risk factor for acquired cholesteatoma – a growth of keratinised skin cells within the middle ear. This can cause hearing loss through ossicular chain disruption or erosion. The imaging of choice for detecting cholesteatoma is CT or MRI.

21 Vascular ischaemia (of the cochlear blood supply) is another theory of sudden sensorineural hearing loss, and may explain the sudden onset nature and the increased prevalence of vasculopaths.

22 Neurofibromatosis 1 (NF1; also known as von Recklinghausen disease) and 2 (NF2) are genetic conditions characterised by the growth of nervous system tumours. NF1 often presents with cutaneous tumours, and has an increased risk of intracranial tumours such as acoustic neuromas and meningiomas. NF2 (central neurofibromatosis) is characterised by bilateral acoustic neuromas. Approximately 5% of acoustic neuromas will be related to neurofibromatosis 1 or 2, with the remaining 95% being unilateral and idiopathic.

23 Multiple sclerosis can present with any constellation of neurological symptoms, including hearing loss (affecting the cochlear nerve) and vertigo (affecting the vestibular nerve).

Examination

- The patient appears **comfortable** [1]. Vital signs are unremarkable.
- **Auscultation of the heart** [2] reveals normal heart sounds with no added sounds.
- **Auscultation of the lungs** [3] reveals normal vesicular breath sounds.
- Otoscopy reveals a normal external ear and auditory canal with no **vesicles** [4] and no **swelling/discharge** [5].
- The tympanic membrane is **translucent** [6] and **mobile** [7] on pneumatic otoscopy, with no **perforation** [6] or **retraction pockets** [8].
- The visible **middle ear structures** [9] appear normal.
- **Anterior rhinoscopy** [10] reveals no nasal masses.
- Cranial nerve (CN) examination is as follows:
  - **CN I** [11]: intact.
  - **CN II** [12]: normal visual fields and acuity in all quadrants. Normal colour vision.
  - **CN III, IV, VI** [13] normal extra-ocular movements, normal accommodation reflex, normal pupillary light reflex.
  - **CN V** [14]: mildly decreased sensation of right V1–V3, **right corneal reflex absent** [15], no atrophy of muscles of mastication. Left side normal.
  - **CN VII** [16]: no facial nerve weakness (House–Brackmann Scale grade 1)
  - **CN VIII** [17]: Weber lateralises to left, Left Rinne positive, Right Rinne positive. **Poor speech discrimination** [18]. **Head impulse test** [19] is normal. There is no appreciable **nystagmus** [20]. **Test of skew** [21] is negative.
  - **CN IX, X** [22]: normal palate movement. No uvular deviation.
  - **CN XI** [22]: no sternocleidomastoid (SCM) or trapezius deficit.
  - **CN XII** [22]: no tongue deviation or atrophy.
- **Upper and lower limb neurological examination** [23] is normal.
- There are no notable **stigmata of neuro-fibromatosis** [24] on examination of the body.

1 General inspection provides information regarding the patient's overall state of unwellness.

2 Auscultation of the heart is important to assess for potential cardiac abnormalities (e.g. valvular heart disease) that may pose a significant peri-operative risk. If abnormalities are discovered on cardiac examination, these should be investigated where pertinent to identify the cause (as they may impact on the patient's fitness for surgery, or they may need to be addressed prior to surgery).

3 Auscultation of the lungs is important to assess for evidence of pulmonary disease. It is also of particular importance peri-operatively, where any form of lung disease significantly affects peri-operative fitness.

4 Vesicles in the external auditory canal likely represent herpes zoster oticus. This is a varicella reactivation in the geniculate ganglion of the facial nerve, and can present with hearing loss along with facial numbness and weakness.

5 Swelling and discharge in the external ear usually indicate otitis externa. If hearing loss is present due to otitis externa alone, this should be conductive in nature, as the inflammation is limited to the external ear.

6 A translucent and mobile tympanic membrane indicates an aerated middle ear cleft with no effusion or other middle ear pathology.

7 A perforation in the tympanic membrane may cause conductive hearing loss. If present, it is important to characterise the type of perforation (e.g. central vs. marginal) and determine the cause.

8 Retraction pockets are indicative of negative middle ear pressure. This is usually due to Eustachian tube dysfunction or recurrent tympanic membrane trauma (e.g. perforations, grommets). Retraction pockets may be prone to accumulation of squamous cells and development of cholesteatoma.

9 Through a translucent tympanic membrane, several middle ear structures can be seen including the lateral process and manubrium of the malleus, the long process of the incus and the stapes. Pathology causing erosion in the middle ear (e.g. cholesteatoma) may disrupt these structures and may be visible through the tympanic membrane.

10 Anterior rhinoscopy is useful to exclude nasal masses which may be causing Eustachian tube obstruction and middle ear effusion.

11 The olfactory nerve is rarely affected, and thus rarely tested. If necessary, smelling salts such as coffee will suffice.

12 The optic nerve is rarely implicated in posterior cranial fossa tumours; however, it may be affected in systemic neurological processes such as multiple sclerosis or NF. Signs of early optic neuritis (red desaturation, foggy vision and reduced night vision) may be due to multiple sclerosis.

13 The oculomotor, trochlear and abducens nerves control the extraocular eye movements. A temporal bone pathology (e.g. cholesteatoma, petrous apicitis) may present with an abducens palsy due to the proximity of the abducens nerve passing by the petrous apex of the temporal bone.

14 The trigeminal nerve may be compressed by a cerebellopontine angle (CPA) tumour if large enough. This generally occurs at approximately 3cm in diameter, and may cause paraesthesia or hypaesthesia. If long-standing compression occurs, atrophy of the muscles of mastication may occur.

15 The afferent limb of the corneal reflex resides in the V1 division of the trigeminal nerve. Absence of the corneal reflex may indicate damage or compression of the trigeminal nerve.

16 Assessment of the facial nerve should be standardised using the House–Brackmann Scale (where 1 = normal, and 6 = complete loss of function). Weakness or loss of function of the facial nerve may occur early in acoustic neuroma due to the proximity of the facial nerve to the vestibulocochlear nerve in the internal acoustic canal. If facial nerve weakness is present, close attention should be paid towards the eyes' ability to close fully. If the eyelids are unable to fully oppose, the patient will be at risk of corneal ulceration and should be given preventive measures such as regular artificial tears and taping the eye closed at night.

17 Assessment of the 8th cranial nerve is divided into assessment of the cochlear nerve and assessment of the vestibular nerve. The mainstay of assessment of the cochlear nerve is tuning fork tests. In this situation, tuning fork tests are consistent with a right-sided sensorineural hearing loss.

18 Poor speech discrimination can be assessed at the bedside but is ideally assessed objectively during audiometry. It is a hallmark of retrocochlear pathology (as discussed above).

19 Head impulse test assesses the vestibulo-ocular reflex and is an indicator of vestibular function. It is performed by sharply rotating the patient's head whilst watching for a corrective saccade in the eyes. When abnormal, it can be helpful in differentiating peripheral vertigo (e.g. vestibular neuritis, acoustic neuroma) from central vertigo (e.g. posterior circulation stroke).

20 Nystagmus is a flickering/beating movement of the eye. The type of nystagmus can indicate the type of vertigo (e.g. central vs. peripheral) and if peripheral, can sometimes localise the nystagmus to a particular semicircular canal. Peripheral vertigo is generally unidirectional, whereas central vertigo is more commonly bidirectional.

21 Positive test of skew is a sign of a central neurological lesion (e.g. stroke, tumour) and is also known as dysconjugate gaze. Together with the head impulse test and the nystagmus test, these bedside tests form the HINTS exam (**H**ead **I**mpulse, **N**ystagmus, **T**est of **S**kew), a series of tests with a specificity of 96% for the presence of a central lesion.

22 Lower motor neurone dysfunction of the lower cranial nerves (IX, X, XI, XII) is collectively known as bulbar palsy, and often occurs together due to the proximity of these nerves when originating from the medulla. A large CPA tumour may cause compression into these nerves, or alternatively evidence of a bulbar palsy may indicate an alternative rarer cause (e.g. CN X neuroma).

23 Upper and lower limb neurological examination is a key component of any cranial nerve examination. Although an acoustic neuroma will generally not cause any upper or lower limb neurological deficits, if the tumour enlarges enough it may eventually cause compression onto the 4th ventricle, developing signs of hydrocephalus such as long tract signs (e.g. hyperreflexia, positive Babinski test, positive Hoffman test) and ataxia.

24 NF1 requires at least 2 out of 7 diagnostic criteria including ≥6 café au lait spots, axillary or inguinal freckles, ≥2 neurofibromas, optic nerve glioma, ≥2 Lisch nodules (on slit lamp examination), sphenoid dysplasia or a first-degree relative with NF1.

Investigations

- **FBE** [1] reports a normal Hb, normal white cell count and normal platelets. **UEC** [1] results demonstrate normal electrolytes and an estimated glomerular filtration rate (eGFR) of >90ml/min/1.73m^2.
- **Coagulation studies** [2] are within normal limits.
- **CT head with contrast** [3] demonstrates a 3cm CPA tumour with **widening of the right internal acoustic canal** [4].
- **MRI head** [5] reveals a right-sided 3cm tumour arising from the internal acoustic canal and **mushrooming into the right cerebellopontine angle** [6].
- **Pure tone audiometry** [7] reveals down-sloping right-sided hearing loss of 30dB with **no air–bone gap** [8]. The left side is normal.
- **Speech discrimination** [9] demonstrates a peak of 85% speech intelligibility with **reduced intelligibility at greater intensities** [10].
- **Vestibular function testing** [11] (caloric testing) shows a right-sided unilateral weakness of 30%.

1 FBE and urea, electrolytes and creatinine (UEC) are often considered baseline tests (especially in preoperative patients) as they effectively screen for many conditions (either acute or pre-existing) that may have an impact on the patient's presentation or potential management. It is important to ensure the patient is not anaemic, thrombocytopenic and does not have pre-existing renal impairment, all of which pose a potential peri-operative risk and need to be addressed prior to surgical intervention.

2 Abnormalities found on coagulation studies (along with platelet count) are important in any surgery with high intraoperative and postoperative bleeding risk, including intracranial surgery, and need to be addressed prior to surgery. An INR of <1.4 and platelets of >100 x 10^9/L is generally considered safe for surgery, although this will vary depending on surgeon, patient and type of operation.

3 CT and MRI together make up the initial diagnostic imaging studies for investigation of CPA tumours. Both modalities provide different crucial information. CT provides excellent information regarding the bony structures of the head and neck, including the temporal bone, middle ear cleft and ossicles. However, it is not well suited to detecting intracranial tumours (especially small tumours <1.5cm), and this aspect of imaging has largely been superseded by MRI. Despite this, CT is still necessary in surgical planning, where multiple approaches to a CPA tumour need to be considered to achieve the best outcome for the patient.

4 Widening of the internal acoustic canal is a characteristic finding of acoustic neuroma. This is due to the origin of the tumour from the vestibular nerve within the internal acoustic canal causing slow bony expansion. With further growth, the tumour eventually extends into the CPA, causing compressive symptoms onto surrounding structures.

5 MRI has excellent sensitivity and specificity for the detection of intracranial tumours, especially small intracanalicular tumours. MRI can also reliably differentiate between different types of posterior fossa masses, helping to dictate management and surgical approach.

6 The mushrooming appearance is a hallmark of an acoustic neuroma. This is because most acoustic neuromas originate from within the internal acoustic canal, as opposed to other CPA tumours (e.g. meningiomas, epidermoids).

7 Pure tone audiometry measures the severity and characterises the nature of hearing loss. A down-sloping or flat audiogram associated with sudden sensorineural hearing loss is a poor prognostic sign for recovery of hearing.

8 The absence of an air–bone gap on audiometry indicates a sensorineural hearing loss and implies pathology at the inner ear (cochlear) or cochlear nerve (retrocochlear).

9 Speech discrimination is measured through speech audiometry. A peak of 85% indicates that the patient can only understand 85% of one-syllable words regardless of intensity of sound. Reduced speech discrimination out of proportion to hearing loss is a hallmark of a retrocochlear pathology.

[10] The presence of rollover phenomenon (reduced speech discrimination at higher intensities) is also a sign of retrocochlear pathology; however, it is not particularly sensitive.

[11] Vestibular function testing includes a wide array of tests to assess the cause and severity of vestibular dysfunction. The caloric stimulation test is the most useful in assessment of acoustic neuroma. Cold and warm water is irrigated into the external auditory canal, causing involuntary nystagmus. The severities of left and right nystagmus are compared, and unilateral weakness >30% is indicative of an ipsilateral vestibular lesion.

Management

Immediate

Seek advice [1] from the ENT team. Counsel the patient [2] regarding the diagnosis and their options.

Short-term

Present the case at a base of skull MDT meeting [3] . Consider watchful waiting [4] and stereotactic radiation [5] . If surgery is indicated, consider the surgical approach [6] . After the surgery, auscultate the lungs [7] and examine the lower limbs [8] . Reassess the hearing [9] using bedside tests. Monitor for immediate postoperative complications [10] . The patient may be discharged [11] if the vitals remain stable and there are no signs of postoperative complications.

Long-term

Re-present the patient at the MDT meeting [12] . Follow up the patient in the outpatient clinic [13] regularly.

[1] Acoustic neuromas are managed by ENT surgeons in conjunction with neurosurgeons. As a highly specialised area of surgery, acoustic neuromas and other base of skull tumours will often be managed by a combined base of skull team including both ENT surgeons (otologists) and neurosurgeons.

[2] It is important to educate patients regarding their diagnosis, as the discovery of an intracranial tumour can be extremely stressful and many patients do not have prior understanding or knowledge of the condition. Acoustic neuromas are benign, often slow-growing tumours and can be actively managed (through surgery or radiotherapy) or serially monitored (with regular imaging and hearing assessment).

[3] Most CPA tumours and other base of skull tumours will be managed through the multidisciplinary approach with both ENT surgeons and neurosurgeons. This provides varied experience and a vast knowledge base to allow for the most appropriate management of the patient.

[4] Watchful waiting is a viable strategy for managing small tumours or in patients who may be deemed high surgical risk (due to difficult anatomical or surgical factors, e.g. high riding jugular bulb, or due to patient comorbidities increasing the risk of long surgery). Often this option will be chosen if the tumour is small and there is no appreciable functional deficit yet (e.g. no hearing loss, no vestibular dysfunction, etc.). Although the decision for surgical intervention is tailored

to the patient, a rapidly growing tumour (>2.5mm per year) often warrants active intervention.

[5] Radiation therapy is a viable alternative that has been used for patients with small tumours (<3cm) or with high surgical risk. Although some regimens can result in excellent tumour control rates (>95%), radiation therapy has a significantly higher overall risk of long-term complications including hearing loss, facial nerve palsy and tumour growth.

[6] If surgical resection is decided, then the surgical approach needs to be considered. When managing acoustic neuromas, there are several surgical approaches including translabyrinthine, retrosigmoid and middle fossa. Each has advantages and disadvantages and these should be discussed with the patient in order to select the best approach for the patient. Aspects to consider include whether hearing preservation is important, size of tumour, risk of complications and risk of facial nerve palsy.

[7] Posterior cranial fossa surgery is a long and intensive surgery, and postoperative medical complications are not uncommon, especially in the older population. HAP is a common and easily avoidable medical complication that, if present, should be detected and managed early.

[8] DVT is also an important complication, especially following long surgery. The calves should be inspected for swelling, redness and tenderness, and if there is suspicion of DVT, a calf ultrasound should be ordered.

9 If a hearing-preserving surgical approach is used, it is important to assess whether this was successful. This can easily be performed with bedside tuning fork testing, which should be compared with preoperative results, and formal audiometry results.

10 The potential postoperative complications will differ depending on the surgical approach taken. Complications to look out for include headache, venous sinus thrombosis, CSF leak, meningitis, facial nerve injury and corneal insensitivity (and possible corneal ulceration).

11 If the postoperative period goes without complication, most acoustic neuroma patients will be discharged from hospital within 5–7 days. This extended stay will allow for ample monitoring for postoperative complications.

12 Once the final histopathology results are published, the patient's case should be discussed again at an MDT meeting to decide on further course of action. Occasionally, the final diagnosis is unexpected (e.g. malignant tumour) and further intervention with radiotherapy may be required. However, in most cases, once resection has been performed no further intervention is required.

13 Follow-up is integral to all surgical patients, and in particular those who have had an invasive procedure or operation. The patient should be reassessed for any complications of inpatient management or surgery (e.g. wound infection, CSF leak, facial nerve injury). Formal reassessment of the hearing is usually performed at the same time as outpatient follow-up. This allows for a new baseline hearing to be established following surgery, and also assesses for complications such as hearing loss if hearing-preserving surgery was undertaken. Formal vestibular function reassessment is also necessary to establish a new baseline and assess for complications. Although resection of a benign acoustic neuroma is considered curative, recurrence is possible. This is often due to incomplete resection from difficult surgical exposure, intraoperative complications or regrowth from microscopic residual tumour. Thus, regular monitoring for recurrence is necessary. This is often done with regular MRI (usually 6-monthly or yearly) and clinical assessment. Due to the slow-growing nature of acoustic neuromas, extended follow-up of up to 10 years is often necessary.

CASE 12: Acute bacterial parotitis

History

- A **67-year-old** [1] **male** [2] presents with a 2-day history of left **cheek pain** [3] and **swelling** [4].
- He has associated **trismus** [5], and complains of a **foul taste in the mouth** [6].
- The pain is **worse on eating** [7].
- He denies any **right-sided symptoms** [8], **viral prodrome** [9], **weight loss or loss of appetite** [10], **night sweats** [11] or **dry eyes** [12].

- He has had a **recent elective right total hip replacement** [13] 4 weeks ago and has a past history of **type 2 diabetes mellitus** [14] (diet controlled), mild **chronic kidney disease** [15] and depression, for which he takes **citalopram** [16].
- He emigrated from **Myanmar** [17] to the UK 5 years ago.
- He denies **smoking or alcohol intake** [18].

[1] Parotitis most commonly occurs in the 40–70-year-old age group, although it can occur in all age groups.

[2] Parotitis has a slight male predilection, although Sjögren's syndrome (an autoimmune condition of glands), like other autoimmune conditions, has a strong female predisposition of 9:1.

[3] The parotid gland is a bilateral salivary gland (the largest of the three major salivary glands) located in the face anterior to the auditory canal and superficial to the masseter muscle. It produces predominantly serous saliva (as opposed to mucous saliva of the submandibular gland).

[4] Swelling in the parotid is a non-specific sign that must be interpreted within the clinical context. Although enlargement may indicate infection in the right context, there are many non-acute causes of parotidomegaly (e.g. alcoholism, inflammatory, tumour).

[5] Trismus is a common presenting symptom of parotitis due to inflammation of the adjacent muscles of mastication. However, trismus can also be present in severe deep neck space infections, and thus these conditions need to be ruled out before the trismus is presumed to be due to parotitis alone.

[6] Foul taste in the mouth often indicates purulent discharge into the mouth. This may arise from several locations (e.g. dental abscess, quinsy), and in this case, is likely from purulent discharge from Stensen's duct.

[7] Pain on eating is a common symptom of salivary gland infection, due to excretion of saliva causing irritation of the parotid gland. It can also occur in sialolithiasis due to obstruction causing postprandial salivary colic without infection.

[8] Bilateral parotitis secondary to bacterial infection is rare, and presence of bilateral parotitis should make the clinician suspicious for a viral cause (the classic cause being mumps due to paramyxovirus) or other systemic/inflammatory condition.

[9] Viral prodrome (myalgias, malaise, headache, etc.) may indicate a viral cause for parotitis. This includes mumps (paramyxovirus) Epstein–Barr virus (EBV), cytomegalovirus (CMV) and other upper respiratory tract viruses.

[10] Loss of weight and loss of appetite are non-specific symptoms, but may be concerning for malignancy. In patients presenting with facial pain and swelling, this may be due to malignancy in the parotid region (e.g. salivary gland malignancy), malignancy with spread to peri-parotid lymph nodes (e.g. cutaneous head and neck malignancy) or even lymphoma with enlarged peri-parotid lymph nodes.

[11] Loss of weight, night sweats and fevers are also characteristic features of TB, which should be considered as a differential for all patients from endemic countries. As the patient has recently emigrated from Myanmar, this possibility should be considered.

[12] Dry eyes and dry mouth (causing parotitis) are the hallmark symptoms of Sjögren's syndrome. Sjögren's syndrome may also have systemic symptoms such as arthralgias, thyroid problems and chronic cough.

[13] Studies have shown incidence of parotitis is higher in patients following surgery, and significantly higher in patients receiving major surgery (e.g. major joint replacement or abdominal surgery). This is due to dehydration in the acute postoperative setting, and is most common in the 2 weeks immediately post operation. In this setting, the patient's recent surgery likely plays a role in his dehydration causing parotitis.

14 Diabetes is a risk factor for developing parotitis (and other bacterial infections) due to immunodeficiency from poorly functioning white blood cells.

15 Chronic kidney injury is a known risk factor for parotitis. This may be due to altered salivary biochemistry (raised levels of calcium, phosphorus, urea, sodium and potassium) increasing the risk of sialolithiasis.

16 Whilst depression itself is not a risk factor for parotitis, medications with anticholinergic effects (including citalopram, a selective serotonin reuptake inhibitor (SSRI)) reduce saliva production, increasing the risk of parotitis and sialolithiasis.

17 Myanmar (a south-east Asian country), along with many other countries, is endemic with TB. Although TB is primarily a pulmonary disease, 20% of TB cases are extra-pulmonary, and they may occasionally present as enlarged lymph nodes in the head and neck region. Enlarged peri-parotid lymph nodes may be tender and can be mistaken for parotitis.

18 Although smoking and alcohol intake are not direct risk factors for parotitis, they are associated with poor dental hygiene (which is a risk factor for parotitis). Furthermore, they are a strong risk factor for head and neck mucosal malignancy, which may present with peri-parotid lymph node metastases.

Examination

- The patient appears in **discomfort** [1].
- There are **no signs of respiratory distress** [2].
- Vital signs reveal a heart rate of **110bpm** [3] and a temperature of **38.2°C** [4].
- **Skin turgor** [5] is reduced and **mucous membranes** [5] are dry. **Urine output** [5] is low.
- **Auscultation of the heart** [6] reveals normal heart sounds with no added sounds.
- **Auscultation of the lungs** [7] reveals normal vesicular breath sounds.
- **Examination of the hip** [8] is unremarkable, and the lower limbs **reveal no swelling or tenderness** [9].
- The left preauricular area is **tender to palpation** [10] with **warmth and induration** [11] of the overlying skin.

- On oral examination there is 3-finger trismus and **poor dental hygiene** [12].
- There are no lumps on **bimanual oral palpation** [13], but doing so results in **purulent discharge from Stensen's duct** [14].
- Cranial nerve examination demonstrates **normal facial nerve function bilaterally** [15].
- **Examination of the right face** [16] is unremarkable.
- There is no **palpable mass** [17] or **thrombophlebitis of the jugular vein** [18].
- There is no **discharge or erythema on examination of the ears** [19].

1 Extreme discomfort may be correlated with a particularly unwell patient. It also provides insight into the urgency of the problem.

2 Respiratory distress (e.g. stridor, accessory muscle use) may indicate a potential or partially obstructed airway. Whilst most presentations of parotitis do not threaten the airway, if there is extension into the deep neck spaces, obstruction is possible.

3 Tachycardia can be attributed to multiple aetiologies. In parotitis, when tachycardia is present it is usually secondary to infection or dehydration due to poor oral fluid intake. If due to dehydration, it is important to implement prompt fluid rehydration. In the setting of recent surgery (especially joint surgery), the possibility of occult pulmonary embolism (PE) needs to be considered, and if tachycardia does not resolve with simple fluid rehydration, this avenue should be investigated and ruled out.

4 Fevers are a feature of most infective processes (in particular bacterial). In this case, it is consistent with the diagnosis of parotitis.

5 Skin turgor, mucous membrane appearance and urine output are all indicators of overall fluid status. Dehydration is a common cause of parotitis due to the salivary stasis, leading to a retrograde bacteria migration in Stensen's duct or stone formation. Reduced urine output is a surrogate marker for reduced end organ perfusion, and if present, other markers of reduced end-organ perfusion should be examined for (e.g. reduced mental status, cool peripheries, capillary refill time, chest pain, lactate levels).

6 Auscultation of the heart is important to assess for potential cardiac abnormalities (e.g. valvular heart disease) that may pose a significant peri-operative risk.

7 All febrile patients should be thoroughly investigated for a source of sepsis. The commonest locations would be pulmonary and urinary. Auscultation of the lungs is an important part of assessing this, and also assesses for evidence of pulmonary disease which is of particular importance in smokers, where COPD is extremely common, which significantly affects peri-operative fitness.

8 In all recently postoperative patients, the possibility of postoperative complications related to the initial procedure should be at the forefront of the clinician's mind. For example, in this patient, common complications of hip surgery would be wound infection, joint infection or DVT.

9 Examination of the lower limbs is important in any postoperative patient to assess for DVT. This is particularly important following major lower limb joint surgery (e.g. hip or knee surgery).

10 Tenderness to palpation is the most common finding for parotitis. However, this is not specific to parotitis, as most other infective conditions will cause the same.

11 Warmth and induration indicate an inflammatory process is occurring. Again, this is not specific to parotitis.

12 Oral examination is important to assess for presence of deep neck space infection or abscess (either as a primary diagnosis or as a complication from the parotitis). Poor dental hygiene is a risk factor for parotitis, but also raises the possibility of a dental abscess with spread into the buccal or masticator space, which can present similarly with preauricular tenderness, swelling and induration.

13 Bimanual palpation aims to directly palpate the parotid gland. This allows the clinician to assess for lumps/collections but also to attempt to express saliva from Stensen's duct, adjacent to the 2nd upper molar.

14 Purulent discharge from Stensen's duct is essentially diagnostic of acute bacterial parotitis in the appropriate clinical context.

15 The facial nerve courses through, and is intimately related to the parotid gland. Its function (motor function to the face through its five terminal branches) should be thoroughly assessed in all parotid pathology. Loss of facial nerve function is rare in parotitis, and if present, should prompt the clinician to thoroughly investigate for another cause of facial nerve paralysis (e.g. parotid tumour causing mass effect, malignancy with perineural invasion, Bell's palsy). If no other cause is found, then the facial paralysis is presumed to be due to perineuritis; however, close monitoring and follow-up are required to ensure the facial nerve returns to full function soon after the infection has resolved.

16 Unilateral symptoms are more consistent with a bacterial cause for parotitis, whereas bilateral symptoms may indicate a viral or other systemic cause (e.g. autoimmune conditions, lymphoma).

17 The parotid gland is the most common location for salivary gland tumours.

18 Internal jugular vein thrombophlebitis (Lemierre's syndrome) is a rare and potentially fatal complication of many deep neck space infections. It usually presents with sore throat, fever and neck pain, and represents spread of infection to the internal jugular vein, resulting in possible distant infective thromboemboli, often to the lungs and joints. Lemierre's syndrome has a documented mortality rate of up to 10%.

19 Discharge or erythema of the ears may indicate spread of infection superiorly and possible erosion through the external auditory canal causing otitis externa.

Investigations

- FBE reports a moderately **raised WCC** [1].
- UEC results demonstrate a **mild hypernatraemia** [2], and an **eGFR of 45ml/min/1.73m^2** [3].
- **CRP is raised** [4].
- **Serum amylase is raised** [5].
- **Mumps, EBV and CMV serology** [6] are negative.
- **Rheumatoid factor, antinuclear antibody, anti-SSA and anti-SSB antibody** [7] tests are all negative.
- **Capillary blood glucose level (BGL)** [8] is 7.8mmol/L.
- **Serial mycobacterial sputum culture and QuantiFERON-TB Gold interferon gamma release assay** [9] are both negative.
- **Urine dipstick** [10] is normal. **CXR** [10] is normal.

- **Ultrasound** [11] of the left parotid gland reveals a **diffusely enlarged, hypoechoic and hyperaemic parotid gland** [12].
- A **2mm sialolith** [13] can be seen in the proximal Stensen's duct.
- There is no **parotid abscess** [14] or **mass** [15].
- **CT head and neck** [16] confirms an enlarged left parotid gland and sialolith with **contrast enhancement and adjacent fat stranding** [17].
- There is no cervical lymphadenopathy, **dental abscess** [18] or **deep neck space abscess** [19].
- Bacterial culture of the purulent discharge from Stensen's duct reveals a heavy growth of *Staphylococcus aureus* [20].

1 Infection and inflammation are common causes of an elevated white cell count (WCC). In this patient, the presence of parotitis is the likely cause.

2 Hypernatraemia may be consistent with a state of dehydration, which should be corrected with fluid rehydration. If the hypernatraemia does not correct following adequate fluid rehydration, other causes of hypernatraemia should be considered.

3 Low eGFR may be consistent with the patient's past history of chronic kidney injury, or this may be a superimposed acute kidney injury (possibly from dehydration). It is important to compare this eGFR to the patient's baseline.

4 CRP is an acute phase reactant that becomes elevated during inflammatory conditions. It is commonly raised in many infective conditions including parotitis.

5 Serum amylase (a digestive enzyme secreted in saliva) is raised in both parotitis and pancreatitis.

6 Mumps (paramyxovirus), EBV and CMV are all viral causes of parotitis. It is usually not necessary to investigate for these conditions unless there is clinical suspicion to do so (e.g. bilateral parotitis).

7 Rheumatoid factor, ANA, anti-SSA and anti-SSB antibodies are all investigations that are elevated in inflammatory autoimmune conditions. Whilst rheumatoid factor and ANA are relatively non-specific, anti-SSA and anti-SSB antibodies are often specific for Sjögren's syndrome (although they can be raised in other conditions, e.g. systemic lupus erythematosus (SLE)).

8 It is important to assess and monitor BGL in all diabetic patients regardless of cause for admission; diabetic patients are frequently susceptible to complications from the presenting condition (e.g. worsening of infection, spread to other structures) and also complications from diabetes itself (e.g. hypo- or hyperglycaemia). Strict glycaemic control is important to reduce these risks.

9 Mycobacterial sputum culture and the QuantiFERON-TB Gold interferon gamma release assay are tests for TB. These should be considered in all patients from endemic countries.

10 Urine dipstick and CXR are part of a standard screen for infection in all patients with infection and possible sepsis. As parotitis causing serious sepsis is uncommon, it is prudent to investigate patients for other sources of infection in order to rule out these more common sources.

11 Ultrasound of the parotid gland is generally well tolerated and provides good anatomical resolution of the parotid gland and its surrounding structures. When a stone is suspected, ultrasound has a sensitivity of up to 94% for detecting sialolithiasis, and can also detect collections that may require drainage, or unexpected tumours.

12 The classic appearance of parotitis on ultrasound is a diffusely enlarged, hypoechoic and hyperaemic gland.

13 Stones are the most common disorder of major salivary glands. Stones are most commonly formed in the submandibular gland, with the parotid gland being second most common. They are believed to be caused by dehydration and salivary stasis, leading to deposition of salts and formation of the stone. This can cause obstruction and eventual inflammation of the salivary gland. In the parotid gland, stones often form at the hilum or at the proximal duct, making these stones difficult to definitively manage with conservative measures alone.

14 Parotid abscesses are a complication of parotitis that does not improve with conservative management alone and requires surgical drainage.

15 Parotid tumours are relatively common, and are often found incidentally during imaging. They are the most common location for salivary gland tumours, comprising up to 70%. Although mostly benign (e.g. pleomorphic adenoma), the parotid gland can develop invasive malignancies such as adenoid cystic carcinoma and mucoepidermoid carcinoma (compared to the submandibular gland which is approximately 50:50 benign vs. malignant).

16 CT provides excellent anatomical resolution of the parotid and is also great for detecting sialolithiasis. It is often used as an alternative to ultrasound, and also provides information about deeper anatomical structures to rule out deep neck space abscesses or dental abscesses.

17 CT findings for parotitis include contrast enhancement (compared to the contralateral side) and fat stranding with loss of fat plane definition (an indication of inflammation). It is important to look for and rule out a parotid abscess, as the presence of this would usually necessitate surgery.

18 Dental abscesses in the buccal or masticator space may mimic parotitis; however, the management of these is very different. In most cases, tooth extraction is necessary, with the possibility of open drainage being required as well. Most dental abscesses should be managed by a maxillofacial surgery team or by the dental team in conjunction with ENT.

19 Deep neck space abscesses may result from extension of parotitis, or may be the primary issue. If present, these almost always require surgical drainage and immediate airway assessment and management.

20 Although obtaining cultures and Gram stain is not always necessary in parotitis, it can be helpful to guide antibiotic therapy in difficult to treat parotitis that is not responding well to empiric antibiotics. However, it is important to recognise that due to the location of the duct, culture samples may easily be contaminated with normal oral flora. The most common bacteria causing sialadenitis (salivary gland infection) are *Staphylococcus aureus* and less commonly anaerobic bacteria (e.g. *Fusobacterium* and *Peptostreptococcus*).

Management

Immediate

Assess the airway [1] and ensure there are no signs of respiratory distress. Obtain IV access and **administer IV antibiotics** [2] . **Administer IV rehydration** [3] . **Seek advice** [4] from the ENT team.

Short-term

Start the patient on **sialogogues** [5] and recommend **frequent massage of the gland** [6] . **Cease anticholinergics** [7] . **Provide oral analgesia and local heat application** [8] . If there is no improvement after 48 hours of IV antibiotics, consider **surgical intervention with incision and drainage** [9] . **The patient may be discharged once the infection is clinically improving and the vitals are stable** [10] . Antibiotics can be changed to **target the cultured organism** [11] .

Long-term

Follow up [12] the patient in the outpatient clinic. Assess for postoperative complications. Consider **sialoendoscopy** [13] or **superficial parotidectomy** [14] for definitive management of the parotid stone. Refer the patient for **dental review** [15] .

[1] Ensuring a patent airway is a particularly important step when assessing any patient with a head and neck condition, and the clinician should take deliberate note of the presence of any signs of respiratory distress and address them first and foremost.

[2] IV antibiotics are a common immediate management in many infective conditions. Studies have shown that in patients presenting with sepsis, overall mortality increases significantly for every hour after the first hour that IV antibiotics are not administered. Antibiotics should be targeted to the most common causative organisms; in the case of parotitis, the most appropriate empirical antibiotic is flucloxacillin (to treat *Staphylococcus aureus*).

[3] IV fluid replacement should be administered in all patients with parotitis, as dehydration is one of the main causes of parotitis. Adequate hydration is important to increase saliva production (acting to drain pus), and improve the acute renal failure that is likely due to dehydration.

[4] Parotitis is primarily an ENT surgery condition and usually requires admission to hospital. Management should be directed by the ENT team, including antibiotic therapy, performing an incision and drainage if necessary, and ensuring post-procedure management and follow-up.

[5] Sialogogues are agents that increase saliva production (e.g. lemon drops or orange wedges). This is a simple and easy treatment, with the increased salivary production acting to increase pus drainage. It is thus a mainstay of management in acute bacterial parotitis.

[6] Parotid massage also acts to increase pus drainage through manual expression.

[7] Anticholinergics should be ceased if possible (as these reduce saliva production, which increases the risk of parotitis) and alternative agents should be considered, especially in cases of recurrent acute parotitis.

[8] Analgesia is important in all painful conditions, and local heat application (with heat packs) is very effective at providing analgesic effect as well.

[9] Although surgical intervention is not usually necessary for simple parotitis, it should be considered if there is no significant improvement in the patient's clinical condition after 48–72 hours of IV antibiotic therapy. Before considering surgical intervention, repeat imaging should be obtained to assess whether a collection that can be drained is present. If present, an incision and drainage is recommended (with or without leaving a drain tube), with ongoing IV antibiotics until the patient demonstrates significant clinical improvement.

[10] Once the patient is afebrile and improving clinically, they may be discharged. Most simple cases of parotitis require 1–2 days in hospital, although if surgical management was required then this will be longer. If a postoperative surgical drain tube was placed (to prevent re-collection of pus), the drain should be removed (once 24-hour drainage is below an acceptable threshold) prior to discharge.

[11] Continuation of antibiotics (orally) to complete a full course is routine upon discharge for patients with bacterial parotitis. If an organism has successfully been cultured, antibiotic therapy can be targeted towards the organism's sensitivity.

[12] Follow-up aims to serve several purposes: ensuring the patient's acute illness has resolved, ensuring the patient has not suffered any late complication from the procedure (e.g. poor wound healing, re-collection of abscess, facial nerve injury), providing reassurance to the patient that the acute illness has resolved and finally, providing a management plan for possible future events.

13 Sialoendoscopy is a relatively new technique that involves inserting an endoscope though the cannulated papilla of a salivary gland (e.g. Stensen's duct). Stones can be visualised and removed with a wire basket, or if too big, may be fragmented with laser lithotripsy. This technique has significantly altered management of sialolithiasis through gland-preserving techniques, and has a success rate of 80–100%. Sialoendoscopy, however, is a treatment usually reserved for elective management and not recommended for acute management of stones, as the instrumentation and manipulation of acutely inflamed ducts may be complicated by high risk of stricture.

14 The parotid is anatomically divided into superficial and deep lobes separated by the facial nerve (functionally there is no division, as the entire parotid acts as a single gland). Superficial parotidectomy (removal of the superficial parotid) may occasionally still be necessary for management of large stones or stones that were not amenable to endoscopic treatment. Due to the intimacy of the facial nerve, the procedure is associated with a small risk of facial nerve injury, which may result in permanent facial nerve paresis. Thus, for the treatment of sialolithiasis, the procedure is usually only reserved for severe cases not managed by medical or endoscopic treatment.

15 Poor dental hygiene has been linked to many head and neck infections (including parotitis, deep neck space abscess and sinusitis). Thus when poor dentition is noted, dental referral should be recommended.

CASE 13: Acute otitis media

History

- A **4-year-old** [1] **Caucasian** [2] **boy** [3] presents with a 2-day history of right **ear pain** [4] and **hearing loss** [5].
- He has associated **sensation of blocked ear** [6] and has recently had **nasal congestion** [7], **clear nasal discharge** [7] and **sneezing** [7].
- He denies any **left-sided symptoms** [8], **tinnitus** [9], **vertigo** [10], **ear discharge** [11], **fevers** [12], **facial pain** [13], **diplopia** [14], **headaches** [15] or **neck stiffness** [15].

- The boy has a past history of successful **cleft palate surgery** [16] and **recurrent ear infections** [17].
- He attends **day care** [18] regularly.
- **Immunisations** [19] are up to date.
- His parents are **smokers** [20].
- There has not been any noticeable **speech or language delay** [21].

[1] The peak incidence for acute otitis media (AOM) occurs in the 6–18-month age group, and declines following that (with a small increase between 5 and 6 years of age). This is due to a number of factors including anatomy and immature immunology.

[2] Some racial minority groups (e.g. indigenous populations and children in developing countries) have a significantly increased risk of AOM (with some studies indicating a prevalence of >90%). For these at-risk groups, early active treatment (i.e. antibiotics) and intervention should be considered.

[3] Acute otitis media is slightly more prevalent in males than females.

[4] Ear pain (otalgia) is the best predictor of acute otitis media. It is also one of the features differentiating AOM from otitis media with effusion (OME). These two conditions, whilst thought of separately, probably constitute a spectrum of disease, with acute otitis media being characterised by acute onset of effusion in the middle ear accompanied by signs of inflammation (e.g. otalgia, irritability, fever, redness of the tympanic membrane). On the other hand, OME is characterised by the presence of middle ear effusion without features of inflammation.

[5] Hearing loss in acute otitis media is common, and most often is due to conductive hearing loss secondary to the middle ear effusion. This can be assessed using tuning forks and confirmed with audiology. Conductive hearing loss due to middle ear effusion in acute otitis media should be monitored until it has resolved.

[6] Sensation of blocked ear often occurs as a result of hearing loss and subsequent autophony (the sensation

of loud hearing of one's own voice). This is usually due to a conductive hearing loss (in the case of AOM, likely from middle ear effusion).

[7] In the case of AOM, a recent upper respiratory viral infection usually acts as a precedent, causing inflammatory oedema of the upper respiratory tract (the nose, nasopharynx and Eustachian tube). This inflammation causes obstruction of the Eustachian tube and subsequent loss of ventilation of the middle ear, which leads to accumulation of secretions into the middle ear.

[8] Although bilateral AOM can (and often does) occur, especially in at-risk patients, the presence of bilateral symptoms should prompt the clinician to be wary of systemic causes of otalgia (e.g. autoimmune conditions such as relapsing polychondritis, dermatitis, referred otalgia from dental or tonsillar pathology).

[9] Tinnitus is a non-specific symptom that usually occurs with hearing loss, and usually localises a pathology to the ear. Tinnitus often occurs following loud noise exposure (temporary hearing threshold shift), but can occur with any hearing loss.

[10] Vertigo can occur due to central (e.g. stroke, brainstem pathology) or peripheral causes (e.g. vestibular neuritis, benign paroxysmal positional vertigo, Ménière's disease). Peripheral causes of vertigo are all localised to the vestibular apparatus of the inner ear, which can be affected by inflammation or crystal formation.

[11] Otorrhoea is often an indication of an ongoing inflammatory process. Purulent otorrhoea is often due to bacterial otitis externa and is not necessarily a feature of otitis media, although it can occur following perforation of the

tympanic membrane due to raised middle ear pressure from middle ear effusion.

12 Fevers are not necessarily common following AOM. When present, they likely indicate a more severe course of disease (and the possible need for antibiotics).

13 Facial pain is also a non-specific symptom that may indicate a number of pathologies including acute bacterial rhinosinusitis or dental infection/abscess (with referred otalgia).

14 Acute diplopia (in particular horizontal diplopia secondary to abducens palsy) accompanied by fever and facial pain is extremely concerning for Gradenigo syndrome. Gradenigo syndrome (petrous apicitis) is a severe complication of otitis media characterised by inflammation of the petrous apex of the temporal bone, and can result in intracranial complications such as meningitis or cavernous sinus thrombosis. The horizontal diplopia is due to inflammation of the abducens nerve (CN VI) as it passes the petrous apex of the temporal bone on its way to the clivus.

15 Headaches and neck stiffness are signs of meningism, and when paired with AOM should alert the clinician to the possibility of intracranial complications (e.g. meningitis). Intracranial complications can be severe and life-threatening, and it is important to investigate thoroughly (usually with CT brain or MRI brain) and if present, treat with high dose and prolonged antibiotic therapy. The possibility of acute surgery (e.g. myringotomy or mastoidectomy) to reduce bacterial load should also be considered.

16 In children with cleft palate, the muscles and tendons that open the Eustachian tube (tensor palatini and levator palatini) have abnormal origins. This leads to a poorly functioning or non-functioning Eustachian tube, increasing the risk of AOM.

17 Recurrent AOM (defined as ≥3 episodes in 6 months or ≥4 episodes in 12 months) is common in childhood, and this usually resolves with age (often at 3–4 years of age). Recurrent acute otitis media is one of the most common reasons for tympanostomy tube insertion.

18 There is a discernible increase in the incidence of AOM in children of day care age due to the transmission of bacterial and viral pathogens in day care centres.

19 The impact of serious AOM has reduced following the introduction of pneumococcal vaccines into the routine immunisation schedule in the UK; however, AOM of other aetiology still presents a large burden on the health system.

20 Exposure to tobacco smoke (and other environmental pollutants) significantly increases the risk of AOM, although the pathogenesis is unclear.

21 Hearing is crucial for proper speech and language development in the child, and studies have shown lower speech and language skills in children with prolonged middle ear effusion.

Examination

- The patient appears in discomfort but is alert and oriented.
- He is **tugging on his right ear** [1].
- **Vital signs** [2] are age-appropriate. Temperature is 36.2°C.
- Examination of bilateral external ears is unremarkable, with no **pinna erythema** [3] or **swelling** [3].
- There is no postauricular/**mastoid tenderness** [4], **erythema** [4] or **swelling** [5] and the pinna is not **pushed forward** [5].
- On otoscopy, there is no **narrowing** [6] or **erythema** [7] of the external auditory canal, no **vesicles** [8], and no **purulent discharge** [9] or **fungal debris** [10].
- The right tympanic membrane is **opaque** [11],

white [11], **bulging** [12] and **erythematous** [13], with middle ear fluid visible behind the eardrum.
- There is mild **tympanosclerosis** [14], but no **perforation** [15] or **bullae** [16] in the tympanic membrane.
- On pneumatic otoscopy, the **right eardrum is immobile** [17].
- On **tuning fork testing** [18], **Weber lateralises to the right** [19], and **Rinne is negative on the right ear, and positive on the left** [20].
- On examination of the eyes, there is no **conjunctivitis** [21] or **ophthalmoplegia** [22].
- The **facial nerve** [23] is intact.
- There is no **neck stiffness** [24] or **photophobia** [24]. Orofacial examination shows scars consistent with past history of repaired cleft palate.

1 Tugging on the ear is an indicator of middle ear pain and is a classic sign of AOM. Although not always present, this sign can be useful to localise the problem in younger patients who often present with more systemic features, and who may not yet be able to verbalise the problem.

2 It is important to be aware that paediatric patients have different ranges of normal vital signs from adults. The Paediatric Early Warning Score (PEWS) outlines objective clinical manifestations that may indicate rapid deterioration in the younger patient. It has standardised ranges for different paediatric age groups, and may be accompanied by a visual tracking observations chart to easily identify trends.

3 Pinna erythema or swelling may indicate a number of infective conditions causing otalgia, such as pinna cellulitis, perichondritis or acute otitis externa.

4 Mastoid tenderness and erythema both indicate possible mastoiditis, an uncommon complication of otitis media where infection spreads into the mastoid process.

5 Mastoid swelling or protrusion of the pinna may be due to subperiosteal abscess of the mastoid process (where infection has eroded through the bone and into the skin).

6 Narrowing of the external auditory canal may be due to acute inflammation (e.g. acute otitis externa) or chronic conditions (e.g. exostoses).

7 The presence of erythema in the external auditory canal would usually indicate acute inflammation (likely from acute otitis externa); however, occasionally other pathologies are the cause (e.g. dermatitis, Ramsay Hunt syndrome).

8 Vesicles in the auditory canal are a sign of Ramsay Hunt syndrome (herpes zoster oticus – reactivation of the varicella zoster virus in the geniculate ganglion of the facial nerve). The other features of Ramsay Hunt syndrome are variable but include facial paralysis, ear pain and loss of taste on the anterior two-thirds of the tongue (via the chorda tympani).

9 Purulent discharge from the auditory canal may be due to acute otitis externa (infection of the external auditory canal) or due to AOM with tympanic membrane perforation.

10 Fungal debris from fungal otitis externa is most commonly seen in immunosuppressed patients (e.g. diabetics). Fungal otitis externa comprises approximately 10% of otitis externa (with the other 90% from bacterial infection), and classically presents with itchiness rather than pain.

11 The colour and opacity of the tympanic membrane provide clues to the pathology in the eardrum or in the middle ear. In the normal state, the tympanic membrane appears grey or pink. An opaque white or yellow eardrum may indicate purulent middle ear effusion. Amber or blue may indicate non-infected fluid (i.e. OME).

12 The position of the tympanic membrane can be described as retracted, neutral, full or bulging. A bulging tympanic membrane is a hallmark feature of AOM, and can be used to differentiate AOM from OME.

13 An erythematous or haemorrhagic eardrum may indicate inflammation of the eardrum; however, a hyperaemic eardrum is usually related to vasodilation from crying, fever or manipulation of the external auditory canal.

14 Tympanosclerosis (whitish plaques of calcium that form on the tympanic membrane) is indicative of previous injury or inflammation to the tympanic membrane. This may be from previous AOM, tympanostomy tube placement or previous perforation.

15 Perforation of the tympanic membrane is a common sequela of AOM, occurring in approximately 7% of cases. When present, the perforation will spontaneously heal >90% of the time. When perforation and purulent otorrhoea is persistent for >6 weeks, this is termed chronic suppurative otitis media.

16 Haemorrhagic bullae of the tympanic membrane indicate bullous myringitis (inflammation of the tympanic membrane). This occurs with AOM and is characterised by increased pain. However, the bacteriology, treatment and prognosis of bullous myringitis is the same as AOM without bullae.

17 Pneumatic otoscopy is the gold standard for detection of middle ear effusions. An immobile tympanic membrane is essentially diagnostic of a middle ear effusion; however, this does not differentiate whether the fluid is infected, and thus other clinical features (colour of fluid, the presence of pain or fever, etc.) are needed to differentiate AOM from OME. It is important to note that all bulging tympanic membranes are inherently immobile, thus pneumatic otoscopy is not warranted when a bulging eardrum is seen.

18 Tuning fork tests (Weber and Rinne tests) are useful screening tests to determine whether hearing loss is present. If hearing loss is present, Rinne and Weber tests are interpreted in combination to help differentiate conductive from sensorineural hearing loss. In this situation, this would be consistent with a conductive hearing loss in the right ear (likely due to the middle ear effusion and tympanic membrane perforation).

19 Weber test is performed by placing the tuning fork on the forehead and determining which side the tone lateralises to. This bypasses any conductive defect and assesses the inner ear function. A midline lateralisation is normal.

20 Rinne test compares air conduction of sound to bone conduction of sound and can be performed a variety of ways. A negative test (air conducting sound better than bone) is normal due to the sound amplification qualities of the middle ear.

21 Conjunctivitis of the ipsilateral eye with otitis media is known as conjunctivitis-otitis media syndrome. This occurs in up to 25% of patients presenting with conjunctivitis.

22 Ophthalmoplegia (particularly abducens palsy) is concerning for Gradenigo syndrome, as discussed above.

23 Facial nerve palsy is a rare complication of AOM and is presumably related to perineuritis of the nerve. If present, patients should be treated with antibiotics and corticosteroids, and the function of the facial nerve should be closely monitored until complete recovery. Alternatively, presence of facial nerve palsy may indicate Ramsay Hunt syndrome, and should prompt the clinician to look for vesicles in the external auditory canal.

24 Neck stiffness and photophobia might indicate meningitis or other intracranial complication (as discussed above).

Investigations

- FBE reports a moderately **raised WCC** [1].
- UEC is normal. **CRP is raised** [2].
- **CT of the head and neck** [3] demonstrates **fluid within the right middle ear** [4].
- The **mastoid air cells are opacified with fluid** [5] without signs of **coalescence** [6] or **abscess** [7].
- The **petrous apex** [8] is also well aerated.
- There is no **erosion of the tegmen tympani** [9] or **sigmoid sinus thrombosis** [10].

- **MRI head and neck** [11] reveals no meningitis or intracranial abscess.
- **Audiometry shows an air–bone gap of 15dB** [12] resulting in mild hearing loss in the right ear, with normal hearing in the left ear, and **tympanometry reveals a type B tympanogram** [13] (tympanometric width >350daPa).

1 Infection and inflammation are common causes of an elevated WCC. In this patient, the presence of AOM is the likely cause.

2 CRP is an acute phase reactant that becomes elevated during inflammatory conditions. It is commonly raised in many infective conditions including AOM.

3 Imaging is normally not indicated in cases of simple AOM, and any form of radiation should be strongly avoided in paediatric populations. Occasionally, however, imaging is necessary to investigate for potential complications. Where mastoiditis or other intratemporal complications of AOM are suspected, CT is the ideal modality due to its enhanced bony resolution and relatively wide availability.

4 Fluid in the middle ear on CT imaging is consistent with middle ear effusion, and thus some form of otitis media. However, as with detecting middle ear effusions on otoscopy, this needs to be interpreted with other findings on clinical assessment to diagnose AOM.

5 Fluid within the mastoid air cells is often seen on cross-sectional imaging. The presence of fluid alone in the mastoid air cells does not make a diagnosis of mastoiditis – there must be some indication of inflammation (e.g. erythema, tenderness, subperiosteal abscess).

6 Coalescence (the erosion of cell walls in the mastoid air cells), if present on imaging, represents a more aggressive form of mastoiditis.

7 The most common complication of mastoiditis is the subperiosteal abscess (caused by erosion of the lateral wall of the mastoid). Erosion and abscess formation can occur elsewhere less commonly, including erosion through the sigmoid plate (causing epidural abscess), erosion medially into the SCM (causing Bezold abscess) or erosion anteriorly into the digastric (causing Citelli abscess).

8 The petrous apex (a part of the temporal bone) is pneumatised in 30% of the population. When infected, this can lead to Gradenigo syndrome.

9 The tegmen tympani (the roof of the mastoid and middle ear cavity) is a thin plate of bone that separates the middle ear from the intracranial cavity. Erosion through this thin plate may result in intracranial abscess.

10 The sigmoid sinus drains the transverse sinus into the jugular bulb. It runs in close proximity to the middle ear and the mastoid air cells. Thrombosis can present with headache, nausea and vomiting, and variable neurological deficits.

11 When investigating for intracranial complications of AOM, MRI is the imaging modality of choice. It is excellent at detecting meningeal enhancement and intracranial abscesses.

12 Audiometry (hearing test) should be undertaken for all patients with hearing loss to provide an objective baseline and also to track changes over time. An air–bone gap (i.e. a difference in air and bone hearing threshold) of <30dB is expected from purely conductive hearing loss with no sensorineural component.

13 Tympanometry (measurement of sound compliance through the eardrum) is often conducted with audiometry.

Tympanometry gives insight into the flexibility of the eardrum and is graphed on a tympanogram. There are a number of characteristic shapes of tympanogram that correspond with different disease processes (e.g. type A – normal tympanogram). A type B tympanogram (with no identifiable peak compliance) is consistent with a middle ear effusion, and is the most common type of tympanogram seen in cases of otitis media.

Management

Immediate

Assess the severity of the patient [1] and consider inpatient vs. outpatient management. Initiate analgesia. **Consider observation for the first 48–72 hours** [2] . If the patient will be observed in the outpatient setting, ensure close **follow-up within 48–72 hours** [3] .

Short-term

If there is no improvement in symptoms after 48–72 hours (or the patient severity is deemed high), initiate **antibiotic therapy** [4] . If infection persists despite broad-spectrum antibiotics, consider **tympanocentesis** [5] and culture of middle ear fluid.

Rarely, more **invasive surgical intervention** [6] is required (e.g. mastoidectomy, drainage of intracranial abscess). **The patient may be discharged once the infection is clinically improving and the vitals are stable** [7] . **Antibiotics can be changed to target the cultured organism** [8] .

Long-term

Follow up [9] the patient in the outpatient clinic. **Repeat audiometry and tympanometry to ensure resolution** [10] . Consider insertion of **tympanostomy tubes** [11] (grommets). Consider **adenoidectomy** [12] .

[1] AOM is a condition that can most of the time be managed in the outpatient setting. Occasionally, patients will require inpatient management for IV antibiotics, and this usually occurs when complications are present (e.g. mastoiditis, intracranial abscesses) or in high risk patients (e.g. immunocompromised, extremes of ages).

[2] The majority (>90%) of uncomplicated AOM is self-limiting. For this reason, most guidelines would recommend a 48 to 72-hour period of watchful waiting prior to the initiation of antibiotic therapy. Occasionally, immediate commencement of oral antibiotics is recommended, and this usually occurs in high risk groups (e.g. <2 years of age, at-risk minorities, immunosuppressed patients) or in cases of severe infection (e.g. fevers, lethargy, severe pain).

[3] If the patient is to be observed in the outpatient setting, a follow-up appointment should be made after 48–72 hours, allowing the clinician to reassess the need for antibiotics.

[4] If antibiotic therapy is used to treat AOM, in most cases this will be with oral antibiotics in the outpatient setting. This most commonly occurs if symptoms are not improving after an initial observation period. Empirical antibiotic therapy should be targeted at the common causative agents (*Streptococcus pneumoniae* and *Haemophilus influenzae*) and thus amoxicillin is most often recommended as the first-line agent. In patients with severe disease or complications requiring inpatient treatment, IV antibiotics should be administered. Ampicillin is the empirical drug of choice (or ceftriaxone if penicillin-allergic).

[5] Tympanocentesis (needle aspiration of the middle ear effusion) or myringotomy (incision of the tympanic membrane to allow aspiration of middle ear fluid) is not commonly used to treat AOM. However, when complications are present, or when initial antibiotic therapy fails despite broad-spectrum antibiotics, this procedure is relatively easy to perform, safe and can help to reduce bacterial load and also provide a culture sample to direct antibiotic therapy.

[6] Rare complications such as coalescent mastoiditis not responding to IV antibiotic therapy or intracranial abscess requires invasive surgical procedure. The procedure required depends on the type of complication (e.g. mastoidectomy for coalescent mastoiditis), and further imaging of some form is almost always necessary. If intracranial complications are present, a neurosurgical unit must be consulted, and invasive intracranial operation may be required.

[7] Once the patient is afebrile and improving, they may be discharged from hospital. Most cases of AOM (and even mastoiditis) will resolve without surgical intervention. However, if surgical management was required then close postoperative monitoring will necessitate a longer in-hospital stay.

8 A 10-day course of antibiotic treatment is routine for AOM (if antibiotics are given). If tympanocentesis and culture of fluid demonstrates a bacterial growth, antibiotics can be targeted towards a specific organism.

9 Follow-up is integral to all surgical patients, and in particular those who have had an invasive procedure or operation. Follow-up aims to serve several purposes: ensuring the patient's acute illness has resolved and that they have not suffered any late complication from the procedure (e.g. poor wound healing, facial nerve injury), providing reassurance to the patient that the acute illness has resolved and finally, providing a management plan for possible future events.

10 If audiometry and tympanometry performed at the initial assessment detected abnormalities, they must be repeated upon resolution of the AOM to ensure return to normal. If return to normal does not occur following sufficient recovery from the acute illness, this should prompt the clinician to investigate for a possible underlying cause (e.g. cholesteatoma causing recurrent AOM and persistent conductive hearing loss).

11 Tympanostomy tubes (grommets) should be considered in children with recurrent AOM (defined as ≥3 episodes in 6 months or ≥4 episodes in 12 months) and in whom preventive and medical treatment have failed. The procedure is most commonly performed under general anaesthetic with an operating binocular microscope, and promotes ventilation of the middle ear and drainage through the tympanostomy tube. Most tympanostomy tubes are temporary (with extrusion times ranging from 3 months to permanent).

12 The adenoidal pad is located in the nasopharynx and can cause obstruction of the Eustachian tubes (increasing the risk of recurrent AOM). With age, the adenoids usually atrophy and do not pose any issues. Adenoidectomy (with or without tonsillectomy) has been shown to reduce rates of AOM in children. This procedure is reserved as a backup surgical procedure if the initial procedure (insertion of tympanostomy tubes) has failed, due to the associated morbidity (pain, bleeding).

CASE 14: Acute rhinosinusitis

History

- A 45-year-old male presents to the ED with a **10-day history** [1] of **facial pain** [2].
- He also complains of **nasal congestion** [3], **purulent nasal discharge** [4] and **loss of smell** [5] (anosmia).
- He reports that whilst his illness was initially mild, he has significantly **worsened over the past 2 days** [6], with **left periorbital oedema** [7] and **fevers** [8].

- He denies **neck stiffness** [9], **photophobia** [9], **epistaxis** [10], **diplopia** [11], **loss of visual acuity** [12] or **painful ophthalmoplegia** [13].
- He has a past history of **allergic rhinitis** [14] (hay fever) but otherwise no significant past medical history or family history.
- He has a **20 pack year smoking history** [15], and smokes 1 pack per day.

[1] Sinusitis can be acute or chronic in nature, and the clinical presentation and underlying pathologies are quite different. Generally, acute sinusitis results from an infective process (usually viral, but occasionally bacterial), and by definition lasts <3 months. On the other hand, chronic sinusitis is usually an inflammatory process, and by definition lasts >3 months.

[2] Facial pain is one of the diagnostic features of sinusitis (both acute and chronic) and is included in the diagnostic criteria for acute sinusitis (from the European Position Paper on Sinusitis).

[3] Nasal congestion (or nasal obstruction) is a hallmark feature of sinusitis, along with nasal discharge (either anteriorly or posteriorly – see below). According to the diagnostic criteria, at least one of these two symptoms must be present for a diagnosis of acute sinusitis to be given.

[4] Purulent nasal discharge (often described as green and malodorous) can be either anterior or posterior. The location may provide clues as to which sinus is affected (e.g. sinuses that drain to the middle meatus are more likely to cause anterior nasal discharge, whereas those that drain to the superior meatus are more likely to cause posterior nasal discharge). The presence of nasal discharge is one of two core criteria for making a diagnosis of acute sinusitis (see above).

[5] Loss of smell (anosmia) is another of the diagnostic features of sinusitis. A diagnosis of acute sinusitis can be made when there is acute onset (<3 months) of either nasal congestion or purulent nasal discharge, along with either facial pain/pressure or hyposmia/anosmia.

[6] Worsening of the illness after an initial mild period (known as 'double sickening') is a feature of acute bacterial sinusitis, and generally causes a more serious illness. The other features of acute bacterial sinusitis are purulent nasal discharge, fever, severe pain and raised inflammatory markers;

with ≥3 of these features present, a diagnosis of acute bacterial sinusitis can be made.

[7] Spread of infection into the orbital and periorbital tissues is one of the potentially serious complications of acute sinusitis. Any suggestion of orbital manifestations should be taken seriously, as infection can quickly cause long-term visual complications.

[8] Fevers are a feature of most infective processes (in particular bacterial). It is included as one of the diagnostic criteria for acute bacterial sinusitis (discussed above).

[9] Neck stiffness and photophobia together suggest the presence of meningism. In any patient this would be concerning for meningitis. This is particularly true of patients with sinusitis, as several of the paranasal sinuses form the skull base (anterior and posterior ethmoids, frontal sinus, sphenoid sinus) and are in extremely close proximity to meningeal layers. As with orbital complications, intracranial complications of sinusitis can be serious, and any suggestion of their presence should be investigated thoroughly.

[10] Epistaxis is a red flag when assessing patients with possible sinusitis. This is concerning for a friable bleeding mass, which may represent a sinonasal tumour. If causing obstruction of the natural ostia, it may also present with classic sinusitis symptoms (e.g. purulent nasal discharge, facial pain).

[11] Diplopia generally indicates some form of ophthalmoplegia (uncoordinated eye movements). In sinusitis, this may be due to orbital complications (e.g. orbital abscess or post-septal cellulitis) and should be taken seriously.

[12] Loss of visual acuity, like diplopia, raises concern for orbital complications of sinusitis. Alternatively, due to the anatomical proximity of the optic chiasm to the sphenoid sinus, sphenoid sinusitis or other sphenoid sinus-related

pathology can cause visual symptoms (e.g. pituitary mass compressing the optic chiasm, resulting in bitemporal hemianopia).

13 Painful ophthalmoplegia, along with other eye symptoms, is again concerning for orbital complications (e.g. orbital abscess, subperiosteal abscess).

14 Allergic rhinitis is a common condition affecting 10–20% of people, and is an IgE-mediated immune response towards

allergens, causing non-infectious rhinitis. Given the many overlapping symptoms (e.g. nasal congestion, discharge) this can be confused with sinusitis. However, allergic rhinitis usually has a history of symptoms in response to exposure to allergens and/or a seasonal pattern. Whether or not allergic rhinitis predisposes a patient to sinusitis is still a subject of debate.

15 There is some evidence to suggest smoking is a risk factor for developing acute sinusitis.

Examination

- The patient appears fatigued but is **alert and oriented** [1].
- Vital signs are unremarkable apart from a temperature of **38.2°C** [2].
- Auscultation of the heart reveals normal heart sounds with no added sounds. Auscultation of the lungs reveals normal vesicular breath sounds.
- Palpation of the sinuses reveals **left maxillary tenderness** [3].
- Anterior rhinoscopy reveals bilateral **mucosal oedema and erythema** [4], with **purulent nasal discharge arising from the middle meatus** [5].

- The **nasal septum is moderately deviated** [6] to the left with **grade 1 nasal polyposis bilaterally** [7].
- Examination of the eyes reveals left **periorbital swelling and erythema** [8].
- There is no **ophthalmoplegia, proptosis or loss of visual acuity** [9]. The globe itself appears normal on both sides. Flexible nasoendoscopy confirms the above anterior rhinoscopy findings, but otherwise is normal.
- There is no evidence of **laryngopharyngeal reflux** [10].

1 General inspection provides information regarding the patient's overall state of unwellness. Cognitive status is important, especially in patients with signs of meningism, as this may indicate an intracranial complication.

2 Fevers are a feature of most infective processes (in particular bacterial). It is included as one of the diagnostic criteria for acute bacterial sinusitis (discussed above).

3 Tenderness on palpation allows localisation of the sinus that is inflamed. Furthermore, the presence of tenderness often indicates more severe disease and the need for antibiotics to treat acute bacterial sinusitis.

4 Mucosal oedema and erythema are non-specific findings in all types of rhinitis and rhinosinusitis (both infectious and non-infectious). As the nasal and sinus mucosa is continuous, evidence of rhinitis is always a feature of sinusitis.

5 Purulent nasal discharge is an indicator of acute bacterial rhinosinusitis. Purulent drainage from the middle meatus indicates pathology originating from either the maxillary, frontal or anterior ethmoid sinuses (as these sinuses all drain into the middle meatus).

6 The presence of nasal septal deviation and other anatomical factors (e.g. Haller cells, choanal atresia, nasal polyps) have been associated with acute sinusitis. This is presumably due to the narrower anatomy of the

infundibulum allowing for easier obstruction due to congestion.

7 Nasal polyposis occurs as a result of ongoing inflammation within the sinonasal mucosa. This is usually secondary to chronic rhinitis or rhinosinusitis, but also predisposes patients to acute sinusitis.

8 Orbital complications are the most common complications of acute sinusitis and are associated with the ethmoid, maxillary and frontal sinuses in decreasing frequency. It is important during assessment to attempt to discern whether there is presence of orbital infection (post-septal cellulitis).

9 The presence of the following features is extremely concerning for orbital infection: ophthalmoplegia, proptosis or loss of visual acuity. If concerned, the advice of a specialist ophthalmologist should be sought to facilitate objective assessment of proptosis, orbital pressure, visual acuity and eye movements.

10 The link between laryngopharyngeal reflux and acute sinusitis is unclear; however, some studies have suggested a significant association.

Investigations

- **FBE** [1] reports a white cell count of 14.3 x 10⁹/L. UEC results demonstrate normal electrolytes and an eGFR of >90ml/min/1.73m².
- **CRP** [2] is 143mg/L.
- **Coagulation studies** [3] are within normal limits.
- **Urine dipstick is negative** [4]. **CXR is clear** [4].
- **CT sinuses and orbits** [5] reveals **opacification of the left maxillary sinus with air fluid level** [6], **mucosal thickening** [7] and **periodontal bone loss surrounding the 1st left upper molar** [8].
- There is no **double-density sign** [9].
- There is no other **bony destruction** [10] or **intracranial extension** [11].

- The moderate **nasal septal deviation** [12] is confirmed, and there is also a **left concha bullosa** [13]. The other sinuses are clear.
- There **is preseptal soft tissue swelling** [14] but no **post-septal soft tissue swelling** [15], **intra-orbital abscess** [15] or **cavernous sinus thrombosis** [15]. MRI confirms the mucosal thickening of the left maxillary sinus with fluid.
- There is no **fungal mass** [16] or **absent mucosal enhancement** [17].

---

1 Raised white cell count is consistent with inflammation/infection. This is consistent with sinusitis.

2 CRP is an acute phase reactant that rises with inflammation/infection. A raised CRP is more consistent with a bacterial infection such as acute bacterial sinusitis.

3 Coagulation studies should be considered in all potential operative candidates (and especially in those considered high risk for bleeding). An INR of <1.4 and platelets of >100 x 10⁹/L is generally considered safe for surgery, although this will vary depending on surgeon, patient and type of operation.

4 Urine dipstick and CXR are part of a standard screen for infection in all patients with infection and possible sepsis. As acute bacterial sinusitis causing serious sepsis is uncommon, it is prudent to investigate patients for other sources of infection in order to rule out these more common sources.

5 CT is the best first-line modality for imaging the sinuses, as X-ray does not provide adequate resolution or anatomical detail. However, CT findings alone are not diagnostic, as imaging findings can be seen in up to 40% of asymptomatic patients. Thus, any imaging findings should be interpreted with the clinical presentation.

6 On a CT sinus, the sinuses are normally well aerated. When inflammation occurs, this produces exudate (pus). Furthermore, whilst a normal sinus would usually drain the pus through normal mucociliary clearance, when inflamed this mechanism becomes ineffective. The end result is a build-up of purulent fluid in the sinus, causing opacification on the CT scan. It is important to note, however, that opacification may also be due to other pathologies (e.g. mucocele, tumours).

7 Mucosal thickening in the paranasal sinuses indicates inflammation (i.e. sinusitis).

8 Odontogenic sinusitis (sinusitis from dental origin) causes up to 20% of maxillary sinusitis. It can often result from

recent dental surgery (causing oroantral fistula) or be due to dental disease with apical periodontitis. The tooth of origin is most often the first or second molar. Odontogenic sinusitis should be suspected if there is unilateral maxillary sinusitis (especially for >12 weeks) or the patient has had recent dental surgery.

9 Double-density sign (hyperintense and hypointense material in the sinuses) indicates possible chronic fungal sinusitis. Fungal sinusitis does not respond well to medical treatment and usually requires surgical intervention.

10 Bony destruction is a poor prognostic sign if seen on CT; this indicates infection causing erosion of the bone and spread to other areas. The most common areas of spread for sinusitis are the orbits and intracranially.

11 Intracranial extension is the second most common complication of sinusitis (behind orbital complications).

12 Nasal septal deviation (if severe enough) is a risk factor for sinusitis. This is due to narrowing of the infundibulum that drains the anterior ethmoids, maxillary and frontal sinuses, increasing the risk of obstruction.

13 Presence of concha bullosa (aerated middle turbinate) is also a risk factor for sinusitis. The aerated bulky turbinate causes narrowing of the infundibulum (similar to with septal deviation), and thus affects the same sinuses (anterior ethmoids, maxillary and frontal).

14 Preseptal soft tissue swelling is caused by inflammation of the eyelid and conjunctiva (the tissues anterior to the orbital septum). It is consistent with a diagnosis of preseptal cellulitis. It can also be seen in dacrocystitis (infection of the lacrimal sac), facial cellulitis, or as a result of URTI). In the setting of concurrent sinusitis, this is likely a complication of the adjacent sinusitis spreading into the preseptal tissues. Clinically, there is usually no proptosis or restriction of eye movements.

15 Post-septal cellulitis/orbital cellulitis, intra-orbital abscess and cavernous sinus thrombosis are serious complications of sinusitis. These usually present with chemosis, proptosis, ocular pain and ophthalmoplegia with pain, and any suggestion of post-septal complications should necessitate imaging to confirm this (usually CT). This requires aggressive treatment with IV antibiotics and consideration of surgery to manage the source of infection. They are all classified under orbital complications of sinusitis and are graded according to the Chandler classification (Grade 1: preseptal cellulitis with normal visual acuity and extra-ocular eye movement; Grade 2: orbital cellulitis with diffuse orbital oedema; Grade 3: subperiosteal abscess; Grade 4: orbital abscess; Grade 5: cavernous sinus thrombosis).

16 MRI is usually not indicated in the investigation of straightforward sinusitis. However, it can be useful to differentiate acute bacterial sinusitis from fungal sinusitis (where it will demonstrate a fungal mass with low intensity on T2 phase). It is also useful to assess for intracranial complications when suspected.

17 Absent mucosal enhancement on contrast-enhanced MRI indicates mucosal necrosis. This most often occurs from acute invasive fungal sinusitis, a severe form of fungal sinusitis that occurs in immunocompromised patients (e.g. diabetics, patients on immunosuppressants).

Management

Immediate

Monitor vital signs [1] and perform **regular visual assessments** [2]. **Seek advice from the ENT team** [3]. **Seek advice from the ophthalmology team** [4]. **Seek advice from the dental team** [5].

Short-term

Administer **intranasal corticosteroids** [6]. Obtain IV access and consider administering **IV antibiotics** [7]. Consider **adjunct oral corticosteroids** [8]. Consider **nasal decongestants** [9]. If no improvement after 24–48 hours on IV antibiotics, **surgical drainage** [10] may be warranted. Postoperatively, continue to monitor the **vital signs and perform regular visual assessments** [11]. The patient may be discharged if the sinusitis and preseptal cellulitis is **clearly improving** [12] and the vitals remain stable.

Long-term

Follow up [13] the patient in the outpatient clinic and assess for postoperative complications.

1 Severe bacterial infections (e.g. severe acute bacterial sinusitis) can result in septic shock which may be reflected in the vital signs by a hypotension and tachycardia with warm peripheries. A patient with unstable vital signs or vital signs outside of normal limits warrants closer monitoring and swifter management.

2 Regular visual assessments (visual acuity, extra-ocular movement assessment) are crucial when orbital complications are present, as these may progress quickly and cause permanent vision loss or ophthalmoplegia. Any deterioration in visual assessments should be flagged to the treating team and the ophthalmologists.

3 Sinusitis is primarily an ENT condition. Initial management, including antibiotic choice, should be directed by their advice. The recommendation whether to admit a patient or not will also be guided by the ENT team.

4 The ophthalmology team should always be involved whenever an orbital complication is present. This allows for objective assessment of proptosis (using an exophthalmometer), orbital pressure (using a tonometer), visual acuity, colour vision and eye movements.

5 If odontogenic sinusitis is suspected or confirmed, dental treatment is necessary to manage or eliminate the source of infection. This may involve dental treatment or tooth extraction, and should be guided by the dental team in discussion with the ENT surgeons. If the dental source of infection is not managed, recurrent acute sinusitis or chronic sinusitis is likely to occur, as the source of infection has not been removed.

6 Intranasal corticosteroids work to reduce mucosal inflammation, allowing for increased drainage from the sinuses. They are generally well tolerated with very few side-effects. Intranasal corticosteroids are recommended for treatment in all cases of moderate or severe acute sinusitis, and this has been supported by several studies. Intranasal corticosteroids have been shown to be superior at improving symptoms when compared to antibiotics alone and placebo.

7 Antibiotics are generally only recommended for severe cases of acute sinusitis, as 80% of patients treated without antibiotics will improve within 2 weeks. Furthermore, the majority of cases of acute sinusitis are viral in origin, and thus will not respond to antibiotics. Current guidelines recommend considering antibiotics if there is suggestion of acute bacterial sinusitis with three of the following criteria: double sickening, fever, raised inflammatory markers, purulent nasal discharge or severe facial pain. Otherwise, antibiotics can be considered if a patient is not improving after 7 days of illness, or if there are complications of sinusitis present. Choice of antibiotics should be targeted towards the most common causative agents (*Streptococcus pneumoniae* and *Haemophilus influenzae*); oral amoxicillin or IV ceftriaxone represent good options.

8 There is poor evidence for oral corticosteroids in the treatment of acute sinusitis; however, when used as an adjunctive therapy with antibiotics, they may provide short-term symptom relief (e.g. headache, facial pain). Long-term steroid use has well documented and recognised side-effects, and thus should be avoided where possible.

9 Nasal decongestants (e.g. oxymetazoline) are often very effective at improving symptoms. They work by decreasing congestion and aim to improve sinus ventilation and drainage. Although there is theoretical benefit, most studies do not show a significant change in clinical course when nasal decongestants are used for treatment. Furthermore, long-term use of nasal decongestants can cause rebound nasal congestion (rhinitis medicamentosa), and thus most nasal decongestants have a recommended use of 3–5 days maximum.

10 Functional endoscopic sinus surgery (FESS) is a common procedure performed for difficult-to-treat chronic sinusitis.

It aims to widen the natural ostia of the sinuses to allow for easier drainage and aeration, and can be targeted specifically to the affected sinus. Although rarely required in acute sinusitis, indications for sinus surgery include sinusitis with orbital or intracranial complications that progress despite IV antibiotic therapy, or failure to improve despite IV antibiotics.

11 FESS is generally a very well tolerated surgery with low complications. When performed electively, most patients will be discharged the next day after surgery. In the acute setting, intraoperative complications (e.g. intraconal haematoma, breach of skull base) are more likely and thus postoperative monitoring should include assessing for progressive proptosis or change in cognition, as well as more general complications (e.g. epistaxis, pain).

12 Once clinical improvement is seen, the patient can be discharged with the expectation that oral antibiotics will continue to treat the residual infection.

13 Long-term follow-up is routine for all postoperative patients. Although FESS is usually well tolerated, a few delayed complications can occur (synechiae, hyposmia, epiphora or closure of natural ostia) which need to be assessed for in the clinic. Follow-up for patients following a FESS procedure usually entails a 2–3-week postoperative appointment and another appointment at the 3-month mark. If postoperative complications are present, further surgery may be warranted to manage these.

CASE 15: Epistaxis

History

- A **75-year-old** [1] male presents with 4-hour history of intractable **epistaxis** [2], initially **left-sided** [3] but now **bilateral** [4].
- He reports an **estimated blood loss** [5] of 500ml, and has some associated **light-headedness** [6] and **nausea but no vomiting** [7].
- He reports an **upper respiratory tract illness** [8] 1 week ago.
- He denies recent **facial trauma** [9], **digital nasal trauma** [10], **nasal obstruction** [11], **otalgia** [12], **hearing loss** [12], **dyspnoea** [13] or **chest pain** [13].

- He has a past history of **recurrent epistaxis** [14], **hypertension** [15] and atrial fibrillation for which he takes **warfarin** [16].
- He denies any **intranasal drug use** [17].
- He does not have any past history or family history of **hereditary haemorrhagic telangiectasia** [18] (HHT) or other **bleeding diathesis** [19] (e.g. haemophilia) and has never required **nasal surgery** [20] or **medical intervention** [21] for epistaxis.
- He tried **applying pressure to the nose** [22] several times with no effect.

1 Age is a risk factor for epistaxis and has a bimodal distribution, with peaks at the young (2–10 years) and old (50–80 years) ages.

2 Epistaxis (or nosebleed) is a common and easily treatable ENT condition. Due to the nasal cavity's abundant vascular supply, bleeding is common, and can occasionally be profuse. 90% of epistaxis is anterior, with the majority of these originating from Little's area (Kiesselbach's plexus) on the anterior septum. The other 10% of epistaxis are classified as posterior, and are usually more difficult to treat.

3 It is important to specify which side of the nasal cavity was initially bleeding, as it will guide the clinician toward the culprit side that is actively bleeding on assessment.

4 Bleeding from both nostrils is common; however, this is usually due to bleeding on one side (the left side) overflowing past the nasopharynx onto the contralateral nasal passage (the right side), or through a septal perforation. Occasionally, there may be active bleeding from bilateral nasal cavities, or a posterior epistaxis bleeding equally into both nasal passages.

5 Estimating blood loss is important in all bleeding conditions, as this will provide information on the rate of blood loss and also the potential relative hypovolaemia. This information is important to dictate the severity of the presentation, the pace at which management is implemented and escalated, and also to guide the amount and rate of fluid rehydration.

6 Light-headedness may indicate hypovolaemia resulting in hypotension, and needs to be investigated and addressed. Alternatively, it may be due to a vasovagal response to bleeding, which can be common.

7 Nausea and/or vomiting during epistaxis is often due to the patient swallowing large amounts of blood. Thus, the vomitus is usually blood-stained. Along the same lines, the patient may present with melaena several days later, often being confused for an acute upper GI bleed.

8 Recent upper respiratory tract illness is a risk factor for epistaxis, as it increases nasal mucosal dryness, and also increases the amount of trauma to the nasal lining (from constant wiping of the nose).

9 Facial trauma (in particular nasal trauma) is a relatively common cause of epistaxis in the younger age group. Whilst most non-traumatic epistaxis originates from Little's area, nasal trauma can cause bleeding from many areas. One of the most significant is bleeding from the anterior ethmoid artery (often due to fracture of the nasoethmoid complex) which presents as epistaxis originating from the nasal vault. Bleeding from the anterior ethmoid artery does not respond well to conservative management techniques, and thus often requires surgical intervention (anterior ethmoid artery ligation).

10 Digital nasal trauma is another risk factor for epistaxis, often from Little's area on the anterior septum where there is a very superficial confluence of several prominent arteries.

11 Nasal obstruction may indicate URTI (a risk factor for epistaxis) but rarely may imply an obstructive lesion or mass which is bleeding (e.g. juvenile nasopharyngeal angiofibroma, nasopharyngeal carcinoma).

12 Ipsilateral otalgia and hearing loss may relate to Eustachian tube blockage (causing ipsilateral middle ear effusion). When accompanied by ipsilateral nasal obstruction, this points to an obstructing mass in the nasopharynx, and is particularly concerning for nasopharyngeal carcinoma causing compression on the Eustachian tube.

13 Dyspnoea or chest pain in a bleeding patient is concerning for severe anaemia and resultant cardiac demand ischaemia. If present, a troponin and ECG should be performed promptly, and blood transfusion should be administered as soon as possible.

14 Recurrent epistaxis is common, and may reflect a simple predilection towards epistaxis, or may hint at a bleeding diathesis (such as HHT, haemophilia or von Willebrand disease – see below).

15 Hypertension is common in patients with epistaxis, due to vascular fragility from long-standing disease.

16 Warfarin (and other anticoagulants and antiplatelets) greatly increase the risk of epistaxis, especially with minimal trauma. It is important to ascertain the reason for anticoagulants/antiplatelets and whether this can be ceased (either in the short term or permanently), as continuing these will make managing the epistaxis significantly harder.

17 Intranasal drug use (e.g. cocaine) often irritates the sensitive lining of the nasal cavity, causing bleeding.

18 HHT is a rare genetic condition characterised by improperly developed blood vessels (telangiectasias).

These telangiectasias can occur anywhere, but often occur in mucous membranes, the lungs, liver and the brain. It is inherited in an autosomal dominant fashion and the telangiectasias often bleed spontaneously, causing frequent and heavy blood loss.

19 Haemophilia and other bleeding disorders (e.g. von Willebrand disease) increase a patient's risk of bleeding, worsen the severity of bleeding and also make bleeding more resistant to intervention. Whilst epistaxis is usually easily managed, epistaxis in a bleeding disorder patient can become extremely difficult and complicated.

20 Recent nasal surgery increases the risk of bleeding, and often results in bleeding that is difficult to manage due to the location of bleeding. Often this requires re-intervention to stop the bleeding, and this comes at the risk of altering the outcomes of the original surgery.

21 It is important to know if a patient has required invasive medical intervention in the past to manage epistaxis, as this serves as a guideline to roughly how difficult the epistaxis is to treat, and what treatment path to take.

22 Many patients have erroneous ideas as to how to apply nasal pressure to manage epistaxis. Ascertaining whether the patient utilised effective epistaxis first aid may alter whether it is attempted again in the hospital setting or whether to move on to the next, more invasive measure.

Examination

- The patient appears **pale and lethargic** [1] but is still **alert and oriented** [2] .
- There are **no signs of respiratory distress** [3] .
- Vital signs reveal an irregularly irregular heart rate of **130bpm** [4] and a blood pressure of **90/60mmHg** [5] .
- **Skin turgor** [6] is reduced, **mucous membranes** [6] are dry and he has **not passed urine** [6] for the past 6 hours.
- A **bladder scan** [7] reveals 60ml of urine in the bladder.
- **Auscultation of the heart** [8] reveals normal heart sounds with no added sounds. Auscultation of the lungs reveals normal vesicular breath sounds.
- The left nostril is bleeding **profusely** [9] , with some blood from the right nostril.

- On **anterior rhinoscopy** [10] , the bleeding seems to be originating from the anterior septum at Little's area.
- On **oral examination** [11] , there is active bleeding into the oropharynx. The rest of the oral examination is normal.
- Examination of the external ear is normal. Otoscopy demonstrates a normal external auditory canal and a normal **tympanic membrane** [12] .
- **Flexible nasoendoscopy** [13] cannot be performed due to the amount of bleeding.
- Further examination shows **pallor of the palmar creases and conjunctiva** [14] .

1 General inspection provides information regarding the patient's overall state of unwellness. In the bleeding patient, pallor indicates a potentially significant amount of blood loss has already occurred. Furthermore, the accompanying lethargy implies a moderate level of severity already, warranting speedy resuscitation and management of the problem.

2 Alertness and orientation are important to take note of. If a patient is drowsy and confused, this may be an indicator of hypovolaemic shock and subsequent under-perfusion of end organs.

3 Respiratory distress (e.g. stridor, accessory muscle use) may indicate a potential or partially obstructed airway. Whilst most presentations of epistaxis do not threaten the airway, if there is a significant rate and amount of bleeding, it can occur either due to direct obstruction of the airway, or due to significant hypovolaemic shock and subsequent reduced conscious state. Thus, it is important to address this issue immediately, prior to addressing the epistaxis, in order to prevent an airway emergency situation.

4 Tachycardia can be attributed to multiple aetiologies; however, in epistaxis the majority of cases will be due to hypovolaemia. In the setting of acute blood loss, the central tenet is that "blood should be replaced with blood" – acute blood loss of any cause should prompt the strong consideration of blood transfusion (especially is there is profuse active bleeding, pre-existing cardiac comorbidities or pre-existing anaemia).

5 Hypotension may be subsequent to severe hypovolaemia, which generally presents with cool pale peripheries. Identifying this and implementing timely management (e.g. fluid rehydration, blood transfusion) is crucial.

6 Skin turgor, mucous membrane appearance and urine output are all indicators of overall fluid status. A normal urine output is generally accepted as 30ml/hour or 0.5ml/kg/hour. Epistaxis may lead to excessive blood loss and hypovolaemia, causing reduced end-organ perfusion. Reduced urine output is a surrogate marker for reduced end-organ perfusion, and if present, other markers of reduced end-organ perfusion should be examined for (e.g. reduced mental status, cool peripheries, capillary refill time, chest pain, lactate levels).

7 Poor urine output may be due to poor urine production (oliguria/anuria), of which severe hypovolaemia is of particular concern in epistaxis, or it may be due to urinary retention (e.g. due to obstruction). Bladder scan is a simple bedside ultrasound test that can approximate the volume of urine in the bladder and can be used to differentiate between the two (e.g. in this case, the urine output is 60ml over 6 hours, or 10ml/hour – clearly oliguric).

8 Hypovolaemia causes cardiac stress by reducing stroke volume, thus causing a reflexive increase in heart rate to maintain cardiac output. If the patient has a pre-existing heart condition (e.g. valvular heart disease, congestive cardiac failure), this may precipitate cardiac failure. Auscultation of the heart is important to ascertain whether there may be an element of structural heart abnormality. Furthermore, it is an important part of the surgical work-up to assess for operative fitness, and incidental findings on a routine preoperative cardiac examination warrant further investigation.

9 It is important to attempt to quantify the rate at which the bleeding is occurring – a stream of blood from the nose needs to be addressed much more rapidly than a slow trickle.

10 Proper anterior rhinoscopy of both nasal cavities is the crux of a good epistaxis assessment. It is important to actively inspect all elements of the nasal cavity that can be viewed, including turbinates, nasal vault, nasal septum and nasal floor. If bleeding is visualised, it is important to document specifically from which of these elements there is bleeding. If the source of bleeding cannot be visualised, this is equally important to document, as this indicates that the bleeding is by definition posterior in nature.

11 Active streaming of blood into the oral cavity is common but also important to assess. Often, the bleeding from the nose seems to have ceased; however, it is only bleeding posteriorly into the nasopharynx instead (with the patient swallowing the blood). The epistaxis can only be said to have stopped when there is no further blood loss from the nose or into the oropharynx.

12 Otoscopic examination of the tympanic membrane may be indicated if the patient is complaining of otalgia or hearing loss, as this may represent a bleeding mass in the nasopharynx causing obstruction of the Eustachian tube and subsequent middle ear effusion. Such masses include juvenile nasopharyngeal angiofibroma (a highly vascular tumour almost exclusive to adolescent males) or nasopharyngeal carcinoma.

13 Flexible nasoendoscopy can sometimes be useful to assess posterior bleeding that is not visualised on anterior rhinoscopy. However, often in practice the bleeding is too rapid to provide an adequate view and is not useful.

14 Pallor of the palmar creases and pallor of the conjunctiva are both signs of anaemia.

Investigations

- **ECG** [1] is consistent with the patient's known atrial fibrillation.
- FBE reports a **Hb of 89g/L** [2] , and **platelets** [3] are normal.
- UEC results demonstrate an **eGFR of 45ml/min/1.73m^2** [4] .

- On coagulation studies the **INR is 3.0** [5] .
- **LFTs and liver ultrasound** [6] are normal.
- A **blood group and hold** [7] is taken.
- **CT of the head and neck with angiogram** [8] reveals active contrast extravasation in the left anterior nasal septum and no masses.

1 A baseline ECG is necessary in any patient with known long-standing arrhythmia (e.g. atrial fibrillation) to confirm the arrhythmia and to assess for any other complications (e.g. demand ischaemia due to hypovolaemia). This is also an important preoperative investigation, especially in the elderly.

2 Haemoglobin count is important to assess in every patient with active bleeding. Anaemia due to active blood loss should be corrected, particularly in the preoperative patient, or those at increased risk of cardiac complications due to pre-existing cardiac comorbidities (e.g. history of ischaemic heart disease). It is also important to realise that in very acute blood loss, the Hb may not be low, as the intravascular Hb concentration is unchanged. Thus, in a patient with large volume losses, strong consideration of transfusion should be made even with a normal Hb, as this is likely to fall over the coming hours, especially with IV fluid resuscitation.

3 Platelets are essential to activating the clotting pathway, the body's natural mechanism for arresting bleeding. If the patient is thrombocytopenic (due to pre-existing or acute haematological conditions), they are at increased risk of developing spontaneous bleeding, and this bleeding is usually significantly harder to arrest. In these situations, the cause of thrombocytopenia needs to be considered, as well as how to improve the platelet count (e.g. through platelet transfusions) and thus improve the patient's self-clotting ability.

4 eGFR is an estimate of renal function, and in this situation is likely reduced in the setting of an acute kidney injury secondary to hypovolaemia and shock. The acute kidney injury needs to be addressed (usually with IV fluid rehydration) to prevent long-term kidney damage.

5 Warfarin is a common medication for treatment of atrial fibrillation and other disorders where development of a thrombus is likely and is usually measured using the INR. Although prescribed as a treatment for atrial fibrillation, it greatly increases the risk of bleeding and makes managing this bleeding much harder. When managing a bleeding patient on anticoagulation, consideration needs to be given to the reason for anticoagulation and the severity of the bleeding. An active decision bearing these factors in mind needs to be made whether to continue the medication or cease it (and/or possibly reverse it).

6 The proteins necessary for the clotting pathway all originate from the liver – thus patients with reduced synthetic liver function often have raised INR and subsequent bleeding diathesis. In a patient with a raised INR of unknown cause, liver cirrhosis should be investigated and ruled out.

7 Blood group and hold is an essential investigation for all bleeding patients, and should be taken as soon as possible, in case transfusion is necessary. Whilst it is ideal to cross-match blood as well prior to transfusion (to reduce as much transfusion reaction risk as possible), in an extreme emergency, packed red blood cells with type O negative can be given.

8 CT of the head and neck +/– angiogram is in most cases not necessary when dealing with simple epistaxis. However, if a mass is visualised or expected based on the history, it may help investigate the cause prior to biopsy (which may precipitate massive haemorrhage in juvenile nasopharyngeal angiofibroma).

Management

Immediate

Assess the airway [1] and ensure there are no signs of respiratory distress. Obtain IV access. Consider the need for **blood transfusion** [2] . Monitor **vital signs** [3] and **urine output** [4] . Administer **topical vasoconstrictors** [5] (e.g. phenylephrine spray) or IV **tranexamic acid** [6] . Determine whether the bleeding is anterior or posterior in nature. Initiate **epistaxis first aid** [7] . If the bleeding point is visible, attempt **nasal cautery** [8] . **Withhold or reverse anticoagulants and antiplatelets** [9] if possible. **Seek advice** [10] from the ENT team.

Short-term

If epistaxis first aid and nasal cautery fail, move on to **nasal packing** [11]. Consider the need for **contralateral nasal cavity packing** [12] or **posterior nasal packing** [12] as well. If ongoing bleeding occurs despite this, plan for surgical intervention with **examination under anaesthesia (EUA), nasal cautery and/or sphenopalatine artery ligation** [13]. If surgical intervention fails, refer the patient for **percutaneous angioembolisation** [14].

Long-term

Once bleeding has ceased, advise patient to **maintain a cool diet, avoid nose blowing and sleep upright** [15]. Cautiously **reinstate anticoagulants or antiplatelets** [16]. The patient may be discharged if they have recommenced all of their regular medications and have not had any **further epistaxis** [17] for a reasonable amount of time (12–24 hours is standard). Follow the patient up in an **outpatient clinic** [18].

1 Ensuring a patent airway is the first step when assessing all patients. It is a particularly important step when assessing any patient with a head and neck condition, and the clinician should take deliberate note of the presence of any signs of respiratory distress and address them first and foremost.

2 Blood transfusion should be considered in all patients with acute blood loss (especially those with large volume loss). This decision should be clinically based, and not dependent on the Hb count (which may not reflect the acute hypovolaemia due to blood loss). If time is critical, O negative blood can be given instead of type-matched blood.

3 Blood loss in epistaxis can be massive, especially in patients with a bleeding tendency (either congenital or medication-induced, e.g. warfarin), and severe bleeding can result in hypovolaemic shock which may be reflected in the vital signs by a hypotension, tachycardia and cool, shut-down peripheries. A patient with unstable vital signs or vital signs outside of normal limits warrants closer monitoring and swifter management.

4 Urine output is a good indicator of overall fluid status. Low urine output in epistaxis usually reflects acute dehydration and end-organ hypoperfusion.

5 Topical vasoconstrictors (e.g. phenylephrine spray) act locally to reduce bleeding. These are often combined with topical anaesthetic agents to ease pain/discomfort on examination and increase patient compliance (particularly with flexible nasoendoscopy). Most EDs and ENT teams will have this readily available for administration.

6 Tranexamic acid is an antifibrinolytic agent that can be administered topically (to the nose), orally or intravenously. It is often used to prevent and reduce blood loss and has been shown to reduce death due to bleeding. It is usually well tolerated, and side-effects are rare.

7 Epistaxis first aid consists of several simple-to-implement measures that, when used properly, are very effective at managing epistaxis without resorting to invasive intervention. The measures include: sitting upright, leaning forward, applying constant pressure with the finger and thumb to the soft part of the nostrils (not the bridge) for a minimum of 10 minutes without releasing, ice to suck on, cool pack to the back of the neck. These measures combined work to reduce blood flow and blood pressure in the nose, and encourage coagulation within the bleeding artery, and are effective in 65–70% of epistaxis cases.

8 In cases where epistaxis first aid fails, the next step is usually to attempt nasal cautery with silver nitrate. Nasal cautery can only be attempted when the location of bleeding can be directly visualised and thus by definition, can only be used for anterior bleeds. When implemented correctly, nasal cautery has a documented success rate of up to 80%. In the case of bilateral epistaxis, caution should always be taken to never cauterise the same or close-by areas on each side of the septum. As the cartilaginous nasal septum receives its blood supply from the overlying mucosa, cautery to both sides of the septum at similar locations may cut off blood to this area, possibly causing ischaemic necrosis and eventually a septal perforation.

9 Epistaxis due to anticoagulation and antiplatelet agents is extremely common, especially in the elderly (where epistaxis is more common and anticoagulant or antiplatelet agents are more common). Although most epistaxis can be managed without resorting to withholding or reversing these agents, occasionally this may be difficult or impossible, and in these cases, the benefits of ceasing anticoagulation need to be considered (in the short and long term). Requiring reversal of anticoagulation to manage epistaxis is rare.

10 Although the majority of epistaxis is well managed by GPs and ED physicians, epistaxis is primarily an ENT condition. If the epistaxis is not being controlled by simple measures implemented by these clinicians, help from the ENT team should be sought to provide further advice and ongoing specialised management.

11 Nasal packing is often used when first aid and nasal cautery fail. There are a variety of choices (e.g. Rapid Rhino, Merocel, nasal packing gauze); however, they all aim to do the same thing – provide prolonged and sustained pressure to the bleeding area and promote coagulation to halt the bleeding. The Rapid Rhino balloon nasal pack is commonly found in EDs, and is made of carboxymethylcellulose which acts to promote platelet aggregation. Insertion is often very painful, and thus topical anaesthetic spray is administered prior to attempting nasal packing. The most significant complication with nasal packing is migration of the pack. Rare case reports of aspiration have been documented, and thus packs should always be secured to the patient in some fashion if possible. Other complications include septal necrosis, foreign body reaction and staphylococcal toxic shock syndrome. The use of prophylactic antibiotics (usually cephalexin) has not been adequately studied, but should be considered in patients with prolonged anterior packing (>48 hours) or in all patients with posterior packing. Removal of nasal packing usually occurs 24–48 hours after insertion, and occasionally may precipitate bleeding again. If this occurs, strong consideration should be made toward surgical management.

12 Occasionally, due to anatomical factors unilateral packing may not be sufficient to apply pressure to the bleeding location. A contralateral pack may be inserted to provide counterpressure to the septum and initial pack, and may succeed where the unilateral packing failed. If the bleeding location was not adequately visualised, and packing is not successful in stopping the bleeding, the clinician should consider the possibility that this is a posterior bleed. If contralateral packing is also unsuccessful, posterior nasal packing is the next step.

13 When nasal packing fails, surgical intervention is usually warranted. This usually entails an EUA with rigid endoscope to visualise the bleeding. Once the bleeding is visualised, direct nasal electrocautery can be applied to coagulate the bleeding vessels. If this fails to stem the bleeding, the surgeon may attempt to ligate the sphenopalatine artery – the main feeding artery to Little's area.

14 Percutaneous angioembolisation provides an alternative option to manage epistaxis. This procedure has a reported success rate of 87–93%; however, it is accompanied by the risk of cerebrovascular ischaemia, soft tissue necrosis and facial nerve paralysis. For these reasons, angioembolisation as a treatment for epistaxis is usually reserved for patients in whom surgical management has failed or peri-operative risk has been deemed too high.

15 This advice aims to reduce blood flow and pressure to the nose, and avoid disruption of blood clots that may lead to recurrent bleeding.

16 If anticoagulation or antiplatelet agents have been ceased, these usually will need to be reinstated. This is best done in a hospital setting, where frequent close monitoring can occur, and immediate management can be implemented if bleeding recurs.

17 Once the epistaxis has been managed and bleeding has ceased for a reasonable amount of time (generally 12–24 hours), the patient can be safely discharged. A reasonable amount of time will vary from patient to patient (e.g. in a patient with very high risk of re-bleeding, the astute clinician may opt to monitor the patient for 24–36 hours after cessation of epistaxis before discharging them).

18 Follow-up is integral to all surgical patients, and in particular those who have had an invasive procedure or operation. The patient should be assessed for any complications of inpatient management or surgery (e.g. soft tissue necrosis, septal perforation, anosmia). Although recurrent epistaxis is common, this may warrant further investigation for coagulopathy or friable bleeding mass.

CASE 16: Foreign body

History

- An **80-year-old** [1] male presents with a **3-hour history** [2] of sudden onset severe **dysphagia** [3] and **odynophagia** [4] after eating chicken.
- He has associated **drooling** [5], **hypersalivation** [6] and **blood-stained saliva** [7].
- He is able to **tolerate liquids** [8] but unable to swallow solids.
- He denies **fevers** [9], **dysphonia** [10], **dyspnoea** [11], **cough** [12], **neck pain** [13], **regurgitation** [14], **retrosternal fullness** [15], **chest pain** [16] or **abdominal pain** [17].
- He has a past medical history of **gastro-oesophageal reflux disease** [18] and previous **stroke** [19].
- He denies **eosinophilic oesophagitis** [20], **psychiatric illness** [21] or **intentional ingestion** [22] of dangerous or illegal substances.
- He drinks **5–7 units of alcohol per day** [23], and denies smoking or other drug use.
- Following the onset of pain, he unsuccessfully attempted to relieve his symptoms with **cola** [24].

[1] Foreign bodies are significantly more likely to occur at the extremes of ages. In children, foreign bodies are relatively common, and can occur in the ear, nose or throat. In adults, however, foreign bodies are relatively rare, and are most often related to food.

[2] The onset of symptoms associated with an ingested foreign body are typically extremely acute.

[3] Dysphagia is the most common symptom associated with an ingested foreign body, indicating its impaction in the digestive tract (as opposed to the airway). The most common site of impaction for a food bolus is within the oesophagus, often due to a pre-existing stricture or ring. Other common oesophageal locations for impaction are at sites of physiologic narrowing such as the upper oesophageal sphincter, at the level of the arch of aorta crossing the oesophagus, and at the diaphragmatic hiatus.

[4] Odynophagia with a food bolus is uncommon, and may be due to oesophageal spasm, but may also indicate ulceration or perforation. When a sharp foreign body is expected, odynophagia is a common symptom.

[5] Drooling may be a concerning sign for complete oesophageal obstruction and the inability to swallow saliva. Alternatively, drooling may be related to odynophagia and reluctance to swallow.

[6] Hypersalivation is a physiologic response to a foreign body in the GI tract.

[7] Blood-stained saliva likely indicates some mucosal trauma associated with the foreign body. This may be due to a sharp foreign body or due to ulceration from a long-standing food bolus or other non-sharp object.

[8] Typically, patients presenting with a foreign body are able to tolerate liquids but not necessarily solids. If a patient is unable to tolerate liquids (including their own saliva), this may indicate complete oesophageal obstruction, and is a strong indication for emergency endoscopy to relieve the obstruction.

[9] Fevers are not common in acute presentations, and likely indicate an infective complication of a foreign body, usually as a result of perforation. Depending on the site of perforation, this may present as acute intrathoracic sepsis or acute abdominal sepsis.

[10] Dysphonia may indicate the foreign body has fallen into the airway. This is very uncommon in fit and healthy adults; however, it can occur in patients with long-standing poor swallowing coordination or reduced pharyngeal sensation. These situations most often occur following a stroke or other neurological conditions. If dysphonia is present, the foreign body can usually be localised to within the larynx.

[11] Dyspnoea may indicate a foreign body has progressed past the larynx into the lower airways. Obstruction of a main or lobar bronchus may occur, and if left for some time, may result in complications such as collapse, infection or perforation.

[12] Cough may be another indicator of lower airway foreign body resulting in collapse or infection.

[13] Neck pain is not typical following acute foreign body impaction. If this symptom is present, it may indicate perforation.

[14] Regurgitation (especially of undigested food) is a common symptom following impacted oesophageal foreign body.

15 Retrosternal fullness may help localise an impacted foreign body to the thoracic oesophagus (as opposed to the cervical oesophagus).

16 Chest pain (especially in the presence of dyspnoea or sepsis) is a concerning sign for oesophageal perforation (Boerhaave syndrome). This can present with acute and severe sepsis with chest pain and SOB, and commonly occurs following a bout of vomiting.

17 Abdominal pain (especially if acute) is concerning for an intrabdominal perforation. This pain may radiate to the shoulder (reflecting the shared innervation of the diaphragm and the shoulder tip: C3–5), and may be accompanied by rebound tenderness, guarding and generalised peritonism. Onset of pain and subsequent sepsis can develop rapidly within several hours.

18 Gastro-oesophageal reflux disease (GORD) and other functional oesophageal disorders (e.g. strictures, webs, diverticula) increase the risk of oesophageal foreign body.

19 Patients with previous history of stroke (along with other neurological disorders affecting swallowing function and coordination, e.g. Parkinson's disease and multiple sclerosis) are at significantly increased risk of foreign body impaction of all types. Many of these patients will have recurrent foreign body impaction due to ongoing issues with dysphagia and incoordinated swallow.

20 Eosinophilic oesophagitis is a common but under-recognised oesophageal dysmotility disorder due to allergic eosinophil infiltration of the oesophagus. It is estimated up to 50% of patients with oesophageal food impaction will have underlying eosinophilic oesophagitis.

21 Psychiatric disorder of all types is a risk factor for foreign body ingestion. This may be incidental or as a result of purposeful self-harm. In these situations, foreign bodies may be objects other than food (e.g. magnets, coins, batteries, paperclips).

22 Occasionally, impacted foreign bodies are illegal substances that patients are attempting to conceal for the purposes of drug trafficking. If this is suspected, it is important to ascertain what type of substance and the amount, as inadvertent rupture of the container and spillage of contents may quickly result in drug overdose or other illness.

23 Alcohol intoxication causes incoordination in all areas including the swallow, and can predispose an individual to foreign body impaction similar to other swallowing coordination disorders.

24 Several studies have supported the use of cola (or other fizzy drinks) to disimpact oesophageal soft food bolus obstruction with encouraging results. However, this has no effect when managing sharp foreign bodies (e.g. fish or chicken bones). Furthermore, most impacted sharp foreign bodies will require attempted endoscopic retrieval, and the presence of liquids in the stomach increases the risk of aspiration and complicates anaesthetic measures. Thus, it is not recommended unless one can be sure that the impacted object is a soft food bolus only, and contains no bones or unchewed meat.

Examination

- The patient appears in **marked discomfort** [1] but is alert and oriented.
- Vital signs are within normal limits, in particular **respiratory rate is 20 per minute** [2] , and **SpO$_2$ is 99%** [2] on air.
- There are no **signs of respiratory distress** [3] .
- Auscultation of the heart reveals normal heart sounds with no murmurs, and **auscultation of the lungs** [4] is unremarkable.
- **Palpation of the abdomen** [5] is soft and non-tender.
- When asked to **indicate where the pain is** [6] , the patient points to the right anterior triangle, at the level of the hyoid bone.
- Inspection of the oral cavity reveals **upper and lower dentures** [7] .
- **Upon removal of the dentures** [8] , no foreign body or other abnormality is noted.
- The **oropharynx** [9] appears normal with bilateral grade 1 tonsils, and no **pharyngeal swelling, erythema or postnasal drip** [10] .
- Palpation of the head and neck reveals no **crepitus** [11] , **tenderness** [12] or **swelling** [12] .
- On **flexible nasoendoscopy** [13] , the nasal passages and nasopharynx are unremarkable.
- The oropharynx including the **tonsillar crypt, tongue base and valleculae** [14] are normal.
- Within the **hypopharynx** [15] a long sharp foreign body can be seen impacted into the **right aryepiglottic fold** [16] .
- There is no **ulceration** [17] visible.
- The **larynx and vocal folds** [18] are unremarkable, with normal vocal fold movement and no obstruction of the airway.

1 Discomfort may be correlated with a particularly unwell patient. It also provides insight into the urgency of the problem (i.e. a very unwell patient generally requires swifter diagnosis and management than a relatively well-looking patient).

2 A normal respiratory rate and oxygen saturation does not exclude the possibility of airway obstruction.

3 Signs of respiratory distress (increased work of breathing, accessory muscle use, stridor, etc.) should alert every clinician to the possibility of airway obstruction. Although most ingested foreign bodies become impacted in the oesophagus, occasionally (and especially in patients with pre-existing swallowing issues) impaction in the airway can present with signs of airway obstruction. Airway assessment and management becomes the first priority in managing this patient.

4 Assessment of the lungs is an important part of the peri-operative work-up to screen for any pathologies. Furthermore, in patients with dysphagia, inadvertent aspiration is common and can lead to aspiration pneumonia, complicating management of the patient.

5 Palpation of the abdomen may elicit tenderness, guarding or peritonism and may be indicative of an intra-abdominal perforation.

6 Often patients are able to localise accurately where the level of impaction is. This may provide some insight to which team is most appropriate to manage the foreign body. In this situation, the location of the pain is roughly at the level of the hypopharynx or larynx.

7 Patients with dentures are at higher risk of sharp foreign body ingestion due to the inability to feel bones in the mouth.

8 When dentures are in place it is important to have these removed to allow inspection of the entire oral cavity including the maxillary and mandibular alveolar ridges. The oral cavity itself is an uncommon site for foreign body impaction.

9 The oropharynx (the tonsils in particular) is one of the most common sites for sharp foreign body impaction. When suspecting a sharp foreign body ingestion, it is important to always document inspection of the tonsils.

10 Occasionally, patients with pharyngitis or postnasal drip will complain of dysphagia or globus pharyngeus (sensation of foreign body in throat). These conditions may mimic an impacted foreign body, and should be considered especially when a patient presents with clinical history not consistent with an acute foreign body ingestion (e.g. vague onset of pain, subacute presentation).

11 Crepitus in the neck is concerning for perforation with cervical subcutaneous emphysema. If present, urgent imaging and endoscopy is required, as sepsis (especially mediastinitis) can quickly occur.

12 Tenderness or swelling in the neck may be indicative of a deep neck space infection or abscess. The most common cause of retropharyngeal abscess is an ingested foreign body (likely causing erosion or excoriation of the posterior pharyngeal wall). If there is concern for a deep neck space abscess, this should be investigated promptly with a CT of the head and neck with IV contrast.

13 Flexible nasoendoscopy is essential in all potential foreign body ingestions. The entire upper aerodigestive tract can be visualised from the nasopharynx to the hypopharynx and larynx, and often the foreign body itself can be seen.

14 The tonsils, tongue base and valleculae are the three most common sites for impaction for sharp foreign bodies within the oropharynx (and for sharp foreign bodies in general). If impaction occurs in the oropharynx, this can often be removed at the bedside using long forceps if the patient is compliant, eliminating the need for anaesthetic and endoscopy.

15 The hypopharynx is the second most common site for impaction of ingested sharp foreign bodies. Occasionally secondary signs of foreign body impaction can be seen despite not being able to visualise the foreign body itself. These signs include erosion and pooling of saliva.

16 The aryepiglottic folds are folds of mucosa bridging between the arytenoid processes and the epiglottis. They form the lateral borders of the laryngeal inlet and separate the larynx from the piriform sinus.

17 Presence of ulceration indicates a foreign body has been present for a relatively long time. Ulceration increases the risk of perforation and other complications such as deep neck space abscess.

18 Although uncommon, laryngeal/airway foreign bodies can occur, causing obstruction and an airway emergency. It is good practice to routinely assess the airway, including vocal fold function and overall patency of the airway, during every flexible nasoendoscopy.

Investigations

- FBE reports a **normal WCC** [1] . UEC is normal. CRP is normal.
- **Lateral and anteroposterior neck X-ray** [2] reveals no foreign body and no thickening of the **prevertebral tissues** [3] .
- On **CXR** [4] the lung fields are unremarkable, with no consolidation.
- There is no **foreign body** [5] , **subdiaphragmatic gas** [5] , or **free mediastinal gas** [6] , **mediastinal air fluid level** [6] or **mediastinal widening** [6] .

- **Abdominal X-ray** [7] reveals no foreign body.
- **CT neck** [8] confirms a small sharp radiopaque pointed object impacted in the right aryepiglottic fold with some associated soft tissue oedema.
- There is no associated **collection** [9] or **cervical subcutaneous emphysema** [9] .
- The imaged **mediastinum** [10] and **airspaces** [10] are unremarkable.

[1] Raised inflammatory markers (white cell count, CRP) is uncommon when dealing with a simple ingested foreign body due to the acute presentation. If raised inflammatory markers are present, this should alert the clinician to the possibility of a complication from the foreign body (e.g. perforation, ulceration, deep neck space abscess, aspiration).

[2] X-ray of the neck should always include lateral and antero-posterior (AP) views, as some ingested objects do not project well on the overlying neck soft tissues. Although neck X-rays are a widely available and simple investigation, they are poorly suited to assessing for foreign bodies, as many ingested foreign bodies (including some bones) are not radio-opaque. Furthermore, neck X-rays can be difficult to interpret due to multiple overlapping soft tissue densities and calcific cartilaginous structures.

[3] Thickening of the prevertebral tissues (defined as prevertebral tissue thickness >7mm at C2 or >2cm at C7 in adults) is indicative of retropharyngeal abscess, the most common cause of which is ingested sharp foreign body causing erosion and subsequent infection.

[4] CXR is important to rule out aspiration related to dysphagia. The classic features of aspiration on CXR are consolidation in the right middle or lower lobes.

[5] CXR also assesses for the presence of an aspirated foreign body and free subdiaphragmatic gas, a hallmark sign of abdominal hollow organ perforation.

[6] Features of mediastinitis on CXR include mediastinal gas, air fluid level and mediastinal widening. The presence of mediastinitis is a poor prognostic sign, and cardiothoracic surgery involvement is necessary. Mediastinitis itself has a mortality of 30–40%.

[7] Abdominal X-ray may be useful if the foreign body has progressed into the abdomen. The majority of foreign bodies that reach the stomach (including sharp foreign bodies) will pass without issues. If the object is a high risk object (e.g. sharp object, battery, magnet) and is still retrievable or within 24 hours of ingestion, an attempt should be made to retrieve the object via endoscopy. If this is not possible, or if endoscopy was attempted and failed, the object should be tracked to ensure progression through the GI tract.

[8] If an ingested foreign body is suspected, CT of the neck is the imaging modality of choice. CT imaging can detect radio-opaque objects with a sensitivity of 98%, although this is lower for non-radio-opaque objects. Important aspects to assess include location of foreign body, shape, size, depth and presence of complications.

[9] CT is also excellent for assessing for complications such as deep neck space infections which may require further surgical management, or perforation evidenced by subcutaneous emphysema, oedema, fluid. Although CT is highly sensitive for the detection of gas bubble locules in the soft tissues indicating the presence of a perforation, it is a poor modality for accurately localising the site of perforation.

[10] CT neck does image part of the mediastinum (mostly the superior mediastinum), and routine assessment of the imaged mediastinum is prudent. However, if mediastinal complications are suspected (thoracic oesophageal perforation, mediastinitis), formal imaging of the mediastinum by CT chest with IV contrast is required. Likewise, if intra-abdominal complications are suspected (intra-abdominal perforation), a formal CT abdomen and pelvis is required.

Management

Immediate

Assess the airway [1] and determine the need for **definitive airway management** [2]. **Avoid positioning the patient** [3]. **Keep the patient fasted** [4]. **Seek advice** [5] from the ENT team or the gastroenterology team.

Short-term

Perform an **endoscopic retrieval** [6] of the foreign body, as well as a **panendoscopy** [7] to inspect for any complications. Following the procedure, keep the patient in hospital for **monitoring** [8]. **Auscultate the lungs** [9]. **Re-examine the oral cavity and re-perform flexible nasoendoscopy** [10]. **Reassess the swallow** [11]. **The patient may be discharged** [12] if vital signs remain stable, they can tolerate oral intake, and there is no evidence of postoperative complications.

Long-term

Follow up [13] the patient in the outpatient clinic if necessary, to monitor for postoperative complications. Consider **repeat endoscopy** [14] to reassess mucosal healing. Refer to speech pathology for **swallowing exercises** [15]. Prescribe **proton pump inhibitors** [16].

---

[1] Assessment of the airway is the first step in managing any patient. In most patients, this will be as simple as confirming that the patient can speak (airway is patent) and that there are no signs of respiratory distress or airway obstruction (e.g. stridor, accessory muscle use). In circumstances where a compromised airway is suspected, a more comprehensive airway assessment must be undertaken – this usually includes flexible nasoendoscopy to visualise the airway and review by either the ENT team or the anaesthetics team, or preferably both.

[2] If a compromised airway has been discovered, the need for a definitive airway must be assessed. This should occur before any other intervention and should not be delayed by imaging or other investigations. A definitive airway is defined as a tube placed in the trachea with a cuff inflated below the vocal folds. In most situations this will be an awake fibreoptic endotracheal tube (ETT). However, in the presence of a potential obstructing airway foreign body, an attempt to first remove the foreign body via direct laryngoscopy may be made if the patient is stable enough. Rarely, if the obstructing foreign body is unable to be removed and an ETT is unable to be passed, a surgical airway may be required. This will usually take the form of an emergency cricothyroidotomy to establish a quick, safe and secure means of ventilation. The process of establishing a definitive airway should be a discussion between the ENT surgery team, the anaesthetic team and the intensive care team, and will depend on the clinical state of the patient, the extent of airway obstruction and the likely plan for management. The plan for definitive airway should include where the attempted insertion will take place (e.g. operating theatre vs. ED), who will be available, what airway will be attempted first, who will make the attempt (the anaesthetist vs. ENT surgeon) and what the backup plan is (usually emergency cricothyroidotomy).

[3] In cases of airway obstruction, patients often adopt the tripod posture (leaning forward and supporting the upper body with both hands) and the 'sniffing the morning air' position (flexion of the neck at the cervicothoracic junction and extension at the atlantoaxial junction – this aligns the oral cavity, pharynx and larynx, allowing for the least turbulent flow of air). The patient should never be positioned against their will, as this may cause complete airway obstruction (this includes lying flat for CT scan).

[4] Keeping the patient fasted is crucial in the preoperative management of the patient. It reduces the risk of aspiration in the setting of anaesthesia. Ideally, patients should be fasted off solid foods for 6 hours prior to anaesthetic. In the emergency setting and if time is critical, RSI is an alternative to reduce the risk of aspiration (especially so in patients who are not fasted).

[5] Ingested foreign bodies can be managed by both the ENT team or the gastroenterology team. Generally, sharp foreign bodies and airway foreign bodies will be managed by the ENT team, whereas impacted food boluses, oesophageal foreign bodies and more distal foreign bodies will be managed by the gastroenterology team. In this case of a sharp foreign body located in the right aryepiglottic fold, a referral to the ENT is appropriate. Care of the patient, including airway management and definitive foreign body management, should be directed by them.

[6] A retrieval attempt should at least be considered for all ingested foreign bodies. Sharp foreign bodies and airway foreign bodies should always be retrieved. Retrieval should happen as soon as possible, and should not be delayed, in order to reduce risk of ulceration, perforation or subsequent infective complications such as retropharyngeal abscess and mediastinitis. Endoscopic retrieval in this situation may be a simple laryngoscopy and removal with forceps; however,

oesophageal or airway foreign bodies may require more advanced techniques and equipment such as gastroscopy and snare retrieval. At the same time as the retrieval, an examination of the surrounding structures should be made again to inspect for complications such as perforation.

7 Depending on the likelihood of complications and the location of the foreign body, a panendoscopy (combined laryngoscopy, bronchoscopy and oesophagoscopy) may be warranted to inspect the full upper aerodigestive tract for complications or other impacted foreign bodies.

8 Monitoring is essential for all post-procedure patients to look for post-procedure complications. The length of monitoring is variable, and depends on the clinical status of the patient and the condition being treated. In the case of an acute foreign body impaction with a very short history (3 hours), the postoperative monitoring period may only be several hours. However, in cases with a longer history, the clinician must be more aware of the possibility of complications.

9 Aspiration is a common complication of any patient presenting with dysphagia, and this risk is increased after patients are anaesthetised. HAP is important to recognise early, to prevent poor outcomes.

10 Given the relatively inaccessible location of the foreign body in many cases, clinical examination can only be performed with flexible nasoendoscopy. Monitoring for postoperative complications, such as perforation and abscess, is required for all foreign body ingestions.

11 Swallow should be assessed (either by bedside testing or with formal assessment by speech pathologists) prior to reinstatement of oral intake. This is to ensure that risk of aspiration has resolved.

12 The patient may be discharged if all parameters are improving. Often, if the presentation is acute (as in this case) and the risk of postoperative complications is low (including complications from the foreign body as well as anaesthetic complications), patients may be discharged the same day with the expectation that the recovery process will be uncomplicated. However, clinicians should have a low threshold for monitoring patients overnight if they pose a higher postoperative risk.

13 Follow-up is integral to all surgical patients, and in particular those who have had an invasive procedure or operation. Follow-up aims to serve several purposes: ensuring the patient's acute illness has resolved, ensuring they have not suffered any late complication from the procedure (e.g. persistent dysphagia), providing reassurance to the patient that the acute illness has resolved and finally, providing a management plan for possible future events.

14 Patients who encountered complications should be considered for repeat endoscopy to ensure resolution. This is particularly useful in patients suffering from recurrent foreign body impaction, to assess for an underlying swallowing disorder such as eosinophilic oesophagitis.

15 Swallow exercises decrease the risk of aspiration and can also help in cases of persistent dysphagia (which may predispose a patient to recurrent foreign body impaction). Common causes of persistent dysphagia include stroke, neurological disorders such as Parkinson's disease and multiple sclerosis, and oesophageal disorders such as GORD and eosinophilic oesophagitis.

16 Given this patient's known history of GORD, follow-up can also serve as an opportunity to assess for common related conditions and treat these simultaneously.

CASE 17: Oropharyngeal cancer

History

- A **40-year-old** [1] female presents to the **outpatient department** [2] with a **6-week history** [3] of enlarging left-sided **non-tender neck mass** [4].
- She also reports a **muffled voice** [5] in the past 3–4 days and **4kg weight loss** [6] in the past 2 months.
- She denies **dysphagia** [7], **odynophagia** [7], **otalgia** [8], **hearing loss** [9], **tinnitus** [9], **nasal obstruction** [10], **epistaxis** [11], **haemoptysis** [12], **shortness of breath** [13], **fevers** [14] or **night sweats** [14].

- She denies **past history of head and neck surgery** [15], **thyroid disease** [16] or **excessive sun exposure** [17].
- She has a **20 pack year smoking history** [18] and **drinks 2 units of alcohol per day** [19].
- She denies having a **human papillomavirus (HPV) vaccination** [20].
- She reports having **multiple sexual partners** [21].

1 Age is a risk factor for almost all head and neck cancers. The majority of adults over 40 years of age presenting with neck masses will have malignancy.

2 Most neck masses will not present acutely to the ED. For this reason, it is important to assess patients comprehensively, and order all necessary investigations in a timely manner to avoid diagnostic delay and management delays, which can worsen prognosis. Diagnostic delay is a particularly concerning problem in head and neck cancers, with some studies regularly documenting delays of up to 180 days.

3 Any neck mass that is present for >2 weeks should be considered malignant until proven otherwise. Whilst there are benign causes of neck masses (e.g. infective lymphadenitis, congenital cysts) these are uncommon in adults, and pursuing these diagnoses leads to delays in diagnosis and management, which worsens prognosis.

4 Most acute inflammatory conditions that cause neck masses (e.g. lymphadenitis, infected branchial cleft cyst) will present with painful or tender lymphadenopathy. Thus, any new neck mass that is non-tender is extremely concerning for malignancy with likely local lymph node metastasis.

5 Muffled voice ('hot potato' voice) is often characteristic of peritonsillar abscess; however, it can be present in any condition causing oropharyngeal crowding. In the absence of any infective symptoms, 'hot potato' voice is concerning for an oropharyngeal mass.

6 Loss of weight in any patient is concerning for malignancy, and is associated with poorer treatment outcomes (e.g. wound healing, postoperative recovery) due to relative malnutrition. Recent weight loss is particularly problematic in the management of head and neck cancers, due to the effects of treatment on a patient's swallow. Surgical resection often renders oral intake difficult

or impossible in the short term, further exacerbating malnutrition, and radiotherapy poses a similar risk, and often causes long-term dysphagia.

7 Dysphagia and odynophagia in the presence of a new neck mass indicate a likely mucosal tumour. This may originate from the oral cavity (e.g. tongue, floor of mouth), oropharynx (e.g. tonsil, pharyngeal wall, vallecula), or the hypopharynx (e.g. piriform fossa, postcricoid region). Occasionally, laryngeal tumours may grow large enough to cause surrounding mass effect and dysphagia or odynophagia as well.

8 Otalgia may indicate a primary middle ear tumour; however, middle ear malignancy is extremely rare. Most often, otalgia with malignancy is due to a cutaneous malignancy (e.g. squamous cell carcinoma or melanoma), or is referred otalgia from the tonsillar fossa (via the tympanic branch of the glossopharyngeal nerve), hypopharynx (via the superior laryngeal branch of the vagus nerve) or larynx (via the superior laryngeal or recurrent laryngeal branches of the vagus nerve).

9 Hearing loss and tinnitus indicate a primary ear pathology. This may be a primary ear malignancy, but if unilateral and present with nasal obstruction, may indicate Eustachian tube obstruction with middle ear effusion – a hallmark constellation of symptoms very suggestive of a nasopharyngeal tumour (e.g. nasopharyngeal carcinoma).

10 Nasal obstruction may be related to rhinosinusitis or other benign anatomical obstruction; however, in the setting of a new neck mass, this would be concerning for a sinonasal or nasopharyngeal tumour (e.g. nasopharyngeal carcinoma).

11 Epistaxis is a poor sign when assessing a patient for malignancy – this is very concerning for sinonasal malignancy or nasopharyngeal malignancy.

12 Haemoptysis indicates bleeding occurring along the airway. Although this is usually associated with lower airway pathology (either malignant, e.g. lung cancer, or non-malignant, e.g. pneumonia), the bleeding may also originate from the larynx and may be indicative of a laryngeal tumour or other laryngeal pathology.

13 Shortness of breath may relate to a lower airway pathology; however, the possibility of airway obstruction needs to be considered and ruled out.

14 Fevers and night sweats (together with weight loss) are known as B symptoms and are suggestive of lymphoma. If B symptoms are present, a haematological examination including palpation of all lymph node groups in the body is necessary. It can be difficult to diagnose or exclude lymphoma as a diagnosis based on history and examination alone – often biopsy is necessary.

15 A history of previous head and neck malignancy significantly increases the risk of recurrence or a second primary, often in the same site or an adjacent structure. Furthermore, previous head and neck surgery alters the lymphatic drainage of the surrounding structures and can change the location of likely lymph node metastatic spread. This can change management of neck disease (e.g. which levels are dissected, unilateral vs. bilateral).

16 Most lateral neck lumps in adults will be cervical lymphadenopathy or another congenital cyst. If a neck lump is present anteriorly, this is likely to be located in the thyroid.

17 Excessive sun exposure is a strong risk factor for skin cancer. Rates of skin cancer are increasing faster than any other cancer in the UK, with figures doubling every 10–20 years – many of these will occur on the head and neck (in particular the external ears, cheeks and nasal tip).

18 Smoking is a risk factor for many tumours of the head and neck, particularly mucosal SCCs. Besides this, smoking places most patients at a higher peri-operative risk (through its associated lung conditions) and postoperative complication risk (e.g. poorer wound healing, higher risk of postoperative wound infections and hospital-acquired infections), making this something to consider when counselling patients regarding their options.

19 Alcohol intake is also a strong risk factor for mucosal SCCs, and has a synergistic effect with smoking. If dependency or liver disease is present, this can create issues surrounding peri-operative risk and postoperative care (e.g. managing withdrawal).

20 The overall incidence of oropharyngeal cancer is on the rise due to the marked increase of HPV-related oropharyngeal cancer. Furthermore, HPV-related oropharyngeal cancer patients often do not fit the stereotype of patients with malignancy, and are frequently younger, non-smoking males who often present with massive cervical lymphadenopathy with asymptomatic primary tumours. Although HPV vaccination in the UK does target the most common oncogenic types (i.e. type 16 and 18), HPV-related oropharyngeal cancer is still a significant cause of malignancy.

21 A higher number of sexual partners (in particular oral sex) is strongly linked with an increased risk of HPV-related oropharyngeal cancer.

Examination

- The patient appears **comfortable** [1].
- There are **no signs of respiratory distress** [2]. Vital signs are unremarkable.
- **Examination of the ear reveals** [3] no masses or infection, and no middle ear effusion.
- **Anterior rhinoscopy** [4] reveals no masses.
- **Examination of the oral cavity** [5] reveals **enlarged left-sided grade 3 tonsil with an ulcerated surface** [6]. The rest of the oral cavity is unremarkable.
- **The oropharynx** [7] is not erythematous or swollen.
- **Palpation of the neck** [8] demonstrates left-sided cervical lymphadenopathy at levels II and III.
- The lymph nodes are **firm** [9] and **non-tender** [10], and are **not fixed to the skin or underlying tissue** [11].
- The **thyroid gland** [12] is not enlarged and no nodules are palpable.
- Examination of the face and external ears reveals no **cutaneous lesions** [13].
- On **flexible nasoendoscopy** [14] there are no masses in the nasopharynx. The oropharynx again demonstrates the enlarged left-sided tonsil with ulcerated surface.
- The **hypopharynx** [15] and **larynx** [16] are un-remarkable, with normal **vocal fold movement** [17].

1 General inspection provides information regarding the patient's overall state of unwellness. Often malignancy will present slowly and insidiously, in an otherwise well-looking patient.

2 Respiratory distress (e.g. stridor, accessory muscle use) may indicate a potential or partially obstructed airway. Whilst most patients presenting with a neck lump do not have a threatened airway, if there is significant narrowing of the airway due to mass effect from a primary tumour, there is a possibility of acute obstruction. Thus, it is important to address this issue immediately to prevent an airway emergency situation. This usually would indicate a direct admission to hospital.

3 A complete ear, nose and throat examination is warranted in cases of possible malignancy. A brief otoscopy is useful to exclude external auditory canal infection (otitis externa) or malignancy, middle ear tumours, middle ear effusion (from nasopharyngeal tumour).

4 Anterior rhinoscopy is useful to exclude nasal masses and potential sinusitis. Sinus masses are poorly assessed by examination, and almost always require imaging.

5 It is important to assess every aspect of the oral cavity when assessing for a possible malignancy. This includes the lips, floor of mouth, tongue (including superior and inferior surface), vestibule (between the gums and the cheek), the alveolar processes and the tonsillar pillars. If dentures are present, these should be removed to properly assess the alveolar processes.

6 Asymmetry of the tonsils is very concerning for a tonsillar tumour. Other possibilities are quinsy or parapharyngeal mass/abscess causing medial tonsil displacement. Ulceration on the surface of a tonsil is very concerning for malignancy, especially in an enlarged and non-painful tonsil. Alternatively, tonsillar ulcers may be caused by herpangina, a viral infection.

7 The oropharynx includes the soft palate, tonsillar pillars, the tonsils, the posterior one-third of the tongue, the vallecula, the lingual surface of the epiglottis and the posterior and lateral pharyngeal walls. Erythema and swelling are signs of inflammation that may indicate an infective cause.

8 The neck is divided into six levels, each describing lymph node regions, with the midline being the central dividing line between left and right. Emphasis should be placed on accurately documenting the location of cervical lymphadenopathy.

9 Firm lymph nodes are more consistent with malignancy.

10 Reactive lymph nodes (i.e. lymphadenopathy due to infection) tend to be tender (due to the inflammatory response within the lymph node). Non-tender lymphadenopathy is usually concerning for malignancy.

11 Fixation to skin or underlying tissue is an ominous sign. This indicates the possibility of tumour spread outside the capsule of the lymph node and into the surrounding tissues. This is termed clinically overt extranodal extension and implies a late stage of disease and thus poor prognosis.

12 Whilst a lateral neck mass is often lymphadenopathy (especially in adults), a thyroid nodule or enlarged thyroid gland is also a possibility. The pathophysiology and management of thyroid gland is vastly different from the management of mucosal head and neck tumours.

13 Skin cancer is becoming more common in the UK and occurs particularly often on the sun-bearing areas of the face, head and neck. Thus, a cutaneous examination of the head and neck is essential to rule out this very common condition.

14 Flexible nasoendoscopy is the most common way to visualise the nasopharynx (which cannot be properly assessed with anterior rhinoscopy). Nasopharyngeal tumours (e.g. nasopharyngeal carcinoma) are uncommon and often asymptomatic until late in the disease. The classic nasopharyngeal carcinoma presents with unilateral hearing loss with middle ear effusion and ipsilateral nasal obstruction. It is much more common in males of Asian or African descent.

15 The hypopharynx includes the piriform sinus, the hypopharyngeal walls and the postcricoid area.

16 The larynx includes the cartilaginous structures (thyroid cartilage, cricoid cartilage, epiglottis (laryngeal surface), arytenoids, cuneiforms and corniculate cartilages, the aryepiglottic folds and the vocal folds. It is further divided into the supraglottis, the glottis and the subglottis.

17 Loss of vocal fold movement may be due to intrinsic pathology of the vocal fold (e.g. vocal fold tumour, granulomas), pathology at the arytenoids (e.g. cricoarytenoid dislocation, posterior glottic stenosis from interarytenoid scar), or pathology along the neural supply (e.g. recurrent laryngeal nerve injury or paresis from mass effect in the neck or perineural invasion).

Investigations

- **FBE** [1] reports a normal Hb, normal white cell count, and normal platelets. **UEC** [1] results demonstrate normal electrolytes and an eGFR of >90ml/min/1.73m^2.
- **HPV serology** [2] is negative.
- **Coagulation studies** [3] are within normal limits.
- A **group and hold** [4] is performed.
- **ECG** [5] shows normal sinus rhythm.

- CXR reveals normal lung fields and **no lung masses** [6].
- **Pulmonary function test** [7] is unremarkable.
- **CT of the head and neck with IV contrast** [8] demonstrates left tonsillar tumour with **invasion into the left glossotonsillar sulcus** [9].
- **The mass is 3cm in diameter** [10].
- There are **3cm lymph nodes in level II and III** [11].

- **CT of the chest** [12] demonstrates no mediastinal lymphadenopathy and no emphysematous lung disease.
- **PET scan** [13] reveals marked avidity in the left tonsil and vallecula but shows no distant metastases.
- **FNA** [14] of the left cervical lymphadenopathy is consistent with SCC with negative **p16 immunohistochemistry** [15].

[1] FBE and UEC are often considered baseline tests (especially in preoperative patients) as they effectively screen for many conditions (either acute or pre-existing) that may have an impact on the patient's presentation or potential management. In this situation, where the patient may require surgical management, it is important to ensure the patient is not anaemic or thrombocytopenic and does not have pre-existing renal impairment, all of which pose a potential peri-operative risk and need to be addressed prior to surgical intervention.

[2] HPV has strongly increased the incidence of oropharyngeal cancer despite reduced rates of smoking (see discussion above).

[3] Abnormalities found on coagulation studies (along with platelet count) are important in any surgery with high intraoperative and postoperative bleeding risk (e.g. thyroidectomy) and need to be addressed prior to surgery. An INR of <1.4 and platelets of >100 x 10⁹/L is generally considered safe for surgery, although this will vary depending on surgeon, patient and type of operation.

[4] Blood group and hold is an essential investigation for all preoperative patients at high risk of bleeding (either due to surgical risk or pre-existing patient factors).

[5] A baseline ECG is a necessary and simple test for most preoperative patients (in particular the elderly) to screen for pre-existing cardiac disease/arrhythmia.

[6] Pulmonary masses on CXR need to be investigated further as part of the peri-operative work-up of the patient. In this setting, this may be due to metastasis of tumour to the mediastinal lymph nodes; however, in the setting of known long-standing smoking history, it may represent a primary lung tumour.

[7] Pulmonary function tests (PFTs) are a useful investigation to assess lung function and to stratify peri-operative risk for patients undergoing long, invasive surgery. It is especially important in this patient, given her long smoking history and no known diagnosis of lung disease.

[8] CT with IV contrast provides excellent cross-sectional anatomical detail of all structures in the head and neck region. It also confirms lymphadenopathy and location of lymph nodes, and often detects subclinical lymphadenopathy (enlarged nodes not picked up on initial examination), which frequently changes staging and management.

[9] Invasion of the tumour into surrounding structures is important to document. Although this does not influence the T staging of the tumour (unless involving distant structures, e.g. larynx, extrinsic muscles of tongue, hard palate), it does influence which structures need to be removed to achieve oncological clearance.

[10] Tumour size is one of the criteria that influences T staging in oropharyngeal cancer (and many other cancers). A tumour size of 3cm indicates a T2 category.

[11] Nodal staging in oropharyngeal cancer depends on the laterality of the nodes to the primary tumour, the number of nodes present and the size. 3cm lymph nodes in levels II and III (without extranodal extension) correlate with a nodal stage of N2b.

[12] CT chest may be indicated to investigate for superior mediastinal lymphadenopathy (level VII lymph nodes). It may also be indicated to investigate lung disease prior to major surgery, or if lung masses are suspected on CXR.

[13] PET scan (with FDG) is a highly sensitive scan for head and neck malignancy. Its current use in primary mucosal head and neck malignancy is limited to detecting recurrent tumours post treatment, detecting tumours in patients with malignant lymphadenopathy of unknown primary, or detecting metastases in patients at high risk of metastatic disease (either due to cancer type or staging). However, PET-fused CT is playing an increasingly greater role in the primary work-up of head and neck cancers.

[14] Fine needle aspiration (FNA) is a first-line investigation for most neck lumps. It is a relatively well tolerated and low risk procedure that can be performed under ultrasound guidance, and provides histological sample to confirm a suspected diagnosis. According to meta-analysis, fine needle aspiration has an overall accuracy of 93.1% in neck masses of all types.

[15] p16 immunohistochemistry positivity is strongly associated with HPV-related oropharyngeal cancer. p16 positive oropharyngeal cancer carries a significantly better prognosis than p16 negative oropharyngeal cancer, and is increasingly being treated as a separate condition to p16 negative oropharyngeal cancer, with alternative staging and treatment pathways.

Management

Immediate

Assess the airway [1] and ensure there are no signs of respiratory distress. Assess the patient for **peri-operative fitness** [2] and organise any necessary **supplementary investigations** [3] in a timely manner. **Seek advice** [4] from the ENT team. **Counsel the patient** [5] regarding the diagnosis and their options.

Short-term

Perform a **panendoscopy and biopsy** [6]. Present the case at a **head and neck cancer MDT meeting** [7]. Perform a **radical tonsillectomy** [8] with **left neck dissection** [9]. Following the procedure, **monitor the patient** [10] for postoperative complications. **Auscultate the lungs** [11] and **examine the lower limbs** [12]. The patient may be discharged if the **vitals remain stable** [13], **the patient is tolerating oral intake** [14] and there are no signs of postoperative complications.

Long-term

Re-present the patient at the MDT meeting [15]. Follow up the patient in the **outpatient clinic regularly** [16]. Depending on the final histopathology and staging, consider **adjuvant radiotherapy** [17] and/or **chemotherapy** [17]. **Monitor for recurrence** [18].

[1] Ensuring a patent airway is the first step when assessing all patients. It is a particularly important step when assessing any patient with a head and neck mass, and the clinician should take especial note of the presence of any signs of respiratory distress and address them first and foremost.

[2] The mainstay of treatment of the majority of malignancies is surgical resection, and this is also true of tonsillar malignancies. Consciously assessing peri-operative fitness during the first assessment is a good habit for all surgical clinicians to develop.

[3] Whilst supplementary investigations may not be necessary in all cases, often they are required to ensure that a surgical operation can be performed safely (e.g. investigating lung function with PFTs prior to general anaesthetic, echocardiogram if the patient has potential cardiac disease).

[4] Tonsillar malignancies are managed primarily by ENT surgeons. In most hospitals, management decision will be made jointly by an MDT, with an ENT surgeon usually acting as the head and mediator.

[5] Counselling patients about diagnoses, expected progress and management options is a crucial skill in the surgeon's repertoire. Being able to adequately explain conditions, appropriately consent patients for procedures, and provide reassurance helps patients in what is definitely a stressful period.

[6] Panendoscopy and biopsy is a surgical procedure that combines direct pharyngoscopy, laryngoscopy, rigid oesophagoscopy and rigid bronchoscopy to comprehensively examine the upper aerodigestive tract. This is most often performed to obtain a biopsy sample for difficult-to-reach tumours.

[7] Surgical management of cancers is usually best done through a multidisciplinary approach. In the case of oropharyngeal cancers, this usually involves a head and neck surgeon, an oncologist, a radiation oncologist, a radiologist, a pathologist and other allied health staff. These clinicians discuss cases to provide a combined experienced opinion on the most appropriate management for the patient.

[8] Radical tonsillectomy differs from standard tonsillectomy by the inclusion of the tonsillar fossa within the resection. This is performed in order to obtain clear oncological margins; however, it is associated with an increased risk of post-tonsillectomy bleeding.

[9] Neck dissection involves removing the lymph node chains in the neck. Not all oropharyngeal malignancies will require a neck dissection in conjunction with excision of the primary; the decision to perform the neck dissection (and which lymph node groups to remove) will depend on whether or not there are clinically evident lymph node metastases, and if not, the risk of lymph node metastases occurring without a neck dissection. As oropharyngeal malignancies are often midline structures (e.g. the vallecula, posterior pharyngeal wall), bilateral neck dissection may be indicated.

[10] The most common postoperative complication of radical tonsillectomy is post-tonsillectomy bleeding. This can be rapid and profuse, and can occur up to 2 weeks postoperatively. Any significant amount of bleeding (more than a tablespoon) should be monitored in hospital.

[11] Hospital-acquired complications (e.g. HAP) are common, particularly following a long surgery. Preventive measures such as deep breathing exercises should be implemented. If a hospital-acquired infection occurs, this should be managed early.

12 DVT is also an important complication, especially following long surgery. The calves should be inspected for swelling, redness and tenderness, and if there is suspicion of DVT, a calf ultrasound should be ordered.

13 Vital signs (heart rate, respiratory rate, oxygen saturation and BP) should be assessed in all patients daily, as they have been shown to directly correlate with a patient's progress in hospital. A patient with unstable vital signs or vital signs outside of normal limits should alert the clinician, warranting closer monitoring and swifter management, even if the cause is unclear.

14 If the postoperative period goes without complication, the pain is adequately controlled (tonsillectomy is notoriously painful), and the patient can tolerate oral intake, the patient can be discharged from hospital. In most cases of tonsillectomy alone, this will be the following day. If the surgical operation is more extensive (e.g. tonsillectomy with left neck dissection), the postoperative length of stay will be longer.

15 Once the final histopathology results are published, the patient's case should be discussed again at an MDT meeting to decide the further course of action. Whether a patient will receive radiotherapy, chemotherapy, immunotherapy or all of the above will depend on the tumour biology, the patient's postoperative recovery and the surgical margins.

16 Follow-up is integral to all surgical patients, and in particular those who have had an invasive procedure or operation. The patient should be reassessed for any complications of inpatient management or surgery (e.g. wound healing, post-tonsillectomy bleeding). Follow-up also serves to continue the patient management through the outpatient setting – as the surgery is only the first step in the management of most cancer patients. The final recommendations from the MDT discussion can be relayed to the patient, and any further referrals for ongoing treatment or management can be made from there.

17 Radiotherapy and/or chemotherapy can be given as adjuvant therapy (usually in the presence of poor prognostic features such as extranodal extension, perineural invasion, lymphovascular invasion). Alternatively, due to the difficulty of resecting some forms of oropharyngeal malignancy, chemoradiotherapy can be used as the primary treatment modality.

18 Monitoring for recurrence is an unfortunate necessity for all cancer patients, and the method of monitoring depends on the type of tumour. In the case of oropharyngeal cancer (as with most other mucosal head and neck malignancies), monitoring can be achieved through regular clinical assessments (usually 3-monthly for the first year) and examination with flexible nasoendoscopy. Recurrence is common in head and neck malignancy, and especially so in smokers who develop a 'field effect' across broad areas of the oropharynx, hypopharynx and larynx, which is particularly susceptible to dysplastic changes and subsequent malignancy.

CASE 18: Peritonsillar abscess

History

- A **16-year-old** [1] male presents with **severe** [2] **left-sided** [3] **throat pain** over the past **4 days** [4].
- He has associated **fevers** [5], **odynophagia** [6], **dysphagia** [7], **altered voice** [8], **difficulty opening his mouth** [9] and **left-sided ear pain** [10].
- He has a past history of **recurrent tonsillitis** [11] but is otherwise fit and healthy with no surgical history.

- He has a **1 year pack history of smoking** [12] and drinks alcohol occasionally.
- He denies any **neck stiffness/pain** [13], **dental pain** [14] or **breathing difficulty** [15].

[1] Peritonsillar abscess (quinsy) is a relatively common condition with an incidence of approximately 1:10 000, making it the most common deep neck space abscess. Although it can occur in any age group, it is most common in adolescence. It occurs equally in males and females.

[2] Severe throat pain is an indicator of pharyngeal inflammation and is a hallmark of a peritonsillar abscess; however, it is also characteristic of many other oropharyngeal conditions such as tonsillitis, pharyngitis and dental abscesses. Differentiating between these clinical entities depends on accurate history taking and examination.

[3] Peritonsillar abscesses are usually unilateral, causing the pain to localise to one side. Although the possibility of a bilateral peritonsillar abscess causing bilateral throat pain should be kept in the back of the mind, it is a rare occurrence.

[4] Peritonsillar abscess is an acute condition that usually develops over several days. A condition that has occurred within several hours is unlikely to be a peritonsillar abscess, as it generally takes 1–2 days for a collection to develop. Similarly, a peritonsillar abscess is unlikely to present after weeks due to the acuity and severity of the condition. In these cases (relatively short or relatively long history of presenting complaint), the clinician should have a low threshold for considering other diagnoses.

[5] Fever is a common complaint in many infective or inflammatory conditions. Although the absence of fever does not rule out an infective cause such as a peritonsillar abscess, the presence of a fever makes an infective cause much more likely.

[6] Odynophagia (painful swallowing) is another hallmark of peritonsillar abscess. Similar to throat pain, it is an indicator of pharyngeal inflammation, and thus is present in other conditions.

[7] Dysphagia (difficulty swallowing) often occurs in peritonsillar abscess secondary to the altered anatomy due to the peritonsillar swelling causing pharyngeal crowding.

[8] Altered voice (dysphonia) is also a classic symptom of peritonsillar abscess. Although there are many forms of dysphonia (e.g. breathy, rough, strained), the classic dysphonia in peritonsillar abscess is described as a 'hot potato' voice in which the speech has a muffled quality. 'Hot potato' voice is uncommon in other causes of throat pain (e.g. tonsillitis, simple pharyngitis) and thus is a good differentiating factor between these conditions.

[9] Difficulty with mouth opening (trismus) is another classic symptom of peritonsillar abscess. When due to peritonsillar abscess, it represents inflammation in the muscles responsible for mouth opening (pterygoids) and is another reliable differentiator between peritonsillar abscess and other pharyngeal conditions. However, trismus can also be caused by some dental abscesses or deep neck space abscesses other than peritonsillar abscess.

[10] Pain is often referred to the ipsilateral ear, reflecting their joint innervation by the glossopharyngeal nerve (CN IX).

[11] Peritonsillar abscess is generally thought to be the final stage of the tonsillitis disease progression (from tonsillitis to peritonsillar cellulitis to peritonsillar abscess). Although it may present during the first episode of tonsillitis, most patients will have a history of recurrent tonsillitis before developing an episode of peritonsillar abscess.

[12] Smoking has been associated with a significantly increased risk for peritonsillar abscess. Furthermore, smoking is a risk factor for peri-operative complications and wound healing complications.

[13] Neck stiffness is not a typical presenting complaint for patients with peritonsillar abscess, and its presence should prompt the clinician to explore the possibility of other deep

neck space abscesses (e.g. retropharyngeal/parapharyngeal abscess) which are usually associated with significantly worse outcomes.

14 Dental pain is also not a typical presenting complaint for patients with peritonsillar abscess; however, it is the hallmark of dental abscesses. Dental abscesses have varied locations and presentations, and some can present very similarly to peritonsillar abscess. Occasionally, dental abscesses can be life-threatening (e.g. Ludwig's angina, retropharyngeal or

parapharyngeal abscess), and poor dental hygiene or recent dental work increase this possibility.

15 Breathing difficulty in any patient necessitates the consideration of potential airway obstruction. Airway obstruction is extremely rare in peritonsillar abscess, and may indicate potential spread into the parapharyngeal space, or possibly an alternative diagnosis (e.g. retropharyngeal abscess, Ludwig's angina, epiglottitis, tracheitis). Further assessment and management are vital to avoid the possibility of complete airway obstruction.

Examination

- The patient appears **uncomfortable** [1] ; however, he is **alert and oriented** [2] with no signs of respiratory distress or **drooling** [3] .
- Heart rate is **115bpm** [4] and regular.
- The patient is **normotensive** [5] .
- Temperature is **38.0°C** [6] .
- **Skin turgor** [7] is appropriate, **mucous membranes** [7] are moist and he is producing adequate **urine output** [7] .
- Examination of the external ear reveals no **discharge** [8] or **erythema** [9] , and no **mastoid tenderness** [10] .
- Otoscopy demonstrates a normal **external auditory canal** [11] and a normal **tympanic membrane** [12] .
- **Weber test** [13] lateralises to the midline and **Rinne test** [13] is positive bilaterally.
- On anterior rhinoscopy there is no **discharge** [14] or **swelling** [14] .

- Oral examination reveals **two-finger trismus** [15] .
- A **bulging, non-pulsatile left soft palate** [16] [17] with a **deviated uvula** [18] to the right can be seen with **grade 3 tonsils** [19] bilaterally.
- The oropharynx is **erythematous** [20] but there is no **purulent exudate** [21] .
- There is no **floor of mouth, retropharyngeal or parapharyngeal swelling** [22] .
- **Dental hygiene** [23] is adequate.
- Neck examination demonstrates moderately **enlarged level II lymph nodes** [24] which are tender and mobile.
- There is no **stiffness or restricted neck movements** [25] .
- On palpation of the abdomen, there is no **hepatomegaly or splenomegaly** [26] .
- **Flexible nasoendoscopy** [27] is normal with no abnormalities detected and no **foreign bodies** [28] .

1 General inspection provides information regarding the patient's overall state of unwellness. Extreme discomfort may be correlated with a particularly unwell patient. It also provides insight into the urgency of the problem (i.e. a very unwell patient generally requires swifter diagnosis and management than a relatively well-looking patient).

2 Alertness and orientation are important to take note of. If a patient is drowsy and confused, this may be an indicator of severe sepsis and subsequent under-perfusion of end organs (e.g. the brain).

3 Drooling is a cardinal sign of epiglottitis and should alert the clinician to be extremely cautious. It represents a patient who is unable to tolerate swallowing their own saliva due to severe inflammation of the epiglottis, which may progress to rapid airway obstruction. If the diagnosis of epiglottitis is suspected, airway management is a priority, and should not be delayed for further flexible nasoendoscopy or imaging.

4 Tachycardia can be attributed to multiple aetiologies. In peritonsillar abscess, when tachycardia is present it is usually

secondary to infection or dehydration due to poor oral fluid intake. If due to dehydration, it is important to implement prompt fluid rehydration.

5 Blood pressure is an important vital sign when assessing the sick patient. Hypotension may represent septic shock due to inflammatory cytokines causing widespread peripheral vasodilation. This may be accompanied by warm peripheries (which is uncommon in other forms of shock). Hypotension may also be subsequent to severe dehydration. In either setting, identifying the issue and implementing timely management (e.g. fluid rehydration, antibiotics, vasopressors) is crucial.

6 Fever is a characteristic feature of most infections, including peritonsillar abscess.

7 Skin turgor, mucous membrane appearance and urine output are all indicators of overall fluid status. Dehydration is common in peritonsillar abscess due to the associated severe throat pain, leading to a reduced oral intake. Reduced urine output is a surrogate marker for reduced end-organ perfusion, and if present, other markers of reduced end-organ perfusion should be examined for (e.g. reduced mental status, cool peripheries, capillary refill time, chest pain, lactate levels).

8 Aural discharge in the presence of otalgia may indicate otitis externa or otitis media with perforated tympanic membrane.

9 Erythema of the external ear with otalgia may indicate pinna cellulitis or perichondritis.

10 Mastoid tenderness is an indicator of mastoiditis, an uncommon but potentially severe condition which usually arises from an otitis media.

11 The external auditory canal may demonstrate purulent discharge, erythema, swelling or fungal debris, all of which are indicators of otitis externa (bacterial or fungal).

12 The tympanic membrane (eardrum) is the lateral border of the middle ear. Abnormalities in the tympanic membrane (e.g. bulging, opacity, redness, bullae) may indicate a middle ear pathology such as otitis media.

13 The Weber and Rinne tests are complementary tests that are performed and interpreted in conjunction with each other. When interpreted accurately, these are fairly reliable screening tests for many ear pathologies causing hearing loss (either sensorineural or conductive).

14 Nasal discharge or swelling of the structures in the nasal cavity (e.g. the turbinates) may indicate an infective process such as sinusitis or a viral URTI. Whilst anterior rhinoscopy in the absence of nasal symptoms is not always necessary, it is part of a complete ENT examination.

15 Trismus is a hallmark sign of peritonsillar abscess due to inflammation of the pterygoid muscles (the muscles of mastication); however, it can also be present in other conditions.

16 A bulging soft palate is the classical finding in peritonsillar abscess (which usually collects superolaterally to the tonsil). The bulge is caused by the collection of pus developing in the potential peritonsillar space.

17 Although rare, internal carotid artery aneurysms or ectatic internal carotid arteries can cause a bulging in the parapharyngeal space and can appear similar to a peritonsillar abscess. Usually there will be an absence of infective symptoms (fever, chills, sore throat); however, there may still be aerodigestive symptoms related to the mass effect from the artery (e.g. dysphagia). The patient may have significant cardiovascular comorbidities or neurological manifestations related to decreased cerebrovascular perfusion.

18 The uvula often deviates to the contralateral side in peritonsillar abscess. This is caused by mass effect due to the swelling in the soft palate, and may sometimes be easier to appreciate compared to palatal swelling (which can be subtle).

19 Enlarged tonsils are common in tonsillitis (the precursor to peritonsillar abscess). Persistently enlarged tonsils may also play a factor in obstructive sleep apnoea (especially in younger children). Tonsil size is graded from grade I (smallest) to grade IV (largest).

20 Pharyngeal erythema indicates some element of pharyngitis (pharyngeal inflammation) of which tonsillitis is a specific, localised type.

21 Purulent exudate in the pharynx or tonsils (exudative pharyngitis/tonsillitis) is an indicator of infection (either viral or bacterial). Two common causes of exudative tonsillitis are EBV and group A beta-haemolytic streptococcus (GABHS).

22 Floor of mouth, parapharyngeal or retropharyngeal swelling point to a cause of sore throat that is not simply peritonsillar abscess (e.g. Ludwig's angina, parapharyngeal abscess, retropharyngeal abscess). If any of these are present, further investigation should be undertaken to exclude these conditions, as they can be serious and life-threatening.

23 Poor dental hygiene is a risk factor for peritonsillar abscess. Furthermore, poor dental hygiene is a nidus for a multitude of dental infections and abscesses that can cause sore throat and mimic peritonsillar abscess (e.g. retromolar abscess).

24 Enlarged lymph nodes are common secondary to infective processes in the head and neck, and these are usually tender and mobile. The tonsillar fossa is classically described as draining to the level II cervical nodes; however, it is not uncommon to have multiple enlarged cervical lymph nodes. Furthermore, the presence of cervical lymph nodes is not limited to peritonsillar abscess nor necessarily even an infective process, so their presence must be interpreted within the greater context of the patient's signs and symptoms.

25 Stiffness or restricted neck movements is not common for a simple peritonsillar abscess and indicates a possible alternative pathology, such as retropharyngeal abscess, or extension of the peritonsillar abscess into the parapharyngeal space.

26 Hepatomegaly and splenomegaly are common features of EBV infection (as are fatigue and malaise), which commonly causes tonsillitis.

27 Flexible nasoendoscopy is a simple, well-tolerated bedside examination that may be performed to better examine the nasopharynx, oropharynx, hypopharynx and larynx if an alternative pathology is suspected or needs to be excluded.

28 Foreign bodies can mimic a wide range of painful conditions depending on where the foreign body is trapped. Usually, however, this is accompanied by a fairly characteristic history of swallowing an object (e.g. chicken or fish bone) and immediately developing pain and the sensation of a foreign body.

Investigations

- FBE reports a significantly **increased WBC count** [1].
- **UEC results** [2] are normal.
- **LFT results** [3] are normal.
- **CRP is elevated** [4].
- **Antistreptolysin O titre (ASOT) is elevated** [5].
- **EBV serology** [6] and **monospot test** [7] is negative.
- **Throat culture** [8] demonstrates growth of GABHS.
- A **CT scan of the neck** [9] with contrast confirms a left superolaterally-based **rim-enhancing collection** [10] in the **peritonsillar space** [11] consistent with a peritonsillar abscess with bilateral enlarged level II cervical lymph nodes.
- There is no **parapharyngeal extension** [12].
- There is no **dental abscess** [13].
- There is no **internal jugular vein thrombophlebitis** [14].

[1] Infection and inflammation are common causes of an elevated WBC count. In this patient, the presence of peritonsillar abscess is the likely cause.

[2] UECs are important to identify reduced renal function. This may be as a result of dehydration or as a pre-existing condition and may be a contraindication for IV contrast with CT scanning. Furthermore, electrolyte imbalances are important to investigate in the setting of extended poor oral intake.

[3] Liver function tests are not routine when peritonsillar abscess is the main differential diagnosis; however, they should be considered if EBV tonsillitis is suspected, or if hepatomegaly or splenomegaly are present.

[4] C-reactive protein is an acute phase reactant that becomes elevated during inflammatory conditions. It is commonly raised in many infective conditions including peritonsillar abscess.

[5] ASOT is an antibody made against streptolysin O (an exotoxin produced by many species of streptococcus). An elevated ASOT is indicative of streptococcal infection, and in the presence of sore throat, likely indicates streptococcal pharyngitis (strep throat) or streptococcal tonsillitis.

[6] EBV serology measures both immunoglobulin M (IgM) and immunoglobulin G (IgG). Raised IgM indicates recent or current infection, whereas raised IgG indicates previous infection.

[7] Monospot test is a rapid test for active EBV infection. Although quick and highly specific, its sensitivity is only 70–92%, and thus it is not commonly used, with the EBV serology test taking its place.

[8] Although throat culture can accurately determine the causative bacterial agent of a pharyngeal infection, it is rarely used due to the high false negative rate and long culture time, and given the usually self-resolving nature of most causes of pharyngitis. In the setting of peritonsillar abscess, pus is usually easily obtained during the treatment process (aspiration or incision and drainage) which can be cultured if deemed necessary (in the majority of cases, the causative agents for peritonsillar abscesses are streptococci, in particular *Streptococcus pyogenes*). This may be useful in directing antimicrobial therapy.

[9] CT scan of the neck should always be performed with IV contrast if possible, for better soft tissue differentiation. It is the main imaging modality in suspected infective processes in the head and neck as X-ray does not provide a sufficiently detailed anatomical picture in most cases. CT is not routine in the investigation of peritonsillar abscess if the clinical picture is characteristic; however, clinicians should have a low threshold for imaging if an alternative pathology is suspected (e.g. other deep neck space infection, cervical lymphangitis, retained foreign body).

[10] The classical findings for an abscess on CT are a fluid collection with an enhancing rim during the IV contrast phase.

[11] The peritonsillar space is a potential space between the superior pharyngeal constrictor muscle laterally and the tonsillar capsule medially. Pus collects in this potential space in peritonsillar abscess.

[12] Simple peritonsillar abscesses are confined to the peritonsillar space; however, extension into other deep neck spaces is uncommon but possible, and can be potentially more dangerous. These spaces include the parapharyngeal space, submandibular space and the masticator space. Extension into these spaces may be suspected on clinical assessment; however, this should prompt the clinician to further investigate with CT imaging.

[13] Dental abscesses can commonly mimic peritonsillar abscess and can be differentiated through cross-sectional CT imaging.

[14] Internal jugular vein thrombophlebitis (Lemierre's syndrome) is a rare and potentially fatal complication of many deep neck space infections, including peritonsillar abscess. It usually presents with sore throat, fever and neck pain, and represents spread of infection to the internal jugular vein, resulting in possible distant infective thromboemboli, often to the lungs and joints. Lemierre's syndrome has a documented mortality rate of up to 10%.

Management

Immediate

Assess the airway [1] and ensure there are no signs of respiratory distress. Monitor **vital signs** [2] and urine output. Provide **analgesia** [3]. Obtain IV access and **administer antibiotics** [4]. Consider **IV fluid replacement** [5]. Consider administering a **corticosteroid anti-inflammatory** [6]. **Seek advice** [7] from the ENT team.

Short-term

Perform an **incision and drainage** [8]. Following the procedure, keep the patient in hospital for monitoring [9]. The patient should be encouraged to **eat and drink** [10]. If the patient is **haemodynamically stable, clinically improving and tolerating oral intake** [11], they may be discharged.

Long-term

Follow the patient up in an **outpatient clinic** [12]. Strongly consider booking the patient for an **elective tonsillectomy** [13] in several weeks, once the acute infection has resolved.

[1] Ensuring a patent airway is the first step when assessing all patients. It is a particularly important step when assessing any patient with a head and neck condition, and the clinician should take deliberate note of the presence of any signs of respiratory distress and address them first and foremost.

[2] Many severe infections can result in septic shock, which may be reflected in the vital signs by a hypotension, tachycardia and tachypnoea. A patient with unstable vital signs or vital signs outside of normal limits warrants closer monitoring and swifter management.

[3] Oropharyngeal inflammation (due to pharyngitis, tonsillitis or peritonsillar abscess) is particularly painful and analgesia is an important part of the immediate and short-term management. Unmanaged pain may cause tachycardia which may be misinterpreted as a worsening in clinical condition, or it may prevent the patient from adequate oral intake.

[4] IV antibiotics are a common immediate management in many infective conditions. Studies have shown that in patients presenting with sepsis, overall mortality increases significantly for every hour after the first hour that IV antibiotics are not administered. Whilst IV antibiotics alone are unlikely to be sufficient to manage a peritonsillar abscess, they will help prevent deterioration in the patient's overall clinical status due to septicaemia. Antibiotics should be targeted to the most common causative organisms; in the case of peritonsillar abscess, the most appropriate antibiotic is benzylpenicillin. If the patient is allergic to penicillin, clindamycin is an appropriate alternative.

[5] IV fluid replacement should be administered in most patients with peritonsillar abscess, as they are likely to be dehydrated due to the infection, and poor oral intake from odynophagia. Adequate hydration is important to prevent acute renal failure, as discussed above. It may also reduce the risk of contrast nephropathy if given before and after IV contrast administration.

[6] Corticosteroids provide good analgesic effect, may help improve trismus, and significantly reduce inflammation which may reduce the risk of airway obstruction. Dexamethasone is a commonly used corticosteroid in ENT.

[7] Peritonsillar abscess, whilst a relatively common presentation, is primarily an ENT surgery condition. Management should be directed by the ENT team, including antibiotic therapy, performing the incision and drainage, and ensuring post-procedure management and follow-up.

[8] Incision and drainage (or aspiration) is the mainstay of treatment in peritonsillar abscess (as with most other abscesses). This reduces the overall bacterial load and allows the IV antibiotics and the body's own immune system to treat the residual infection. The procedure is usually performed with local anaesthetic infiltration only, and is generally very well tolerated. Alternatively, a 'hot' tonsillectomy (with active infection) may be performed. This is generally undesirable as the surgery requires a general anaesthetic, is much more invasive, and significantly more difficult due to the active ongoing inflammation, leading to significantly increased risk of post-tonsillectomy bleeding. However, 'hot' tonsillectomy may be necessary if incision and drainage is unsuccessful due to patient non-compliance, poor access due to severe trismus, or difficult location of abscess.

[9] Monitoring is essential for all post-procedure patients to look for post-procedure complications. The length of monitoring is variable, and depends on the clinical status of the patient and the condition being treated. Although the definitive treatment has been performed (incision and drainage), the patient is still susceptible to sepsis, acute renal failure, or re-collection of the abscess warranting further action.

10 Ensuring the patient can eat and drink is an important step in the post-procedure clinical assessment. This is important to prevent dehydration and malnutrition in the short term. Failure to tolerate adequate oral intake may indicate insufficient analgesia or persistent collection that was not managed by the initial incision and drainage. Furthermore, the physical action of swallowing acts to massage the oropharyngeal tissues and continue to express any residual pus, helping to prevent re-collection.

11 If the patient remains haemodynamically stable, is clinically improving and is tolerating oral intake, they may be discharged (usually with a course of oral antibiotics). Most straightforward cases of peritonsillar abscess can be managed and discharged within 12–24 hours after the incision and drainage procedure.

12 Follow-up is integral to all surgical patients, and in particular those who have had an invasive procedure or operation. Follow-up aims to serve several purposes: ensuring the patient's acute illness has resolved, ensuring the patient has not suffered any late complication from the procedure, providing reassurance to the patient that the acute illness has resolved and finally providing a management plan for possible future events (e.g. recurrent peritonsillar abscess) or recommendations (e.g. tonsillectomy).

13 Strong consideration should be given to tonsillectomy for all patients presenting with peritonsillar abscess, as this will eliminate the possibility of further peritonsillar abscesses. The peritonsillar recurrence rate is between 10% and 20%, and the difficulty of the surgery increases significantly with each episode. This is due to inflammation and subsequent scarring of the tonsillar capsule which increases the post-tonsillectomy bleed rate. Whilst there is no strict guideline for adults regarding tonsillectomy following peritonsillar abscess, most clinicians would strongly consider it after the second episode of peritonsillar abscess. In those under 18 years of age, the Paradise criteria provide a good guideline for when tonsillectomy should be considered. Tonsillectomy can be performed in a number of ways including: cold steel, electrocautery (monopolar, bipolar), coblation, ultrasound/harmonic scalpel and microdebridement. It is most often performed as a day surgery or an overnight surgery, and is known for being particularly painful, especially in the 2-week postoperative period. The most significant complication of tonsillectomy is post-tonsillectomy bleeding, which may occur up to 2 weeks postoperatively and has an overall incidence of 5–15%. The bleeding may be significant and may require return to theatre, so any bleeding should be properly assessed, and the need for admission for monitoring should be considered.

CASE 19: Retropharyngeal abscess

History

- A 45-year-old male presents with a 4-day history of severe progressive **dysphagia and odynophagia** [1].
- He has associated **SOB** [2], **neck stiffness** [3], **fevers** [4] and **lethargy** [5].
- For the past week, he has recently had **nasal congestion, clear nasal discharge and sneezing** [6].
- He denies any **change in voice** [7], **otalgia** [8], **facial pain** [9], **headaches** [10] or **chest pain** [11].

- He denies any recent **dental surgery** [12], **ingested foreign body** [13] or other **trauma** [14].
- He has a past history of **type 2 diabetes mellitus (T2DM)** [15] and previous **tonsillectomy** [16].
- He has a **20 pack year smoking history** [17] and drinks **alcohol** [18] socially.
- He denies any **IV drug use** [19].

[1] The presenting features of retropharyngeal abscess depend highly on the primary cause of the infection. Severe dysphagia (difficulty swallowing) and odynophagia (painful swallowing) are common due to the swelling and inflammation of the posterior pharyngeal wall and subsequent irritation with each swallow. This can be so severe that the patient is unable to tolerate their own saliva, causing drooling.

[2] Shortness of breath can occur from a problem anywhere along the respiratory tract. When caused by a potential airway obstruction, this is usually a late and very concerning symptom indicating impending obstruction.

[3] Neck stiffness and pain on neck movements are usually only present in deep neck space infections that involve the neck. Neck stiffness may also be caused by meningitis (a potential complication of other deep neck space infections with spread to the CNS).

[4] Fevers are a feature of most infective processes (in particular bacterial). In this situation, the fever is likely due to the deep neck space abscess.

[5] Lethargy is a very non-specific symptom; however, it does provide information as to the severity of the condition. Extreme lethargy in any potentially infective condition is a poor sign.

[6] The presence of recent coryzal symptoms indicates a recent viral URTI. In the case of retropharyngeal abscess, a viral URTI usually acts as a precedent, causing inflammation of retropharyngeal lymph nodes and subsequent lymphadenitis. In rare cases, this develops into retropharyngeal abscess.

[7] If change in voice (dysphonia) is present, this may indicate quinsy (the classic 'hot potato' voice) or inflammation of the laryngeal structures (e.g. supraglottitis, laryngitis).

[8] Otalgia is not a common symptom of retropharyngeal abscess; however, it may be present due to the cause of the retropharyngeal abscess (e.g. otalgia from rhinosinusitis, foreign body) or it may indicate another pathology (e.g. tonsillitis).

[9] Retropharyngeal abscesses can either develop from direct spread (e.g. parapharyngeal space infection to retropharyngeal space infection) or from distant spread (e.g. rhinosinusitis or odontogenic infection with retropharyngeal lymphadenitis). Facial pain in the presence of retropharyngeal abscess usually is due to the primary infection, thus helping localise the initial infection that spread to the retropharyngeal space (e.g. parotid abscess).

[10] In the presence of neck stiffness, headaches may indicate meningitis (as a primary diagnosis or as a subsequent complication of a deep neck space infection).

[11] The retropharyngeal space extends into the superior mediastinum in the chest (the inferior extent being T2 vertebral body). Chest pain and shortness of breath in the context of retropharyngeal abscess may indicate mediastinitis. This generally presents with dyspnoea, pleuritic chest pain on deep breathing, tachycardia and hypoxia, and is a feared complication of retropharyngeal abscess.

[12] Recent dental surgery (and poor dental hygiene with chronic infection) is a common source of contamination for deep neck space infections. When implicated in retropharyngeal abscess, infection either needs to spread via multiple neck spaces along fascial planes or cause retropharyngeal lymphadenitis to reach the retropharyngeal space. A common scenario for spread would be lower molar tooth infection, to submandibular space infection, to parapharyngeal space infection, to retropharyngeal space infection.

13 Ingested or impacted foreign body (especially those that are sharp in nature) is an uncommon cause of retropharyngeal abscess caused by direct trauma to the posterior pharyngeal wall. This can also occur with recent instrumentation (e.g. endoscopy, intubation).

14 Other penetrating trauma to the head or neck can also rarely cause deep neck space infection (including retropharyngeal abscess). It is important to consider what microorganisms may be implicated (e.g. *Staphylococcus* spp.) if recent penetrating trauma has occurred, as skin flora differs largely from oral flora and this may direct antibiotic choice.

15 Diabetes is a risk factor for developing all types of bacterial infections due to the immunodeficiency from poorly functioning white blood cells. It is also a complicating factor in the management of any acute patient, requiring close monitoring of BGLs to prevent complications.

16 Quinsy (peritonsillar abscess) is the most common deep neck space infection and can rarely result in spread to the parapharyngeal space and subsequently the retropharyngeal space. In a patient with previous tonsillectomy, they theoretically are unable to develop a quinsy (although incomplete/subtotal tonsillectomy is possible).

17 Smoking increases peri-operative risk of all types and thus should be noted prior to any surgery. Furthermore, smoking is a strong risk factor for mucosal head and neck cancer (especially oral, oropharyngeal and laryngeal cancer). Although most deep neck space infections are caused by primary infections with spread to deep tissues, approximately 5% of deep neck space infections are caused by malignant necrotic lymph nodes with an asymptomatic primary tumour. This may especially be the case in patients with recurrent deep neck space infection.

18 Alcohol (as with smoking) is a strong risk factor for the development of mucosal head and neck cancer.

19 IV drug use (especially injecting into neck vessels) is a strong risk factor for a wide range of infections. It is important to ascertain when and where the drugs were injected, and also to consider the possibility of bloodborne diseases which may pose complications to the medical staff (if needle-stick injury is a risk, e.g. if surgery is required) or the patient (bloodborne diseases, e.g. HIV and hepatitis, cause immunodeficiency which may present with rapidly progressing illness or uncommon microbiology).

Examination

- The patient appears in **marked discomfort** [1] but is alert and oriented.
- Vital signs are unremarkable, particularly a **normal respiratory rate and SpO$_2$** [2].
- He has markedly increased **work of breathing** [3], with **tripod posturing** [4], **accessory muscle use** [5] and **supraclavicular retraction** [6].
- An audible **inspiratory stridor** [7] can be heard.
- Palpation of the neck and face reveals some **generalised neck tenderness** [8] but no **fluctuance** [9] and no **crepitus** [10].
- There is no swelling or purulent discharge on **examination of the ear** [11].
- There is no swelling or purulent discharge on **anterior rhinoscopy** [12], and no foreign body.
- On examination of the mouth there is **one-finger trismus** [13].
- The **floor of mouth** [14] is soft with no swelling.
- The **tongue is not protruding** [15].
- **Dentition** [16] is generally poor, but there is no **alveolar swelling** [17].
- **Bimanual palpation** [18] of Stensen's and Wharton's ducts expresses normal saliva with no purulent discharge.
- **Visualisation of the oropharynx** [19] reveals posterior pharyngeal wall erythema and swelling. The lateral pharyngeal walls look unremarkable.
- **Examination of the eye** [20] is unremarkable.
- **Cranial nerve examination** [21] demonstrates normal intact function of all cranial nerves.
- **Flexible nasoendoscopy** [22] reveals marked swelling of the posterior pharyngeal wall with 70% occlusion of the upper airway, and significant **pooling of saliva** [23] in the piriform fossa.
- **Vocal fold function** [24] is intact.
- **Auscultation of the heart** [25] reveals normal heart sounds with no murmurs, and **auscultation of the lungs** [26] is unremarkable.

1 General inspection provides information regarding the patient's overall state of unwellness. Extreme discomfort may be correlated with a particularly unwell patient. It also provides insight into the urgency of the problem (i.e. a very unwell patient generally requires swifter diagnosis and management than a relatively well-looking patient).

2 A normal respiratory rate and oxygen saturation does not exclude the possibility of airway obstruction and does not eliminate the need for airway assessment. Desaturation does not typically occur until the airway is completely occluded, and when desaturation from airway obstruction develops, the oxygen saturation drops rapidly.

3 Increased work of breathing should alert every clinician to the possibility of airway obstruction. Airway assessment and management become the first priority in managing this patient.

4 Tripod posturing (leaning forward and supporting the upper body with both hands) is a clear indicator of respiratory distress. It acts to increase air flow by taking advantage of accessory muscles of breathing.

5 Accessory muscle use is another indicator of respiratory distress. Muscles such as the sternocleidomastoid and the scalene muscles can be seen contracting in the neck with each inspiration to assist in elevating the ribcage and increasing air flow.

6 Supraclavicular retraction (along with intercostal and suprasternal retraction) is another indicator of respiratory distress. This is the indrawing of skin above the clavicle (or between ribs/above the sternum) caused by high negative intrathoracic pressure associated with heavy breathing.

7 Stridor is a high-pitched audible sound on respiration caused by turbulent air flow through the larger upper airways (compared with wheeze, which is generated in the lower airways). The phase of respiration in which the stridor is present (i.e. inspiratory, expiratory or biphasic) indicates where in the upper airway the obstruction is – inspiratory indicates obstruction above the vocal folds, expiratory indicates obstruction below and biphasic indicates obstruction at the level of the vocal folds. The presence of stridor should be taken seriously in every patient, and assessment of the airway and possible definitive management become the first priority. In the setting of retropharyngeal abscess, obstruction occurs above the level of the vocal folds in the pharyngeal soft tissues, thus causing an inspiratory stridor.

8 Palpation of the neck may elicit tenderness to one specific area, helping to localise the infection (e.g. right-sided neck tenderness may indicate a right parapharyngeal abscess as opposed to a retropharyngeal abscess). However, physical examination alone misidentifies the involved space and number of involved spaces in up to 70% of cases, and thus imaging is necessary to confirm any suspicions.

9 Fluctuance is rare on physical examination due to the deep nature of the fascial planes involved. If palpable, this may indicate a superficial component to the abscess.

10 Crepitus on palpation is indicative of subcutaneous emphysema. This air may originate from the airways (e.g. tracheal injury, traumatic pneumothorax) or may be secondary to gas-producing bacteria.

11 A quick otoscopic examination should be performed to look for swelling, erythema and purulent discharge (signs of infection). If absent, an ear infection can be essentially excluded from the list of differentials.

12 A quick rhinoscopic examination should also be performed to look for signs of infection and foreign body.

As with the otoscopic examination, if absent, a sinonasal infection can essentially be excluded.

13 Trismus (difficulty opening the mouth) is a sign of inflammation of the muscles of mastication (pterygoids, masseters) and is measured in fingerbreadths. Trismus can occur in multiple deep neck space infections (e.g. quinsy, masseteric space abscess, parapharyngeal abscess, retropharyngeal abscess) and can help detect if a deep neck space infection has spread to another compartment. For example, if a submandibular space abscess presents with trismus as well, this may indicate spread of infection of the parapharyngeal space.

14 The floor of the mouth contains three spaces – the sublingual space, the submandibular space and the submental space (known as the mandibular spaces). Infection of these spaces is usually due to dental infection or occasionally submandibular gland infection. If all three spaces bilaterally become infected, this is known as Ludwig's angina, and is characterised by gross swelling, and protrusion of the tongue.

15 Tongue protrusion (as seen in Ludwig's angina and other mandibular space abscesses) can quickly cause airway obstruction due to swelling and the posterior displacement of the tongue. If present, this can quickly proceed to death.

16 Poor dentition with apical infection is one of the commonest causes of deep neck space infections. The location of the infected tooth will determine the location of the deep neck space infection. Occasionally, these infections can be managed by tooth extraction and drainage of pus through the exposed root. However, if this is not possible, then surgical drainage must be achieved another way if necessary.

17 Alveolar swelling may indicate apical tooth infection or vestibular space abscess. If present, these should be addressed by the dental or oral and maxillofacial surgery team.

18 Bimanual palpation allows for palpation of the masticator and buccal spaces to assess for abscesses. It also allows palpation of the salivary glands and their ducts to examine for obstructed stones or purulent discharge indicating sialadenitis and possible salivary gland abscess.

19 Proper direct visualisation of the oropharynx is crucial when assessing a patient with odynophagia and airway distress. The clinician should make clear note of the posterior pharyngeal wall, the lateral pharyngeal walls, the tonsils and tonsillar pillars, any signs of inflammation (e.g. erythema, purulent discharge) as well as any asymmetry. Swelling and erythema of the posterior pharyngeal wall would indicate a pathology in the retropharyngeal space, consistent with a retropharyngeal abscess.

20 Deep neck space infections (particularly in the face) can occasionally spread to the orbits via the facial and ophthalmic veins. Thus, an orbital examination needs to be performed to rule out orbital inflammation of abscess. Painful ophthalmoplegia or absent light reflexes is a concerning sign and imaging with ophthalmological review is warranted.

21 Cranial nerve neuropathy is an uncommon complication of deep neck space abscesses. The particular cranial nerve involved will depend on the location of the infection. For example, parotid infections may involve the facial nerve, and parapharyngeal infections may involve the vagus nerve.

22 Visualisation of the upper airway is necessary in all patients with potential airway obstruction. This is usually performed with flexible nasoendoscopy. Similar to assessment of the oropharynx, clinicians should make clear note of the visible structures including the posterior and lateral pharyngeal walls, epiglottis, arytenoids, aryepiglottic folds, vocal folds and piriform fossa. Any pathology should be clearly documented, and if the airway is narrowed, a rough estimation of the remaining airway should be given.

23 Pooling of saliva is a common sign of severe odynophagia where it tends to pool in the piriform fossa,

and is seen in conditions such as retropharyngeal abscess, epiglottitis and supraglottitis.

24 In a normal patient, the vocal folds are the narrowest point in the upper airway. Visualising movement of the vocal folds serves to assess the recurrent laryngeal nerve (a branch of the vagus nerve) and also to ensure that any airway obstruction is not originating from the vocal folds themselves.

25 Certain deep neck space infections can extend into the thorax (e.g. retropharyngeal abscess) and even into the abdomen (e.g. danger space abscess, prevertebral space abscess). When extension into the thorax occurs, the main concern is mediastinitis (infection of the mediastinum), which can lead to severe sepsis and cardiac tamponade.

26 Assessment of the lungs is an important part of the peri-operative work-up to screen for any pathologies. Furthermore, in patients with dysphagia, inadvertent aspiration is common and can lead to aspiration pneumonia, complicating management of the patient.

Investigations

- FBE reports a **moderately raised WCC** [1].
- UEC is normal. **CRP is raised** [2]. BGL is 8.5mmol/L.
- **Orthopantomogram (OPG) X-ray** [3] reveals no apical lucencies or salivary stones.
- **Lateral neck X-ray** [4] demonstrates thickening of the prevertebral tissues at levels C2–C7.
- **CXR** [5] demonstrates normal lung fields with no aspiration pneumonia and no mediastinal gas.
- On **CT of the head and neck with IV contrast** [6], **soft tissue swelling** [7] with **a rim-enhancing** [8]

collection with **air–fluid level** [9] is seen in the retropharyngeal space extending from C1 to T2.
- Small bilateral **cervical lymphadenopathy** [10] without **necrosis** [11] can be seen.
- **MRI of the head and neck** [12] reveals no intracranial infection and no **internal jugular vein thrombus** [13].

[1] Infection and inflammation are common causes of an elevated WBC count. In this patient, the presence of retropharyngeal abscess is the likely cause.

[2] CRP is an acute phase reactant that becomes elevated during inflammatory conditions. It is commonly raised in many infective conditions including retropharyngeal abscess.

[3] OPG X-ray is a common radiograph to examine the teeth and alveolar processes. It has the benefit of being quick and easy and is relatively good at detecting dental root infections. However, if a collection is suspected, a CT is indicated to delineate the location of the abscess and surrounding anatomy. As a side benefit to OPG, occasionally salivary stones (>5mm) can be seen as well.

[4] Lateral neck X-rays are useful for a quick assessment of the upper aerodigestive tract to screen for retropharyngeal abscess or epiglottitis. Thickening of the prevertebral tissues

(defined as prevertebral tissue thickness >7mm at C2 or >2cm at C7 in adults) is indicative of retropharyngeal abscess. Thickening of the epiglottis (known as thumbprint sign) can also occasionally be seen on lateral X-ray and indicates epiglottitis (more common in children) or supraglottitis (more common in adults).

[5] CXR is important to rule out aspiration related to dysphagia or descending mediastinitis secondary to the retropharyngeal abscess. The classic features of aspiration on CXR are consolidation in the right middle or lower lobes. Features of mediastinitis on CXR include mediastinal gas and mediastinal widening. The presence of mediastinitis is a poor prognostic sign, and cardiothoracic surgery involvement is necessary to consider thoracotomy and open drainage. Mediastinitis itself has a mortality of 30–40%.

[6] CT with IV contrast is the standard imaging modality for all deep neck space infections. It is almost always indicated,

as clinical assessment alone is extremely unreliable (physical examination alone misidentifies the involved space and number of spaces in 70% of cases). CT with IV contrast provides excellent anatomical detail, allows the clinician to localise the primary infection and any involved neck spaces, and also assists in surgical approach and planning.

7 Soft tissue swelling in the retropharyngeal space is a sign of inflammation secondary to infection.

8 Although CT is an excellent imaging modality in deep neck space infections, CT alone does not reliably differentiate between phlegmon (inflammatory oedematous tissue) and abscess collection, and both conditions may have rim enhancement.

9 An air–fluid level is a reliable sign of a fluid (pus) collection (as opposed to a phlegmon). Definitive evidence of purulent abscess formation is an absolute indication for surgical exploration and drainage.

10 Cervical lymphadenopathy is common and likely reactive in any head and neck infection. If detected, it should be followed up with repeat imaging (ultrasound is appropriate) once the acute infection has resolved, to ensure the cervical lymphadenopathy has also resolved. If lymphadenopathy is persistent despite resolved infection, this should be further investigated.

11 Necrotic lymph nodes may be secondary to a simple primary infection (e.g. lymphadenitis) but occasionally occur as a result of malignancy, other rare pathology (e.g. TB), or are actually congenital cysts (e.g. branchial cleft cyst). When necrotic lymph nodes are detected, the clinician should consider the possible differentials, and excisional biopsy may be warranted.

12 MRI of the head and neck is not routinely used in deep neck space infections. Obtaining an MRI is often time-consuming and less likely to be tolerated in patients having trouble maintaining their airway (especially supine). It does, however, provide superior information in select circumstances (e.g. suspected CNS involvement such as intracranial infection or prevertebral infection, assessing neck vessels with MR angiography).

13 Internal jugular vein thrombophlebitis (Lemierre's syndrome) is a rare and potentially fatal complication of many deep neck space infections, including retropharyngeal abscess. It usually presents with sore throat, fever and neck pain, and represents spread of infection to the internal jugular vein, resulting in possible distant infective thromboemboli, often to the lungs and joints. Lemierre's syndrome has a documented mortality rate of up to 10%.

Management

Immediate

Assess the airway [1] and determine the need for **definitive airway management** [2]. **Avoid positioning the patient** [3]. Administer **supplemental oxygen** [4] and **nebulised adrenaline** [5]. Obtain IV access and administer **IV corticosteroids** [6], **IV antibiotics** [7] and **IV fluid rehydration** [8]. **Admit the patient to ICU** [9]. **Monitor vital signs and urine output** [10]. **Keep the patient fasted** [11]. **Seek advice** [12] from the ENT team.

Short-term

Perform a **surgical drainage of the abscess** [13] and **culture of fluid** [14]. Following the procedure, keep the patient in hospital for **monitoring** [15]. **Auscultate the lungs** [16]. **Review the surgical site** [17] and **re-examine the oral cavity and reperform flexible nasoendoscopy** [18]. **Reassess the swallow** [19]. **The patient may be discharged** [20] if they have been extubated, vital signs remain stable, the patient can tolerate oral intake, and if a drain was inserted, the drain output is negligible and can be removed.

Long-term

Follow up [21] the patient in the outpatient clinic if necessary for continuing wound management and monitoring for postoperative complications.

1 Assessment of the airway is the first step in managing any patient. In most patients, this will be as simple as confirming that the patient can speak and that there are no signs of respiratory distress or airway obstruction. In the case of this patient with retropharyngeal abscess, there is clear evidence of respiratory distress and possible airway obstruction. In these circumstances, a more comprehensive airway assessment must be undertaken – this usually includes flexible nasoendoscopy to visualise the airway and review by either the ENT team or anaesthetics team, or preferably both.

2 Once a compromised airway has been discovered, the need for a definitive airway must be assessed. This should occur before any other intervention and should not be delayed by imaging or other investigations. A definitive airway is defined as a tube placed in the trachea with a cuff inflated below the vocal folds. This is most often an awake fibre-optic ETT; however, uncommonly a tracheostomy will be required. Whether a definitive airway will be required should be a discussion between the ENT surgery team, the anaesthetic team and the intensive care team, and will depend on the clinical state of the patient, the extent of airway obstruction and the likely plan for management. The plan for definitive airway should include where the attempted insertion will take place (e.g. operating theatre vs. ED), who will be available, what airway will be attempted first, who will make the attempt (the anaesthetist vs. ENT surgeon) and what the back-up plan is (usually emergency cricothyroidotomy and proceeding directly to tracheostomy).

3 In cases of airway obstruction, patients often adopt the tripod posture (leaning forward and supporting the upper body with both hands) and the 'sniffing the morning air' position (flexion of the neck at the cervicothoracic junction and extension at the atlantoaxial junction – this aligns the oral cavity, pharynx and larynx, allowing for the least turbulent flow of air). The patient should never be positioned against their will, as this may cause complete airway obstruction (this includes lying flat for CT scan).

4 Supplemental oxygen is necessary even in patients with normal saturation on air, as airway compromise can occur rapidly, and desaturation is a late sign of airway obstruction.

5 Nebulised adrenaline acts to reduce upper airway oedema by causing vasoconstriction. It is an effective airway management tool in the short to medium term, and is often used in conjunction with corticosteroids.

6 IV corticosteroids act to reduce oedema of the upper airway and increase airway patency. Dexamethasone is a commonly used corticosteroid in ENT.

7 IV antibiotics are a common immediate management in many infective conditions. Studies have shown that in patients presenting with sepsis, overall mortality increases significantly for every hour after the first hour that IV antibiotics are not administered. Antibiotics should be targeted to the most common causative organisms; in the case of retropharyngeal abscess, most infections are polymicrobial with a combination of Gram-positive and Gram-negatives without anaerobes. An appropriate empirical antibiotic is intravenous amoxycillin and clavulanic acid.

8 Many patients with deep neck space abscesses become dehydrated due to poor oral intake from severe odynophagia. Furthermore, many patients are relatively intravascularly depleted due to the widespread vasodilatory effects of circulating inflammatory cytokines. Dehydration may result in acute kidney injury or hypovolaemic shock, adding complications to an already severe infection. Most patients will benefit from 1–2L of crystalloid infusion.

9 Whether or not a definitive airway is placed, all potential airway patients should be monitored in a critical care setting until the risk of airway compromise is resolved. This can be in the ED for the initial assessment but is usually the ICU for ongoing monitoring. The ICU provides close nursing and staff trained in airway skills, should the patient suddenly become obstructed.

10 Monitoring the vital signs and urine output provides an indication of the patient's clinical progress, especially in sedated and intubated patients where history taking is impossible, and clinical examination of the oropharynx is extremely difficult.

11 Keeping the patient fasted is crucial in the preoperative management of the patient. It reduces the risk of aspiration in the setting of anaesthesia. Ideally, patients should be fasted off solid foods for 6 hours prior to anaesthetic. In the emergency setting and if time critical, RSI is an alternative to reduce the risk of aspiration (especially so in patients who are not fasted).

12 Retropharyngeal abscess is managed by the ENT team and care (including airway management and surgical drainage) should be directed by them.

13 Although surgical drainage is not always required (in mild infections), it is often necessary. The following circumstances should be absolute indications for surgical drainage: when air–fluid level or gas-producing organisms are present, when airway obstruction is a concern, or when there is no improvement after 48–72 hours of empirical antibiotics. The surgical approach to drainage can be either transoral or transcervical, depending on the location of the abscess. Occasionally, both will be used together to facilitate better drainage. A surgical drain may be left to encourage ongoing drainage.

14 Infected pus or fluid should be cultured to advise antibiotic therapy. The presence of MRSA or other resistant organisms will often indicate a change in antibiotic therapy (e.g. adding vancomycin) and a possible extended duration. Antibiotic choices in infections with complicated microbiology will often be guided by the infectious diseases team.

15 Monitoring is essential for all post-procedure patients to look for post-procedure complications. The length of monitoring is variable, and depends on the clinical status of the patient and the condition being treated. Although the definitive treatment has been performed (incision and drainage), the patient is still susceptible to sepsis, acute renal failure, or re-collection of the abscess warranting further action.

16 Following placement of a definitive airway, a phenomenon known as post-obstructive pulmonary oedema may occur. This is characterised by frothy airway secretions and increased peak airway pressures. Continually assessing the lungs will allow for early detection and management.

Most cases will typically resolve with diuresis and positive pressure mechanical ventilation.

17 Review the surgical site to assess for ongoing drainage. Once the cavity has been fully drained (evidenced by minimal ongoing drain tube outputs), the drain tube can be removed. If the surgical drainage site closes prematurely, this may cause re-collection and may indicate the need for reoperation.

18 Regular examination of the oral cavity and flexible nasoendoscopy are necessary to monitor the swelling and airway obstruction to ensure resolution.

19 Swallow should be assessed (either by bedside testing or with formal assessment by speech pathologists) prior to reinstatement of oral intake. This is to ensure that risk of aspiration has resolved.

20 The patient may be discharged once they have been extubated, vital signs remain stable, and they can tolerate oral intake, and if a drain was inserted, the drain output is negligible and can be removed. Given the severe nature of these infections, many patients will require up to a week or longer in hospital before being deemed well enough to be discharged.

21 Follow-up is integral to all surgical patients, and in particular those who have had an invasive procedure or operation. Follow-up aims to serve several purposes: ensuring the patient's acute illness has resolved, ensuring the patient has not suffered any late complication from the procedure (e.g. poor wound healing, re-collection of abscess, persistent dysphagia), providing reassurance to the patient that the acute illness has resolved and finally, providing a management plan for possible future events. Recurrent events of deep neck space infections should be thoroughly investigated, and any pathology discovered during the acute infection (e.g. cervical lymphadenopathy, poor dentition) should be addressed.

CASE 20: Thyroid cancer

History

- A **67-year-old** [1] **Caucasian** [2] **female** [3] presents to the **outpatient department** [4] with a **3-month history** [5] of a lump in the neck.
- The lump is located **anteriorly** [6] and is **painless** [7].
- She also complains of some recent **hoarseness of voice** [8] and **dysphagia** [9], with some occasional **aspiration** [10].
- She denies any recent **change in weight** [11], **change in appetite** [12], **heat or cold intolerance** [13], **odynophagia** [14] or **dyspnoea** [15].

- She has a past history of **breast cancer** [16] 10 years ago, but denies past history of **radiation exposure** [17], or **multiple endocrine neoplasia (MEN) syndrome** [18].
- She has no notable **family history** [19].
- She has a **15 pack year smoking history** [20] and **drinks alcohol socially** [21].

1 Unlike most malignancies, in differentiated thyroid cancer (e.g. not anaplastic thyroid cancer) age is an independent predictor of prognosis and is incorporated into the American Joint Committee on Cancer (AJCC) staging guidelines.

2 Thyroid cancer is more prevalent in Caucasian and Asian patients.

3 Thyroid cancer has a 3:1 female to male predilection. The reason for this is not fully known.

4 Most thyroid cancers and other neck masses will not present acutely to the ED. For this reason, it is important to assess patients comprehensively, and order all necessary investigations in a timely manner to avoid diagnostic and management delays which can worsen prognosis.

5 Thyroid cancers (as with most cancers) often present with a slow, insidious history of onset, compared to acute conditions. However, rapid onset associated with a tumour is an ominous sign.

6 Thyroid tumours often present as a palpable neck mass as the only symptom. If this is located anteriorly, it is usually the primary thyroid tumour. If presenting with a lateral neck mass, this may indicate a nodal metastasis or alternative neck mass (e.g. branchial cleft cyst, parotid tumour).

7 Thyroid malignancies are usually painless, compared to neck masses of reactive/infective origin (e.g. reactive lymph nodes, infected cysts).

8 Hoarseness of voice is a very nebulous and poorly defined term that will have different meanings to different patients. This should prompt the clinician to further clarify what the patient means by "hoarse". In the setting of a neck mass, there should be significant concern for mass effect

causing compression and palsy of the recurrent laryngeal nerve, or a tumour of the larynx/pharynx directly affecting functions of the vocal fold.

9 Dysphagia is a non-specific symptom that can arise in many acute and subacute conditions presenting in the head and neck region. The concern in this case is that a mass may be causing significant mass effect to alter the patient's swallow.

10 The primary function of the vocal folds is to protect the airway and prevent aspiration, with phonation being a secondary function. Occasional aspiration in this situation gives the clinician insight into the possibility that the vocal folds may be compromised, either due to recurrent laryngeal nerve palsy or due to mass effect directly to the vocal folds themselves.

11 Weight change may be indicative of over-/underactive thyroid disease, or may be a symptom of malignancy.

12 Change in appetite may also be indicative of over-/underactive thyroid disease, or may be a symptom of malignancy.

13 Heat or cold intolerance may be indicative of over-/underactive thyroid disease.

14 Odynophagia (together with dysphagia) should alert the clinician to a potential pharyngeal issue. Malignancy would be of particular concern in a patient presenting with dysphagia, odynophagia and a palpable neck mass.

15 Dyspnoea due to a neck mass is extremely concerning for a compromised airway. Although rare, advanced malignancy of the thyroid or other head and neck tumours can occasionally expand or erode into the airway, causing obstruction. If this is discovered in the outpatient setting, strong consideration should be made toward admitting the patient directly to hospital and taking steps to secure the airway (either through a debulking procedure or other definitive airway).

16 Breast cancer survivors (especially those diagnosed at a younger age, and those diagnosed in the past 5 years) have a higher risk of thyroid cancer. The reason for this is still being investigated.

17 Radiation exposure (especially at a young age) is a well documented risk factor for thyroid cancer (in particular papillary and follicular). This includes any previous therapeutic radiation (e.g. radiation therapy for some forms of lymphoma).

18 MEN syndrome is a syndrome presenting with tumours of endocrine glands. These are inherited in an autosomal dominant fashion and include head and neck tumours such as parathyroid hyperplasia (MEN I, MEN IIa) and medullary thyroid cancer (MEN IIa and MEN IIb).

19 Family history plays an important role in any head and neck tumour, and particularly in thyroid cancer.

Approximately 25% of medullary thyroid cancer cases have a genetic cause (often linked to the RET proto-oncogene), and are identified as familial medullary thyroid cancer. Furthermore, family history of precancerous polyps in the colon increases the risk of papillary thyroid cancer.

20 Smoking is a risk factor for many tumours of the head and neck, particularly mucosal SCCs. Interestingly, some studies have shown that smoking reduces the incidence of thyroid cancers, although the reason for this is unknown. Besides this, smoking places most patients at a higher peri-operative risk (through its associated lung conditions) and postoperative complication risk (e.g. poorer wound healing, higher risk of postoperative wound infections and hospital-acquired infections), making this something to consider when counselling patients regarding their options.

21 Alcohol intake is also a risk factor for mucosal SCC. If dependency or liver disease is present, this can create issues surrounding peri-operative risk and postoperative care (e.g. managing withdrawal).

Examination

- The patient appears **comfortable** [1] and **appropriately dressed** [2].
- There are **no signs of respiratory distress** [3]. Vital signs are unremarkable.
- **Auscultation of the heart** [4] reveals normal heart sounds with no added sounds.
- **Auscultation of the lungs** [5] reveals normal vesicular breath sounds.
- Examination of the neck reveals a **3cm anterior neck mass** [6] in the left lobe of the thyroid.
- It is **non-tender and firm** [7] but is **not fixed** [8] to the trachea or overlying skin.
- The mass does **not move on protrusion of the tongue** [9].

- There are bilateral palpable, **non-tender and enlarged level III cervical lymph nodes** [10].
- Examination of the ear, nose and throat reveals no abnormality.
- On flexible nasoendoscopy, the **left vocal fold is paralysed** [11] in a **lateral position** [12], although the right is mobile. There is no other abnormality on flexible nasoendoscopy, no visible mass and the airway looks patent.
- On assessment, the patient's voice is **weak and breathy** [13].

1 General inspection provides information regarding the patient's overall state of unwellness. Often malignancy will present slowly and insidiously, in an otherwise well-looking patient.

2 A patient's clothing may indicate cold or heat intolerance – a clue to possible under-/overactive thyroid.

3 Respiratory distress (e.g. stridor, accessory muscle use) may indicate a potential or partially obstructed airway. Whilst most patients presenting with a neck mass do not have a threatened airway, if there is significant narrowing of the airway due to mass effect, there is a possibility of acute obstruction. Thus, it is important to address this issue

immediately to prevent an airway emergency situation. This usually would indicate a direct admission to hospital.

4 Auscultation of the heart is important to assess for potential cardiac abnormalities (e.g. valvular heart disease) that may pose a significant peri-operative risk. If abnormalities are discovered on cardiac examination, these should be investigated where pertinent to identify the cause (as they may impact on the patient's fitness for surgery, or they may need to be addressed prior to surgery).

5 Auscultation of the lungs is important to assess for evidence of pulmonary disease. In this patient's situation, recurrent aspiration may lead to infective changes that need to be addressed. It is also of particular importance in smokers, where COPD is extremely common, which significantly affects peri-operative fitness.

6 Anterior neck masses are likely to be related to the thyroid (e.g. thyroid malignancy, thyroid nodule, thyroglossal cysts). The size and location of the neck mass is crucial to assess and document accurately. This allows for contrasting and comparing between clinicians' assessments, which provides further insight into the progress of the condition (e.g. is the lump enlarging? Are there multiple lumps?).

7 Thyroid malignancy is typically non-tender and firm (as opposed to an infected cyst which is usually tender and fluctuant).

8 Fixation of a lump to overlying or underlying tissues can be an ominous sign. This indicates loss of tissue planes between structures and in the case of thyroid malignancy, implies extrathyroidal extension into either the trachea, strap muscles or other surrounding structures. According to the 2018 AJCC guidelines, this is automatically T category T3 and above (on TNM staging), a relatively advanced T stage.

9 Movement of a thyroid lump on protrusion of the tongue is a hallmark sign of a thyroglossal cyst. This remnant congenital cyst sits posterior to the body of the hyoid bone and represents the embryological tract (from the base of tongue to the anterior neck) along which the thyroid tissue descends. It is a benign condition and can be surgically removed (Sistrunk procedure).

10 As above, tenderness of lateral cervical lymph-adenopathy usually indicates inflammation due to an infective process. In the head and neck, enlarged lymph nodes are generally defined as diameter >10mm. Non-tender lymphadenopathy is more consistent with malignancy with lymph node metastases.

11 The recurrent laryngeal nerve (a branch of the vagus nerve) travels in the tracheo-oesophageal groove adjacent to the thyroid gland. Loss of function of this nerve causes paralysis of the ipsilateral vocal fold (thus causing dysphonia). This loss of function is an uncommon but significant feature to identify – it may simply be due to mass effect impinging the nerve, or it may signify tumour invasion into the nerve (perineural invasion), which is associated with a poorer prognosis. Furthermore, this may have implications on the surgery performed (as the recurrent laryngeal nerve may need to be resected to gain clear oncological margins) and thus how the patient is counselled and consented.

12 The vocal fold can sit in several positions when paralysed and these will have different corresponding features on assessment which will give clues as to the position prior to visualisation. When sitting laterally, there is no apposition of the two vocal folds, producing a weak and breathy voice and placing the patient at risk of aspiration. When sitting in a midline position, good vocal fold apposition can be achieved, producing a fairly normal voice; however, the airway is permanently narrowed, and may cause stridor or respiratory distress. In the paramedian position, there may be a mix of symptoms, and the voice may become strained, as the hypopharynx and contralateral vocal fold attempt to compensate for lack of glottal (vocal fold) closure.

13 A weak and breathy voice in this patient reflects the position of the left vocal fold (in the lateral position). Although there are procedures to assist this issue (e.g. medialisation thyroplasty), this is best addressed electively and at a later date, after more concerning issues have fully been resolved. (i.e. the thyroid mass).

Investigations

- **FBE** [1] is unremarkable. **UEC** [1] results demonstrate normal electrolytes and an eGFR of 80ml/min/1.73m^2.
- **Coagulation studies** [2] are within normal limits.
- **Thyroid function tests** [3] are within normal limits.
- **Serum calcitonin** [4] and **serum carcinoembryonic antigen (CEA)** [5] levels are very high.
- **Serum calcium** [6] is normal.
- **Parathyroid hormone levels** [7] are normal.
- CXR reveals **mildly hyperexpanded lung fields** [8] but **no masses** [9].
- **Pulmonary function tests (PFTs)** [10] reveal a post-bronchodilator FEV$_1$/FVC ratio of 0.62 (with FEV$_1$ 85% predicted).
- **Radioactive iodine uptake test** [11] shows normal even uptake.

- On **ultrasound of the neck** [12], a 4.1cm solid, hypoechoic smooth mass with microcalcifications can be seen in the left lobe of the thyroid.
- **CT of the head and neck with IV contrast** [13] confirms the thyroid mass.
- There is no **extrathyroidal extension** [14] into the surrounding strap muscles or trachea.
- Prominent **cervical lymph nodes** [15] are seen bilaterally in level III and IV, and in level VI.
- **Fine needle aspiration and cytology** [16] is performed at the time of the ultrasound, confirming a diagnosis of **medullary thyroid carcinoma** [17].
- **PET scan** [18] shows marked avidity in the left thyroid mass and the corresponding cervical lymphadenopathy, but is negative for **distant metastases** [19].

1 In this situation, where the patient may require surgical management, it is important to ensure they are not anaemic or thrombocytopenic and do not have pre-existing renal impairment, all of which pose a potential peri-operative risk and need to be addressed prior to surgical intervention.

2 Abnormalities found on coagulation studies (along with platelet count) are important in any surgery with high intraoperative and postoperative bleeding risk (e.g. thyroidectomy) and need to be addressed prior to surgery. An INR of <1.4 and platelets of >100 x 10⁹/L is generally considered safe for surgery, although this will vary depending on surgeon, patient and type of operation.

3 The thyroid gland is responsible for producing thyroid hormone under the influence of thyroid-stimulating hormone (TSH) on a negative feedback loop. Some conditions (e.g. multinodular goitre) may produce thyroid nodules/ lumps that excessively secrete thyroid hormone, resulting in hyperthyroidism, or predispose patients to developing thyroid cancers (e.g. Graves' disease). However, malignant thyroid masses generally do not cause hyperthyroidism, thus thyroid function tests would be normal.

4 Calcitonin is a hormone produced by the C cells in the thyroid and is responsible for reducing serum calcium (in opposition to parathyroid hormone). In humans, it has a weak effect and does not need to be replaced upon removal of the thyroid gland. As medullary thyroid cancer also originates from C cells, this causes calcitonin levels to rise.

5 CEA is also produced by medullary thyroid cancer cells and can be used as a screening tool for recurrent disease. A baseline value is recommended as part of the additional work-up of medullary thyroid cancer.

6 Although serum calcitonin levels are high in patients with medullary thyroid cancer, this usually does not translate into low serum calcium levels, due to calcitonin's weak activity in the human body, and also the systemic resistance to high calcitonin levels.

7 The parathyroid glands (four in total) sit posterior to the thyroid gland, and can be very difficult to differentiate from thyroid tissue. What is initially thought to be a thyroid nodule may in fact be a very rare parathyroid carcinoma (which may result in hyperparathyroidism). Generally, this would be accompanied by high serum calcium levels due to high parathyroid hormone levels.

8 Hyperexpanded lung fields is consistent with a diagnosis of COPD due to a long-standing history of smoking. This should prompt the clinician to consider PFTs to assess the patient's fitness for surgery and peri-operative risk.

9 Pulmonary masses on CXR need to be investigated further as part of the peri-operative work-up of the patient. In this setting, this may be due to metastasis of tumour to the mediastinal lymph nodes; however, in the setting of known long-standing smoking history, it may represent a primary lung tumour.

10 PFTs are a useful investigation to assess lung function and to stratify peri-operative risk for patients undergoing long, invasive surgery. It is especially important in this patient, given her long smoking history and no known diagnosis of lung disease. Post-bronchodilator FEV_1/FVC ratio of <0.70 is consistent with an obstructive defect that does not respond to bronchodilators (i.e. COPD). FEV_1 85% predicted indicates a mild level of obstruction (according to GOLD criteria).

11 Radioactive iodine uptake test is a nuclear medicine imaging modality using a radioisotope of iodine and measuring uptake of iodine into the thyroid at a later interval. The uptake amount and evenness help to identify any areas that are hyper- or hypofunctional. In this setting, although a lump in the left lobe is palpable, the radioactive iodine uptake test shows no abnormal uptake, indicating that the lump is not overactive (i.e. a 'cold' nodule) which would be consistent with a diagnosis of malignancy.

12 Ultrasound is a useful and easy-to-access first-line investigation for all thyroid masses. It provides decent anatomical information, given the thyroid's relatively superficial location on the neck. Thyroid nodules can be described using the TI-RADS reporting system (a useful systematic reporting system recommended by the American College of Radiology). This patient scores 5 points, for an overall TI-RADS category of TR4 (solid – 2, hypoechoic – 2, smooth – 0, microcalcifications – 1), which indicates need for further biopsy (via FNA) if >1.5cm in diameter. The risk of malignancy has also been validated using the TI-RADS scale (TR4 has a 9.1% malignancy rate).

13 CT with IV contrast (or MRI with IV contrast) provides further cross-sectional detail and may provide important information about deeper structures which may be difficult to visualise on ultrasound (e.g. extrathyroidal extension, presence of level VII nodes). CT imaging is not always necessary for all thyroid masses, as ultrasound is generally very good.

14 Extrathyroidal extension is a poor prognostic marker if seen on imaging. It indicates spread of a tumour outside of the thyroid glandular tissue and into surrounding structures (e.g. surrounding strap muscles, trachea, connective tissue) and indicates a T category of at least T3 (on TNM staging).

15 The presence of prominent lymph nodes on imaging indicates lymph node metastases (another poor prognostic marker). If present, this necessitates incorporating a neck dissection (clearing the cervical lymph nodes) into the surgical plan to gain oncological clearance, significantly increasing the morbidity of the procedure.

16 FNA is a first-line investigation for thyroid masses (as well as most other neck lumps including cysts and lymphadenopathy). It is a relatively well tolerated and low risk procedure that can be performed under ultrasound guidance, and provides histological sample to confirm a suspected diagnosis. According to meta-analysis, FNA has an overall accuracy of 93.1% in neck masses of all types.

[17] Medullary thyroid carcinoma is a subtype of thyroid cancer and makes up approximately 3% of thyroid cancers. It is the third most common subtype of thyroid cancer (behind follicular and papillary thyroid cancer). It is associated with a poorer prognosis than follicular or papillary thyroid cancer, but better than anaplastic thyroid cancer, with an overall 5-year survival rate of 80–90%.

[18] PET scan (either with FDG or Ga-68 DOTATATE in the setting of medullary thyroid cancer) is a highly sensitive scan for thyroid malignancy. Its use in primary thyroid malignancy is limited to detecting asymptomatic metastases in patients at high risk of metastatic disease (either due to cancer type or staging).

[19] Distant metastases indicate late stage disease in thyroid cancer, and if present, rule out the possibility of a surgical clearance. In this situation, radiotherapy, chemotherapy or immunotherapy become first-line options, with palliative surgical debulking becoming an option.

Management

Immediate

Assess the airway [1] and ensure there are no signs of respiratory distress. Assess the patient for peri-operative fitness [2] and organise any necessary supplementary investigations [3] in a timely manner. Screen for other associated conditions [4]. Seek advice [5] from the ENT team or the endocrine surgery team. Counsel the patient [6] regarding the diagnosis and their options.

Short-term

Present the case at a head and neck or thyroid cancer MDT meeting [7]. Perform a total thyroidectomy [8] with anterior and bilateral neck dissection [9]. Following the procedure, monitor the patient [10] for postoperative complications. Reassess the voice [11]. Start the patient on thyroxine replacement therapy [12]. Monitor the calcium and PTH levels [13]. The patient may be discharged if the vitals remain stable and there are no signs of postoperative complications [14].

Long-term

Re-present the patient at the MDT meeting [15]. Follow up the patient in the outpatient clinic regularly [16]. Depending on the final histopathology and staging, consider adjuvant radiotherapy [17]. Monitor TSH levels and adjust thyroxine replacement dose [18] as necessary. Monitor for recurrence with regular assessments and calcitonin levels and CEA levels.

[1] Ensuring a patent airway is the first step when assessing all patients. It is a particularly important step when assessing any patient with a head and neck mass, and the clinician should take deliberate note of the presence of any signs of respiratory distress and address them first.

[2] The mainstay of treatment of the majority of malignancies is surgical resection, and this is also true of thyroid malignancies. Consciously assessing peri-operative fitness during the first assessment is a good habit for all surgical clinicians to develop.

[3] Whilst supplementary investigations may not be necessary in all cases, often they are required to ensure that a surgical operation can be performed safely (e.g. investigating lung function with PFTs prior to general anaesthetic) and also to ensure that certain specific aspects of a condition can be investigated. In the setting of medullary thyroid carcinoma, 25% of medullary thyroid carcinoma is associated with a RET proto-oncogene mutation (which is inheritable) – thus the patient and their family should be screened for this mutation.

[4] Medullary thyroid cancer is associated with parathyroid adenomas, phaeochromocytomas, Marfan syndrome (all through MEN syndrome).

[5] Thyroid cancers can be managed by ENT surgeons or endocrine surgeons. In many hospitals, both of these teams will perform thyroid operations. Specialised investigations and further management should be driven by these surgeons.

[6] Counselling patients about diagnoses, expected progress and management options is a crucial skill in the surgeon's repertoire. Being able to adequately explain conditions, appropriately consent patients for procedures, and provide reassurance helps patients in what is definitely a stressful period.

[7] Surgical management of cancers is usually best managed through a multidisciplinary approach. In the case of thyroid cancers, this usually involves a head and neck or endocrine surgeon, an oncologist, a radiation oncologist, a radiologist, a pathologist and potentially others. These

clinicians discuss cases to provide a combined experienced opinion on the most appropriate management for the patient.

8 In the majority of thyroid malignancies, a total thyroidectomy is performed. This involves removing the entire thyroid gland whilst leaving the parathyroid glands. This is most often done through the open neck approach; however, new techniques with endoscopic and robotic equipment are being developed.

9 Neck dissection involves removing the lymph node chains in the neck. Not all thyroid malignancies will require a neck dissection in conjunction with the thyroidectomy, and the decision to perform the neck dissection (and which lymph node groups to remove) will depend on whether or not there is clinically evident lymph node metastasis, and if not, the risk of lymph node metastases occurring without a neck dissection.

10 The most feared postoperative complication of thyroidectomy is the post-thyroidectomy haematoma. This can develop rapidly, and cause compression on the trachea and eventual airway obstruction and respiratory arrest. For this reason, a thyroid kit (including a scalpel and suction) should be at the bedside of all thyroidectomy patients postoperatively, in case emergency evacuation of a haematoma is necessary.

11 The other uncommon but well recognised complication of thyroidectomy is recurrent laryngeal nerve injury. This may be accidental (as the recurrent laryngeal nerve runs directly adjacent to the thyroid gland) or part of the nerve may need to be resected along with the thyroid gland due to it being involved in the tumour (which may be the cause of the patient's initial dysphonia).

12 Thyroxine replacement should start immediately following total thyroidectomy. Most hospitals will have an established protocol for initiation of thyroid hormone replacement.

13 Although the parathyroid glands are usually identified and reimplanted during a total thyroidectomy, parathyroid hormone (PTH) levels may still fall due to misidentification or failure of the parathyroid glands to reactivate. Most hospitals will have a protocol surrounding PTH and calcium level monitoring, and also a calcium replacement protocol if necessary.

14 If the postoperative period goes without complication, and the postoperative calcium and PTH monitoring is within normal limits, most thyroidectomy patients can be discharged from hospital the following day. If the surgical operation is more extensive (e.g. total thyroidectomy with anterior and bilateral neck dissection), the postoperative length of stay will be longer.

15 Once the final histopathology results are published, the patient's case should be discussed again at an MDT meeting to decide the further course of action. Whether a patient will receive radiotherapy, chemotherapy, immunotherapy or all of the above will depend on the tumour biology, the patient's postoperative recovery and the surgical margins.

16 The patient should be reassessed for any complications of inpatient management or surgery. Follow-up also serves to continue the patient management through the outpatient setting – the surgery is only the first step in the management of most cancer patients. The final recommendations from the MDT discussion can be relayed to the patient, and any further referrals for ongoing treatment or management can be made from there. In the case of medullary thyroid cancer, monitoring can be achieved through regular clinical assessments (usually 3-monthly for the first year) and annual serum CEA and calcitonin levels. Additional imaging (e.g. regular ultrasound) may also be helpful.

17 Adjuvant radiotherapy is rarely recommended for medullary thyroid cancer unless there are grossly incomplete tumour resection margins, and further attempts at surgical resection are not warranted.

18 Thyroxine replacement dosing can be managed by the operating surgeon, the oncologist or the GP. Thyroid function testing should occur approximately 3-monthly, with dosage adjustments made until the appropriate dosing schedule is maintained.

CASE 21: Abdominal trauma

History

- A **25-year-old** [1] male with **no known past medical history** [2] is brought into the ED following a motor vehicle accident **1 hour ago** [3].
- His **car collided front-on with another vehicle** [4], both travelling at 70km (43 miles) per hour.
- His **GCS was 10** [5] when **paramedics provided him with analgesics** [6] during transit to hospital.
- He is now **able to respond to questions** [7].
- He complains of **diffuse abdominal pain** [8].
- The **pain does not radiate** [9] anywhere else.
- There is **no pain elsewhere** [10] including the head, arms, groin or legs.
- The patient feels **light-headed** [11].
- He denies **losing consciousness, nausea or vomiting** [12].
- There is **no pain in his back or neck** [13].
- The patient has no **allergies** [14] and no regular medications.
- He **does not smoke** [15] and **denies alcohol intake today** [16].
- The patient has **never had past surgeries** [17].

[1] The age of the patient is important to note. Those who are old are more likely to have medical comorbidities while those who are young are more likely to be healthy. This is useful when assessing patients who cannot provide a medical history.

[2] Past medical history is important in determining fitness for surgery and any illnesses or diseases that must be addressed in the setting of abdominal trauma (e.g. coagulopathy).

[3] The timeline of the trauma must be documented. For patients who are bleeding, an injury that occurred a long time ago would place them at risk of hypovolaemic shock.

[4] Abdominal trauma patients are difficult to assess due to the wide range of potential injuries and other factors such as altered mental status. Hence, the mechanism of injury is extremely important as it will guide the history, focused examination and investigations. In relation to abdominal trauma, it will assist in categorising the injury as either blunt or penetrating trauma. The main causes of blunt abdominal trauma include motor vehicle accidents (MVAs), motorcycle accidents, pedestrian vs. vehicle impacts, falls and assaults. MVAs are the most common cause, contributing to 75% of blunt abdominal injuries. The most common penetrating injuries are gunshot wounds or stab wounds.

[5] The Glasgow Coma Scale (GCS) is a neurological scale used to record the state of a person's consciousness. It considers eye response, verbal response and motor function. A score of 15/15 indicates a fully conscious person whereas a score of 3/15 (lowest score) indicates deep unconsciousness.

In general, patients with a score of <8 should be considered for intubation.

[6] Being aware of what medications (and doses) have been given to the patient prior to arrival at the hospital is crucial, so that important medications are not missed or not given in higher doses than appropriate.

[7] When patients are unable to provide a history, collateral history should be sought from the ambulance officers, any witnesses and family/friends. Collateral history will help to identify any factors that may place the patient's life at risk if unaddressed (e.g. past medical history, medications, allergies).

[8] Abdominal pain raises the suspicion of intra-abdominal injuries. The location of the pain may give clues as to which organs may be affected. For example, pain in the upper left quadrant is associated with splenic injury; however, this is not specific and hence requires further investigation. Up to 90% of visceral injuries present with local or general abdominal tenderness. The absence of abdominal pain or tenderness does not rule out the presence of significant intra-abdominal injury. Any evidence of extra-abdominal injury calls for assessment of intra-abdominal injuries even if the patient is haemodynamically stable.

[9] Kehr's sign is radiation of abdominal pain to the left shoulder or neck which is associated with a spleen injury. Similarly, liver injury can cause referred pain to the right shoulder.

[10] It is important to ask if pain is felt anywhere else, as there may be multiple injuries that have not yet been identified.

Other injuries associated with MVAs include long bone fractures, head injuries and chest trauma.

11 Presyncope (light-headedness) may indicate hypovolaemia due to haemorrhage. Haemorrhagic shock is an urgent consideration in patients involved in major trauma.

12 Loss of consciousness and nausea/vomiting may indicate a raised intracranial pressure (ICP) secondary to intracranial haemorrhage.

13 During an MVA, intense forces can cause spinal injury and fractures. If there is any reason to suspect an injured cervical spine (e.g. pain in the neck), then a cervical collar needs to be put on the patient immediately to prevent further injury.

14 Any allergies must be elicited from the patient or from collateral history.

15 Smoking is associated with an increased risk of peri-operative respiratory, cardiac and wound-related complications. It is important to assess the patient's peri-operative risk whilst taking a history. Also ask about any previous exposure to general anaesthetic, and any allergies.

16 History about alcohol use is important in ruling out intoxication as a cause of altered mental status and more specifically in this case, whether alcohol was involved in the accident.

17 A history of past surgeries is useful for surgeons to know in terms of what procedures the patient has tolerated and whether past surgeries complicate any near future procedures (e.g. bowel adhesions which would slow an exploratory laparotomy).

Examination

- The patient appears **pale and uncomfortable but is able to respond** [1].
- There is **no sign of respiratory distress** [2].
- Heart rate is **110bpm** [3] and regular.
- BP is **100/70 mmHg** [4].
- Temperature is **37.3°C** [5].
- **Pupils are 3mm, equal and reactive** [6].
- The patient's capillary refill time is **<2 seconds** [7].
- The **patient is exposed** [8] appropriately.
- **Seat belt sign** [9] is seen on his chest and abdomen.
- Heart sounds are dual with **no murmurs** [10].
- Auscultation reveals vesicular breathing sounds and **equal air entry** [11].

- On inspection of the abdomen, there is **bruising seen around the umbilicus** [12].
- The abdomen appears moderately **distended** [13].
- There is no evidence of **surgical scars** [14].
- On palpation, there is **tenderness localised in the right upper quadrant** [15].
- No abdominal **rigidity** [16] or **rebound tenderness** [17] is felt.
- The **liver is normal in size and the spleen and kidneys cannot be palpated** [18].
- **Bowel sounds are present** [19].
- There are no **skin changes, deformities or tenderness of the pelvis, perineum and legs** [20].

1 As discussed in *Case 9*, the primary survey begins immediately, concurrent with resuscitation. As the patient is able to respond, it can be determined that the airway is patent. It is also noted that the patient is pale. In the context of abdominal trauma, this is likely to be secondary to haemorrhage which must be identified and treated urgently. When assessing a trauma patient, the primary survey is important in identifying, prioritising and treating immediate and delayed threats to life.

2 Respiratory distress in a patient may reflect hypoxia due to hypovolaemia (haemorrhage) or injury to the lung (pneumothorax). It is not a diagnosis in itself but should prompt the clinician to urgently determine the cause for respiratory distress and treat appropriately. Dyspnoea may also be due to diaphragmatic injury. This is more common in upper abdominal injuries. Delayed treatment may result in hernia or strangulation.

3 Tachycardia can be attributed to multiple aetiologies. Pain, anxiety and hypoxia are important causes to further investigate. Be sure to check the patient's other vital signs, including temperature, and feel the pulse for regularity.

4 Hypotension is often a result of haemorrhage from a solid organ injury or damage to intra-abdominal vessels. However, other sources of potential bleeding must be looked for as well (e.g. scalp, thorax, long bones). The most important thing to determine in a patient with hypotension is if the patient is in shock. If so, fluid resuscitation and identifying the cause of shock are imperative. Other features that are highly suspicious of shock include abnormal mental state, tachycardia, oliguria, tachypnoea, metabolic acidosis and hyperlactataemia.

5 Fever is a characteristic feature of most infections. If present, peritonitis and sepsis must be suspected and treated immediately with antibiotics.

6 In the setting of an MVA, pupils must be checked for size, shape and reaction to light, as abnormal results may indicate raised ICP. Pupils should be equal and reactive and around 3.5mm in diameter. If the pupils are not equal or are sluggish or non-reactive (fixed), this is concerning for brain or nerve injury or a mass effect secondary to a bleed.

7 An adequate capillary refill time indicates the patient is perfusing well and thus would likely have preserved end-organ perfusion. In addition, it suggests the patient is adequately hydrated. Other signs of adequate hydration are warm peripheries, normal skin turgor, moist mucous membranes and normal urine output.

8 The patient's body should be adequately exposed to identify injuries. In an MVA, anything can be injured due to the large force impacts on the body. Other sources of bleeding apart from the abdomen include long bones, thoracic cavity and brain. A concomitant femur fracture is a distracting injury often seen among pedestrians struck by vehicles.

9 Seat belt sign is bruising across the chest and/or abdominal area in the distribution during a high impact collision. Due to inertia, an abrupt halt of the vehicle means that the upper body will continue moving forward with high force. This exerts high pressure on the chest and abdomen which can cause abrasion and internal organ damage. Those with seat belt sign should be investigated for a Chance fracture (spinal fracture due to flexion-distraction injury) and bladder and bowel perforation. Around 30% of patients with seat belt sign will have some sort of intra-abdominal injury. A lap belt is associated with mesenteric or intestinal injury.

10 Abnormal heart sounds may indicate injury or a pathology of the heart. For example, muffled heart sounds in combination with a raised JVP may prompt further investigation for cardiac tamponade. Heart murmurs may suggest pre-existing valvular disease or a new valvular injury secondary to trauma.

11 A respiratory exam is performed to look for any signs of rib fractures, pneumothorax and haemothorax. Bowel sounds heard in the chest may suggest diaphragmatic rupture.

12 Cullen's sign is periumbilical ecchymoses while Grey Turner's sign is flank ecchymoses. Cullen's sign points to haemorrhage in the peritoneum, while the latter indicates retroperitoneal haemorrhage. These findings are sometimes difficult to appreciate in the acute resuscitation setting.

13 Blood or air in the peritoneum causes abdominal distension and peritoneal irritation.

14 Evidence of previous surgeries introduces the risk of postoperative abdominal adhesions. Adhesions increase the risk for complications in future surgeries in the form of difficult abdominal access due to loss of tissue planes and distorted anatomy, the inability to perform laparoscopic surgery, unintentional small bowel, bladder or ureter damage, increased blood loss and surgery time.

15 The location and character of tenderness elicited on the abdomen must be noted. Pain in the right upper quadrant (RUQ) is likely to be a liver injury whereas pain in the left upper quadrant could be a splenic injury. Splenic injury should be suspected if there is injury to the left lower ribcage. 30% of splenic injuries will present with hypotensive shock.

16 Abdominal rigidity is the involuntary contraction of abdominal wall muscles in an attempt to protect inflamed organs. It is a common manifestation of peritonitis, which can occur in a bowel perforation due to blunt abdominal trauma. Patients often stay still, as any movement exacerbates the pain.

17 Rebound tenderness, also known as Blumberg's sign, is another sign of peritonitis. Peritoneal irritation can also be tested by percussing the abdomen.

18 Blunt abdominal trauma can cause injury to solid organs. Solid organs include the liver, spleen, pancreas and kidneys. These injuries can range from insignificant lacerations to severe haemorrhage requiring immediate surgical management. Blunt abdominal trauma can also damage hollow organs such as the stomach, bowel, gall bladder and urinary bladder. Bowel injuries require surgical repair to prevent peritonitis, sepsis and shock.

19 Irritation and chemical peritonitis (due to haemorrhage or perforation) lead to ileus, which is seen as decreased bowel sounds.

20 Inspection of the pelvis, genitals, perineum and lower limbs is essential in identifying the presence of any other injuries that are life-threatening and/or contributing to the patient's hypotension (e.g. bleeding from a pelvic or femur fracture).

Investigations

- FBE reports a significantly **decreased haemoglobin and haematocrit** [1] and a mildly **raised WCC** [2].
- **UEC results are within normal limits** [3].
- **LFT results are within normal limits** [4].
- A **urine dipstick is normal** [5].
- A **venous blood gas (VBG)** [6] shows raised lactate.
- **Serum lipase** [7] and **coagulation tests** [8] are normal.
- **Blood cultures are negative** [9].

- A **FAST scan reveals free fluid** [10] in the hepatorenal recess.
- CXR shows **no fractures, hernias or free gas under the diaphragm** [11].
- **CT scan of the abdomen** [12] reveals a Grade III hepatic laceration and free fluid. There are thickened segmental loops of small bowel suspicious for a small bowel injury.

[1] Haemoglobin (Hb) and haematocrit (Hct) must be observed, as any falling value is concerning for haemorrhage which may require urgent blood transfusion. Haematocrit <30% is concerning for major haemorrhage. The mechanism of injury, extent of haemorrhage, time since injury and any administration of fluids/blood transfusion must be considered when interpreting anaemia. A normal haematocrit does not rule out internal haemorrhage in the acute trauma patient.

[2] Infection and inflammation are common causes of an elevated WBC count (e.g. peritonitis). WCC may also be elevated from catecholamine release due to trauma.

[3] UECs are important in the setting of a surgical emergency. Firstly, it identifies any electrolyte abnormalities that most often need correction prior to surgery. Secondly, it assesses renal function and fitness for IV contrast in the setting of imaging (such as a CT abdomen and pelvis), as well as serving as a prognosticator for postoperative recovery.

[4] In patients with abdominal trauma, liver function tests can be used to identify and monitor liver injury.

[5] A urine sample may reveal gross haematuria which is suggestive of serious renal injury. If present, further investigation is required. A urine dipstick can be used as a screening tool in low risk patients. A finding of microscopic haematuria increases the likelihood of having significant intra-abdominal injury.

[6] A venous or arterial blood gas provides useful information on partial pressure of gases, oxygen saturation, pH, bicarbonate and lactate levels. An elevated lactate can indicate sepsis or tissue ischaemia. In hypovolaemic shock, base deficit becomes more negative before pH changes occur. A base deficit of <–6 is associated with intra-abdominal haemorrhage.

[7] Pancreatic enzymes, such as serum amylase and lipase, can be measured to look for pancreatic injury. Normal pancreatic enzyme levels cannot exclude injury to the pancreas, therefore if suspected, a CT scan is required.

[8] Coagulation tests should be ordered to ensure the patient does not have a coagulopathy that may be predisposing him to haemorrhage or worsening any current haemorrhage. It is also important to order this in patients who are taking anticoagulant medication.

[9] Blood cultures should be ordered if peritonitis is suspected. This can aid in antibiotic treatment.

[10] A focused assessment with sonography in trauma (FAST) scan is a series of ultrasound scans performed to look for bleeding in the abdomen. Any free fluid found in the hepatorenal recess (Morrison's pouch), splenorenal recess, pouch of Douglas or pericardium is assumed to be haemoperitoneum in the context of trauma. Ultrasound will only identify peritoneal free fluid if >500ml is present; hence a negative FAST scan does not rule out intra-abdominal bleeding. An extended FAST (eFAST) scan is now the standard of care. It has an additional view of the pleura which is used to identify any pneumothorax.

[11] An erect CXR allows for identification of free gas under the diaphragm. This indicates perforation of an organ that contains air, most commonly the bowel. Other hollow organs that can be damaged include the urinary bladder and gall bladder. Rib fractures and diaphragmatic hernias may also be identified on a CXR. In the context of trauma, it is important to note that if the patient is in spinal precautions, it may not be possible to perform an erect CXR in the early stages.

[12] A CT scan is the most common and accurate diagnostic method for abdominal injury. Due to the time required for a patient to undertake a CT scan, the test is only appropriate for patients who are haemodynamically stable. The clinician must also be wary of any potential spinal cord injuries that should be protected during positioning and transfer for imaging. Patients who are not cooperative will interfere with imaging results and place themselves at risk of further injury. Due to radiation exposure, only patients who are likely to benefit from imaging should undergo a CT scan. Unstable patients may benefit from angiography which can identify areas of haemorrhage and stop bleeding through embolisation. However, angiography can be time-consuming compared to laparotomy and requires coordination with interventional radiology services, which may not be available.

Management

Immediate

Stabilise the patient and monitor vital signs [1] and urine output [2] . Keep the patient fasted [3] . Obtain IV access [4] and administer analgesics and fluids [5] . Insert a gastric tube [6] . Seek advice [7] from the general surgery team.

Short-term

Perform an emergency laparotomy [8] . Haemoperitoneum and a bleeding laceration to the left liver lobe are found. All other organs appear normal and intact. The bleeding is controlled [9] and the haemoperitoneum is evacuated. Following the procedure, keep the patient in ICU for monitoring [10] . Correct the patient's parameters [11] and administer IV fluids [12] as appropriate. Review the patient's surgical site [13] and perform an abdominal examination [14] . Auscultate the lungs [15] and examine the lower limbs [16] . The patient may be discharged if vital signs remain stable [17] , they can tolerate oral intake and are back to their premorbid level of function [18] .

Long-term

Follow the patient up in an outpatient clinic [19] if necessary, for continuing wound management and monitoring for postoperative complications.

[1] Addressing the ABC (airway, breathing and circulation) is the first step in managing a trauma patient. Ensure the patient remains haemodynamically stable prior to operative treatment. In the setting of an MVA, we are concerned with haemorrhage and hypovolaemia. Any haemodynamic instability calls for an exploratory laparotomy.

[2] Urine output is an indicator of fluid balance. Poor urine output may indicate acute renal failure due to hypovolaemia. Urinary catheterisation allows accurate measurement of urine output. A urinary catheter is contraindicated in trauma patients suspected of urethral injury. Signs of urethral injury include blood at the urethral meatus or a genital/perineal haematoma.

[3] Keeping the patient fasted is crucial in their preoperative management. It allows the patient to have bowel rest, as well as reducing the risk of aspiration in the setting of anaesthesia. Ideally, patients should be fasted off solid foods for 6 hours and clear fluids for 2 hours, prior to induction of anaesthesia.

[4] Two large-bore cannulas should be inserted in the patient for fluid resuscitation, blood transfusions or administration of medication. Any violation of the peritoneum or retroperitoneum requires prophylactic antibiotics which must cover gut flora.

[5] Intravenous fluid is integral in fluid resuscitation and stabilisation of circulation; the choice (crystalloid vs. blood products) may differ from patient to patient. A general principle of trauma is that blood should be replaced with blood, therefore any patient with suspicion of large amounts of bleeding should be replaced with packed red blood cells. A systolic blood pressure of >90mmHg should be maintained.

[6] A nasogastric tube is used to decompress the stomach of fluid, air or blood. This reduces the risk of vomiting or aspiration, especially in this setting where ileus is present. Bloody aspirate from the tube suggests stomach injury. A nasogastric tube is contraindicated in patients suspected of a base of skull fracture.

[7] Exploratory laparotomy falls under the general surgeon's domain, and care should be directed by their advice. They will usually come to assess the patient themselves and consent the patient for an exploratory laparotomy if possible.

[8] Indications for exploratory laparotomy in the context of trauma include haemodynamic instability, signs of peritonism, suspected/known diaphragmatic injury, bowel or rectal perforation and a positive FAST scan. Haemorrhage control is of utmost importance. During an exploratory laparotomy, all organs and vessels should be checked for bleeding. Packing all four abdominal quadrants can help the surgeon in establishing initial haemorrhagic control. Blunt trauma involving the liver can be managed conservatively if the patient is haemodynamically stable, has no signs of peritonitis and is not requiring excessive transfusions.

[9] An injured solid organ, such as the spleen or kidney, should be resected if the haemorrhage is uncontrollable. Haemorrhage from the liver can be controlled in a variety of ways, such as with electrocautery, bipolar devices, topical haemostatic agents or sutures. If there is major haemorrhage, manual compression, hepatic packing, vessel ligation or hepatic vascular isolation may be used. Injury to the spleen requires immediate laparotomy if there is haemodynamic instability, an expanding haematoma or the patient is on blood thinners or has coagulopathy. Damaged parts of the spleen are removed or the whole spleen can be removed. In patients who have undergone splenectomy, vaccinations against pneumococcus, meningococcus and *Haemophilus influenzae* type B should be given. Angioembolisation is

useful in patients with persistent arterial bleeding after damage control procedures.

10 Patients must be monitored postoperatively for any immediate complications of surgery. These include signs of shock (septic or hypovolaemic), infection, reaction to anaesthesia, DVT and PE, urinary retention or renal failure, and postoperative ileus. A tertiary survey (repeated secondary survey) should be performed to ensure there are no other missed injuries. Further deterioration requires laparotomy or interventional radiology.

11 The goal is to manage the 'lethal triad' of metabolic acidosis, hypothermia and coagulopathy. This combination is commonly seen in major trauma patients and significantly increases mortality rate. The patient should be given warm blankets and fluids and have their blood volume and Hb restored. Calcium should be replaced if depleted (as it is involved in the coagulation cascade) and transfusion products should be administered if appropriate.

12 Patients are nil by mouth prior to surgery and so maintenance fluids are essential in keeping the patient adequately hydrated. Following this, ensure the patient is on a fluid chart in order to monitor fluid input and output.

13 Review the surgical site to ensure adequate closure, as well as the amount of ooze and any signs of infection from the wound. Determine if the patient's pain is in proportion to the surgical wound. Review the wound two weeks after the surgery when sutures are removed. The larger the wound, the higher the risk of wound dehiscence. The patient should avoid forceful coughing, sneezing, bending over and straining with bowel movements as these actions increase the risk of wound dehiscence.

14 Palpate the abdomen again to examine for clinical recovery of liver laceration, any signs of peritonitis and any missed injuries. Absence of bowel sounds may indicate postoperative ileus.

15 Listen for any crepitations. The presence of crackles in the lung may indicate either atelectasis or pneumonia.

16 Recent surgery and subsequent immobilisation in bed postoperatively are major risk factors for the development of DVT. Inspect the calves for unilateral swelling and erythema. Palpate the calves to ensure they are not tender.

17 If the patient remains afebrile, is haemodynamically stable and looks well, they are generally well enough to be discharged home.

18 The patient should ideally be able to function at the level that they were able to prior to becoming ill. If unsure, refer to the allied health team (primarily physiotherapy, occupational therapy and social work) for further assessment on fitness for discharge home at a functional level.

19 Follow-up visits with the general surgeons are important to ensure adequate recovery and identification of any missed injuries. For example, injury to the pancreas is rare and may present weeks to months later with vague symptoms of abdominal pain or loss of appetite. On imaging, a pancreatic pseudocyst secondary to trauma may be found as the cause of such symptoms.

CASE 22: Acute cholecystitis

History

- A **45-year-old** [1] **female** [2] with **a history of type 2 diabetes mellitus** [3] presents with **constant** [4] **right upper quadrant abdominal pain** [5] radiating to the right shoulder, worsening over the **past 12 hours** [6] .
- She also notes **nausea, loss of appetite** [7] and **fever** [8] .
- She **last ate 9 hours ago** [9] .
- She **does not smoke** [10] and does not drink alcohol.
- She has previously had **self-limiting right upper quadrant pain associated with fatty meals** [11] .
- She is **not on any anticoagulants** [12] and has **no significant surgical history** [13] .
- She has no **allergies** [14] .

[1] Gall bladder disease is more common with increasing age.

[2] Female sex is also a predisposing factor for gall bladder disease.

[3] A diagnosis of T2DM increases the risk of gall bladder disease. In addition to considering the role of the past medical history in ascertaining causative and contributing factors towards a probable diagnosis and differential diagnoses, past medical history is also significant for determining fitness for surgery. In the case of diabetic patients, relevant further history includes their usual glycaemic control, any complications (both microvascular and macrovascular) and current treatment (ranging from lifestyle modification to insulin).

[4] Constant, worsening pain is typical of inflammatory causes. Occurring in the right upper quadrant (RUQ), key differential diagnoses are acute cholecystitis or cholangitis, rather than the classical biliary colic pain which waxes and wanes.

[5] RUQ pain is most commonly associated with gall bladder disease. Pain may also radiate to the right shoulder or the back. Importantly, keep in mind that gall bladder disease may also present with epigastric pain. Hepatitis and right lower lobe pneumonia/embolism are also associated with RUQ pain. Pancreatitis, gastritis and acute coronary syndrome are important differential diagnoses for upper abdominal pain more generally, while renal colic and appendicitis should be considered as differential diagnoses for right-sided abdominal pain.

[6] Pain associated with acute cholecystitis generally persists and may worsen over several hours, as opposed to the self-limiting pain of biliary colic. Patients may report that this pain is worse with deep inspiration, or with ingestion of food.

[7] Acute cholecystitis is also associated with nausea and anorexia, although these symptoms are non-specific if in isolation.

[8] Persistent fever may suggest complications such as abscess formation or perforation. Acute cholangitis should also be considered as an important differential diagnosis in patients with fever and RUQ pain – fever, RUQ pain and jaundice are the classical triad of acute cholangitis (eponymously known as Charcot's triad).

[9] Fasting status is important to ascertain in any patient who may require an emergency operation, to determine timing of surgery.

[10] Smoking may increase risk of gall bladder disease, and is also significant for increased risk of complications from anaesthetic, and its adverse impact on wound healing. For elective surgeries, it is recommended that patients reduce their smoking and, if possible, cease smoking entirely as long as possible before surgery.

[11] This symptomatology is classically associated with biliary colic. Fatty food ingestion usually precipitates biliary colic, and may also be associated with onset of acute cholecystitis. Cholelithiasis is implicated in 90% of cases of cholecystitis, and cholecystitis in turn can affect up to 10% of patients with symptomatic cholelithiasis, as the most frequent complication of cholelithiasis. Uncommonly, acalculous cholecystitis can occur (cholecystitis in the absence of cholelithiasis). Acalculous cholecystitis is generally associated with certain comorbidities, such as total parenteral nutrition, diabetes mellitus or other conditions predisposing patients to gall bladder ischaemia and stasis.

[12] All anticoagulants, as well as antiplatelet medications, need careful management peri-operatively. Depending on risk, surgery may sometimes proceed for a patient on aspirin, but patients on other antiplatelet agents or who are

therapeutically anticoagulated usually require reversal or withholding for a period of time before they are fit to proceed to surgery.

13 Past surgical history is likewise important when planning for an operation. Specifically, a history of abdominal surgery will indicate if the patient has already had a cholecystectomy, which rules out cholecystitis as a diagnosis, as long as the cholecystectomy was complete, and the patient gives an accurate history. A patient with previous abdominal surgeries may also have adhesions, which increases operative risk and makes surgery more difficult – this risk is increased with the number and complexity of previous abdominal surgeries.

14 In this patient, a history of drug allergies is particularly relevant to antibiotic choice. Penicillin allergies are relatively common, and anaphylactic reactions to penicillin preclude the use of cephalosporins.

Examination

- On examination, the patient appears **uncomfortable** [1] but **not acutely unwell** [2] and is **haemodynamically stable** [3] .
- She is **not clinically jaundiced** [4] .
- She is **febrile** [5] .
- Her **abdomen is soft** [6] , with **moderate tenderness in the RUQ** [7] .

- **Murphy's sign is positive** [8] , and there is **no palpable abdominal mass** [9] .
- There is also **no crepitus** [10] over the RUQ, and on auscultation, **bowel sounds are present** [11] .

1 The review of every patient must begin with general inspection. Expect a patient with acute cholecystitis to be uncomfortable, but if a patient has had adequate analgesia, they may appear settled. Hence, do not be deceived into dismissing the history of pain. They may also be lying very still on the examination table, as pain associated with peritonitis will be aggravated by movement.

2 In a critically unwell patient in whom cholecystitis is suspected, consider complications such as perforation, or alternative diagnoses, such as cholangitis.

3 Begin with an assessment of vital signs – airway, breathing and circulation. Be particularly wary of tachycardia or tachypnoea which may be due to sepsis, especially if not resolving with analgesia. Sepsis may also be suggestive of gangrenous cholecystitis, the most common complication of cholecystitis. Hypotension is a later sign of sepsis.

4 Jaundice in the presence of fever and RUQ pain is suggestive of acute cholangitis, rather than acute cholecystitis. In acute cholangitis, obstruction of the biliary tree is complicated by infection, a potentially life-threatening condition.

5 In a febrile patient with RUQ pain, the most likely diagnosis will be acute cholecystitis, or acute cholangitis, rather than biliary colic. This is consistent with a systemic inflammatory response.

6 On abdominal examination, consider if the abdomen shows signs of peritonism. Guarding, rigidity and rebound tenderness are the major findings associated with peritonism.

Localised peritonism is consistent with acute cholecystitis, with inflammation of the parietal peritoneum. Generalised peritonism is suggestive of perforation, and is associated with high mortality.

7 Tenderness in the RUQ is again consistent with inflammation of the parietal peritoneum, consistent with acute cholecystitis.

8 Pain with deep inspiration while the examiner palpates the RUQ adjacent to the liver edge is a positive Murphy's sign, which is classically associated with cholecystitis, though its sensitivity and specificity are variable.

9 A distended, tender gall bladder may be palpable, as may a pericholecystitic abscess.

10 Emphysematous cholecystitis is caused by infection secondary to gas-forming organisms, typically *Clostridium* species. Emphysematous cholecystitis makes up a small proportion of cases of acute cholecystitis, but carries significantly higher risk of gangrene, perforation and mortality.

11 Gallstone ileus may arise from passage of a gallstone into the small bowel through a cholecystoenteric fistula, causing a bowel obstruction.

Investigations

- On FBE, the **haemoglobin and platelet count are within normal limits** [1], but **WCC is elevated** [2].
- **CRP is elevated** [3].
- **UEC is unremarkable** [4].
- LFT demonstrates **elevated ALP and GGT, but normal ALT, bilirubin and albumin** [5].
- **Lipase is normal** [6].
- **HCG is negative** [7].

- An erect CXR demonstrates **no free gas under the diaphragm** [8].
- On **abdominal ultrasound** [9], there is a finding of **cholelithiasis** [10], with an **impacted gallstone in Hartmann's pouch** [11], a **positive sonographic Murphy's sign** [12], a **thickened, hyperaemic gall bladder wall** [13], **pericholecystic fluid** [14] and a **normal calibre common bile duct** [15].

[1] Haemoglobin and platelet count are important considerations for operative planning in any surgical patient. Packed red blood cells or platelet transfusion may be necessary preoperatively, as well as investigation for the underlying cause, for anaemia or thrombocytopenia respectively.

[2] Elevated WCC is consistent with systemic infection or inflammation.

[3] C-reactive protein is an acute phase reactant. Elevated CRP is consistent with a systemic inflammatory response.

[4] Renal function is also significant for operative planning, but should be unaffected in patients with acute cholecystitis, except in cases of severe sepsis or dehydration.

[5] Elevated ALP and GGT is consistent with an 'obstructive' pattern of LFT derangement, and suggests biliary pathology, whereas elevated alanine aminotransferase (ALT) and GGT would be consistent with a 'hepatitic' pattern of LFT derangement, usually associated with hepatitis or other causes of liver disease. It is important to establish whether bilirubin is elevated in patients with RUQ pain and fever – if so, this is suspicious for cholangitis, secondary to choledocholithiasis (biliary obstruction secondary to a gallstone in the common bile duct). Be aware that patients may have both acute cholangitis and acute cholecystitis.

[6] Lipase should be performed in every patient presenting with upper abdominal pain. Elevated lipase is associated with pancreatitis, which is also commonly associated with gallstone disease.

[7] HCG should also be performed in every woman of childbearing age. Pregnancy is relevant both for differential diagnosis of abdominal pain, as well as for management. Anaesthesia inevitably involves some risk of miscarriage, depending on the stage of pregnancy, and this must be discussed with the pregnant woman as part of the process of consent for an operation. Depending on gestational age, the operation may also be made more challenging technically due to the gravid uterus.

[8] Erect CXR is a useful initial imaging modality in any patient with abdominal pain concerning for perforated viscus. The classic finding of free gas under the diaphragm is ominous, and generally requires urgent surgical management. This finding usually correlates clinically with generalised peritonitis.

[9] Abdominal ultrasound is the radiological investigation of choice for the initial work-up of RUQ pain. Ultrasound is inexpensive, widely available and not associated with ionising radiation. However, it may also be limited by obesity or bowel gas overlying the gall bladder.

[10] Ultrasound is highly sensitive and specific for the detection of gallstones. The absence of cholelithiasis does not exclude cholecystitis (a proportion of individuals may have acalculous cholecystitis, as discussed earlier), but makes it less likely. If ultrasound findings are equivocal for cholecystitis, a HIDA scan (cholescintigraphy) may be indicated to determine whether the cystic duct is patent. The Technetium-labelled HIDA is extracted by hepatocytes and excreted into bile. Persistent non-filling of the gall bladder is consistent with acute cholecystitis. A HIDA scan is also useful to detect bile leak postoperatively. Additionally, abdominal CT may be sometimes obtained to rule out other causes of undifferentiated abdominal pain, or to evaluate for complications such as gall bladder perforation, emphysematous cholecystitis or gallstone ileus.

[11] Hartmann's pouch is an outpouching of part of the gall bladder between the gall bladder neck and the cystic duct, which is often a site of gallstone impaction. Obstruction of the cystic duct causes acute cholecystitis, while compression of the common hepatic duct may result in obstructive jaundice, otherwise known as Mirizzi syndrome. This is occasionally complicated by a fistulous connection between the infundibulum of the gall bladder and the common hepatic or common bile duct.

[12] The sonographic Murphy's sign is similar to the clinical Murphy's sign in palpation of the RUQ but is here associated with tenderness on palpation of the gall bladder with the ultrasound probe. This is a more accurate sign than the clinical Murphy's sign, as the position of the gall bladder is sonographically correlated with the point of tenderness.

13 Gall bladder wall thickening (>4mm) or oedema may be suggestive of acute cholecystitis, though may also be due to elevated portal or systemic venous pressure, in conditions such as renal failure, cardiac failure or liver cirrhosis. Hyperaemia of the gall bladder wall may be seen on Doppler ultrasound, and is associated with inflammation.

14 The presence of pericholecystic fluid also supports a diagnosis of cholecystitis.

15 The assessment of the common bile duct is critical. A dilated common bile duct (>7mm) may be associated with choledocholithiasis, which results in bile stasis and can result in secondary infection and cholangitis. Uncommonly,

other causes of biliary obstruction may be implicated in common bile duct dilatation, such as carcinoma of the head of the pancreas. Choledocholithiasis is most often managed by endoscopic retrograde cholangiopancreatography (ERCP), which is both diagnostic and therapeutic, prior to cholecystectomy. Alternatively, depending on availability, cholecystectomy can be performed in some centres with transcystic exploration of the common bile duct to retrieve any stone(s). Where bilirubin is elevated or there is a dilated common bile duct on ultrasound, magnetic resonance cholangiopancreatography (MRCP) may be considered to assess the biliary tree and determine whether there is also choledocholithiasis.

Management

Immediate

Monitor **vital signs** and **perform resuscitation if required** [1]. **Admit** [2] the patient to hospital. Keep the patient **fasted** [3]. Give IV **fluids** [4] and **antibiotics** [5]. Give appropriate **analgesia** [6]. **Liaise with the anaesthetics team** [7] regarding planning for theatre.

Short-term

At the **earliest opportunity** [8] during the acute admission, perform a **laparoscopic**

cholecystectomy [9] with consideration of **intraoperative cholangiography** [10]. Postoperatively, if the patient is stable, they may be transferred to the ward. Review the **surgical sites** [11] and examine the **abdomen** [12]. The patient may be discharged when they have been **afebrile for 24 hours** [13], with **stable vital signs** [14], **mobilising** [15], and **tolerating normal diet** [16].

Long-term

Follow up the patient in an **outpatient clinic** [17] to review histopathology and the wounds.

1 Resuscitate the patient if necessary. This should occur at your first encounter with the patient and take place as you consider the vital signs.

2 Ensure that your planned disposition is appropriate (e.g. assess the need for intensive care, or transfer to a higher acuity hospital). Ensure that facilities are available for acute, unplanned surgical intervention.

3 Prior to the induction of anaesthesia, patients should be fasted for 6 hours to minimise risk of aspiration.

4 IV fluids are essential for resuscitation, as well as for fluid maintenance in the fasting patient. Urine output is a valuable indicator of hydration status and should be measured strictly. Be aware that maintenance fluid requirements are increased by sepsis. A patient who is hypotensive or tachycardic will require rapid fluid resuscitation with crystalloid solution (normal saline and Hartmann's solution are widely used). Also ensure that fluid losses are replaced – is the patient vomiting? Yet also be wary of fluid overload secondary to overly aggressive fluid resuscitation in the patient with comorbid renal or cardiac failure – seek advice if necessary.

5 IV antibiotics are fundamental to the management of sepsis, and in uncomplicated acute cholecystitis, to reduce risk of complicating gall bladder empyema, pericholecystic abscess or sepsis. Activity should preferably include aerobic Gram-negative bacteria as well as anaerobes. For sepsis originating from an intra-abdominal source, ampicillin, metronidazole and gentamicin in combination are recommended; if gentamicin is contraindicated, piperacillin/tazobactam can be used as monotherapy; while in the case of non-severe penicillin allergy, ceftriaxone and metronidazole is also an alternative. For uncomplicated acute cholecystitis without the presence of sepsis, the addition of metronidazole may not be necessary.

6 Analgesia may include non-steroidal anti-inflammatory drugs (NSAIDs) (if not contraindicated) or opioids.

7 In order to book this patient for an emergency operation, the general surgery team will need to coordinate with anaesthetics. Ensure that the anaesthetist is aware of the patient's comorbidities, haemodynamics and fasting status, so that they can assess the patient's suitability for a general anaesthetic, and plan for an operation within an appropriate time frame.

8 Complications such as gall bladder necrosis, perforation, emphysematous cholecystitis, intractable pain or septic shock may indicate emergency cholecystectomy. Otherwise, unless contraindicated due to comorbidity, cholecystectomy should be performed early within the acute admission. Early cholecystectomy reduces peri-operative morbidity and mortality in patients with acute cholecystitis. Dissection becomes more difficult after the first three days following onset of symptoms, due to increased inflammation. However, in patients who would be at high operative risk for cholecystectomy, consider a trial of conservative management with antibiotics with or without percutaneous cholecystostomy to drain the gall bladder. For these patients, consider cholecystectomy electively to eliminate risk of recurrent symptoms.

9 Laparoscopic cholecystectomy is the standard surgical approach for acute cholecystitis and is associated with less morbidity and mortality than an open approach. A minority of cases are not able to be completed laparoscopically and require conversion to open; patients should be warned about this risk when they are consented.

10 Intraoperative cholangiography characterises the biliary anatomy to identify anatomical variants, which may prevent injury to the extrahepatic biliary tract. Intraoperative cholangiography also detects occult choledocholithiasis. However, practice varies on whether intraoperative cholangiography is performed routinely or selectively for cases of suspected choledocholithiasis only.

11 Surgical sites should be reviewed to ensure closure, and to check for signs of wound infection, such as surrounding erythema, or discharge. The risk of dehiscence is greatly reduced by laparoscopic technique compared to laparotomy, as the wound sites are much smaller.

12 Expect the postoperative abdominal examination to demonstrate a degree of tenderness over the operative sites. Nevertheless, be alert for peritonism or disproportionate abdominal tenderness which may suggest bile leak, bleeding or another complication.

13 Patients who become febrile again postoperatively should be worked up for causes of postoperative fever or ongoing sepsis.

14 Monitor patients postoperatively for complications. Haemodynamic instability should prompt urgent review. It is important not to miss medical causes in the work-up such as pulmonary embolism or a cardiac event.

15 Elderly and comorbid patients are particularly vulnerable to functional decline associated with hospital admission and acute illness. Allied health teams provide valuable input to ensure that patients are safe to discharge from a functional point of view, or otherwise to facilitate inpatient rehabilitation if required.

16 Postoperative ileus is much less common in cholecystectomy than in bowel surgeries, but it is important to ensure that your patients are tolerating diet and passing flatus, if not opening bowels, prior to discharge.

17 Review of postoperative patients should include histopathology review, as well as review of wounds to ensure that they have healed. Generally, if patients are well at this point and there are no unexpected findings on histopathology, they can then be discharged from the clinic. If review in the outpatient clinic is not going to take place for a number of weeks, consider referring the patient back to their GP to have the wounds reviewed in 1–2 weeks postoperatively.

CASE 23: Acute pancreatitis

History

- A **55-year-old female** [1] with **a history of infrequent biliary colic** [2] presents with **abrupt onset** [3] **severe epigastric pain** [4], **nausea and vomiting** [5] for **the past 9 hours** [6].
- The pain **radiates to her back** [7] and is **relieved by bending forward** [8].
- She also has a history of **obesity** [9] and **type 2 diabetes mellitus** [9] managed with metformin.
- She denies any **recent trauma** [10].
- She has no **history of surgical procedures** [11] and has **no other regular medications** [12].
- She has **no family history of pancreatitis** [13], and indicates that she **drinks alcohol socially** [14], with an average of 2.5–4 units three times a week.

[1] Gallstone pancreatitis is more common in middle-aged women, whilst alcoholic pancreatitis is more common in young men. Advanced age is also associated with complications.

[2] Gallstones are the most common cause of pancreatitis. However, pancreatitis only affects a small minority of patients with gallstone disease.

[3] Characteristically, gallstone pancreatitis has a more abrupt onset, whereas alcoholic pancreatitis or pancreatitis related to metabolic causes arises over a longer time period.

[4] Persistent severe epigastric pain is the classic clinical picture associated with acute pancreatitis, although it can sometimes present with pain in the RUQ. It is usually described as stabbing in character. Be sure to consider other differential diagnoses for epigastric pain as well, including peptic ulcer disease, biliary disease and cardiac ischaemia.

[5] Most patients with pancreatitis also have associated nausea and vomiting.

[6] Generally, patients with acute pancreatitis present within a day of onset of symptoms.

[7] In many patients with pancreatitis, epigastric pain radiates through to the back.

[8] Pain associated with pancreatitis may improve with sitting or leaning forwards.

[9] Obesity and T2DM increase the risk of complications associated with pancreatitis. Diabetes mellitus also requires management of hypoglycaemics, both oral and injectable during the acute setting, as well as control of blood sugar levels, particularly in the setting of decreased oral intake.

[10] Abdominal trauma is an uncommon cause of acute pancreatitis.

[11] Acute pancreatitis can also occur rarely in patients undergoing ERCP; this is more common in the setting of a difficult, complex or prolonged procedure. Surgical history is also significant for surgical planning for a future laparoscopic cholecystectomy in the case of gallstone pancreatitis.

[12] Rarely, some medications can cause acute pancreatitis, including sulfonamides, diuretics, azathioprine and steroids.

[13] A minority of patients with acute pancreatitis have no discernible aetiology on investigation; many of these may have some genetic risk factors.

[14] A pattern of binge drinking over ≥5 years may be associated with alcohol-related pancreatitis; ethanol is a direct insult to the pancreas. Generally, alcohol is unlikely to be causative without this pattern of binge drinking over a period of time, so alcohol consumption must be clarified in the history.

Examination

- On examination, the patient is uncomfortable, but **alert and oriented** [1] .
- She does not **appear critically unwell** [2] and is **hypertensive and mildly tachycardic, but haemodynamically stable** [3] .
- She is clinically **moderately hypovolaemic** [4] .
- She is **afebrile** [5] .

- Her abdomen is **soft** [6] , with **moderate tenderness in the epigastrium** [7] and **voluntary guarding** [8] .
- She has **hypoactive bowel sounds** [9] on auscultation.
- She has **no periumbilical or flank ecchymoses** [10] .
- She is not **jaundiced and has no scleral icterus** [11] .

[1] Confusion or decreased conscious state is a concerning finding suggesting organ dysfunction secondary to sepsis or hypovolaemia, in this case, and requires an urgent response.

[2] Consider sepsis, pancreatic necrosis or organ failure as potential complications in a critically unwell patient with acute pancreatitis. Begin resuscitation if required.

[3] Hypertension may arise from pain, while hypotension may arise from late sepsis or severe hypovolaemia. Tachycardia may be associated with any of these but would be expected to respond to analgesia if pain-related and would generally improve with fluid resuscitation if related to sepsis or hypovolaemia. Hypoxia may be due to ARDS, secondary to a systemic inflammatory response.

[4] Hypovolaemia manifests clinically as decreased urine output, dry mucous membranes, decreased skin turgor and prolonged capillary refill; when more severe, patients will become tachycardic then hypotensive. In pancreatitis, hypovolaemia may arise from vascular leak as well as vomiting.

[5] Fever suggests a systemic inflammatory response, and is an indicator of more severe pancreatitis, with poorer prognosis. Fever may also be associated with infected

pancreatic necrosis, although this is usually later in the disease course.

[6] Peritonism – characterised by rebound tenderness, guarding or rigidity – suggests necrotising or complicated acute pancreatitis.

[7] Increasing severity of epigastric tenderness in acute pancreatitis usually correlates with the severity of disease.

[8] Voluntary guarding may be present, as the patient voluntarily contracts their abdominal musculature to avoid pain with palpation.

[9] Bowel sounds may be hypoactive, and the abdomen distended secondary to ileus, which commonly occurs in acute pancreatitis.

[10] Cullen's sign (periumbilical ecchymoses) and Grey Turner's sign (flank ecchymoses) are associated with retroperitoneal bleeding, which can occur in severe pancreatitis as a complication of pancreatic necrosis.

[11] Jaundice and scleral icterus are clinical signs of hyperbilirubinaemia, which can arise from choledocholithiasis and biliary obstruction. In combination with a systemic inflammatory response, consider whether cholangitis might be present.

Investigations

- On FBE, the **haemoglobin is within normal limits** [1] , **white cell count is elevated** [2] and **haematocrit is elevated** [3] .
- **CRP is elevated** [4] .
- UEC demonstrates **elevated urea** [5] and **normal electrolytes** [6] .
- VBG shows **normal acid–base status** [7] and a **normal lactate** [8] .

- **LFT is normal, including bilirubin** [9] .
- **HCG is normal** [10] .
- **Lipase is elevated** [11] .
- **Serum calcium is normal** [12] .
- **Serum triglycerides are normal** [13] .
- An **abdominal ultrasound shows cholelithiasis and no choledocholithiasis** [14] .

[1] Haemoglobin may be decreased in haemorrhagic pancreatitis, although this is a late complication. Baseline haemoglobin should also be established as part of preoperative work-up.

[2] Elevated white cell count suggests systemic inflammatory response and may indicate infection.

[3] Elevated Hct is consistent with hypovolaemia.

4 Elevated CRP, like elevated white cell count, is indicative of a systemic inflammatory response. A grossly elevated CRP also correlates with more severe pancreatitis.

5 Elevated urea is also consistent with hypovolaemia, which may cause an acute kidney injury.

6 Electrolytes should be checked and replaced as needed.

7 Metabolic acidosis may arise secondary to hypovolaemia and acute kidney injury, or sepsis; alternatively, prolonged vomiting can cause metabolic alkalosis.

8 Elevated lactate is an indicator of organ dysfunction, which may be secondary to hypovolaemia or sepsis.

9 Liver function testing should be performed, both to assess for hepatobiliary causes of upper abdominal pain, and to establish whether there is biliary obstruction. Elevated bilirubin suggests choledocholithiasis; this may lead to cholangitis as well as pancreatitis.

10 HCG should be checked in all women of childbearing age; pregnancy presents unique challenges in management of any condition and will likely require consultation with the obstetrics unit.

11 Elevated lipase is sensitive but not specific for acute pancreatitis. Lipase elevation arises from leakage of pancreatic enzymes into the systemic circulation. Typically, acute pancreatitis causes lipase elevation of more than three times the upper limit of normal. In patients with epigastric pain in whom pancreatitis is suspected, lipase elevation is diagnostic. Note that serum amylase level is also not sensitive for pancreatitis, and as it has a short half-life, has therefore less utility in the diagnostic work-up of suspected acute pancreatitis.

12 Hypercalcaemia is a rare cause of pancreatitis.

13 Triglyceride level of >11mmol/L is also an uncommon cause of acute pancreatitis; the hypertriglyceridaemia may be primary or secondary to other metabolic disease.

14 Abdominal ultrasound should be performed in all patients with pancreatitis; cholelithiasis is the most common cause of pancreatitis. Abdominal ultrasound will also assess for choledocholithiasis. Further abdominal imaging with CT is unnecessary if the diagnosis of pancreatitis is already established.

Management

Immediate

Monitor **vital signs** [1] and resuscitate as required. **Admit** [2] the patient to hospital. Keep the patient **fasted** [3]. Give IV **fluids** [4] and appropriate **analgesia** [5]. Correct **any electrolyte, triglyceride or acid–base disturbance** [6].

Short-term

Continue to **monitor and replace electrolytes** [7] during the acute admission. Control the patient's **blood glucose level** [8]. **Titrate IV fluid rate** [9] to urine output. If the patient has **hypercalcaemia or trigliceridaemia** [10], correct these. Depending on symptoms, **diet can be introduced early** [11] and progressively upgraded as tolerated. **Monitor for sepsis or deterioration** [12], which may suggest **infection or**

pancreatic necrosis [13]. If the abdominal ultrasound demonstrates cholelithiasis, **perform a laparoscopic cholecystectomy** [14] once the patient is clinically improved. If alcoholic pancreatitis is suspected, commence a **brief alcohol intervention** [15] in the inpatient setting. The patient may be discharged when they are **haemodynamically stable and afebrile** [16], **functionally independent** [17], **pain-free** [18], **and tolerating normal diet** [19].

Long-term

Give **appropriate prevention advice** [20] according to the underlying cause. If the patient is postoperative, follow up the patient in an **outpatient clinic** [21] to review histopathology and the wounds, and to arrange appropriate ongoing care.

1 As for every patient, commence with an assessment of vital signs – airway, breathing and circulation – and proceed to implement resuscitation if necessary. Tachycardia and hypotension should prompt aggressive fluid resuscitation.

2 All patients with acute pancreatitis should be admitted to hospital under either the gastroenterology or general

surgery unit, depending on institutional protocol. In cases of severe pancreatitis, or in patients who are comorbid or systemically unwell, consider admission to the intensive care unit, and transfer to a major referral centre if needed.

3 Keep the patient nil by mouth initially until pain, nausea and vomiting improve.

4 Begin fluid resuscitation with crystalloids such as normal saline or compound sodium lactate (Hartmann's solution). Ensure that losses are replaced, and adequate maintenance fluids are given; remember that maintenance fluid requirements are increased in sepsis. In patients with cardiac failure or renal failure, be wary of fluid overload and seek specialist advice if needed.

5 Analgesia should be given as required to avoid pain-related haemodynamic instability; opioids will be key to an effective analgesia strategy. Monitor for sedation or respiratory depression if large doses are required.

6 Correct any electrolyte imbalances or acid–base disturbance; seek ICU admission if these are severe. Replacement of potassium and magnesium is also key to resolution of any ileus.

7 Continue to monitor and replace electrolytes during the acute admission.

8 The BGL should be carefully managed to reduce risk of secondary infection. Exercise caution, however, in patients with poor or restricted oral intake. Seek Endocrinology advice if needed.

9 Continue to ensure that losses are replaced, and maintenance fluid requirements are met. Urine output should be measured strictly and is a good guide as to the patient's volume status, although in patients with intrinsic renal disease, be careful not to misinterpret low urine output as hypovolaemia, to avoid causing iatrogenic fluid overload.

10 Correct any hypercalcaemia or hypertriglyceridaemia which could be the underlying aetiology of the acute pancreatitis, and seek Endocrinology advice as necessary.

11 Oral intake should be reintroduced early when nausea and vomiting have resolved, and upgraded as tolerated, providing that abdominal pain is decreasing, and inflammatory markers are downtrending. This can be from clear fluids to free fluids to light ward diet and finally full ward diet, or more rapidly, according to the clinical scenario. If the patient's clinical situation precludes diet from being reintroduced within 5–7 days, consider whether the patient may benefit from enteral or parenteral nutrition.

12 Monitor the patient's vital signs and inflammatory markers, and perform serial abdominal examinations, to detect any developing infection, pseudocysts, collection or necrosis. After the first 3 days, CT abdomen is a useful study to identify the presence of local complications.

13 Infected necrosis may require antibiotic treatment; aspiration or necrosectomy are also interventions which may be considered for the management of infected collections or necrosis.

14 Laparoscopic cholecystectomy should be performed in all patients with gallstone pancreatitis following recovery, to prevent future pancreatobiliary disease. Patients should be pain-free and tolerating normal diet before proceeding to surgery. Cholecystectomy can usually be performed during the index admission, although patients with severe necrotising pancreatitis may need to have surgery delayed and done electively. If there is a high suspicion of choledocholithiasis, ERCP can be done preoperatively; this is both diagnostic and therapeutic for choledocholithiasis.

15 In cases of alcoholic pancreatitis, intervention for alcohol abuse should be commenced during the index admission. Motivational interviewing can be done by any healthcare provider and should determine the patient's readiness for change to establish an appropriate goal with regard to abstinence or reduction of alcohol consumption. The inpatient Addiction Medicine Unit can be involved in this as required and follow-up arranged in the community with the GP or a specialist Drug and Alcohol service.

16 Patients must be haemodynamically stable and afebrile to ensure that they are medically suitable for discharge.

17 Prolonged admissions can cause patients to become deconditioned, and the elderly and comorbid are particularly vulnerable. Involve allied health teams including physiotherapy, occupational therapy and social work to ensure that patients are at pre-morbid level of functioning and safe to be discharged home. Inpatient rehabilitation can be considered if required for additional allied health interventions once a patient is medically cleared.

18 Patients should be pain-free prior to discharge, indicating resolution of their acute pancreatitis.

19 Ensure that patients are also tolerating normal diet before they are discharged; this will signal both that their pancreatitis has resolved, as well as any associated intestinal ileus.

20 Give the patient appropriate prevention advice for future episodes of pancreatitis. In many cases, prevention will be largely achieved during the index admission by cholecystectomy; counselling for alcohol abuse is most relevant for patients presenting with alcoholic pancreatitis. Ensure that patients have appropriate community follow-up, as above.

21 Postoperative patients should be reviewed in the outpatient clinic to check that the wounds have healed. On review in the clinic, check for surrounding cellulitis, fluctuance or discharge to ensure that there is no wound infection. Review the histopathology as well from the excised gallbladder to detect any unexpected findings.

CASE 24: Diverticulitis

History

- A **65-year-old** [1] male with **a history of obesity** [2] presents with **worsening left lower quadrant pain** [3], **nausea and vomiting** [4] for **the past 16 hours** [5].
- He has had **similar pain previously** [6], although less severe, which resolved with oral antibiotics.
- His past medical history is also remarkable for **T2DM** [7] **managed with a basal-bolus insulin regimen** [8].

- He denies any **recent rectal bleeding** [9].
- He has **never had a colonoscopy** [10].
- He **does minimal regular physical activity** [11] and **smokes** [12] 20 cigarettes every day.
- His diet is predominantly **red meat with few vegetables** [13].
- He has **not been tolerating any oral intake** [14] today.

[1] Although only a minority of patients with diverticulosis have complications from their diverticular disease, increasing age is a risk factor both for the occurrence of diverticulitis and for complications associated with diverticulitis.

[2] Obesity is likewise a risk factor for diverticulitis, and sometimes is associated with diverticulitis in younger patients.

[3] Pain associated with sigmoid diverticulitis, which is the most common location of diverticular disease in western, industrialised countries, usually presents in the left lower quadrant. However, Asian countries in contrast have predominantly right-sided disease, and the associated presentation of caecal diverticulitis with right lower quadrant pain can be misdiagnosed as appendicitis.

[4] Ileus may arise from peritoneal irritation associated with diverticulitis, and so many patients with acute diverticulitis also present with nausea and vomiting.

[5] A minority of patients with diverticulitis may present with chronic abdominal pain, but most patients present with a history of acute abdominal pain.

[6] Some patients may have recurrent or a subacute diverticulitis, hence it is important to determine whether there is a history of previous episodes of pain.

[7] History of comorbidities is significant for determining risk for complications, and is a key part of decision-making regarding disposition (whether to admit the patient, and if so, then where), and whether to operate, and if so, in what time frame. In addition, patients with T2DM may have associated problems, such as renal impairment, and will require attention to glycaemic control to minimise the associated additional risk of wound infection or other complications.

[8] The use of insulin in T2DM suggests more advanced disease which has likely been previously inadequately managed with oral hypoglycaemics. Characterise the exact insulin regimen and usual BGLs in order to appropriate titrate insulin as an inpatient, particularly in the context of acute medical stressors and reduced oral intake.

[9] Rarely, diverticular bleeding may occur, which usually presents as rapid onset, painless and large volume haematochezia.

[10] Recent colonoscopy is a valuable aid and may confirm the presence of diverticulosis, as well as excluding the presence of any colorectal cancers.

[11] Risk of symptomatic diverticular disease is increased by sedentary lifestyle, and is decreased by regular exercise.

[12] Smoking is associated with diverticulitis and also increases risk of complications, including abscess and perforation.

[13] Diet that is low in fibre and high in fat, characteristic of highly refined, processed foods, increases risk of symptomatic diverticular disease, as does high intake of red meat.

[14] Patients with diverticulitis may have nausea and vomiting secondary to ileus or bowel obstruction arising from irritation of the peritoneum.

Examination

- On examination, the patient is **alert and oriented** [1] .
- He does not **appear critically unwell** [2] , although he is in obvious pain.
- He is **haemodynamically stable** [3] and clinically **euvolaemic** [4] .
- He is **febrile** [5] .
- His abdomen is **soft** [6] , with **severe tenderness** in the left lower quadrant [7] and **voluntary guarding** [8] .
- There are **no features of peritonism** [9] .
- He has **hypoactive bowel sounds** [10] on auscultation.
- Rectal examination is unremarkable, with **no discernible mass** [11] and **no blood** [12] .

[1] Acute confusion suggests severe systemic illness and may arise secondary to severe hypovolaemia or sepsis.

[2] Expect that a patient with diverticulitis may appear to be uncomfortable; however, if they appear critically unwell, lying still in the bed or in extreme pain, consider whether they may be peritonitic. This may indicate perforation or sepsis.

[3] Severe pain may cause tachycardia and hypertension, whilst hypovolaemia and sepsis will first cause tachycardia then hypotension. A haemodynamically unstable patient may require an urgent resuscitation effort.

[4] Assess the patient's volume status. Reduced tissue turgor, dry mucous membranes, prolonged capillary refill and reduced urine output are signs of hypovolaemia, whilst peripheral oedema or elevated JVP may suggest hypervolaemia, which may result from overly aggressive fluid resuscitation, cardiac or renal disease.

[5] Low grade fever is common in diverticulitis. Persistent fever despite antibiotic treatment may suggest an abscess, while high fever may be associated with sepsis.

[6] In the absence of perforation and peritonitis, expect the abdomen to be soft to palpation. If there is ileus, the abdomen may also be distended and tympanic to percussion.

[7] Left lower quadrant tenderness is consistent with sigmoid diverticulitis.

[8] Voluntary guarding may be present as the patient consciously tightens their abdominal wall musculature to avoid pain associated with palpation.

[9] Assessment of peritonism includes features of rebound tenderness, guarding and rigidity. Peritonism indicates a serious intra-abdominal pathology, which will usually be perforation in the case of suspected diverticulitis.

[10] Bowel sounds may be hypoactive or absent in the setting of ileus or bowel obstruction.

[11] Rectal examination is a mandatory part of the abdominal examination; apart from detecting any rectal cancers, a sigmoid diverticular abscess may be palpable.

[12] Assess for any rectal bleeding; diverticular bleeding is characteristically profuse.

Investigations

- On FBE, the **haemoglobin is within normal limits** [1] and **WCC is elevated** [2] .
- **CRP is elevated** [3] .
- UEC demonstrates **mildly impaired renal function** [4] and **normal electrolytes** [5] .
- VBG shows **normal acid–base status** [6] and a **normal lactate** [7] .
- **LFT and lipase are normal** [8] .
- Urine dipstick shows **leucocytes** [9] .
- **Urine culture is pending** [10] .
- Erect CXR is **negative for pneumoperitoneum** [11] .
- An abdominal CT is consistent with a diagnosis of **acute diverticulitis** [12] complicated by **microperforation** [13] , but **no free perforation or other complications** [14] .

[1] Check for anaemia, which may either be a clue to potentially occult rectal bleeding, or may be a complication in planning an operation.

[2] Mild leucocytosis or normal WCC is consistent with diverticulitis; consider complications such as abscess, perforation or sepsis if WCC is profoundly elevated.

[3] CRP is a marker of systemic inflammatory response; as with WCC, elevation is consistent with acute diverticulitis, although if profound, consider if abscess, perforation or sepsis may be present.

[4] Renal function should be compared with a baseline value to determine if any renal impairment is acute or chronic.

In this patient, chronic kidney disease is likely related to his history of diabetes mellitus, whilst an acute kidney injury could result from severe hypovolaemia or sepsis.

5 Electrolytes should be checked and replaced as required.

6 VBG will rapidly assess acid–base status, as well as haemoglobin and some electrolytes. Metabolic acidosis may arise from hypovolaemia, sepsis or acute kidney injury; metabolic alkalosis may arise from prolonged vomiting.

7 Normal lactate is reassuring; elevated lactate is an indicator of complications such as ischaemia, severe hypovolaemia or sepsis, although non-specific.

8 Liver function testing and lipase should be included as part of the work-up of acute abdominal pain. Although lipase may be slightly elevated in keeping with intra-abdominal inflammation, these results would otherwise be expected to be unremarkable in a patient with acute diverticulitis.

9 Colonic inflammation adjacent to the bladder may cause pyuria. In addition, see whether there is haematuria present, which may raise suspicion of renal or ureteric colic as a differential diagnosis.

10 Urine culture will take over a day to return a result, but should ideally be collected and sent prior to the initial administration of antibiotics. The growth of enteric flora is suggestive of a colovesical fistula, which may complicate acute diverticulitis.

11 Erect CXR can be rapidly facilitated at the bedside to determine if there is any frank pneumoperitoneum, which will appear on a plain radiograph as subdiaphragmatic free gas.

12 CT abdomen is the imaging modality of choice to investigate suspected acute diverticulitis. CT will exclude other causes of acute abdominal pain, confirm the diagnosis of diverticulitis and also determine if any complications are present. CT findings consistent with acute diverticulitis include diverticulosis, peridiverticular fat stranding and local colonic wall thickening.

13 Microperforation is characterised by only a few air bubbles outside the bowel wall; this is importantly distinguished from free perforation, which includes subdiaphragmatic free gas.

14 CT abdomen may demonstrate findings of complicated diverticulitis, including perforation or abscess.

Management

Immediate

Monitor **vital signs** [1] and perform resuscitation if required. **Admit** [2] the patient to hospital. Keep the patient **fasted** [3]. Give IV **fluids** [4] and appropriate **analgesia** [5]. Give IV **antibiotics** [6]. Correct **any electrolyte disturbance** [7]. Consider if there is any **indication for surgery** [8]. Consider **admission to ICU if required** [9].

Short-term

Monitor the patient clinically for any acute deterioration in pain or vital signs [10]. **Monitor and replace electrolytes** [11] during the acute admission. Control the patient's **blood glucose level** [12]. **Titrate IV fluid rate** [13]. **Upgrade diet** [14] progressively as tolerated. **Monitor inflammatory markers** [15]. If there is failure to improve, **consider repeat CT abdomen** [16]. **Manage

any complications** [17] as necessary, or **consider operative intervention** [18]. The patient may be discharged when they are **haemodynamically stable and afebrile** [19], **functionally independent** [20], **pain-free** [21], **tolerating normal diet** [22], and **with downtrending inflammatory markers** [23].

Long-term

Give **dietary and lifestyle advice** [24] prior to discharge. Continue **oral antibiotics** [25]. If the patient is postoperative, follow up the patient in an **outpatient clinic** [26] to review histopathology and the wounds, and to arrange appropriate ongoing care. Otherwise, follow up the patient with a **colonoscopy** [27] after an interval of 6–8 weeks. On review, consider **elective surgery** [28] if symptoms are ongoing or recurrent.

1 Begin your assessment of every patient with an assessment of vital signs and perform resuscitation if required. Basic life support includes management of airway, breathing and circulation, in that order.

2 Some patients with mild, uncomplicated diverticulitis may be managed in an outpatient setting if they are low

risk. However, patients with severe pain, microperforation, fever, sepsis or other complications should be managed as an inpatient, as should patients who are aged >70, comorbid, immunosuppressed or who are not tolerating oral intake.

3 Patients may be fasted or restricted to clear fluids alone, depending on severity, for bowel rest. Patients should also be fasted if emergency surgery is being considered, for at least 6 hours prior to the induction of anaesthesia.

4 IV fluids should be commenced, with consideration of both correcting fluid depletion and maintenance fluid requirements. If the patient is tachycardic or hypotensive, aggressive fluid resuscitation will be required; although in this case, be alert for fluid overload in patients with comorbid cardiac or renal disease.

5 Analgesia should be given as required. Opioid analgesia is effective for the management of severe, acute pain.

6 Commence IV antibiotics. Key antibiotic targets include Gram-negative enteric organisms, as well as obligate anaerobes; for this reason, ceftriaxone and metronidazole in combination are appropriate choices. For patients who are higher risk or with complications, piperacillin-tazobactam as monotherapy is an alternative choice.

7 Any electrolyte disturbance should be corrected, particularly with regard to potassium and magnesium replacement as required.

8 Consider if there is any indication for emergency surgery; most particularly, patients with freely perforated diverticulitis. The objective is to manage peritoneal contamination and resect the diseased segment of colon. The surgical approach for an emergency operation will depend, however, on haemodynamic stability as well as comorbidity and intraoperative findings. A Hartmann's procedure is commonly employed, involving resection of the diseased segment of sigmoid colon, with formation of an end colostomy. In this case, colostomy reversal may be considered after several months, depending on the degree of faecal contamination and patient comorbidities. However, if a patient is too unstable for a definitive colonic resection, a damage control laparotomy can be performed for washout of peritoneal contamination and faecal diversion, with definitive resection delayed to a later time.

9 Consider whether admission to the ICU may be required. Large volume diverticular bleeding, sepsis, haemodynamic instability or comorbidity may be indications for intensive care support, or if required peri-operatively.

10 Review the patient regularly with regular observations and serial abdominal examinations. New or persistent fever may suggest an abscess, whilst peritonitis, tachycardia and hypotension are concerning for perforation. If there is suspicion for acute deterioration, emergency surgery may be indicated, or otherwise erect CXR or repeat CT abdomen can be performed. Patients with failure to improve over 3 days or longer should be re-imaged with a repeat CT abdomen, and even if this is normal, may require exploratory surgery if there is still no improvement over the following days.

11 Electrolytes should continue to be checked and replaced as needed, to promote resolution of any ileus.

12 The patient's BGL should be strictly monitored with adjustment of any oral or injectable hypoglycaemics as required, in accordance with diet status. BGLs may be labile in the setting of acute illness, as well as reduced oral intake.

13 IV fluids should be continued as required for correction of ongoing losses, and for any maintenance fluid requirements not being met orally.

14 Diet can be gradually upgraded from nil by mouth to clear fluids, free fluids, light diet and regular diet. The timing of this will depend on symptoms including pain, nausea and vomiting, serial clinical examination as to vital signs and abdominal tenderness, and laboratory studies, particularly regarding whether the inflammatory markers are downtrending.

15 Serial laboratory studies track the systemic inflammatory response, though it is important to be aware that these may lag behind the clinical findings.

16 Repeat CT abdomen should be considered if there is failure to improve with 2–3 days of IV antibiotic therapy; this will determine whether there is any complicating collection or abscess (particularly if there is persistent fever or pain), any ileus or obstruction (particularly if there is persistent nausea or vomiting), or a fistula (most commonly a colovesical or colovaginal fistula).

17 CT-guided percutaneous drainage can be performed if there is a diverticular abscess or a collection; nasogastric tube insertion and downgrade of diet may be required for ileus or colonic obstruction.

18 Free perforation, a fistula, an abscess which cannot be percutaneously drained, large bowel obstruction and failure to improve after several days of conservative management are all indications for operative intervention. The nature of surgery required will depend on the particular complication but may require a multi-stage procedure including the formation of a diverting colostomy.

19 Haemodynamic stability and absence of any fever signals that the patient is not critically unwell and this is a prerequisite to discharge planning.

20 Functional independence is necessary to consider, particularly for elderly and comorbid patients who may be vulnerable to deconditioning over a prolonged hospital admission. Allied health professionals, including physiotherapists, occupational therapists, social workers and dietitians, are valuable to assess a patient's functional status prior to discharge, and implement any necessary interventions, or otherwise facilitate a referral to inpatient rehabilitation if required. Stomal therapy review is particularly essential for any patients who have had a newly formed stoma, to ensure that they are appropriately resourced and educated to manage this in the community. Stomal education should start early to help the patient to develop these skills in the inpatient setting, and so that this does not become an impediment to discharge when the patient is medically stable.

21 Abdominal pain should have resolved or be substantially controlled prior to discharge, in accordance with resolution of the underlying acute inflammation.

22 Patients must also be tolerating a regular diet prior to discharge, indicating the resolution of any ileus, and so that the patient can easily be managed in the community, without inpatient nutritional and hydration support.

23 Inflammatory markers, WCC and CRP should be downtrending or within normal range prior to discharge, indicating that the systemic inflammatory response is resolving.

24 Give patients prevention advice prior to discharge, to avoid future episodes of diverticulitis. Dietary advice includes encouraging the patient to follow a high-fibre diet, with increased consumption of fruit and vegetables, and to limit intake of red meat. Although patients with diverticulitis were historically advised to avoid nuts and seeds, this is not supported by evidence. Encourage general health measures such as regular physical activity.

25 Oral antibiotics should be continued following discharge, for a total of 10–14 days' total antibiotic treatment (oral and IV). Amoxicillin-clavulanic acid is an appropriate oral choice for broad coverage, including enteric organisms.

26 Postoperative patients need to be reviewed in the outpatient clinic. Wound review should involve verifying that the wound has healed, that there is no cellulitis, fluctuance or discharge indicating a wound infection. Histopathology should also be reviewed, particularly to ensure there are no unexpected findings, such as colorectal cancer, which may require further management.

27 Unless they have had a colonoscopy within the previous year, a colonoscopy should be performed for all patients who present with acute diverticulitis. This serves two functions: to assess the severity of diverticulosis, and importantly, to exclude any colorectal cancer, which can sometimes present similarly to diverticulitis and appear similar radiologically. Delaying the colonoscopy for 6–8 weeks post admission allows time for the inflammation to settle and reduces the risk of colonic perforation.

28 Patients who have high risk of complicated diverticulitis, including immunosuppressed or comorbid, should be considered for elective surgery to resect the diseased segment of colon, to avoid severe morbidity or mortality associated with a recurrent episode. Elective resection should also be considered for patients with ongoing or chronic symptoms who have failed conservative management. In contrast with emergency operations, the resection can usually be done as a single-staged procedure with a primary colonic anastomosis.

CASE 25:   Groin hernia

History

- A **43-year-old** [1] **male** [2] who works as a labourer presents to the ED with a palpable lump in his right groin that **cannot be reduced** [3] following a history of **lifting a heavy object** [4] .
- He is slightly nauseated with pain; however, reports no vomiting, is **passing flatus** [5] and has no other bowel symptoms.
- He reports a dragging pain that extends to his scrotum with **no radiation to his upper thigh** [6] .

- He has a past history significant for hypertension, diet-controlled T2DM and a **history of his father having an inguinal hernia repair** [7] .
- He has **no previous abdominal surgeries** [8] , no regular medications and no allergies.
- He is a current **heavy smoker** [9] .
- He **last ate 6 hours ago** [10] .

[1] While inguinal hernias are quite a common congenital condition and present in infants, in adults increased age is a risk factor for the development of inguinal hernias and indeed all forms of hernias.

[2] There is a male preponderance of inguinal hernias in particular, with a ratio of up to 7:1 compared with females. This is primarily due to the anatomical differences and the structures which pass through the inguinal canal.

[3] In all hernias, it is important to note whether they are reducible. This can indicate either incarcerated or strangulated hernias, which are a surgical emergency.

[4] Any cause of increased intra-abdominal pressure causes an increase in hernias – whether this be on Valsalva manoeuvre, standing upright or on coughing.

[5] When a patient comes in with an irreducible hernia it is important to assess for the presence of any signs or symptoms of bowel obstruction. This would indicate either an incarcerated or strangulated hernia – a surgical emergency. Passing of flatus is a reassuring symptom; however, it is not definitive.

[6] The typical pain described by patients is often not a spot pain but rather a dragging pain that radiates down the path of the canal and to the scrotum. If the pain was extending through to the medial thigh this would indicate that the patient may have a different pathology – a femoral hernia. Femoral hernias are much more common in women and are much more likely to become incarcerated or strangulate and as such are an important differential to consider.

[7] Family history is also a risk factor for inguinal hernias.

[8] Past operations are of particular consideration in this case – recurrent hernias or incisional hernias are also prone to incarcerate, more so than primary ones. This also impacts operative planning and approach – when previous hernias repairs have been open, a laparoscopic approach is preferred in subsequent surgeries if needed.

[9] COPD and chronic cough are associated with hernias – due to chronic elevation of intra-abdominal pressure.

[10] Fasting status and readiness for surgery are important considerations and need to be communicated with the anaesthetic team. In general, the patient needs to be fasting for 6 hours preoperatively in order to reduce the risk of aspiration.

Examination

- The patient **looks uncomfortable** [1] lying in his hospital bed.
- He is **visibly overweight** [2] .
- His vital signs are stable with a **borderline tachycardia of 95bpm** [3] .
- His **abdomen is generally soft on supine examination** [4] and he has a visible lump over his right groin, medial to the inguinal ligament.

- This **does not extend to the scrotum** [5] .
- The lump **cannot be reduced** [6] and is tender on palpation.
- There are **no overlying skin changes** [7] .
- On standing, the lump is slightly increased in size and there is a **cough impulse present** [8] .
- There are **no bowel sounds audible in the lump** [9] .

1 The 'end-of-the-bed-o-gram' is important in clinical medicine. Visible signs of pain or discomfort on passive observation are important signals of the patient's clinical state.

2 Weight of patients is important when assessing anaesthetic risk, surgical difficulty and examination findings. It is more difficult to assess hernias in patients with increased body habitus.

3 Tachycardia can be a sign of hypovolaemia, arrhythmia, or in this case could reflect pain or early sepsis.

4 The absence of peritonism is important in patients with abdominal pathology and can impact operative timing and decision-making. Hernias may be more difficult to identify on supine examination and indeed laying the patient supine can aid in reduction.

5 Inguinal anatomy is important to understand in the setting of examination. The deep inguinal ring lies just medial to the mid-point of the inguinal ligament. By definition, an indirect hernia passes through this point and extends through the canal and can extend all the way to the scrotum. A direct inguinal hernia is a defect in the posterior wall of the canal and occurs in Hesselbach's triangle (formed by the inguinal ligament laterally, the lateral border of the rectus abdominus medially and the inferior epigastric vessels superolaterally). This is more likely an acquired condition, whereas indirect hernias are very common in infants, particularly premature babies, due to the delayed closure of the processus vaginalis. This topic is further discussed in *Case 54* in *Chapter 6*, Paediatric surgery. While differentiating between direct and indirect hernias does not impact management, it does reflect a difference in aetiology and longer-term outcomes. For example, an indirect hernia is much more likely to strangulate.

6 If a hernia cannot be reduced, this can reflect an incarcerated or potentially strangulated hernia.

7 In the presence of pain, it is more likely that the hernia contents are incarcerated or strangulated. If there are overlying skin changes, this again indicates the pathology underlying. In this case, it is not recommended to reduce the hernia. Urgent surgical exploration is indicated.

8 Presence of a cough impulse is diagnostic of a hernia.

9 This is an inexact examination finding; however, it reflects that the presence of bowel sounds is an important consideration when making plans for management.

Investigations

- A routine FBE and UEC were collected which were unremarkable, with **no elevation in WCC or derangement of renal function** [1]. Clotting studies were normal.
- A VBG was also taken, which revealed a **normal lactate of 0.9mmol/L** [2]. Urinalysis was normal.
- The patient was subsequently taken for **groin ultrasound** [3] which showed bilateral inguinal hernias.
- On the right was a **direct inguinal hernia** [4] **containing fat** [5], and on the left was a small indirect inguinal hernia only present on Valsalva.
- There were **no femoral hernias seen** [6].

1 Elevated WCC can indicate infection in the patient or inflammatory response to tissue injury, or is a negative sign in patients with bowel obstruction. In dehydration or sepsis, renal function can become deranged and requires urgent correction.

2 Lactate is a sensitive marker of anaerobic metabolism and is particularly elevated in ischaemic states. While there are other states that cause elevated lactate (including sepsis), in this context a normal lactate is reassuring for the bowel that may be present in the irreducible hernia.

3 The modality of choice is ultrasound, which can identify the contents and anatomy of the hernia. Dynamic studies can also be performed, with and without Valsalva. In situations where there is more uncertainty about the diagnosis or incongruent history or examination, and if access to ultrasound is limited, then CT also is good at demonstrating the contents and size of the hernia and can reflect on the state of the contents, including bowel wall oedema.

4 Direct hernias are less common than indirect and are less likely to strangulate.

5 A fat-containing hernia can still be a painful situation and does run the risk of fat necrosis and the patient becoming unwell with this. However, it is less dangerous than a situation with the hernia containing bowel and being irreducible.

6 Femoral hernias are more likely to strangulate when present. They are more common in women. They are also more difficult to detect clinically unless large.

Management

Immediate

Resuscitate [1] as required. In the absence of pain or other reasons to suspect strangulated hernia, analgesia administration and **attempted reduction is an appropriate first-line approach** [2] . If unsuccessful, admission to hospital and arrangement of emergency theatre is appropriate. Keep the patient **nil by mouth** [3] and as comfortable as possible with IV therapy and analgesia.

Short-term

If the hernia is reducible, the patient should still have a hernia repair as soon as practicable. This can be either open or laparoscopic. The patient should be observed in hospital overnight to ensure there are **no issues with voiding** [4] or postoperative bleeding. Once the patient has been reviewed postoperatively, mobilising, voiding and tolerating diet, they are safe for discharge home.

Long-term

Follow the patient up either through the **surgical outpatient clinic or through their referring GP** [5] .

[1] As always, the priority for every patient is to ensure the ABCs are fully assessed and as stable as possible and then proceed with definitive management.

[2] If a hernia can be reduced, this eliminates the immediate risk of strangulation and incarceration. If there are already signs of these, then proceeding to operative management is the most appropriate course of action.

[3] The patient is most safe when fasted appropriately prior to theatre.

[4] In the immediate postoperative period, urinary retention can occur due to pain, immobility and constipation. This is an important consideration when asked to review the post hernia repair patient.

[5] This would be a routine post-op review for wound review. It is unlikely that a recurrence would occur; however, if the symptoms were to recur surgical evaluation would be recommended. Longer-term side-effects of hernia repair include numbness in the area of the ilioinguinal nerve, and chronic pain can also occur, something that the patient should be made aware of preoperatively.

CASE 26: Large bowel obstruction

History

- A **78-year-old** [1] male **living at home** [2] with **a history of diverticulitis managed conservatively 2 years ago** [3] presents with **worsening colicky, periumbilical abdominal pain** [4] and **obstipation** [5] over the **past 4 days** [6].
- He also feels **bloated** [7] and has noted **unintentional loss of weight over the last month** [8].

- He has been having **increasingly infrequent bowel actions for several months** [9].
- He has **nausea but no vomiting** [10].
- He has **no history of rectal bleeding** [11].
- He **last ate 6 hours ago** [12].
- He has **never had a colonoscopy** [13] and has **no other significant past medical or surgical history** [14].
- He has no **relevant family history** [15].

[1] Large bowel obstruction usually occurs in the elderly.

[2] Institutionalisation is a risk factor for volvulus.

[3] Past medical history is an important clue to determining the aetiology of a suspected large bowel obstruction. Known colorectal malignancy is a risk factor. Diverticular disease, abdominal radiation, past colonic resection, inflammatory bowel disease and episodes of ischaemic colitis are all causes of strictures, which may cause large bowel obstruction. Sigmoid or caecal volvulus may have occurred previously.

[4] The colicky nature of abdominal pain in large bowel obstruction relates to colonic peristalsis. The visceral-type periumbilical pain worsens with colonic distension. Pain becoming constant, focal, and exacerbated by movement, coughing or deep breathing may raise concerns for peritoneal irritation, ischaemia or impending perforation.

[5] Obstipation – when a patient is no longer passing stool or flatus – is characteristic of a complete obstruction. Beware, however; patients may pass faecal matter from colon distal to the obstruction even after the onset of symptoms.

[6] Large bowel obstruction occurring abruptly is usually due to volvulus, whereas a gradual onset suggests other causes, most commonly malignancy.

[7] Bloating will arise from colonic distension and may be more prominent in large bowel obstruction compared to small bowel obstruction.

[8] A history of unintentional, unexplained loss of weight is concerning for underlying malignancy.

[9] Altered bowel habit, particularly worsening constipation, may be related to progressive obstruction secondary to colorectal cancer. Worsening constipation from other causes

may also eventually result in faecal impaction or colonic pseudo-obstruction.

[10] As large bowel obstruction is by definition more distal than small bowel obstruction, nausea and vomiting are consequently less prominent, though they may occur as late symptoms. In particular, a minority of patients with large bowel obstruction may have an incompetent ileocaecal valve, which allows decompression of the obstruction through the small bowel. This may cause symptoms of small bowel obstruction as well – and faeculent vomiting as a late sign.

[11] History of rectal bleeding in the setting of obstipation is concerning for colorectal malignancy.

[12] A patient with bowel obstruction is unlikely to be hungry, and fasting status is important to determine in case an emergency operation is required.

[13] A previous colonoscopy could again be a source of information regarding an aetiology of a suspected large bowel obstruction; a stricture, diverticulosis, a neoplasm or a redundant sigmoid colon are all relevant colonoscopic findings.

[14] Apart from clues to the aetiology of a large bowel obstruction, other relevant risk factors include diabetes mellitus, whereby autonomic dysfunction can be a risk factor for colonic volvulus. Mental illness and laxative abuse are also risk factors for colonic volvulus.

[15] Family history of inflammatory bowel disease and colorectal cancer are particularly relevant.

Examination

- On examination, the patient appears uncomfortable but **not critically unwell** [1].
- He is **haemodynamically stable** [2], but **clinically hypovolaemic** [3].
- He is **afebrile** [4].
- His **abdomen is distended** [5].
- On palpation, there is **moderate generalised tenderness** [6] but **no peritonism** [7].

- There is **no palpable abdominal mass** [8].
- There are **no detectable hernias** [9].
- The abdomen is **tympanic to percussion** [10] and on auscultation, **bowel sounds are increased** [11].
- On rectal examination, the **rectum is empty** [12] and there are no **masses** [12] or **other abnormalities** [12] found.

[1] A critically unwell patient might be peritonitic secondary to perforation, or systemically unwell, requiring urgent management.

[2] Assessment of haemodynamics should include airway, breathing and circulation. Be aware of tachypnoea, tachycardia or hypotension, which may indicate a complicated obstruction, although tachycardia in isolation may relate to hypovolaemia or pain.

[3] Ensure that you assess the patient's volume status, including urine output, mucous membranes, as well as haemodynamic status. Large bowel obstruction may cause hypovolaemia.

[4] Fever may indicate systemic inflammatory response resulting from a complication such as ischaemia or infection.

[5] Abdominal distension is often more prominent in large bowel obstruction compared to small bowel obstruction. Distension will be increased particularly with more distal and more complete obstructions. On abdominal inspection, in a thin patient, peristaltic waves may also be seen and strongly suggest obstruction; these will not be present in ileus, which is characterised by decreased intestinal peristaltic activity.

[6] Generalised tenderness is characteristic of visceral pain secondary to colonic distension. Pain may become more focal in the setting of ischaemia or perforation causing irritation of the parietal peritoneum.

[7] It is critical to assess the patient for signs of peritonism. A patient with large bowel obstruction with guarding, rebound tenderness or rigidity is concerning for perforation and may require urgent intervention.

[8] An abdominal mass may indicate a diverticular abscess or malignancy.

[9] Examination for hernias is also very important. Obstructed hernias are more commonly a cause of small bowel obstruction, but rarely may cause large bowel obstruction. Inspect and palpate for abdominal hernias, including inguinal and femoral hernias.

[10] Gaseous colonic distension may cause the abdomen to be tympanic, or hyperresonant, to percussion.

[11] Bowel sounds are characteristically increased with developing large bowel obstruction, although they may be reduced or absent in late stages with colonic distension.

[12] Rectal examination is critical for this patient. Impacted faeces in the rectum or an obstructing rectal tumour may be a cause of large bowel obstruction, although an empty rectum is the more common finding. Rectal blood may also suggest colorectal malignancy, while soft stool in the rectum may indicate that the obstruction is incomplete.

Investigations

- On FBE, the **haemoglobin and platelet count are within normal limits** [1], and **white cell count is elevated** [2].
- **CRP is elevated** [3].
- **UEC demonstrates elevated urea** [4] and **hypokalaemia** [5].
- **VBG** [6] shows **normal acid–base status** [7] and a **normal lactate** [8].
- **LFT and lipase are normal** [9].

- **CEA is elevated** [10].
- An erect CXR demonstrates **no free gas under the diaphragm** [11].
- On abdomen X-ray, **colonic dilatation is seen** [12], and **no gas in the rectum** [13].
- **Abdominal CT** [14] confirms a **complete large bowel obstruction** [15], secondary to an **obstructing caecal tumour** [16], without **signs of ischaemia** [17].
- **Colonoscopy** [18] confirms a likely caecal malignancy.

1 Haemoglobin and platelet count are important for preoperative assessment. Patients with rectal bleeding may be anaemic, and even with a small amount of rectal bleeding, this may cause anaemia over a long time period. Consider whether packed red blood cells or platelet transfusion are indicated preoperatively, or further investigation for the underlying cause if this is not apparent.

2 Elevated white cell count may suggest complications such as ischaemia, infection, necrosis or perforation.

3 CRP may be elevated, in keeping with a systemic inflammatory response.

4 Hypovolaemia may cause acute kidney injury.

5 Electrolytes should be checked and replaced, particularly potassium and magnesium. These may be deranged by dehydration or fluid shifts, and generally worsen with the duration of obstruction.

6 VBG will allow the rapid assessment of lactate, which can suggest ischaemia if elevated, as well as electrolytes.

7 Metabolic acidosis may result from ischaemia or hypovolaemia.

8 Elevated lactate may indicate ischaemia or sepsis secondary to perforation.

9 LFT and lipase would be expected to be normal, but are necessary to rule out hepatobiliary and pancreatic causes of abdominal pain.

10 Elevated CEA is associated with malignancy and suggests colorectal cancer.

11 Erect CXR is a valuable first imaging modality to assess for perforated viscus; free gas under the diaphragm is the ominous associated finding.

12 Colonic dilatation confirms the diagnosis of large bowel obstruction. Colonic volvulus may also be identified on X-ray in most cases, with a classic coffee bean shape. This may be either a caecal or sigmoid volvulus, depending on whether the colon is rotated to the left or right side, respectively.

13 Gas is usually absent distal to a complete large bowel obstruction.

14 CT abdomen will again confirm the diagnosis, and may indicate the underlying aetiology of the obstruction.

15 CT abdomen will also indicate the grade of the obstruction.

16 In addition to identifying the underlying tumour, CT abdomen will allow assessment of local and regional spread for the purpose of staging.

17 Mural thickening or oedema on CT are signs of colonic ischaemia, whilst intramural air is a late and ominous sign indicating impending perforation.

18 Colonoscopy may be performed in the stable patient to further assess the cause of large bowel obstruction.

Management

Immediate

Monitor **vital signs** and **perform resuscitation if required** [1]. **Admit** [2] the patient to hospital. Keep the patient **fasted** [3]. Give IV **fluids** [4] and **insert a urinary catheter** [5] as well as a **nasogastric tube** [6]. Give appropriate **analgesia** [7]. If **emergency surgery is indicated** [8], **give antibiotics** [9] and **liaise with Anaesthesia** [10] regarding planning for theatre. If the patient has sigmoid volvulus, **flexible or rigid sigmoidoscopy should be performed immediately and a rectal tube inserted** [11].

Short-term

Further management depends on the aetiology of the large bowel obstruction. However, unlike most patients with small bowel obstruction, large bowel obstruction **generally requires operative intervention** [12], if not as an emergency, then usually during the initial admission. If there is a trial of conservative management or a delay in proceeding to operation, then be alert for **deterioration** [13], and if this occurs, emergency operation may be indicated. Postoperatively, if the patient is stable, they may be transferred to the ward. Review the **surgical sites** [14] and examine the **abdomen** [15]. Continue to **check and optimise electrolytes** [16]. Gradually upgrade **diet as tolerated** [17]. Monitor the output of the nasogastric tube; **spigot and then remove this when outputs are minimal** [18]. **Remove the urinary catheter** [19] when the patient is stable and able to mobilise. The patient may be discharged when they have **stable vital signs** [20], are **functionally independent** [21], **opening their bowels (or with an active stoma)** [22] and **tolerating normal diet** [22].

Long-term

Follow up the patient in an **outpatient clinic** [23] to review histopathology and the wounds, and to arrange appropriate ongoing care.

1 Resuscitation should occur at the first encounter with the patient as necessary, according to a systemic approach.

2 If the patient is haemodynamically stable, they can be admitted under Colorectal Surgery unit, or the General Surgery unit if a specialist Colorectal unit is unavailable. If the patient is unstable, consider if they require admission to the ICU or transfer to a higher acuity hospital. Ensure that facilities are available for an emergency operation.

3 Patients with large bowel obstruction should be fasted, both to avoid further colonic distension and in case surgery is required.

4 IV fluids are essential for resuscitation, as well as for fluid maintenance. Patients with large bowel obstruction are likely to be hypovolaemic, and previous losses must be replaced. A hypotensive or tachycardic patient will require a rapid fluid bolus. Be aware that sepsis will also increase maintenance fluid requirements. Normal saline and Hartmann's solution are widely used crystalloid IV fluids; the rate should be according to the level of volume depletion. The choice of IV fluids should be guided by electrolyte status, and electrolyte losses must be replaced intravenously as well. Seek advice if patients have a history of cardiac failure or renal failure and require aggressive fluid resuscitation, as these patients may be vulnerable to fluid overload; diuresis may be required.

5 Strictly monitor urine output and insert an indwelling urinary catheter; urine output is an indicator of volume state.

6 A nasogastric tube should be inserted for decompression. This is normally left on free drainage, with aspiration every four hours – the volume of output should be measured.

7 Analgesia should be prescribed as required in the first instance, with regular analgesia being considered if requirements are high.

8 Urgent surgical intervention is required in patients with perforation or impending perforation; this will likely require irrigation and resection of the perforated colon as a minimum, and will otherwise be directed by the underlying aetiology.

9 Ceftriaxone and metronidazole in combination, or piperacillin-tazobactam monotherapy, are reasonable antibiotic choices to cover for intestinal ischaemia or perforation. Enteric Gram-negative bacilli and anaerobes are key microbes to treat in this scenario.

10 In order to book this patient for an emergency operation, the General Surgery team will need to coordinate with Anaesthetics. Ensure that the anaesthetist is aware of the patient's comorbidities, haemodynamics and fasting status, so that they can assess the patient's suitability for a general anaesthetic, and plan for an operation within an appropriate time frame.

11 Endoscopic decompression with rectal tube insertion under flexible or rigid sigmoidoscopy should be performed as soon as sigmoid volvulus has been performed, provided that there is no complicating ischaemia or perforation necessitating operative intervention. Following rectal tube insertion, repeat abdominal X-ray will confirm that decompression was successful.

12 The surgical management of large bowel obstruction involves resection of the obstructing lesion and compromised bowel. In the case of malignant obstruction, this can be done with curative intent as a single-stage resection with primary anastomosis, or as a multi-stage procedure. Multi-stage procedures may include a diverting colostomy first, followed by resection of the obstructing lesion, followed by restoration of intestinal continuity. The choice of which approach to take is dependent on balancing the risk of anastomotic leak with the morbidity associated with the formation of a stoma. This will depend on the condition of the colon intraoperatively, comorbidities, location of the lesion and life expectancy of the patient. Alternatively, in patients with limited life expectancy and high surgical risk being managed palliatively, a permanent diverting colostomy may be formed. Endoscopic stenting is another approach, either for palliation or to prepare the patient for a definitive procedure, by relieving the acute colonic obstruction.

13 Increasing abdominal distension, worsening pain, nausea or vomiting and particularly peritonism are important signs to be alert for on serial abdominal examination, which may indicate a progression of the large bowel obstruction.

14 Review of the surgical sites postoperatively should check that the wounds are closed, without any erythema, fluctuance or discharge that would suggest infection or dehiscence.

15 Some abdominal tenderness is expected postoperatively; however, increasing abdominal tenderness may indicate a complication such as bleeding (be alert for rectal bleeding as well) or an anastomotic leak. Also, increasing distension may indicate a postoperative ileus requiring downgrade of diet status and nasogastric decompression.

16 Continue to replace electrolyte losses, particularly potassium and magnesium, to support colonic motility.

17 Postoperatively, diet may be upgraded from nil by mouth to sips of clear fluid to clear fluids to free fluids and then light ward diet or regular diet. The upgrade of diet postoperatively is guided by markers of intestinal function – such as passing flatus and opening bowels (or stoma activity) – as well as indicators that ileus may be developing, such as high nasogastric outputs, nausea or vomiting. Operative considerations, such as the complexity and type of surgery, are also relevant.

18 Decreasing nasogastric tube outputs is an indicator that intestinal function is returning to normal, and together with how well the patient is tolerating diet, can guide removal of the nasogastric tube.

19 The urinary catheter can usually be removed when the patient no longer requires it for reasons either of immobility or strict monitoring of urine output.

20 Haemodynamics should be closely monitored, as derangement of these may be the first sign of postoperative complications, including atelectasis, HAP, wound or UTIs, or surgical complications, such as a bleed or an anastomotic leak.

21 In addition to allied health review to ensure that patients are able to mobilise and fulfil activities of daily living at their premorbid level, patients with a new stoma will need education to manage this. If patients are medically stable but requiring further allied health interventions, consider a referral for inpatient rehabilitation.

22 When patients have opened bowels (or have an active stoma) and tolerated regular diet, these are good indicators of a return to intestinal function.

23 Follow-up will depend on the aetiology of the obstruction and the operation performed. In case a multi-stage operation was planned, the timing of any future procedures will need to be decided. In the case of malignant large bowel obstructions, following review of the histopathology, management of the colorectal cancer requires a multidisciplinary approach, and may necessitate referral to Radiation Oncology and/or Medical Oncology for adjuvant radiotherapy or chemotherapy. Common to all postoperative patients, the wounds and abdomen should be examined to ensure that there are no complications from these.

CASE 27: Perianal abscess

History

- A **28-year-old male** [1] presents to the ED with a 3-day history of painful perianal region with a palpable lump and **difficulty defecating secondary to pain** [2] .
- He has a past history significant for **diet-controlled T2DM, hypertension and obesity** [3] .
- He reports subjective fevers at home, but **denies any nausea, vomiting or abdominal pain** [4] . He denies any history of myalgias, arthralgias, mouth ulcers or previous episodes of the same.

- He **denies any perianal exudate or bleeding** [5] .
- He reports a 2-day history of constipation due to very painful defecation but **is still passing flatus** [6] .
- He **last ate 3 hours ago** [7] .
- He reports a **4 pack year history of smoking and currently smokes 10 cigarettes per day** [8] .
- He reports he hasn't been to his GP in about 6 months and **cannot remember the last time he checked his HbA1c or BGLs** [9] .

[1] In terms of perianal disease and perianal abscesses specifically, men are twice as likely as women to have these conditions.

[2] This acute history is suggestive of an infective/inflammatory condition and a new issue rather than a subacute or chronic condition that grumbles along for months to years.

[3] T2DM is a condition that increases the likelihood and severity of skin and soft tissue infections. Knowing more about the patient's diabetes history is important.

[4] This history reveals that he is currently systemically well and doesn't have any symptoms outside of the area of pathology. Symptoms like this would indicate that he is more unwell or there is a multi-system issue occurring – for example inflammatory bowel disease.

[5] This also reflects a system review for a multi-system disease which can be related to perianal disease – Crohn's disease or ulcerative colitis can present with perianal disease. Crohn's disease in particular can have severe and complex perianal disease, including recurrent complicated abscesses and fistulae. Any perianal discharge can also reflect spontaneous drainage of the abscess.

[6] Bowel obstruction is unlikely in this case, given the straightforward history. However, with any constipation or perianal pain there is the possibility of an obstructing lesion which warrants more urgent investigation and management.

[7] Fasting status is important to ascertain in any possible surgical candidate. In emergency situations, anaesthetics can be performed regardless of fasting; however, this increases the risk of aspiration events and is avoided when possible. The sooner the source of the pain and infection is controlled, the better for the patient; however, in this clinical scenario he is well enough to wait until he is as safe as possible for anaesthetic.

[8] Smoking is a risk factor from the point of view of anaesthetics and also wound healing and infection. It reduces wound healing and as such, increases risk of infection.

[9] Further history regarding diabetes, as noted above, is important in terms of reflecting patient understanding of disease, compliance and need for education moving forward. He is not informed about his disease and the need for monitoring early in its course and this may be a chance to impress upon him the importance of preventive healthcare.

Examination

- The patient appears uncomfortable and is lying on his side on the bed.
- **Vital signs are unremarkable, and a random BGL is 11.9mmol/L** [1] .
- His **abdomen is soft and non-tender** [2] although he is uncomfortable supine.
- On per rectum (PR) examination, he is exquisitely tender to examination. At the 3 o'clock position, about 0.5cm from the anal verge is a **large erythematous fluctuant swelling** [3] that is approximately 3 x 4cm in size. There is no exudate but there does seem to be a punctum forming. Internal examination is limited by pain; however, it does not reveal an obvious internal opening or mass. Brown faeces is palpated in the rectum. There is no involvement of the nuchal ridge or more cranially and there are **no obvious pits** [3] .

[1] Whenever assessing a patient, ABCs are the first step. He is speaking and able to give a history, which is a good reflection on his ABCs in general. Specifically, he is maintaining his own airway, has a normal respiratory rate and oxygen saturation. He is not tachycardic or hypotensive and is afebrile. His BGL is elevated which is consistent with his history of diet-controlled diabetes with poor follow-up/compliance to follow-up.

[2] Abdominal examination is still important when there is a perianal pathology. This can reveal previous operations, abdominal extension or peritonism that can lead your differential in a very different direction.

[3] Perianal abscesses, particularly large and under tension, are very painful. It is important to note the distance from the anal verge, the size of the abscess/suspected abscess and presence of any surrounding cellulitis. Some abscesses may be spontaneously expressing which can be purulent or even bloody. Some abscesses can be malignancy-related and a formal internal examination is indicated for this reason and also to attempt to palpate any fistulous tracts which may exist (ridges which can be palpated on the anal wall). The patient should also be examined more cranially and looking at the natal cleft which can be the site of an important differential, pilonidal disease. These form often in hairy people and also form painful abscesses; however, they are located more superiorly and do not involve the perianal region. While perianal abscesses are related to infection of anal glands that are not draining properly, pilonidal abscesses are more cutaneous, and skin related to 'pit' formation and potentially ingrown hairs that become infected that way.

Investigations

- A set of routine bloods reveal a **leucocytosis with neutrophilia** [1] , normal haemoglobin and renal function.
- **CRP is elevated at 150mg/L** [2] . HbA1c is elevated at 8%.
- **No imaging investigations were performed** [3] .

[1] Leucocytosis is consistent with a perianal abscess.

[2] CRP is a marker of systemic inflammatory response; as with white cell count, elevation is consistent with perianal abscess.

[3] A perianal abscess, in the absence of history-related red flags, is a clinical diagnosis that has a straightforward management. If there are any concerns for the severity of the abscess or whether a more complicated pathology exists, CT scan of the pelvis can quickly show the extent of the abscess or any extension, although it may miss small abscesses. MRI scans are extremely sensitive and give a great deal of information, especially in the evaluation of complex perianal disease and particularly fistula formation, identification and management planning. This is more of a long-term management measurement, as the current infection needs control prior to definitive management.

Management

Immediate

Admit the patient to hospital, keep him fasted and commence IV antibiotics. Prescribe sufficient analgesia and IV fluids [1] .

Short-term

Once theatre time is available and the patient is appropriately fasted, proceed to theatre for an **incision and drainage of his perianal abscess** [2] . This includes a thorough examination under anaesthesia to ensure there is no fistulous tract that is being missed which may require further management, for example with a **seton** [3] . Leave the wound open to **heal by secondary intention** [4] .

Long-term

Discharge the patient home with broad-spectrum oral antibiotics. Advise daily dressing changes during the healing process. Review the patient in the **surgical outpatient clinic to ensure complete resolution of symptoms** [5] .

[1] The patient needs an incision and drainage of his abscess. This will relieve his pain and control the source of potential sepsis. Some small procedures can be done in the ED under local anaesthetic; however, perianal disease is generally dealt with under general anaesthesia, which can allow for a thorough examination and evaluation for any fistulous tracts. Broad-spectrum antibiotics will help to treat the causative organism; however, definitive source control is needed to fully solve the problem. As noted earlier, this is a painful condition and sufficient analgesia is important for patient comfort.

[2] The risks and benefits of the procedure were discussed with the patient prior. As with most procedures, the risk of the anaesthetic is discussed, in which the anaesthetist can provide further detail if required. The indication for the procedure is the evacuation of the abscess that is causing the pain and potential worsening and sepsis. The condition could be managed with antibiotics alone; however, there is a very high risk that it will not be treated completely and there can be a chronic infection, increased risk of fistulae and increased risk of perianal sepsis. The risks of the procedure include pain, infection ongoing/related to the procedure, recurrence of the abscess and need for re-operation if there is a significant cavity or severe disease. Given the location of the abscess, there is also the risk of damage to nearby structures, including the internal or external anal sphincters. This holds the risk of faecal incontinence. While this is a rare complication, it is important to include in the consent process because of the seriousness of the impact on the person's life.

[3] The other procedure that can be discussed with the patient is the insertion of a seton if required. A seton is placed in a fistula and remains *in situ* postoperatively. A fistula is an abnormal connection between two areas, in this case the anal canal and the skin in the perianal region. This can be because of internal perianal abscess extending externally and bursting at the skin margin, or through other pathologic means through inflammatory bowel disease. A seton is a ring of plastic that goes through the fistulous tract, maintaining its patency. By doing so it controls the sepsis and the potential for further blockage and abscess formation. It is a temporising measure to control sepsis and allow the infection to settle prior to definitive management (fistulotomy, mucosal advancement flaps).

[4] Surgical wounds are generally said to heal by either primary or secondary intention. Primary intention is when the two sides of epidermis are closely opposed, as in suturing. Secondary intention is when the sides are far apart, and the wound is to heal from the base upwards with granulation and eventual closure. In the setting of active infection and in this area in particular, the abscess cavity is healed through secondary intention and good wound management and dressings.

[5] There is controversy regarding the routine prescription of antibiotics on discharge following incision and drainage of perianal abscesses. A recent study showed that while a course of antibiotics did not reduce the risk of recurrent perianal abscesses, it did reduce the likelihood of fistula formation. Surgeon preference often leads antibiotic choice and duration. Follow-up to ensure resolution and avoidance of complications, such as fistula formation, is important.

CASE 28: PR bleeding

History

- An 84-year-old male presents to the ED with a 2-day history of painless bleeding per rectum (PR). He has a **past history** [1] significant for ischaemic heart disease, atrial fibrillation on warfarin, obesity, ex-smoker with COPD and insulin-dependent T2DM.
- He reports a history of **bright PR bleeding** [2] with clots every 2–3 hours of varying quantity over the last two days, worsened today with increased volume, clots and **associated presyncopal symptoms** [2]. He told his wife and it was she who called the ambulance.
- He denies any **abdominal pain, nausea or vomiting or diarrhoea; has some constipation and has no past history of any abdominal surgeries** [3].
- He lives independently at home, enjoys an active social life and requires **no assistance for mobilisation or activities of daily living** [4].
- He reports having a **colonoscopy in the past** [5]; however, he is not sure when this was or what it found.
- He denies any **family history of colorectal cancer, or any recent loss of weight or fatigue** [6]. He denies previous episodes of PR bleeding.
- He reports he recently started on some **oral antibiotics for an exacerbation of his COPD** [7].

[1] There are a number of relevant points here regarding investigation and management. Ischaemic heart disease reflects that he may not tolerate changes in his haemodynamics or fluid status and will be at risk for demand ischaemia. Having an anticoagulant on board is extremely relevant in someone actively bleeding and knowing the indication means you can make a more informed decision about potential cessation or, in this case, reversal. The knowledge of chronic heart and lung disease also reflects surgical risk.

[2] Quantifying the amount of bleeding is often a difficult task, even with direct observation in the toilet, for example. The colour and presence of clots can give clues as to origin – the dark tarry melaena indicates a more proximal source, while a bright red indicates more distal and less digested blood. The change in symptoms and the reason for presenting to hospital now is important – presyncopal symptoms indicate a compromised haemodynamic state which should ring alarm bells.

[3] He denies any symptoms which may indicate a colitis or infectious cause for PR bleeding. He has no history of surgeries or bowel resection – relatively soon postoperative anastomotic bleeds can occur.

[4] Premorbid history of patients of advancing age is important to ascertain and to note in terms of prognosis, how they will tolerate hospitalisation and potential surgical intervention and indeed, what they would like the limit of care to be.

[5] Given a PR bleed can often be from a pathological source, recent colonoscopy would be informative. Presence of diverticular disease would lead the differential diagnosis more to a diverticular bleed.

[6] Again, risk factors for a pathological cause can be ascertained. While later in life bowel cancers are more likely to be *de novo*, there is still an increased incidence in those with a strong family history.

[7] The relevance of starting a new medication in the setting of warfarin means there can be interactions which increase the efficacy of warfarin and can derange the INR past therapeutic levels.

Examination

- The patient **appears pale** [1].
- His airway is patent. Apart from saturations of 92% on air, his **vital signs are within normal limits** [2]. His GCS is 15 and he **clearly recounts his history for you** [2].
- On **abdominal examination** [3] he is soft and non-tender and there are no palpable lumps. He has no marks of previous surgeries.

- **PR examination** [4] reveals large external haemorrhoids which are non-tender, and not bleeding. The pad is stained with bright red blood. Internal examination does not elicit pain and there are no palpable masses. There is clotted blood with some fresh blood on the glove.

[1] Clinical observation of signs of anaemia can lead to more urgent investigation and management and should not be undervalued.

[2] ABCDE is always an important starting point for patient assessment. He is not tachycardic; however, in patients of this age with cardiac history it is important to also see the medications they are taking – a beta blocker will blunt the tachycardic response to hypovolaemia and means that this vital sign is less reliable acutely. He is getting enough perfusion to his brain to converse with you.

[3] Looking at the patient again for any signs of previous surgeries to align with history is always wise. Non-tender examination again makes an inflammatory colitis as a cause less likely, and absence of peritonism means perforation or extraluminal complications are less likely.

[4] PR examination is both external observation and internal palpation. Haemorrhoids can sometimes be actively bleeding or tender. Evidence of recent PR loss can be evident in the bedspace. If there is a palpable mass then this can guide further investigation somewhat; however, this does not change acute management.

Investigations

- A point of care VBG reveals a **haemoglobin of 75g/L** [1] but is otherwise within normal limits.
- Further investigations on formal bloods reveal a **mild acute kidney injury with an elevated urea** [2]. There is no liver function derangement.

- **INR is elevated at 8** [3].
- CT angiography shows **an active bleed in the descending colon, in the presence of diverticular disease** [4].

[1] Low haemoglobin indicates significant blood loss. This may still be uncompensated in the setting of acute blood loss and with fluid resuscitation, this number may lower further.

[2] Elevated urea occurs in settings of upper GI bleeds, where some breakdown of the red cells has occurred during transit.

[3] The INR being supratherapeutic can sometimes reflect liver disease; however, with normal LFTs and normal albumin it is more likely a clotting cascade specific issue – in this case warfarin therapy.

[4] CT angiography is theoretically able to identify bleeding points when bleeding at greater than 0.25ml/min. This requires active bleeding at the time of scanning, which can sometimes be negative.

Management

Immediate

Admit the patient to hospital, keep him fasted and commence fluid resuscitation [1] . Given his past history of ischaemic heart disease and concurrent anaemia with active bleeding, **blood transfusion is the fluid of choice** [2] . **Reverse his supratherapeutic INR** [3] with reference to local guidelines.

Short-term

Facilitate **transfer to interventional radiology for endoluminal intervention** [4] . Failing this, the patient may need surgical management. **Monitor for complications** [5] post procedure. Keep the patient in hospital with slow upgrade of diet over the next week and assess for recurrence of his symptoms. Restart warfarin **prior to discharge** [6] .

Long-term

Follow the patient up with interval colonoscopy [7] . A note would need to be made in the discharge summary of the supratherapeutic INR in the setting of recent antibiotic use.

[1] This patient could die from his GI bleeding and needs admission. Fluid resuscitation should be instituted and as he will likely require a procedure, he needs to remain nil by mouth to limit risk of potential anaesthetic.

[2] It is safer to assume a patient is unable to handle great volumes of fluid if they are old and have a past history suspicious for it. He still requires fluid but needs close monitoring. The most appropriate fluid to use would be blood, given a history of ischaemic heart disease and active bleeding – he is at higher risk of demand ischaemia, and hence a haemoglobin >80 is generally targeted in these patients. Note should be made of the massive transfusion protocol and potential need for other blood products.

[3] His supratherapeutic INR is definitely contributing to his bleeding and needs to be reversed. He has a high CHA_2DS_2-VASc score, but in the presence of active life-threatening bleeding the risk of exsanguination outweighs the chronic risk of thromboembolic complications of atrial fibrillation. Vitamin K can be used, or Prothrombinex to give clotting factors acutely. Coagulation studies should be rechecked regularly to assess for response.

[4] Angioembolisation is the least invasive way to aim to treat the pathology definitively. The patient needs to be stable enough for transfer and during the procedure. It does not require general anaesthetic.

[5] Potential risks of angioembolisation include complications with vascular access (femoral access, pseudoaneurysm, arterial damage). If the vessel is unable to be identified, the procedure cannot be completed. Sometimes the bleeding has ceased at the time of angiography and cannot be seen again. Once the source has been located and coiled, depending on the vessel and its supply there may be issues with perfusion of nearby structures.

[6] Post procedure, the patient requires a period of observation for complications and to ensure that recommencement of anticoagulation is successful and does not cause recurrence of bleeding. The discharge summary should include reference to the supratherapeutic INR in the setting of new medication. An event like this would also warrant a phone call to the patient's treating GP for a verbal update.

[7] Given his excellent functional status, this patient requires follow-up with interval colonoscopy to confirm the diagnosis of diverticular disease and to ensure there are no other pathologies present that may need further management. It would be appropriate for him to be followed up in the hospital outpatient clinic to ensure this monitoring occurs.

CASE 29: Sigmoid volvulus

History

- An **86-year-old male** [1] from a **high-level care nursing home** [2] is transferred to the ED with vomiting, decreased oral intake and non-specific abdominal pain.
- History from the patient is limited; however, the nursing home notes state that he has been **constipated** [3].

- He has a **past history** [4] significant for Alzheimer's dementia, hypertension, insulin-dependent T2DM, osteoporosis and chronic kidney disease. He has never had abdominal surgery.

[1] Sigmoid volvulus is more common in the older age group and also occurs in men at least twice as many times as in women.

[2] The background social situation of a patient is important to ascertain when making future management decisions and when considering the consent process. This is also relevant when gaining history and trying to elicit signs and symptoms – which is much harder in a patient who is unable to give a history clearly.

[3] These are very non-specific symptoms which can be attributed to multiple conditions. Without history to further guide your diagnosis, it is important to throw a wide net and consider non-surgical causes as important to rule out.

[4] The past history gives more of a picture of the patient and can give further differentials to exclude (e.g. hypoglycaemia, vertebral crush fracture in the setting of osteoporosis, acid–base or electrolyte abnormality, gastroenteritis or bowel obstruction). Investigations need to target and rule out these differentials.

Examination

- The patient is lying in the hospital bed. His airway is patent, his breathing is slightly shallow but non-laboured; **vital signs are unremarkable** [1].
- His **GCS is 13 – he is not oriented to place or time and is confused but obeying commands, with eyes opening to voice** [2].

- His chest is clear. His abdomen is **distended and generally tender** [3]. He has **no scars from previous surgeries** [3] and has **tympanic bowel sounds on auscultation** [3].
- PR examination is unremarkable, with an empty rectum and **no obvious faecal impaction** [4].

[1] First step in examination is ABC. The patient is not clearly shocked at this point and does not need immediate correction of those vitals. You can proceed to the next part of the examination.

[2] GCS is an important vital sign which is often a good reflection of end-organ perfusion. This is confounded in this case by underlying degenerative disease, but knowing his baseline GCS and whether this is a detraction would be useful.

[3] Again, this patient is giving non-specific examination and history findings. There are many causes for a distended abdomen which is diffusely tender. The presence or absence

of abdominal scars is highly relevant, especially when you are given the history of no surgeries. Tympanic bowel sounds, however, indicate that perhaps there is a bowel pathology underlying this presentation.

[4] A PR examination is important, especially in a patient who cannot give a clear history. This is to exclude any distal obstructive cause; however, in this case it does not reveal much.

Investigations

- Investigations ordered by the ED medical staff are initially a **VBG which is largely normal** [1] and an FBE showing an **elevated WCC but normal haemoglobin and platelets** [2].

- **Urea is elevated in proportion to creatinine, and there are no electrolyte abnormalities on UEC** [3].
- A plain abdominal X-ray shows **dilated large bowel loops in a coffee bean sign** [4].

[1] A VBG can give information regarding the patient's acid–base balance, haemoglobin, lactate and glucose levels. The fact that this is largely normal in this case does rule out some of our differentials and is reassuring that the initial test doesn't show a shocked patient.

[2] A confirmatory haemoglobin on a formal blood test is important prior to acting on the venous gas result. An elevated WCC can be affected by vomiting, steroids, pregnancy and infection, among many other causes. In this case you would be suspicious for infection. Platelets are important to consider with bleeding risk and can also be an acute phase reactant (elevated in infection).

[3] The ratio of urea to creatinine can give clues to sources of GI bleeding and also can be a reflection of body mass/ muscle mass. Looking at the patient in conjunction with the blood tests can correlate weird-looking results. He is not suffering abdominal pain from hypercalcaemia or impaired renal function, and so we investigate more.

[4] A plain abdominal X-ray is a good, quick screening test for patients. Often if normal, the patients with unclear diagnoses proceed to CT scan; however, this has a higher radiation load and is more time-consuming than an X-ray. In this case the X-ray shows the classic findings diagnostic of sigmoid volvulus, and the patient would not require further imaging at this stage.

Management

Immediate

Ensure the patient is stable [1]. Insert an **indwelling catheter** [2], a **nasogastric tube (NGT)** [3] and commence strict fluid balance. As this is a large bowel obstruction, an NGT will not decompress the issue – perform **rigid sigmoidoscopy and attempt rectal tube insertion** [3]. If this is unsuccessful, the patient would advance to theatre for **flexible sigmoidoscopy decompression +/– laparotomy + bowel resection** [4].

Short-term

Assess with repeat abdominal X-ray **to confirm detorsion of the volvulus and monitoring for complications relating to the prolonged potential ischaemia** [5]. Gradually upgrade oral intake and once bowels are opening and the patient is feeling well, they are able to discharge home with outpatient follow-up.

Long-term

Depending on patient factors, they can be considered for elective sigmoid resection in order to avoid the possibility of **recurrence of volvulus** [6].

[1] As always, assessment of the patient and ABCs are the first line in any assessment or management.

[2] Regardless of the aetiology of bowel obstruction, the fluid shifts and inability of the GI system to function as it normally would lead to massive fluid deficit and third spacing. Close monitoring of fluid balance, including moderately invasive monitoring, is generally needed. Sigmoid volvulus occurs due to the relative redundancy of the sigmoid colon and the anatomy of its mesentery lending itself to torsion. The obstruction formed is 'closed loop' which can cause

impaired arterial supply and venous drainage and bowel oedema which can quickly proceed to bowel ischaemia.

[3] Nasogastric tubes are a standard of management in small bowel obstructions and help to decompress both the stomach and the more proximal small bowel. In large bowel obstruction, this is slightly less of an immediate effect; however, minimising stasis and build-up of fluid in the bowel aims to maintain physiology and avoid ischaemia or dysfunction of proximal bowel. Rigid sigmoidoscopy involves a PR examination and insertion of a rigid sigmoidoscope with

insufflation. Ideally this will cause devolving and then a rectal tube can remain *in situ* to maintain the anatomy. Operative management is indicated in patients with peritonitis, evidence of bowel ischaemia or perforation or failed non-operative management.

4 Flexible sigmoidoscopy can have a higher success rate given its greater reach; however, sometimes operative management is indicated. In an emergency situation this has a high morbidity and mortality risk. Laparotomy and bowel resection with either primary anastomosis or end colostomy are the definitive treatment.

5 As stated earlier, the patients can have significant fluid shift and in the event of prolonged volvulus with ischaemia can have serious toxic shock, requiring high dependency or intensive care unit management. Close monitoring in the postoperative period for progress is essential.

6 Patients who have successful non-operative management can be monitored and managed on an outpatient basis – elective resection of the redundant sigmoid is often recommended for patients who will tolerate the procedure well.

CASE 30: Small bowel obstruction

History

- A **56-year-old** [1] **female** [2] presents with **nausea and vomiting** [3], **periumbilical, cramping abdominal pain** [4] and **obstipation** [5] over the past **12 hours** [6].
- She reports a **history of right hemicolectomy for colorectal cancer three years ago** [7] and a **previous episode of small bowel obstruction one year ago** [8].

- She also reports **bloating** [9], **loss of appetite** [10] and **fever** [11].
- She **last ate 16 hours ago** [12].
- She **does not smoke** [13] and does not drink alcohol.
- She is **not on any anticoagulants** [14] and has **no other significant past medical history** [15].
- She has no **allergies** [16].

[1] Small bowel obstruction is more common with increasing age, as its usual aetiologies and risk factors, such as prior surgery, hernias and intestinal cancers, increase in incidence with age. It is therefore critical to take a thorough surgical history of all previous abdominal surgeries.

[2] Incidence of small bowel obstruction is similar for males and females.

[3] Nausea and vomiting are common in small bowel obstruction and tend to be earlier and more severe in more proximal obstruction. The character of vomiting may indicate the level of obstruction; faeculent vomiting suggests distal obstruction, while vomiting of gastric contents may suggest gastric outlet obstruction, and bile-stained vomitus may be associated with a proximal small bowel obstruction.

[4] Periumbilical, cramping abdominal pain is characteristic of visceral pain secondary to intestinal peristalsis of an obstructed bowel. More focal pain is suggestive of peritoneal irritation and may indicate ischaemia or strangulation; in the case of sudden onset severe pain, consider intestinal perforation as a possible complication.

[5] Obstipation is the absence of passing flatus or stool and is characteristic of bowel obstruction. It is important to clarify duration of obstipation in the diagnosis of small bowel obstruction.

[6] The time frame of symptoms varies with the grade of a small bowel obstruction. A partial obstruction may manifest over a few days, whilst a complete, high grade obstruction might present over only a few hours.

[7] Mechanical small bowel obstruction is most commonly secondary to adhesions postoperatively, and as a result, history of abdominal surgery is the most important risk factor. Generally, risk of adhesions and associated complications increases with the number and complexity of previous abdominal surgeries. Colorectal surgery, adhesiolysis and gynaecological surgery are variously associated with adhesive small bowel obstruction. However, do not rule out small bowel obstruction in patients without a history of abdominal surgery; adhesions may be congenital or associated with inflammatory bowel conditions (e.g. diverticulitis, inflammatory bowel disease). Other causes of small bowel obstruction may be organised into the categories of luminal (e.g. gallstones, foreign bodies), intramural (e.g. small bowel tumours, strictures, intussusception) and extramural (e.g. other tumours, hernias), for a systematic approach.

[8] Previous episodes of small bowel obstruction also increase risk of recurrent obstruction, and sometimes cause chronic abdominal pain.

[9] Bloating may be associated with constipation (including pseudo-obstruction), ileus or a bowel obstruction; the presence or absence of obstipation, nausea/vomiting and pain differentiates between these.

[10] Characteristically, patients with small bowel obstruction will lose interest in eating and drinking.

[11] Fever is associated with a systemic inflammatory response and, if present, is usually low grade in the case of small bowel obstruction; higher fevers may be suggestive of a complicated small bowel obstruction.

[12] Fasting status is important to ascertain in any patient who may require an emergency operation, to determine timing of surgery.

[13] Smoking is significant for increased risk of complications from anaesthetic, and its adverse impact on wound healing. For elective surgeries, it is recommended that patients reduce their smoking as much as possible and, if able, cease smoking entirely as long as possible before surgery.

14 All anticoagulants, as well as antiplatelet medications, need careful management peri-operatively. Depending on risk, surgery may sometimes proceed for a patient on aspirin, but patients on other antiplatelet agents or who are therapeutically anticoagulated usually require reversal or withholding for a period of time before they are fit to proceed to surgery.

15 Past medical history is significant for anaesthetic risk and operative planning, if needed, as well as management of comorbidities.

16 A history of allergies is important to ascertain in every patient to avoid iatrogenic adverse drug reactions.

Examination

- On examination, the patient appears **in obvious pain** [1] but **not critically unwell** [2].
- She is **tachycardic with a heart rate of 105bpm** [3] but **normotensive** [4].
- She is **clinically hypovolaemic** [5].
- She is **afebrile** [6].
- Her **abdomen is distended** [7].
- There is a healed **midline laparotomy scar** [8].

- On palpation, there is **mild generalised tenderness** [9] but **no peritonism** [10].
- There is **no palpable abdominal mass** [11].
- There are **no detectable hernias** [12].
- The abdomen is **tympanic to percussion** [13] and on auscultation, **bowel sounds are increased** [14].
- On rectal examination, the **rectum is empty** [15] and there are no **masses** [16] or other abnormalities found.

1 As for every patient, begin with general inspection. A patient with small bowel obstruction will most likely have intermittent abdominal pain associated with intestinal peristalsis.

2 In a critically unwell patient, consider whether ischaemia or perforation may complicate the diagnosis of small bowel obstruction.

3 Begin with an ABC assessment of vital signs. Tachycardia in this patient is most likely due to a combination of hypovolaemia and pain, but if refractory to fluid resuscitation and analgesia, may suggest ischaemia or sepsis.

4 Again, hypotension may be due to hypovolaemia, but may also indicate perforation or sepsis.

5 Patients with small bowel obstruction are classically hypovolaemic. Signs of hypovolaemia on examination may include reduced urine output, dry mucous membranes, tachycardia or, in severe cases, hypotension.

6 Fever may suggest ischaemia or infection and indicates a systemic inflammatory response.

7 On abdominal examination, begin with inspection. Distension is a frequent feature of small bowel obstruction, and is more severe in distal obstruction, as the proximal loops of bowel become distended. In thin patients with partial obstruction, visible peristalsis may also be seen.

8 Search for surgical scars, which will suggest a history of previous abdominal surgery, as well as their nature.

9 Mild tenderness is consistent with a simple obstruction; more severe or worsening tenderness may suggest intestinal ischaemia.

10 Consider if the abdomen shows signs of peritonism. Guarding, rigidity and rebound tenderness are the major findings associated with peritonism. Generalised peritonism in this context is suggestive of perforation and is associated with high mortality without urgent intervention.

11 An abdominal mass is uncommon but may suggest malignancy as an underlying aetiology of small bowel obstruction.

12 Examination for hernias is also important. Inspect and palpate for abdominal hernias, including inguinal and femoral hernias, which may be obstructed and thus cause a small bowel obstruction.

13 The abdomen may be tympanic, or hyper-resonant, to percussion secondary to gaseous small bowel distension.

14 Classically, bowel sounds are described as tinkling and high pitched in small bowel obstruction. These will occur simultaneously with the characteristic colicky periumbilical pain. However, bowel sounds may be reduced with progressive distension, or absent, in the case of intestinal pseudo-obstruction.

15 Rectal examination is a mandatory part of this patient's abdominal examination, although is usually normal in the case of small bowel obstruction. Impacted faeces in the rectum may be a cause of large bowel obstruction.

16 A rectal mass may also cause a large bowel obstruction.

Investigations

- On FBE, the **haemoglobin and platelet count** [1] are within normal limits, and **WCC is normal** [2].
- **CRP is elevated** [3].
- **UEC demonstrates elevated urea** [4] and **hypokalaemia** [5].
- **VBG** [6] shows **normal acid–base status** [7] and a **normal lactate** [8].
- **LFTs and lipase are normal** [9].
- **HCG is negative** [10].

- An erect CXR demonstrates **no free gas under the diaphragm** [11].
- On abdominal X-ray, **air–fluid levels and dilated intestinal loops are seen** [12], and **no gas in the rectum** [13].
- **Abdominal CT** [14] confirms a **complete small bowel obstruction** [15], without **signs of ischaemia** [16].

[1] Haemoglobin and platelet count are important considerations for operative planning in any surgical patient. Packed red blood cells or platelet transfusion may be necessary preoperatively, as well as investigation for the underlying cause, for anaemia or thrombocytopenia respectively. For this patient, anaemia may indicate haemorrhage secondary to necrosis.

[2] Elevated WCC is consistent with systemic infection or inflammation. In this case, it may suggest ischaemia, infection and/or necrosis.

[3] CRP is an acute phase reactant. Elevated CRP is consistent with a systemic inflammatory response.

[4] Elevated urea is consistent with dehydration and may indicate the severity of volume depletion. Severe hypovolaemia may result in acute kidney injury. Baseline renal function is also significant for operative planning.

[5] Electrolyte imbalance is also associated with dehydration. Consider whether electrolyte imbalance may in fact be a causative factor in a patient with ileus.

[6] VBG is an inexpensive and rapid blood test to check electrolytes, lactate and acid–base status.

[7] Severe dehydration or ischaemic bowel may result in metabolic acidosis, whilst severe vomiting may alternatively cause a metabolic alkalosis.

[8] Elevated lactate is sensitive but not specific for ischaemia.

[9] LFTs and lipase should be performed for the work-up of acute abdominal pain but would be expected to be normal in the case of suspected small bowel obstruction.

[10] HCG should also be performed in every woman of childbearing age. Pregnancy is relevant both for differential diagnosis of abdominal pain, as well as for management.

[11] Erect CXR is a useful initial imaging modality in any patient with abdominal pain concerning for perforated viscus. The classic finding of free gas under the diaphragm is ominous, and generally requires urgent surgical management. This finding usually correlates clinically with generalised peritonitis.

[12] Air–fluid levels and dilated loops of bowel are characteristic of small bowel obstruction.

[13] Gas is usually absent distal to a complete small bowel obstruction.

[14] Even when confirmed on plain X-ray, if there is no indication for immediate surgery, abdominal CT should be performed to further characterise the obstruction. Abdominal CT will also differentiate large bowel obstruction, small bowel obstruction and ileus, and will determine whether the obstruction is complicated. CT abdomen will also identify a closed loop obstruction, whereby a loop of bowel is obstructed at a single location; this may be due to a hernia, volvulus or adhesions. Closed loop obstruction carries an increased risk of ischaemia and perforation.

[15] The CT findings of small bowel obstruction are similar to those on X-ray, but with greater sensitivity. A transition zone may be identified, and may be an underlying cause of the obstruction, such as a tumour, intussusception or a gallstone.

[16] CT signs of ischaemia include mural thickening or oedema. Intramural air is a late sign which indicates impending perforation.

Management

Immediate

Monitor **vital signs and perform resuscitation if required** [1] . **Admit** [2] the patient to hospital. Keep the patient **fasted** [3] . Give **IV fluids** [4] and **insert an NGT** [5] . Give appropriate **analgesia** [6] . If **emergency surgery is indicated** [7] , give **antibiotics** [8] and **liaise with Anaesthetics** [9] regarding planning for theatre.

Short-term

Perform **serial assessments** [10] of the patient during the acute admission. As the small bowel obstruction **resolves** [11] , **remove the NGT and increase diet as tolerated** [12] . **Gastrograffin follow-through** [13] should be considered after 24 hours. If a trial of conservative management **fails** [14] , or if there is **deterioration** [15] ,

perform **exploratory surgery** [16] . Postoperatively, if the patient is stable, they may be transferred to the ward. Review the **surgical sites** [17] and examine the **abdomen** [18] . Continue to **check and optimise electrolytes** [19] . Whether a patient is being managed conservatively or operatively, they may be discharged when they have **stable vital signs** [20] , are **mobilising** [21] , **opening their bowels**, **and tolerating normal diet** [22] .

Long-term

If the patient is postoperative, follow up the patient in an **outpatient clinic** [23] to review any histopathology and the wounds. Patients who have been conservatively managed successfully can often be discharged to the GP.

---

[1] Resuscitate the patient if necessary. This should occur at your first encounter with the patient and take place as you consider the vital signs.

[2] Ensure that your planned disposition is appropriate (i.e. assess the need for admission to the ICU, or transfer to a higher acuity hospital). Ensure that facilities are available for acute, unplanned surgical intervention.

[3] Patients with small bowel obstruction should routinely be fasted to avoid worsening intestinal distension, although some patients with a partial or early small bowel obstruction may tolerate sips of clear fluids. This also allows patients to remain fasted in case urgent surgery is required.

[4] IV fluids should be commenced for both replacement of fluid deficits and maintenance fluid requirements. Patients with small bowel obstruction may have significant volume depletion, and this must be replaced. Urine output is a valuable indicator of hydration status and should be measured strictly – insertion of an indwelling urinary catheter will enable this. A patient who is hypotensive or tachycardic will require rapid fluid resuscitation with crystalloid solution. The choice of IV fluids should be guided by electrolyte status, and electrolyte losses must be replaced intravenously as well. Seek advice if patients have a history of cardiac failure or renal failure and require aggressive fluid resuscitation, as these patients may be vulnerable to fluid overload; diuresis may be required.

[5] Patients with significant proximal dilatation or who are vomiting should receive an NGT for decompression. This is normally left on free drainage, with aspiration every 4 hours – the volume of output should be measured. Reduced nasogastric output generally indicates improvement.

[6] Analgesia may include NSAIDs (if not contraindicated) or opioids.

[7] Surgical exploration should occur for all patients with small bowel obstruction where there is a suspicion of bowel ischaemia or perforation, and in all patients where there is a correctable aetiology, with the exception of adhesions, as the majority of adhesive small bowel obstructions will resolve with conservative management. In practice, this means that patients with small bowel obstruction and without any history of abdominal surgery should proceed to exploratory surgery. Closed-loop obstruction should also trigger urgent surgery, due to increased risk of complications, as outlined above.

[8] Ceftriaxone and metronidazole in combination, or piperacillin-tazobactam monotherapy, are appropriate antibiotic choices to cover for enteric Gram-negative bacilli and anaerobes, which are the important targets if there is any intestinal ischaemia or perforation.

[9] Liaise with Anaesthetics regarding planning for an emergency operation, including a handover of the patient's comorbidities, haemodynamics and fasting status. Anaesthetics will then assess the patient's suitability for a general anaesthetic and prioritise the operation according to clinical urgency.

[10] Serial abdominal examination and monitoring of urine output, NGT output, nausea, vomiting and abdominal pain will indicate whether the small bowel obstruction is resolving, stable or deteriorating.

[11] Decreasing abdominal distension, resumed passage of flatus and/or stool, decreasing NGT output and increased

urine output, together with improvement of nausea, vomiting and pain, are indicative of a resolving small bowel obstruction.

12 As the patient improves, diet can be gradually upgraded through the steps of clear fluids, free fluids, light ward diet and full ward diet. Ensure that the patient is continuing to improve before continuing to upgrade the diet.

13 Gastrograffin follow-through may accelerate resolution of adhesive small bowel obstruction and is thus therapeutic as well as diagnostic – serial radiographs will demonstrate the passage of gastrograffin through the GI tract. Gastrograffin reaching the colon and rectum indicates high likelihood of resolution with conservative management.

14 Failure to improve with 3–5 days of non-operative management should prompt the consideration of operative intervention, if the patient is a surgical candidate.

15 Increasing abdominal pain or distension, fever, tachycardia, hypotension or other signs of bowel ischaemia or perforation remain indications for emergency surgery in the patient for whom conservative management is being trialled.

16 Operative management of small bowel obstruction generally involves laparotomy and is then directed at the underlying aetiology. If bowel is found to be non-viable, resection may be required, usually with primary anastomosis. However, in select patients with adhesive small bowel obstruction, there may be a role for laparoscopic adhesiolysis.

17 Surgical sites should be reviewed to ensure closure, and to check for signs of wound infection, such as surrounding erythema or discharge. The risk of dehiscence is greatly reduced by laparoscopic technique compared to laparotomy, as the wound sites are much smaller.

18 Expect the postoperative abdominal examination to demonstrate a degree of tenderness over the operative sites. Nevertheless, be alert for peritonism or disproportionate abdominal tenderness which may suggest bile leak, bleeding or another complication.

19 Electrolytes should continue to be monitored and replaced as needed. Pay particular attention to correcting any hypokalaemia and/or hypomagnesaemia.

20 Monitor patients postoperatively for complications. Haemodynamic instability should prompt urgent review.

21 Small bowel obstruction may require a prolonged admission, and elderly and comorbid patients are particularly vulnerable to functional decline. Allied health teams provide valuable input to ensure that patients are safe to discharge from a functional point of view, or otherwise to facilitate inpatient rehabilitation if required.

22 When patients are opening their bowels well and tolerating normal diet, after a period of monitoring for recurrence of symptoms, they may be discharged.

23 Follow-up and prognosis will depend on the underlying aetiology of the small bowel obstruction. Patients with adhesive small bowel obstruction are liable to further episodes, even if adhesiolysis has been performed.

CASE 31: Cauda equina syndrome

History

- A **55-year-old** [1] **overweight** [2] **male** [3] with **a known past medical history of lumbar spinal canal stenosis** [4] **on the background of spinal osteoarthritis (OA)** [4] presents to the ED with **severe low back pain that is shooting in nature** [5].
- He is also feeling a **pins and needles sensation around the groin area and inner thighs** [6].
- He has been a removals man by **occupation for nearly 30 years** [7].
- The low shooting back pain is **different in nature and severity from his usual back pain** [4] [5] and came on **suddenly 4 hours ago when he was lifting a washing machine** [8].

- It is worsening in **severity** [9] and is **currently 8/10 on the pain scale** [9].
- He also notes he has **not urinated in the past 4 hours with loss of the urge to do so** [10] despite a normal amount of fluid intake, and **weakness and numbness in the muscles of both of his legs** [11] that had a similar time of onset. The weakness and numbness began shortly after the heavy lifting.
- He remarked he has been **tripping over his left foot on the ground for the past 4 hours** [12].
- He **does not smoke** [13], and drinks alcohol socially.
- He denies any **recent coryzal symptoms** [14].
- The patient denies any **trauma to his back or falls** [15], **fevers, night sweats or weight loss** [16].

[1] Cauda equina syndrome (CES) is a rare neurosurgical emergency with marked morbidity, characterised by damage or compression to a collection of nerves below the end of the spinal cord known as the cauda equina. It is seen in adults usually after 20 years of age and peaks in people's 40s and 50s. This is due to a greater incidence of disc and spinal pathologies and malignancies in that age group. The age of the patient has significance as CES in an older patient and its surgical outcomes may differ from a younger patient.

[2] Being overweight or obese is not directly a risk factor for CES. However, when combined with spinal canal stenosis and a herniated disc, as seen in our patient, it greatly predisposes to CES.

[3] Males seem to be afflicted slightly more than females. This is due to greater rates of obesity, trauma to the spine, disc pathologies and malignancy metastasising to the spine in males, compared to females.

[4] Our patient's lumbar spinal canal stenosis is known to and managed by his GP. His stenosis can be attributed to the spinal OA as a result of his occupation moving furniture. The vertebrae will undergo degeneration and the resulting osteophytes will compress the nerves, leading to a dull back pain of moderate severity. Sciatica is often an overlapping feature of CES, lumbar spinal canal stenosis and OA. Thus, it is paramount to distinguish the true cause of the sciatica. Nevertheless, if CES is suspected, its investigation and management pathway must be activated. Lumbar spinal canal stenosis on the background of spinal OA is one of the

leading aetiologies of CES. It predisposes to greater rates of herniated discs and narrows an already tight space, increasing the likelihood of cauda equina compression.

[5] The sudden severe low back pain with sciatic features (i.e. travelling from the lower back, down the posterior leg) is different from the usual dull back pain our patient manages every day. Sudden severe low back pain with sciatic features is often a red flag for herniated disc, CES, other types of spinal cord compression and malignancy, especially if other worrying features are present.

[6] The most characteristic symptom that accompanies the severe shooting low back pain is saddle anaesthesia, where the patient experiences pins and needles or numbness of the external genitalia, perineum, anus and inner regions of the thigh. As the cauda equina is compressed, this will affect dermatomes S3–S5, which govern the saddle region and thus result in anaesthesia.

[7] An occupation involving heavy lifting for decades greatly predisposes to disc pathologies and degenerative disease of the spine (OA). This puts him in a high risk category for CES any time there is a disc herniation.

[8] There is a clear aetiology for our patient's sudden severe back pain. This most likely indicates a disc herniation, probably around the L5/S1 area due to his ongoing lumbar spinal canal stenosis. Taken together, they can all compress the cauda equina. If the sudden severe back pain was spontaneous, other aetiologies would be considered such as malignancy or epidural abscess, especially in the presence

of other worrying symptoms (e.g. fever, weight loss, night sweats, night pain).

9 CES often presents with worsening and severe pain out of proportion, due to compression of crucial lumbar and sacral nerve roots, which is consistent with our patient's presentation.

10 Bowel, bladder or sexual dysfunction is the second set of main clinical features that accompany saddle anaesthesia and severe low back pain in CES. Our patient might be demonstrating bladder dysfunction as he has not urinated in the past 4 hours and has lost the sensation to do so. Urinary retention occurs due to compression of the sacral nerve roots (S3–S5) impairing the parasympathetic input to the bladder to ensure relaxation.

11 CES will commonly present with bilateral leg weakness and numbness, following a lower motor neurone (LMN) pattern. The lower motor weakness can be attributed to the compression of cauda equina from a herniated disc.

12 L5/S1 disc herniation is the most common type of disc herniation seen in lumbar spinal canal stenosis, spinal OA and heavy lifting. Disc herniation is also the most recognised and common aetiology of CES. Specifically, an L5/S1 disc herniation will result in the characteristic foot drop.

13 A thorough social, drug and alcohol history is necessary in order to elicit other comorbidities and risks that might affect postoperative outcomes. Smoking is considered a strong risk factor for strokes, hypertension and cranial haemorrhages secondary to strokes and aneurysms. It is associated with an increased risk of peri-operative respiratory, cardiac and wound-related complications.

14 It is important to ask the patient about recent coryzal or flu-like symptoms to rule out communicable diseases. Preceding coryzal symptoms with severe back pain can point to a differential diagnosis of epidural abscess.

15 With CES, it is important to rule out any trauma to the spinal cord. Falls, traffic accidents and sporting injures are some of the culprits that result in spinal cord damage and subsequent CES in young adults. Although our patient suffered trauma in the form of heavy lifting, the resulting insult was a disc herniation that ultimately led to the compression of the cauda equina.

16 If the patient experienced this severe back pain mainly at night with fever, weight loss and night sweats, there should be high suspicion for metastatic malignancy. Fever could also indicate infection/inflammation brewing within the spinal cord.

Examination

- The patient appears **uncomfortable** [1]. Vital signs are unremarkable.
- Heart sounds are dual with **no murmurs** [2]. Auscultation reveals vesicular breathing sounds and equal air.
- Inspection of the back reveals **no wasting, swelling or surgical scars with normal posture** [3].
- **Patient demonstrates unsteady gait with left foot drop** [4].
- Palpation of lower back reveals **normal temperature with mild spasms** [5], but no obvious deformities or fractures.
- All planes of movement (**flexion, extension, twisting and lateral flexion) are limited by pain** [6].
- **Straight leg raise test is positive** [7] on the left side.
- **Schober's test is normal (>5cm change)** [8].
- **Slump test is positive bilaterally** [9] as pain remains despite extension of the neck.
- Lower limb exam reveals **normal muscle bulk with nil fasciculations noted** [10].
- **Hypotonia is noted** [11].
- Power is **4/5** [12] throughout both lower limbs bilaterally.
- Reflexes are symmetrical but **reduced bilaterally** [13].
- Coordination is **slowed** [14].
- Sensory exam reveals impaired **pain sensation via pin prick** [15]. To elaborate, dermatomal testing with pin prick demonstrates **numbness** [15] throughout both legs (anterior and posterior) with **reduced perineal sensation** [15]. **Proprioception is normal** [15].
- **Babinski sign is absent** [16].
- A digital rectal exam (DRE) reveals **reduced anal tone** [17].

1 General inspection of the patient can, at times, guide the clinician's level of concern for the acuity of the patient's pathology. Our patient is uncomfortable due to significant back pain, underscoring the acuity of the situation.

2 Heart murmurs may suggest valvular heart disease or structural heart defects. Important to investigate these peri-operatively to assess fitness for general anaesthetic.

3 With CES, a back exam is crucial to rule out any confounding or masquerading musculoskeletal issues. Previous surgical history is helpful in terms of predicting current surgical outcomes. Wasting is characteristic of LMN disease process but is also seen in CES due to the compression. However, not all patients with CES display wasting, which is the case with our patient. Inspection will reveal the patient's posture; it is important to note any kyphosis or lordosis before the patient is prepped for surgery, as it can impact surgical outcomes.

4 It is important to test gait within the setting of suspected CES on the background of disc herniation. As CES progresses, patients quickly lose their ability to walk and become paraplegic as the weakness transitions to paralysis. The timing of surgery greatly influences morbidity and long-term rehabilitation outcomes. Our patient demonstrates a left foot drop, which is consistent with a L5/S1 disc herniation.

5 Palpation of a patent's back who is suffering from a disc herniation will be difficult due to the pain. However, mild spasms of paraspinal muscles will be present after an injury. High temperature in the local site indicates an infection and is worth checking for in CES, as epidural abscess and other infections have been implicated as potential aetiologies.

6 Testing movement such as flexion and rotation in a back exam is crucial to assess the extent of the injury and subsequent restriction. Due to the severe pain in CES and disc herniation, all planes of movement are usually limited.

7 The straight leg test is the gold standard in determining a herniated disc, especially around the L5 region. It is clear from our patient's left foot drop and heavy lifting preceding the sudden, severe low back, that there is an L5/S1 disc herniation.

8 There is some evidence to perform Schober's test for CES. By measuring the patient's ability to flex the lower back, we can assess for a fixed flexion deformity of the lumbar spine.

9 The slump test induces neural tension and aids in the diagnosis of sciatic nerve impingement. The patient slumps forward, their chin is brought to their chest and their knee is extended. Subsequently, the foot is dorsiflexed. A positive slump test is reproduction of the patient's sciatic symptoms, and is indicative of some form of sciatic nerve pathology.

10 Although LMN symptoms are present in CES, wasting and fasciculations are late-stage symptoms of LMN disease.

Fortunately, our patient presented within 4 hours and would not have any wasting/fasciculations of the lower limb (LL).

11 Hypotonia is a characteristic finding of LMN disease and is often present in CES cases, even at the early stages.

12 Patient demonstrates a power grading of 4/5 throughout both lower limbs for all movements. This power rating indicates movement against gravity and some resistance against the examiner is possible. Onset of weakness in both legs simultaneously is consistent with CES rather than any stroke symptomology which is more likely unilateral.

13 Reflexes are symmetrical and bilaterally present. However, due to the compression, they are reduced in both legs. Without any intervention, the reduced reflexes will transition to areflexia.

14 Coordination of LL is expected to be slowed in CES due to the compression of key nerves.

15 Sensory exam plays a large role in mapping out the sensory deficits in CES. Classically with CES, there will be anaesthesia/analgesia of the entire lower limbs (anteriorly and posteriorly) to pin prick. This is due to impaired neural signalling outflow and damage to the spinothalamic tracts, which govern pain, temperature and vibration. Light touch and proprioception should be somewhat preserved as it is governed by another tract – dorsal column medial lemniscus. If the foot drop occurs in the setting of impaired light touch sensation and proprioception, consider alternative pathologies such as vitamin B12 deficiency polyneuropathy or chronic inflammatory demyelinating polyneuropathy. Additionally, if there is a glove and stocking pattern of impaired light touch and pain sensation along with reduced vibration and damaged proprioception in the LLs, diabetic neuropathy is more likely to be at the top of the differential list. Absent pain sensation in CES is often paired with reduced/altered perineal sensation due to the escape of some sacral nerves from compression.

16 Often, Babinski sign will be absent in CES.

17 Bowel dysfunction is part of the characteristic set of clinical features that form CES. Due to compression of sacral nerve roots, particularly dermatomes S3–S5, there will be reduced anal tone. This can be elicited on DRE.

Investigations

NB. Due to the patient's progressive weakness and urinary retention, these investigations must be performed concurrently with resuscitation. The priority goes to urgently performing spinal decompression.

- An initial bladder scan reveals 900ml of urine. Insertion of a **urinary catheter** [1] reveals absent **catheter sensation** [1].
- **FBE is normal** [2].

- **UEC results are normal** [3].
- **Urine dipstick and MC&S** [4] is unremarkable.
- **ESR and CRP** [5] are within normal limits.
- An ECG shows **normal sinus rhythm** [6].
- **MRI** [7] of the spine **reveals a left lumbar disc herniation at L5/S1 with cauda equina compression** [7], confirming the diagnosis.
- There is no abnormal **hyperintensity or any abscess** [8] on T2 sequence.

1 Urinary dysfunction, particularly urinary retention, is one of the cornerstone clinical features of CES. Due to the compression of sacral nerve roots, patients lose the desire to void and do not anticipate the filling sensation, resulting in retention. The insertion of a urinary catheter can be diagnostic and therapeutic. In CES, there will be absent catheter sensation during insertion due to anaesthesia of the external genitalia.

2 In our patient, FBE is normal. There are no signs of anaemia or infection. An elevated WCC would indicate infection.

3 UECs are important in the setting of a surgical emergency. First, it identifies any electrolyte abnormalities that most often need correction prior to surgery. Secondly, it assesses renal function and fitness for IV contrast, as well as serving as a prognosticator for postoperative recovery.

4 A urine dipstick and further testing with microscopy and culture is an easy test to screen for UTI. An infective process in the setting of a headache AND drowsiness (falling GCS) must be considered.

5 ESR and CRP levels are worth ordering to rule out any inflammatory processes and by extension rule out any infectious causes for CES.

6 An ECG is a simple and non-invasive investigation to assess electrical rhythm, and informs preoperative cardiac risks. It is important to establish sinus rhythm and rule out atrial fibrillation or arrhythmias in the setting of a haemorrhage, to glean whether clotting medications or anticoagulation will be required postoperatively.

7 MRI of the spine is the gold standard investigation to confirm CES. It has high sensitivity and specificity for CES. Our patient's MRI displays a left lumbar disc herniation at L5/S1 with clear cauda equina compression. This confirms the diagnosis of CES.

8 Abnormal hyperintense signals on a T2 sequence of a spine MRI may suggest spinal metastases, an epidural abscess or other spinal cord pathologies such as stenosis.

Management

Immediate

Monitor **vital signs** [1] and potential **urine output within the catheter bag** [2]. Keep the patient **fasted** [3]. Obtain IV access and **commence fluid** [4]. **Seek urgent advice** [5] from the Neurosurgery team. Administer **IV dexamethasone** [6]. **Commence prophylactic IV antibiotics** [7].

Short-term

Perform an **urgent surgical decompression via laminectomy of L5/S1** [8]. Following the procedure, transfer the patient to **ICU for monitoring** [9]. Administer **venous thromboembolism (VTE) prophylaxis** [10] when appropriate. Perform a **post-void bladder scan** [11] to assess for further urinary retention following a trial of void. Review the patient's **surgical site** [12] and perform a **back and neurological examination** [13] once the patient is able to mobilise. The patient may be discharged if **vital signs remain stable** [14], they have **opened their bowels** [15], **urinary retention has resolved** [16], **neurologic deficits have resolved** [17], **they have been cleared by allied health/neurosurgery/neurology** [18] and are back to a satisfactory level of function.

Long-term

The patient may have to be provided with **community rehabilitation** [19]. Follow the patient up in the **outpatient clinic** [20] for monitoring of postoperative complications.

1 Ensure the patient remains haemodynamically stable prior to operative treatment. In particular, blood pressure and heart rate are important to stabilise as they are prognosticators for postoperative recovery.

2 Urine output is an indicator of fluid balance. If urine output dwindles, this may be a sign of acute renal failure, and early recognition is key to effective treatment.

3 Keeping the patient fasted is crucial in their preoperative management. It allows the patient to have bowel rest, as well as reducing the risk of aspiration in the setting of anaesthesia. Ideally, patients should be fasted off solid foods for 6 hours, and clear fluids for 2 hours prior to induction of anaesthesia. This may not always be possible in the acute setting.

4 Intravenous fluid is integral in fluid resuscitation and stabilisation of circulation. Patients are nil by mouth prior to surgery and so maintenance fluids are essential in keeping the patient adequately hydrated. IV fluid management is based around four principles – resuscitation, maintenance, replacement of losses and redistribution.

5 CES warrants urgent neurosurgical evaluation. Surgical decompression by means of laminectomy of the cauda equina must occur without delay. Best practice dictates performing surgery within 6 hours of symptom onset. Despite our patient's CES being in its early stages and his rapid presentation to the ED, he should be advised there is still a 20% chance of poor outcomes, particularly permanent damage to nerves to the bladder and bowel resulting in possibly lifelong bladder/bowel/sexual dysfunction.

6 Commence high dose IV dexamethasone to reduce swelling around the cauda equina.

7 Prophylactic IV antibiotics will be administered to prevent secondary meningitis or any infections from laminectomy.

8 Urgent surgical decompression via laminectomy of L5/S1 discs and cauda equina is the gold standard approach and management in this specific case. It is expected to be a minimally invasive spinal surgery that aims to preserve as much of the surrounding muscle tissue as possible. The laminectomy can also treat his lumbar spinal canal stenosis and relieve some of the OA, which would be a robust preventive measure against future disc herniations and cauda equina compressions.

9 Patients must be monitored postoperatively for any immediate complications of surgery in the ICU. These include signs of shock (septic or hypovolaemic), infection, reaction to anaesthesia, DVT and PE, urinary retention or renal failure and new neurologic deficits.

10 It is not standard procedure to commence subcutaneous (SC) enoxaparin post-decompression, due to the development of potential epidural/paraspinal haematomas. However, the risks of bleeding should be weighed against the risk of clot formation, and be considered in those at high risk of VTE.

11 Perform a post-op post-void bladder scan to ensure resolution of urinary retention. The normal amount of residual urine in the bladder of a 50-year-old male is approximately 80–100ml.

12 Review the surgical site to ensure proper closure, as well as the amount of ooze and any signs of infection from the wound. Particularly after neurosurgery, risk factors for wound dehiscence include coughing, sneezing and straining with bowel movements. Thus, educating the patient about wound dehiscence is important in its prevention.

13 Perform a back and LL neurological exam once the patient is awake and able to mobilise. Once the patient is awake with independent breathing and stable vital signs, they can be transferred to the neurology ward. Compare findings of back and LL neurology exam to initial exam findings from the ED presentation. There should be marked improvements in LL muscle power and resolution of LMN signs. Saddle anaesthesia and absent pain sensation in the LLs and perineum should also resolve. The patient should be able to urinate and defecate without issue and anticipate the sensation to do so within 2–4 weeks. Continuing urinary or bowel issues would require further scans, reviews and therapy.

14 Complex neurosurgical cases on the background of an acute presentation normally take 1–2 weeks before discharge. With respect to CES, discharge hinges on some degree of patient mobility and resolution of neurologic deficits, pain and urinary retention.

15 Opening bowels after surgery and anaesthesia is paramount. The management of post-op constipation is normally conservative, comprising analgesia and nutritional support. However, bowel dysfunction may linger as a permanent complication of CES.

16 Urinary retention must be resolved prior to discharge. If not, the patient may require follow-up in the community for catheter care and subacute trial of void. Urinary dysfunction may linger as a permanent complication of CES.

17 Before the patient can be discharged, improvements must be achieved from a neurological perspective. Any residual weakness and anaesthesia in the lower limbs will progressively and slowly improve over time. If not, these changes may be permanent or require intensive rehab over years to see a return to function.

18 The patient should ideally be able to function at the level that they were able to prior to becoming ill. However, often this does not happen after spinal surgery for CES. As a result, allied health – physiotherapy and occupational therapy – must perform further assessment on fitness for discharge home at a functional level. As part of their discharge plans, each individual team must set up follow-up appointments in their outpatient clinics, update the patient's GP and educate patient and family on CES and a modified lifestyle on the background of any residual disability.

19 Marginal post-op improvements and persistent bladder/bowel dysfunction warrant a transfer to community rehabilitation centre. At the rehab centre, allied health professionals can work on gait, strength, continence and alternative ways to manage activities of daily living (ADLs) in the setting of any remaining neurologic impairments.

20 Lastly, a closing appointment with the neurosurgeon is required to assess for post-op complications such as incidental damage to any of the spinal nerves or other neural structures. If there is persisting bladder/bowel/sexual dysfunction from the cauda equina, referral to other specialty teams may be warranted.

CASE 32: Cervical myelopathy/radiculopathy

History

- A **52-year-old** [1] **male** [2] presents with **difficulty walking** [3].
- He has trouble **writing, buttoning his shirt and using keys** [4].
- He also describes **numbness and tingling in his right hand** [5], **neck and shoulder pain** [6] that is **dull and deep and not well localised** [7] and **intermittent shooting pain down his right arm** [8] that is **relieved with holding arms up above his head** [9].
- He first noticed the symptoms **a few years ago** [10], and they have been **getting worse** [11].
- His **bladder and bowel function have been normal** [12].

- There is no **malaise, fever, anorexia or unexplained weight loss, no past or current history of neoplasm** [13].
- He also denies any **personal or family history of rheumatoid arthritis or ankylosing spondylitis** [14].
- He is not **immunosuppressed** [15] due to underlying diseases or medications.
- He reports no recent history of **trauma** [16] or recent **change in diet or GI symptoms** [17].
- He is **well otherwise** [18].
- He has not had any **surgeries** [19] before.
- He **does not smoke** [20].

[1] The leading cause of spinal cord injury is degenerative cervical myelopathy (DCM), which encompasses a spectrum of degenerative changes in the cervical spine, historically known as cervical spondylotic myelopathy (CSM). It is most prevalent in the middle-aged group, where most patients are diagnosed in their 50s or after. It is uncommon before the age of 40. Consider alternative pathology in younger age groups; e.g. multiple sclerosis (MS) in young adults and acute disseminated encephalomyelitis in children.

[2] Most studies report DCM affects males more than females, at a ratio of about 3:2, and an earlier onset (in their 50s) in males than in females (in their 60s).

[3] Gait disturbance is a common early complaint and one of the hallmark symptoms of cervical myelopathy. It is due to the compression of the corticospinal tract, often with a spastic characteristic.

[4] Clumsiness of the hands and decreased manual dexterity are another hallmark of CSM. These functional declines are sometimes falsely attributed to 'old age'. It is due to the compression of spinocerebellar (disturbing proprioception) and corticospinal tracts.

[5] Paraesthesia of the upper extremities is a common symptom of cervical myelopathy, often diffuse and non-specific. Paraesthesia that follows dermatomal distributions is due to radiculopathy.

[6] Neck and shoulder pain is a common symptom of DCM but can also originate from musculoskeletal structures or be a result of peripheral nerve disease.

[7] This is a typical DCM-type pain due to the irritation of local structures that are sensitive to pain, such as bones. It is often central, deep, aching, with a 'burning' quality, and patients frequently have difficulty describing it. Severe, localised neck pain should prompt suspicion of malignancy or epidural abscess.

[8] Pain of sharp or burning nature radiating from the neck down into the arm following a dermatomal distribution is a feature of radiculopathy (compression of the nerve roots) rather than myelopathy (compression of the spinal cord). It can occur secondary to disc prolapse, osteophytes or spinal instability. Depending on the anatomical structures affected, it can be unilateral or bilateral.

[9] This is also known as the 'shoulder abduction test'. Shoulder abduction can increase the size of the foramen and relieve the compression on nerve roots, hence is a sign for radiculopathy.

[10] An insidious onset over the course of years to decades again implies a degenerative cause such as spondylotic compression – although it can also be subacute or acute following a minor traumatic event to head and neck. Conditions with more acute onset but which can have similar presentation include, but are not limited to, haematoma, tumour, developmental or non-infectious inflammatory pathology. A hyperacute presentation without trauma may suggest a spinal cord ischaemic stroke.

[11] The natural history of DCM is highly variable. Although spondylosis is inevitable with normal ageing, a proportion

of patients never become symptomatic. Among the patients with clinical signs, some remain stable for years, some show stepwise deterioration with intervening stability, while others experience progressive decline in function.

12 Loss of sphincter control is not common in cervical myelopathy. If present, it is often an indicator of severe spinal cord injury. Common complaints are urinary frequency, urgency or hesitancy. Bladder symptoms are more frequent than bowel; however, their presence is not of high diagnostic value because of high prevalence in this age group.

13 Constitutional symptoms help to rule out malignancy as an extramedullary source of compressing the spinal cord. Common primary malignancies include multiple myeloma and plasmacytoma. Metastasis to the cervical spine is relatively uncommon compared to the rest of the spine. Tumours involving vertebral bodies, such as metastatic prostate cancer and multiple myeloma, usually cause bony destruction and severe, unremitting pain. Previous radiation therapy for malignancy treatment may lead to development of myelopathy as a complication.

14 Cervical spinal manifestations are not uncommon in patients with rheumatoid arthritis (RA), with atlantoaxial subluxation involving C1/C2 being the most prevalent; however, it can occur at any and at multiple levels.

15 Immunosuppression, along with fevers, chills and malaise, constitute an infectious picture. Infectious inflammatory causes include epidural abscess, human immunodeficiency-related vacuolar myelopathy, HTLV-1 (human T-lymphotrophic virus) infection and more.

16 Recent trauma may lead to blunt fracture causing impingement or direct trauma to the spinal cord. Cervical sprain may be caused by whiplash injury, which is due to acute hyperextension that may acutely exacerbate CSM. It typically causes central cord compression.

17 Nutritional and metabolic causes are usually further down the differential list. However, they need to be taken into consideration if no structural abnormalities are identified on imaging. Vitamin B12, copper or other mineral deficiency arising from malnutrition or malabsorption can cause subacute combined degeneration of spinal cord, also known as Lichtheim's disease, primarily affecting dorsal columns and lateral corticospinal tracts.

18 Medical conditions such as diabetes can manifest as peripheral neuropathy that may mimic cervical myelopathy.

19 Spinal cord ischaemia is typically present as a complication of aortic aneurysm surgery or stenting.

20 Any form of smoking that contains nicotine is a risk factor for cervical disc degeneration by affecting bone growth and increasing the failure rate of surgery. It also increases the rate of peri-operative complications by slowing down the speed of wound healing by impairing circulation, and causes higher risk of infection. Make sure that patients cease smoking prior to surgery with measures such as nicotine replacement therapy.

Examination

- The patient looks well, and is **alert and oriented** [1].
- When walking, he adopts a **spastic gait** [2].
- His **vital signs are normal** [3].
- On general inspection, there are **no scars** [4].
- No **paraspinal pain** [5] is elicited on palpation.
- **Spine examination as well as full upper and lower limb neurological examination** [6] are performed.
- Neck **range of motion** [7] is limited by painful extension and rotation to the right-hand side.
- Examination of upper limb reveals **3/5 motor weakness of elbow flexion and wrist extension** [8].
- There is **paraesthesia over the right radial forearm, thumb and index finger** [9].
- The **pectoralis reflex** [10] is normal; however, both **biceps and brachioradialis reflexes are diminished** [11] and **triceps reflex is brisk** [12].
- There is **diffuse impairment of sensation to light touch, pin prick and temperature in both hands** [13].
- The symptoms of radiculopathy are **exacerbated when applying downward pressure to an extended and rotated head to the right-hand side** [14].
- Upon **flicking the right middle fingernail, flexion of the ipsilateral thumb and index finger** [15] is observed.
- In addition, with neck flexion, the patient describes an **'electric shock' shooting down the spine and into the limbs** [16].
- He is only able to open and close his hand **10 times in 10 seconds** [17].
- When **tapping on the right distal brachioradialis tendon, there is reflex contraction of the finger flexors** [18].
- Lower limb examination demonstrates **sustained ankle clonus** [19].
- There is also generalised **hypertonia, hyperreflexia and positive Babinski sign** [20].
- Globally, there is **3/5 muscle weakness** [21] and

reduced sensation as with upper limbs.

- **Proprioception** [22] is impaired but **vibratory sensation** [23] is intact.
- He is **unable to maintain balance whilst holding his arms out with his eyes closed** [24].

- The rest of the spine and cranial nerve examination is **unremarkable** [25].

1 Consider intracranial disease or vitamin B12 deficiency that may cause altered cognitive states.

2 Always inspect gait in neurological examination. Here it correlates with the history of an unsteadiness. This is a common early sign of DCM due to the damage to the corticospinal tract. Spasticity is a result of involuntary increased muscle tone, which causes muscles to resist movement due to stiffness and tightness.

3 Fever is present in infectious causes and malignancy. Tachycardia and tachypnoea may indicate severe pain.

4 Scars indicate previous trauma or surgery to the spine that may alter anatomy. Certain conditions are more common following spinal surgery; for example, dorsal cord herniation can occur following laminectomy.

5 Paraspinal pain may indicate muscle stiffness, muscle strain or underlying fracture, tumour or abscess.

6 Generally, in myelopathy, examinations would reveal LMN signs at the level of lesion, and upper motor neurone (UMN) signs below the level of lesion.

7 The mechanism of reduced range of motion is similar to osteoarthritis in other joints. In myelopathy, pain is usually not apparent until later stage of the disease.

8 Power assessment can be limited by pain and is quite subjective. Weakness of elbow flexion and wrist extension reflect a compression on the dorsal root of C6. Bear in mind that neurological findings can be completely normal in patients with radicular pain. Weakness in distal hand and possible interosseous and thenar muscle atrophy suggest cervical myelopathy.

9 This is the dermatomal distribution of C6 nerve root. Beware of possible concomitant ulnar neuropathy or carpal tunnel syndrome which can have referred pain and paraesthesia to arm and forearm.

10 Pectoralis hyperreflexia indicates myelopathy at the level of C2–C4, with reasonable sensitivity (85%) and specificity (96%).

11 Hyporeflexia is an LMN sign which may be seen at the level of spinal cord lesion or in radiculopathy. Here it correlates with the history, pattern of muscle weakness and sensory change, which helps to locate the level of lesion at C6 nerve root.

12 This is an UMN sign of C7 level lesion, indicating the pathology is at C5–C6 interspace or above.

13 This finding indicates damage of the spinothalamic tract. Due to the difference in their level of decussation, pain and temperature are often affected on the contralateral side of the lesion, and proprioception and vibration on the ipsilateral side. Light touch sensation is also affected and follows a dermatomal distribution.

14 This is known as Spurling's test, a provocative manoeuvre to examine patients with suspected radiculopathy. The test is positive when the symptoms of radiculopathy are exacerbated by putting an axial load onto a neck that is extended and rotated to the affected side.

15 This shows presence of Hoffman's sign, also known as the Babinski sign of upper limb, i.e. UMN sign of upper limb. However, the sign is quite subtle and its reliability is debatable.

16 This is a positive Lhermitte's sign. It is a sign of posterior column dysfunction, but is not specific to CSM and may also occur in MS.

17 Grip and release test assesses hand dexterity, where the patient is asked to grip and release their fingers as fast as possible for 10 seconds. Fewer than 20 times is a sign of 'myelopathy hand' due to reduced power in little and ring finger during extension and adduction. Other components of 'myelopathy hand' include intrinsic hand muscle wasting and positive finger escape sign, where there is spontaneous flexion and abduction of the little finger when the patient is asked to hold all digits of the hand in an adducted and extended position. It is due to necrosis of anterior horn cells at the level of C8–T1.

18 Inverted radial reflex suggests compression of spinal cord at the level of C5–C6 and ipsilateral C5 nerve root.

19 Sustained clonus is defined as ≥3 beats; it is a UMN sign of poor sensitivity but nearly 100% specificity.

20 These are all positive UMN signs due to the compression of corticospinal tract. Hyperreflexia may be diminished with concomitant lumbar spine stenosis or peripheral neuropathy.

21 Muscle weakness may indicate an UMN lesion affecting the corticospinal tract.

22 Impaired proprioception suggests a lesion affecting the dorsal column.

23 Loss of sensation to vibration tends to be present in severe, long-standing myelopathy.

24 Positive Romberg's test. It is a sign of posterior column dysfunction.

25 Neurological deficits of lower extremities may be due to a separate insult on the lower segments of the spine. Presence of cranial nerve abnormalities or a hyperactive jaw jerk demonstrate a pathology that is above the cervical level, such as in the brainstem.

Investigations

- **FBE is normal** [1] .
- Serological markers for **rheumatological diseases** [2] are all negative.
- **A lumbar puncture is performed, with unremarkable CSF analysis results** [3] .
- X-ray of the cervical spine depicts no malalignment, but overall **loss of disc height, anterior disc protrusion and osteophyte formation** [4] at the level of **C5–6** [5] .
- **CT of the cervical spine** [6] agrees with the X-ray findings.
- A **T2-weighted sagittal MRI** [7] scan demonstrates **cervical canal stenosis** [8] **and cord compression** [9] with **no signal change** [10] due to **disc protrusion** [11] ,

ventral osteophytosis [12] , ligamentum flavum hypertrophy [13] without **ossification and calcification** [14] , most pronounced at C5–C6 with **diminishing ventral cerebrospinal fluid sleeve** [15] .

- The axial view shows flattening of the cervical cord, with a **compression ratio of 0.6** [16] .
- There are no **signs of inflammation** [17] .
- There is no **visible syrinx** [18] or evidence of **other pathologies** [19] .
- These findings correlate with **examination findings** [20] .
- **MRI of the brain** [21] and the rest of the spine and **electromyography** [22] (EMG) reveals no additional pathology.

1 Anaemia may suggest a nutritional deficiency (such as iron or vitamin B12). Elevated WCC may indicate infection.

2 Biochemical markers for SLE (antinuclear antibody), Sjögren's syndrome (anti-Ro or anti-La antibodies), sarcoidosis (ACE level), RA (rheumatoid factor, anti-CCP) may be performed. However, patients with rheumatological conditions would present with symptoms involving other joints and systems.

3 Alteration in white cell counts, protein and glucose levels would indicate infection. IgG index and oligoclonal bands in the CSF may suggest a diagnosis of MS.

4 X-ray may provide information on spinal alignment, stability and presence of other bony diseases such as RA. Degenerative changes on X-ray are common in the elderly and are not diagnostic of myelopathy, given that a proportion of patients with imaging abnormalities are asymptomatic.

5 C5–6 is thought to be the most loaded level during cervical movement, therefore the most commonly affected.

6 CT is recognised as the optimal imaging modality in detecting cervical spine injury/fracture. It is readily available with high specificity and sensitivity, especially in depicting non-displaced injuries, which may not be demonstrated well on a plain film. In comparison to MRI, CT is superior in evaluating bony structures, therefore can also be used to assess the degree of canal compromise.

7 MRI is the standard diagnostic imaging that is non-invasive and does not involve radiation. It provides superior soft tissue contrast, visualisation of the subarachnoid space and extradural compression, evaluating neural elements and helping identify aetiology and severity of damage. It also provides prognostic information. In those patients who are unable to have MRI, CT myelogram (which involves intrathecal injection of contrast into CSF and visualisation of the subarachnoid space within the spinal canal) can be used.

8 A stenosed spinal canal is estimated to have a diameter of <13mm. It is clear there is a causal relationship between narrowed spinal canal and spinal cord compression.

9 Spinal cord compression is shown as narrowing of the spinal cord. Its calculation not only indicates the severity of compression, but can also be used to evaluate the presence of cord expansion after surgical intervention, which is related to good surgical outcome.

10 The importance of signal change results from the increase in water content in the cord tissue with increasing severity of injury. Therefore, intramedullary change of signal intensity on MRI is related to neural tissue damage, where hyperintensity on T2 indicates myelomalacia and gliosis, and hypointensity on T1 correlates with greater baseline neurological impairment and poor prognosis post surgery.

11 Disc protrusion and herniation most commonly occurs at the level of C5/6 and C6/7, causing C6 and C7 radiculopathy, respectively. The location of neurological structures being compressed has a causal relationship with presenting neurological deficits.

12 Osteophyte formation is a result of dehydration of the nucleus pulposus, leading to uneven distribution of pressure onto the end-plates, which causes bone remodelling and formation of osteophytes. This process may be fast-forwarded with intensive usage.

13 Ligamentum flavum hypertrophy is a response to its infolding secondary to the loss of disc and vertebral height. It may buckle into the spinal canal and causes spinal cord compression.

14 Ossification refers to the formation of ossific-calcific components in the ligament. It is more common in the Japanese population and compresses the spinal cord posteriorly, causing loss of vibration sense and proprioception.

15 CSF appears bright and spinal cord appears dark on T2, therefore effacement of CSF indicates compression.

16 The compression ratio is measured as the ratio between the smallest anteroposterior diameter and the largest transverse diameter of the spinal cord. A ratio <0.4 indicates poor prognosis.

17 Patchy T2 hyperintensities in the spinal cord suggest inflammation. Inflammation can be of non-infectious origin such as neuromyelitis optica or MS.

18 Syringomyelia refers to a fluid-filled cyst within the spinal cord. Its formation has a diverse range of aetiology that influence the CSF flow dynamic. Syringomyelia typically causes central cord lesions, affecting the spinothalamic tracts, leading to reduced sensation to pain and temperature in a cape-like distribution at the level of lesion. Other causes of such central lesions include intrinsic spinal tumour, trauma and demyelination.

19 Other causes that can be ruled out with MRI include malignancy and vascular causes such as spinal cord ischaemia.

20 It is crucial to correlate sensorimotor abnormalities identified on history and examination with imaging findings. A lack of correlation should prompt suspicion of an alternative pathology, such as demyelination due to MS. In such situation, further testing is merited.

21 For MS, an MRI showing a brain lesion, the presence of oligoclonal bands in CSF and abnormal motor-evoked potentials on EMG become important diagnostic adjuncts.

22 EMG serves as a negative diagnostic test in cervical myelopathy to differentiate CSM from conditions such as amyotrophic lateral sclerosis, MS, ulnar neuropathy or carpal tunnel syndrome, the symptoms of which can mimic those of CSM.

Management

Immediate

The patient scores 11 based on the criteria of the **modified Japanese Orthopaedic Association** [1] (mJOA). Consult neurosurgery for **surgical decompression** [2] .

Short-term

Keep the patient **fasted** [3] . Perform an **anterior** [4] **cervical discectomy and fusion (ACDF)**. Following surgery, monitor closely for **complications** [5] and order **postoperative imaging** [6] . Monitor for

postoperative **pain** [7] and **infection** [8] . Administer **VTE prophylaxis** [9] . Educate the patient about **mobility** [10] , adequate **diet** [11] and red flag symptoms, including **progressive neurological deficits and bladder and bowel function** [12] , before discharge.

Long-term

Ensure the patient is followed up in the **outpatient clinic** [13] , to monitor for **postoperative complications** [13] . Additionally, monitor for **adjacent segment disease** [14] .

1 The original JOA is more applicable to the East Asian population (with a component of the ability to use chopsticks). The modified version addresses cultural difference and is widely accepted as a tool to evaluate the clinical severity of compressive cervical myelopathy in the western world. The mJOA scale assesses overall motor deficit, upper limb sensory disturbance and sphincter dysfunction,

sparing sensory dysfunction in lower limbs and the trunk. The myelopathy is considered mild if the score is >13, moderate if between 9 and 12, and severe if <9.

2 Urgent surgical decompression is the gold standard management in moderate, severe or progressive neurological deficits to improve outcomes and halt further deterioration. However, complete reversal of pre-existing damage is unlikely, due to the limited regenerative capacity of the spine. The aim of surgery is to decompress impingement. The decision also needs to be made on whether to maintain or correct cervical misalignment (if any) and fusion. Patients with mild symptoms and no functional compromise may be candidates for non-surgical treatment. Patients presenting with only radiculopathy may also be managed conservatively. Those with symptoms that persist for >6 weeks or showing signs of myelopathy should be referred for imaging and surgery. Non-surgical measures encompass immobilisation with cervical collars to minimise neck motion (thereby reducing nerve irritation), physiotherapy, pain relief with simple analgesia such as NSAIDs and neuropathic agents in cervical radiculopathy, regular clinical follow-up and allied health input.

3 Keeping the patient fasted is imperative to prevent aspiration in the setting of general anaesthetic.

4 ACDF involves removing the herniated or degenerative intervertebral disc and inserting an implant or bone graft to fuse the spine, thereby relieving the pressure on the spinal cord or the nerve root. The type of surgery depends on the severity of compression, the number of vertebral levels involved and the location of the pathology. Prognostic indicators of surgical outcome include patient age, duration of symptoms and neurological status prior to surgery. An anterior approach is preferred when the pathology is most pronounced in the anterior portion, and can also correct kyphosis. The posterior approach includes laminoplasty (reconstruction of the vertebral lamina) and laminectomy (with or without fusion). Posterior approach becomes mandatory if the surgery involves more than two cervical levels, since the failure rate of anterior approach increases. Kyphosis of greater than 13° is a contraindication for any posterior approach. Fusion is indicated for pre-existing instability or if the destruction is extensive. The choice of approach is not always clear-cut.

5 Associated postoperative complications include haematoma, hoarseness (irritation of the recurrent laryngeal nerve causing vocal cord paralysis) and dysphagia (from surgical manipulation of the oesophagus). Haematoma is a potentially serious complication, which may manifest in dysphagia, neck pain, SOB, or even quadriplegia in the setting of spinal cord compression. The need for re-operation should be considered in these cases.

6 A postoperative X-ray serves as baseline to check degree of soft tissue swelling. Sometimes a postoperative CT may be preferred, as it allows for multi-plane assessment of the fusion and fixation.

7 Postoperative pain management is important, as inadequate analgesia administration may delay the patient's ability to mobilise in the early stages. The choice of administration route will be determined by the severity of pain, the patient's premorbid medication history and their compliance.

8 Patients who undergo a posterior approach to their surgery tend to have a higher risk of developing infection. Signs of infection include presence of pus, increased drainage, swelling, increased pain, erythema at the wound site and fever.

9 Postoperatively, it is imperative that VTE prophylaxis is administered. Surgery is a risk factor, as well as the decreased mobility in the peri-operative period. Watch for symptoms such as SOB, chest pain, unilateral calf pain and swelling.

10 Advise the patient to avoid twisting, bending or hyperextending the neck. Allied health input will aid in educating the patient and introducing measures to prevent this.

11 Most patients will experience a degree of dysphagia immediately after the surgery because of local soft tissue swelling and nausea due to anaesthesia or narcotics. Adequate nutrition is important in optimising the healing process. A regular diet should be encouraged.

12 Any worsening of neurology in the upper or lower extremities should be evaluated urgently.

13 Follow-up imaging should be performed to evaluate healing related to grafting (pseudoarthrosis, collapse or fracture), loss of alignment, migration or hardware failure, instability and soft tissue swelling. It would also be an opportunity to monitor for delayed complications after surgery.

14 Adjacent segment disease is defined as the development of radiculopathy or myelopathy of segments above or below the site of previous operation. It is due to accelerated segment degeneration secondary to the loss of mobility of the fused segment and increased mechanical stress posed on adjacent segments. Most commonly, it occurs at the C4–6 level.

CASE 33: CNS tumour

History

- A **64-year-old** [1] **right-handed** [2] **male** [3] presents with **headache** [4] that has been **getting more frequent, more severe and lasting longer** [5] over the **past 3 months** [6] .
- The headache is **generalised but worse on the left side** [7] .
- It is **dull** [8] in nature.
- The patient gives a history of migraines, but states these **headaches are different** [9] .
- The headache is **most prominent in the early morning** [10] , and is **exacerbated by bending down, coughing and sneezing** [11] .
- He also experiences associated **nausea and vomiting** [12] .
- Upon **further questioning** [13] , **his wife** [14] revealed that in the past few weeks, the patient has been having **trouble understanding instructions** [15] .
- He would often **forget about a conversation that had just happened and rarely keep an appointment** [16] .

- Occasionally, he would have **trouble naming objects** [17] and **say things that don't make sense** [18] .
- The patient has been **in a low mood** [19] , and his wife feels he has been a bit **more aggressive than usual** [20] .
- She also recalls him complaining about **objects obscuring his vision in the upper outer quadrant of both eyes** [21] .
- He denies any **history of seizures** [22] .
- He has not had any **fever**, **unintentional weight loss or night sweats** [23] .
- There is no history of **tooth abscess or dental procedure** [24] .
- His past medical history reveals nothing significant. He has not been exposed to **high dose ionising radiation** [25] .
- There is no **personal history of malignancy** [26] and no known **family history of genetic syndromes** [27] .
- He denies a history of **immunosuppression** [28] .

[1] Gliomas constitute about 40% of all primary brain tumours. High grade glioma is more often seen in adults. Low grade cerebellar gliomas, also known as pilocytic astrocytomas, are more prevalent in children and responsible for the greatest number of childhood deaths from primary brain tumour. Medulloblastomas are the most common malignant tumour in the paediatric group. Craniopharyngioma follows a bimodal age distribution with a peak between 5 and 14 years and 50–70 years.

[2] Handedness may aid in determining the dominant hemisphere. Nearly all right-handed individuals are left hemisphere dominant, whereas approximately 70% of left-handed people are left hemisphere dominant. Cognitive dysfunction is more likely observed if tumours develop in the dominant hemisphere.

[3] Brain tumours are slightly more common in men than women, at a ratio of 1.3:1. Glioma occurs in a male to female ratio of 3:2, in contrast to meningioma which is twice as common in females as in males.

[4] Amongst the myriad of clinical manifestations of intracranial tumours, headache is the most common

symptom. However, only about 2% of patients who present with headache have a primary brain malignancy. Headache occurs due to the traction of the structures that are sensitive to pain, such as vascular components, meningeal components and cranial nerves. The brain parenchyma itself is not sensitive to pain. Headache can also be a sign of elevated intracranial pressure or direct irritation of the aforementioned structures. Causes of an elevated ICP include cerebral oedema, hydrocephalus or tumour-related intracranial haemorrhage. Hydrocephalus may arise as a manifestation of posterior fossa tumours that compress the fourth ventricle, therefore obstructing the CSF pathway.

[5] Onset is usually insidious, and progressive headache is a result of mass effect from a growing tumour. Consider vascular causes if the headache is of sudden onset.

[6] The clinical course of patients with intracranial tumour depends on the pattern of growth and location. Over half of the patients with glioblastoma multiforme (GBM) have a prognosis of <3–6 months. In low grade glioma, it may span months to years. Symptoms of glioblastoma cannot reliably differentiate it from other types of glioma. Tumours growing in some regions, such as the right frontal lobe, may remain

clinically silent until reaching a substantial size. In contrast, tumours in the primary motor cortex tend to present early.

7 The location of headache is often generalised, but worse on the side of tumour.

8 The character of the headache in patients with CNS tumour is often dull rather than throbbing; however, pulsatile headaches have been reported. It may resemble common migraine or tension-type headache.

9 Headaches that change character or location should prompt further investigation.

10 Nocturnal or early morning headaches are typical in patients with intracranial malignancy. This is due to nocturnal hypoventilation, with a rise in $PaCO_2$ increasing cerebral blood flow and exacerbating the increased ICP.

11 Valsalva-like manoeuvres cause increases in intrathoracic pressure that will increase ICP and exacerbate a headache that is due to intracranial mass.

12 Nausea and vomiting accompanying headache are common in elevated ICP but not specific; for example, they are common in migraine. In the context of raised ICP, this is due to irritation of the area postrema which is a chemoreceptor trigger zone. The classic triad of increased ICP includes headache, nausea and papilloedema.

13 Gradual changes over time can be subtle and hard to pick up. Acute neurological deficits that wax and wane in female patients aged 20–40 should raise suspicion of MS.

14 Obtaining a collateral history can be important in analysing personality and behavioural changes.

15 Intracranial lesions may lead to Wernicke's or Broca's aphasia. Wernicke's aphasia, also known as receptive aphasia, may arise as a result of lesions located in the dominant posterior temporal lobe. It presents as an impaired ability to process and understand spoken words and sentences. Aphasia can also be expressive due to involvement of Broca's area located in the dominant posterior–inferior frontal lobe, where the patient has an impairment in production of language, but intact comprehension. Other speech and language disturbances include alexia, agraphia, dyscalculia and dysarthria. In particular, alexia, agraphia, right–left disorientation and dyscalculia together comprise Gerstmann syndrome which is due to lesions in the left parietal lobe in the region of the angular gyrus. Cerebellar tumours could manifest with dysarthria owing to difficulty in articulation.

16 Memory deficits are more likely to occur in frontal or temporal lobe lesions. Compromised verbal memory can result from a lesion in the dominant temporal lobe. Damage to the medial temporal lobe impairs both semantic (facts) and episodic (event) learning.

17 Anomic aphasia may occur due to lesions in the dominant temporal or parietal lobe.

18 This may indicate Wernicke's aphasia, where the patient produces fluent speech that does not make sense. It is also referred to as 'word salad' in severe cases.

19 Some of the cognitive manifestations of intracranial tumours may be confused with depression. Examples of these include anhedonia, an inability to concentrate, social retraction, memory difficulties and reduced thinking speed.

20 Deterioration in mental status is the second most common symptom in intracranial tumour. Manifestations include drowsiness, lethargy, personality change and cognitive dysfunction. Personality changes are more common in frontal lobe lesions but are also associated with temporal lobe lesions.

21 The patient is describing a superior homonymous quadrantanopia, sometimes referred to as 'pie in the sky'. It is due to a lesion affecting Meyer's loop in the anterior temporal lobe on the contralateral side of the visual field defect. This can also be due to vascular occlusions in the middle cerebral artery. Occipital lobe tumour would typically induce contralateral hemianopia or quadrantanopia, whereas a parietal lobe tumour would cause inferior quadrantanopia or hemianopia. Bitemporal hemianopia is a result of compression of the optic chiasm, most often at the pituitary region from pituitary adenomas or craniopharyngiomas. Vascular causes such as anterior communicating artery aneurysm could also be considered.

22 Seizure is one of the most common generalised symptoms of brain tumours. However, as with headache, the aetiologies encompass a broad spectrum ranging from idiopathic, cranial infection, trauma, stroke and arteriovenous malformation to systemic disorders such as electrolyte disturbance. In the context of intracranial tumour, seizures tend to occur more often with primary malignancy rather than metastasis, are more prevalent in low grade than high grade tumours, and are less likely to be present in posterior fossa tumours. Seizure can be classified as generalised or focal. Focal seizure means the seizure activity can be attributed to a part of one hemisphere, as opposed to generalised seizure where activity is attributed to both hemispheres. Focal deficits depend on the location of the tumour; signs and symptoms include visual, speech, gait abnormalities, and cranial nerve deficits. Focal seizures can progress to generalised seizures.

23 Constitutional symptoms can be seen in primary CNS lymphoma.

24 Recent dental procedure or history of tooth abscess predisposes a patient to develop brain abscess or meningitis. If brain abscess is suspected, look for chronic fever, recent dental procedure or recent ENT infections.

25 Radiation exposure is the most established risk factor for brain tumours. Common examples are previous exposure to high dose ionising radiation to the head region for childhood leukaemia. Exposure to X-ray in the prenatal period increases the chance of developing childhood brain tumours. Exposure to electromagnetic fields, such as using mobile phones or microwaves, has not been shown to be carcinogenic.

26 Brain metastases are three times more common than primary tumours, most commonly from the lungs. Other primary sites include breast, testicular, thyroid, renal, colorectal and melanoma. Brain metastasis tends to be multiple; however, solitary lesions are sometimes seen, for example in renal cell carcinoma.

27 Several hereditary syndromes have been shown to be related to certain CNS tumours. Examples include neurofibromatosis types 1 and 2 (glioma of optic nerve),

tuberous sclerosis (hamartoma), Turcot syndrome (medulloblastoma or GBM), von Hippel–Lindau disease (haemangioblastoma), and Li–Fraumeni syndrome (medulloblastoma). However, <10% of primary intracranial tumours occur in these syndromes.

28 Immunosuppressed status in individuals is related to the development of primary CNS lymphoma. The immunosuppressed status can be due to HIV or organ transplant. In the setting of immunosuppression, nearly all cells have latent EBV infection. If suspected, additional investigations include lumbar puncture for WCC and lymphoma cytology, HIV testing for CD4 count and viral load, and EBV PCR.

Examination

- The patient appears well. On general inspection, there is **no acromegaly nor cushingoid features of note** [1].
- When walking, the patient shows **no gait disturbance** [2].
- **Eye examination** [3] reveals mild bilateral **swelling of the optic disc** [4], and **bilateral visual field loss in the upper outer quadrant** [5].
- Otherwise, **visual acuity is 6/6 in both eyes** [6] and no **nystagmus** [7] is observed.
- His **pupils are equal and reactive** [8]. He

demonstrates **normal extraocular movements and reports no double vision** [8].
- His **cranial nerve examination** [9] is unremarkable. In particular, his sense of **smell** [10] and **hearing** [11] are intact.
- A **full upper and lower limb neurological examination** [12] is conducted and is unremarkable.
- A **cognitive examination** [13] reveals memory deficits and mild receptive aphasia; however, his ability in **decision-making** [14] is deemed to be intact.

1 General appearance is particularly important in patients with pituitary tumours. Look for physical changes such as acromegaly with changes in digits, coarse facial features and frontal bossing. There may be a characteristic cushingoid appearance which includes central obesity, moon face or buffalo hump.

2 Gait disturbances may include a circumduction gait from increased muscle tone and weakness on the contralateral side of a frontal lobe tumour. Ataxia and incoordination are features of a cerebellar tumour. Gait disturbance due to parietal lobe tumour is often from proprioception deficits.

3 As discussed earlier, visual impairment can be due to a lesion affecting any part of the visual pathway from retinal photoreceptors to the visual cortex.

4 Papilloedema invariably relates to increased ICP but may be absent.

5 As mentioned above, visual field loss such as superior quadrantanopia usually arises from lesions in the contralateral temporal lobe. Inferior quadrantanopia occurs due to lesions in the contralateral parietal lobe. The optic chiasm may be compressed by pituitary adenomas and this leads to

bitemporal hemianopia, whereas occipital lobe lesions result in homonymous hemianopia.

6 Decreased visual acuity may be seen with papilloedema in elevated ICP.

7 Nystagmus may result from a lesion affecting vestibular organs in the inner ear or cerebellum, which controls the central connections of the vestibular system. Nystagmus with vertigo and imbalance suggests lesions in the vestibular system.

8 Pupillary abnormalities and oculomotor abnormalities may be caused by tumours at the skull base, involving the third, fourth or sixth cranial nerve. Increased ICP can also lead to sixth nerve palsy. Restriction of extraocular muscle movements can cause diplopia.

9 Cranial nerve palsies often occur with 'long tract' signs such as hemianaesthesia or hemiparesis in brainstem gliomas. They are commonly accompanied by nystagmus and ataxia.

10 Anosmia, usually unilateral, may occur in frontal lobe lesions.

11 Impaired hearing ability may be seen in tumours of the skull base or those involving the vestibulocochlear apparatus, such as acoustic neuromas and leptomeningeal carcinomatosis. Acoustic neuroma, also known as vestibular schwannoma, features progressive unilateral sensorineural deafness as a result of the compression of CN VIII. It is one of the CPA tumours that are most commonly located in the posterior fossa and are usually benign. Impaired hearing may be accompanied by vertigo, dizziness, unilateral face numbness or weakness and absent corneal reflex.

12 Motor and sensation deficits are common complaints in CNS tumours. It is important to elicit any changes to help localise the lesion.

Intracranial malignancy tends to examine as a UMN lesion with hypertonia, hyperreflexia and positive Babinski sign. Sensory disturbance may be due to lesions in the contralateral parietal lobe where the somatosensory cortex is located. Deficits such as graphaesthesia impairment (inability to interpret a letter written on one's palm without watching), stereoagnosis impairment (inability to determine when an object is placed on one's hand with eyes shut) and diminished sensation to light touch, pain or temperature may be seen as well. Impaired proprioception and sensation to vibration can be attributed to lesions in the cortex or in the brainstem. Muscle weakness, including monoparesis, hemiparesis and paraparesis, can be due to lesions in the contralateral frontal lobe, brainstem, spinal cord or lesions disrupting the corticospinal tract. Muscle weakness may manifest as gait and balance disturbances. The progressive

nature of paralysis in intracranial tumours discriminates it from a cardiovascular event, although acute intratumoural haemorrhage may be seen in high grade glioma. UMN-induced weakness is generally more pronounced in the flexors of the lower extremities and extensors in the upper extremities.

13 Cognitive function is an independent prognostic factor in the survival of glioma patients. In addition, measuring baseline function can guide the goals for neurorehabilitation and determine progression or recurrence. Cognitive screening tools such as the mini mental state examination (MMSE) and Montreal Cognitive Assessment (MOCA) are designed to assess global cognitive decline. In particular, the MOCA includes domain-specific cognitive tests for visuospatial/executive, naming, memory, attention, language, abstraction, delayed recall and orientation. A score of ≥26 out of 30 indicates intact cognition. A comprehensive neuropsychological examination is sometimes desired. However, it can take up to 4 hours to complete and can be fatiguing to patients.

14 Decision-making and capacity are important in obtaining informed consent. Up to 50% of patients with high grade glioma have impaired capacity to make medical decisions. In this event, an appointed medical treatment decision-maker will consent on behalf of the patient.

Investigations

- FBE reports **normal WCC** [1].
- **ESR and CRP are elevated** [2].
- **MRI brain with contrast** [3] shows a large enhancing mass within the **left temporal lobe** [4] that is diffusely **infiltrative** [5] and heterogeneous.

- There is **ring-like enhancement** [6] with extensive **central necrosis** [7] and **peritumoural oedema** [8].

1 White cell count is unlikely to be raised in primary brain malignancy. It is, however, raised in infection. Hence, WCC may guide a clinician to consider different diagnoses.

2 Elevated CRP and ESR are inflammatory markers and can be seen in malignancy, but are also seen in the setting of infection. Consider the inflammatory markers in conjunction with WCC to determine if infection is the primary differential.

3 MRI is the most reliable and efficient way of diagnosing intracranial tumours and excluding other benign aetiologies. MRI is superior to CT in characterising soft tissue, thus can better evaluate the exact location and size of the tumour to guide management. MRI does not provide histological typing. CT with contrast can be used instead if patients could not tolerate MRI due to metallic implants such as ferromagnetic aneurysm clips, cochlear implants or cardiac pacemakers. If there is suspicion of early haemorrhage, CT

without contrast is sufficient, as blood appears hyperdense. CT may also show calcification as an indication of low grade tumour such as oligodendroglioma.

4 Gliomas are usually intra-axial, meaning they grow within white matter. This usually occurs in the supratentorial region of frontal and temporal lobes, but may occur in the cerebellum, brainstem or spinal cord. Primary CNS lymphoma typically appears in the periventricular white matter, basal ganglia and corpus callosum. Meningioma would be extra-axial and dural-based. Brain metastases tend to be found at the junction of white and grey matter, usually surrounded by a zone of oedema.

5 Glial neoplasms tend to be infiltrative. Metastases would appear as rounded, sharply demarcated masses. Meningiomas are usually rounded masses encapsulated by a thin, fibrous tissue.

6 A ring-like enhancement surrounding a mass is characteristic of GBM.

7 Extensive central necrosis may occur if angiogenesis cannot keep up with the growth of the tumour.

8 Peritumoural infiltrative oedema is composed of interstitial water and neoplastic cells which would appear on MRI as hypointense on T1, and hyperintense on T2/FLAIR. It is usually absent in low grade glioma.

Management

Immediate

Ensure the patient is stable. Obtain IV access, and administer **corticosteroids** [1]. Consider the role of **anticonvulsants** [2].

Short-term

Order a preoperative functional **MRI** [3] for surgical planning, then proceed to perform a **surgical resection of the tumour** [4] with intra-operative MRI. Obtain an **intra-operative biopsy** [5] [6] to refine the **treatment plan** [7]. Under the microscope, the cells have **elongated, hyperchromatic nuclei** [8]. Immunohistochemistry stains positive for **glial fibrillary acid** [9] with **marked hypercellularity, pleomorphism and mitotic figures** [10]. Furthermore, there is **endothelial proliferation and palisading necrosis** [11]. The cellular pathology resembles an **IDH-wildtype** [12] **grade IV** [13] **GBM** [14] **with MGMT promoter methylation** [15]. Initiate **radiation therapy** [16] 4 weeks post surgery for 6 weeks with **concurrent chemotherapy** [17]. Commence **antimicrobial prophylaxis for pneumocystis pneumonia** [18]. Monitor **bloods** [19] weekly for the duration of treatment. Order **repeat imaging** [20] after the completion of radiation therapy.

Long-term

Follow up the patient in the community. Continue **tumour surveillance** [21] with regular imaging. Refer the patient to **community palliative care** [22].

1 Corticosteroids are helpful in reducing intracranial oedema. They are indicated in the event of focal neurological symptoms and radiological evidence of peritumoural oedema. IV dexamethasone and mannitol should be given concurrently with signs of severely elevated intracranial pressure. It is also beneficial in patients undergoing radiotherapy (RTx) to reduce headache and nausea attributed to cerebral oedema during treatment. Corticosteroids should be avoided prior to biopsy if CNS lymphoma or infection is on the differential list. The side-effects of steroids are proportionate to the duration of treatment.

2 Anticonvulsants for the purpose of seizure prophylaxis are not recommended.

3 Functional MRI is a type of MRI that detects changes associated with blood flow, thus allowing for delineation of areas that the brain uses for certain actions. This information can be used to minimise surgery-induced neurological dysfunction.

4 Surgery is the most common initial treatment for many tumours including gliomas, meningiomas, primitive neuroectodermal tumours (PNETs) and ependymomas. Tumours can infiltrate into adjacent structures, hence complete resection may not be possible without compromising some neurological function. The goal is therefore to maximally resect the tumour whilst minimising disturbance to neurological function. Debulking may also reduce ICP as an additional benefit in some patient groups.

5 Pathohistological analysis gives accurate diagnosis of tumour type and grade to guide management. It should always be done unless the tumour resembles the appearance of typical grade I astrocytoma that is surgically inaccessible, or if it is a typical diffuse pontine astrocytoma. In either case histological investigation would not alter management.

6 Biopsy should ideally be obtained during surgery. Otherwise, stereotactic biopsy could be performed if the tumour is small or cannot be surgically approached. Stereotactic surgery is subject to sampling error, where the tissue taken does not represent the whole tumour's characteristics. Stereotactic biopsy is usually recommended in CNS lymphoma, since surgical resection would not be offered.

7 Treatment for brain tumours is highly dependent on histological grade and tumour location, and is specific to the patient's age and physical condition. Elderly patients generally are managed less aggressively. An MDT involving neurologists, medical oncologists for chemotherapy, radiation oncologists for radiotherapy, and neurosurgeons should be consulted.

8 These histological findings are typical of an astrocytic tumour. This is in contrast to oligodendrogliomas, where spherical nuclei surrounded by clear halos and calcification would be expected.

9 Glial fibrillary acid protein immunohistochemistry demonstrates the glial nature of the tumour.

10 Nuclear atypia and increased mitotic activity are signs of anaplastic astrocytoma. Minimal mitotic activity is seen in oligodendroglioma.

11 Vascular/endothelial proliferation and pseudopalisading appearance (necrosis surrounded by proliferating tumour cells) are features of grade IV GBMs.

12 GBM can be primary (develops *de novo*) or secondary (evolves from a lower grade astrocytoma). IDH is isocitrate dehydrogenase, a gene implicated in GBM. IDH-wildtype constitutes 90% of GBM, predominantly affecting patients >55 years old. IDH-mutant GBM preferentially affects a younger patient group and carries better survival rate.

13 The World Health Organization (WHO) grades brain tumour from I to IV representing growth potential and aggressiveness. Lower grade (I and II) tumours are slow growing, may be benign, and are associated with better prognosis. Higher grade (III and IV) tumours are malignant, fast growing and infiltrative with metastatic potential and are sometimes associated with central necrosis or tumour-related haemorrhage.

14 GBM is a type of diffuse astrocytoma which is under the umbrella of gliomas; others include pilocytic astrocytomas, ependymomas and oligodendrogliomas.

15 Methyl guanine methyl transferase (MGMT), an enzyme implicated in GBM, is prognostic of improved survival and predicts the response to alkylating chemotherapy.

16 Radiotherapy may be used postoperatively in combination with chemotherapy, or on its own. RTx is an essential adjunct to surgery in malignancies such as GBMs, PNETs and germ cell tumours. Benefits to survival and symptom alleviation need to be carefully balanced against the side-effects, including fatigue, loss of appetite, radiation dermatitis and alopecia. Potential long-term complications include neurocognitive toxicity, leucoencephalopathy and endocrinopathies.

17 Concurrent chemotherapy can work synergistically with radiotherapy and has been proven to prolong survival. Temozolomide is an alkylating agent that targets the O6 position on guanine. The chemotherapy goes on for 5 days every 28 days.

18 *Pneumocystis jirovecii* pneumonia (PJP) is a type of pneumonia caused by an opportunistic yeast-like fungus. It is the most common opportunistic infection in immunosuppressed individuals. In this patient, immunosuppression stems from selective CD4+ T-cell depletion from his chemotherapy.

19 Both chemotherapy and radiotherapy possess side-effects, which require regular monitoring. Haematological toxicity may manifest as thrombocytopenia, lymphopenia and neutropenia. Temozolomide results in mild, self-limiting elevations of serum aminotransferase levels. Radiation-induced liver disease is a potentially fatal side-effect that requires dosage adjustment of radiotherapy, and in some circumstances, halting of treatment.

20 Follow-up imaging by MRI allows assessment of response to treatment, signs of recurrence and local side-effects such as necrosis induced by chemoradiotherapy.

21 Recurrence is demonstrated by gadolinium-enhanced MRI. The frequency of surveillance imaging should be guided by the patient's general health status, residual volume after surgery and recurrence of symptoms. Treatment includes re-operation and second-line chemotherapy. Other agents include bevacizumab which is an anti-angiogenic agent targeting vascular endothelial growth factor (VEGF).

22 Palliative care is almost unavoidable in GBM patients owing to their short life expectancy. Palliative care specialists help to address end of life symptoms such as fatigue, headache, pressure injuries, and bowel and bladder symptoms. They provide patients and their families with physical, psychological, emotional and spiritual support to ensure quality of life and quality of dying.

CASE 34: Extradural haemorrhage

History

- A **24-year-old** [1] **male** [2] with **no known past medical history** [3] presents to the ED after being **knocked unconscious whilst going up for the ball during a local football match, with presumed blow to the head** [4].
- He was roused within one minute but appeared **confused to trainers and complained of a headache** [5].
- He was sent home, and **the confusion quickly resolved** [6]. **At home, he cooked dinner for his partner and appeared normal** [6].
- His partner brought him to the ED due to the **return of his symptoms** [7].
- On presentation he has a **severe constant generalised headache that is worse than his initial headache (collateral from partner)** [8] and associated **severe confusion** [9].
- These symptoms have returned **approximately 5 hours after the initial knock in the morning and are now rapidly progressing** [10].
- Due to his severe confusion and drowsiness, the clinician is unable to take a direct history from the patient and relies on a collateral history. His partner notes he has had one episode of **nausea and vomiting within the past hour** [11], **trouble breathing** [12] and **weakness in his right arm and leg** [13].
- He **does not smoke** [14] and drinks alcohol socially.
- His partner denies that the patient has had any **recent coryzal symptoms** [15].
- His partner also denies **loss of weight** [16] for the patient.

[1] Extradural haemorrhage (EDH) is a neurosurgical emergency and life-threatening condition characterised by an acute bleed in the potential space between the dura mater and the inner surface of the skull. In a healthy adult, this space does not exist. However, due to the traumatic injury as evidenced by a skull fracture and pooling of blood, this space between the dura and skull is prised open. The subsequent accumulation of blood will raise the ICP, compressing surrounding structures. Adult males 20–30 years old present with the highest prevalence of EDH since they are most likely to experience traumatic injury via sporting injuries, assaults, accidents, etc.

[2] EDH is an uncommon complication of a serious and traumatic head injury. There is an evidenced sex bias as more males than females are likely to suffer from EDH due to a greater likelihood of experiencing traumatic brain injuries such as skull fractures.

[3] Past medical history is important in determining fitness for surgery as well as any contributing or causative factors for the patient's acute headache and confusion.

[4] The majority of cases of EDH are complications of head injury caused by falls (sporting injuries), assaults and traffic accidents. The mechanism of injury underlying EDH hinges on skull fractures, which are present in 75% of cases. The area of the skull most subject to a fracture from trauma within the context of an EDH is the temporoparietal area. This is due to a common anatomical fixture known as the pterion. Since it is the fusion point between the parietal, frontal, sphenoid and temporal bones, it is susceptible to trauma and fracture. This is concerning as the middle meningeal artery (MMA) courses underneath the pterion and through the foramen spinosum, making it greatly susceptible to rupture. The rupture of the MMA will lead to a high volume haemorrhage over the cerebral convexity in the middle cranial fossa. It is the cornerstone of EDH and over time the pooling and leaking of this arterial blood strips the dura mater away from the skull. In fact, MMA rupture is classically seen in 75% of cases of EDH, and the accumulation of the massive amount of blood from this artery raises the ICP as it compresses important structures in the brain.

[5] Headache and confusion following an injury to the head in a sporting event that rendered the athlete briefly unconscious raise suspicion of fairly serious concussion. Generally, with EDH, the period of unconsciousness is brief. The initial symptoms of drowsiness, confusion and severe headache immediately following regaining consciousness can be attributed to a ruptured MMA. The pooling of blood will result in a burgeoning haematoma resulting in the initial symptoms of confusion and headache.

[6] A classic presentation of EDH involves a lucid interval. After the head trauma, the initial drowsiness, confusion and any other symptoms may resolve quickly. The patient may

appear normal and seemingly return to their premorbid level of functioning. Symptom resolution does not equal pathophysiological resolution. The duration of lucid interval can be from hours to days, depending on the rate of haemorrhage and compression of structures. Classically it can last 6–8 hours prior to decompensation.

7 Once the lucid interval ceases, there will be rapid deterioration of the patient. The initial symptoms will recur with greater severity.

8 A severe generalised headache is the most commonly reported symptom of EDH. With a severe headache following a lucid interval due to head trauma and accompanying drowsiness, the clinician can place EDH at the top of their differential list. Other types of headaches within different settings are important to keep in mind. For example, a sudden onset severe headache without much of a predisposing cause can point towards subarachnoid haemorrhage (SAH). Moreover, a thorough history (when possible) is required to distinguish the nature, time course and accompanying symptoms of the headache.

9 Severe confusion following a lucid interval in EDH is a common presentation. As arterial blood volume begins to rise in the extradural space, there will be a corresponding increase in ICP. Unabated growth of the haematoma (i.e. uncontrolled increase of ICP) will ultimately lead to thalamic lesions and brainstem injuries via mass effect.

10 The lucid interval can last anywhere from hours to days. Recurrence of symptoms with addition of further positive symptoms following a lucid interval and traumatic injury to the head signifies a rapidly deteriorating EDH.

11 Episodes of nausea and vomiting are quite common in EDH due to the raised ICP from the pooling of the blood. This rise in pressure will activate the chemoreceptor trigger zone in the vomiting centre of the medulla. An urgent CT is warranted to exclude brain tumours and strokes, and confirm the haemorrhage.

12 Irregular breathing can be demonstrated in late stages of several different types of intracranial haemorrhage (ICH). Particularly in EDH, irregular or deep breathing is commonly seen due to a phenomenon known as Cushing's triad. The triad is a physiological response to critically high ICP and consists of irregular/deep breathing, bradycardia and hypertension.

13 Muscle weakness is often seen in EDH due to compression of the primary motor cortex. The growth of the haematoma in the extradural space from a ruptured MMA can also compress the premotor cortex. Evidence suggests that in EDH, weakness nearly always starts on the contralateral side to the haemorrhage. Without urgent treatment at this point, the hemiparesis will progress to the other side of the body (i.e. bilateral) as the ICP continues to rise unabated, signalling brainstem compression.

14 A thorough social and drug and alcohol history is necessary in order to elicit other precipitants for this episode, comorbidities and risks that might dampen postoperative outcomes.

15 It is important to ask the patient about recent coryzal or flu-like symptoms to rule out communicable diseases. Headache in the context of preceding coryzal symptoms suggests a differential diagnosis of meningitis or viral encephalitis.

16 If the patient has experienced unintentional weight loss over a short period of time, urgent exploration following stabilisation is required to rule out a malignant cerebral tumour.

Examination

- The patient appears **drowsy and confused** [1] as he is not **alert to time, person and place** [1].
- His **GCS is 8 – E2V3M3** [2].
- There are **signs of respiratory distress as evidenced by deep and irregular breathing** [3].
- The patient's capillary refill time is **<2 seconds** [4].
- Vital signs are significant for a **pulse rate of 58bpm** [5], **respiratory rate of 10 per minute** [6] and a **blood pressure of 155/95mmHg** [7].
- **Abnormal tone is noted – hypertonia with spasticity** [8].
- **Power is 2/5 on the MRC scale** [9] throughout both upper limbs, **3/5 throughout the L. lower limb** [10] and **2/5 throughout the R. lower limb** [11], mainly due to difficulties testing power against resistance and the patient's inability to obey voice commands.
- Bilateral **symmetrical brisk reflexes (3+)** [12] are present.
- Cranial nerve exam demonstrates a persistently **dilated left pupil** [13] – the right pupil is 2mm and constricts to light, whilst the left pupil is 5mm and does not constrict.
- Visual field and confrontational field testing demonstrate **unclear results** [14] as the patient is not able to consistently keep his eyes open and respond to commands.
- CN III test result yields a **depressed and abducted left eye with ptosis and mydriasis of the left pupil** [15].

- Testing CN IV and VI reveals **unequal pupil constriction in response to light (right eye constricts when light is shone into left eye), with impaired swinging light reflex and impaired accommodation** [16].

- Jaw jerk is absent, but **corneal reflex is present** [17].
- The patient is unlikely to be **able to walk due to drowsiness and weakness** [18].

1 General inspection of the patient can, at times, guide the clinician's level of concern for the acuity of the patient's pathology. For example, a drowsy patient with fluctuating levels of consciousness on the background of traumatic brain injury (TBI) and headache points towards possible neurologic deficits due to an underlying haemorrhage. This raises the triage level of the situation and warrants urgent neurosurgical assessment.

2 With declining levels of consciousness, the GCS is crucial as it helps define the degree of TBI. Our patient within the setting of EDH is unable to open his eyes spontaneously or open them in response to voice commands. He only opens his eyes in response to pain and pressure exerted on his nail bed. When questioned about where he is, our patient responds inappropriately, albeit with discernible words, suggesting marked confusion. In response to pain, he demonstrates abnormal spastic flexion with decorticate posture. As a result our patient has a GCS of 8, suggesting a serious case of EDH.

3 Respiratory distress in a patient may indicate hypoxia or systemic inflammatory response syndrome (SIRS). Our patient is in respiratory distress, as evidenced by his irregular and deep breathing. This is part of the Cushing's triad, which is often seen in EDH due to a physiological response to high ICP. It also signals brainstem involvement, since the breathing/apnoeic centres are located in the medulla.

4 An adequate capillary refill time indicates the patient is perfusing well and thus would likely have preserved end-organ perfusion. In addition, it suggests the patient is adequately hydrated.

5 Bradycardia can be attributed to multiple aetiologies. Ensure to check the patient's other vital signs, including temperature, and feel the pulse for regularity. Consistent with Cushing's triad, our patient is demonstrating bradycardia in response to the high ICP. Possessing any of the symptoms of Cushing's triad is a poor prognostic indicator.

6 Hypoventilation within the setting of EDH may indicate some sort of respiratory depression due to compression of the medulla.

7 In the setting of intracranial haemorrhage, patients may present with hypotension. The most important thing to determine in a patient with hypotension is if the patient is in shock. If so, fluid resuscitation and identifying the cause of shock are imperative. Our young male patient, who does not have a history of essential or secondary hypertension (HTN),

is displaying high BP. This is commonly seen in EDH due to Cushing's triad, where HTN occurs as a response to high ICP.

8 Increased tone would point to a UMN lesion, whilst rigidity would indicate spinal pathology or a movement disorder rife with parkinsonian features. It is important to note these findings overlap with the late stages of EDH.

9 Muscle power is important to test within all planes of movement, to glean the degree or severity of haemorrhage. Power is 2/5 on the MRC scale throughout both upper limbs (UL), which indicates movement is possible, but not against gravity. This indicates the limbs were only tested in the horizontal plane. Our patient's skull fracture and subsequent EDH are left-sided, and hemiparesis generally occurs on the contralateral side to the EDH due to compression of the ipsilateral motor cortex.

10 The left LL of our patient demonstrates a power grading of 3+/5, indicating movement against gravity is possible, but not against examiner resistance. The testing against gravity might suggest our patient can still understand some verbal commands despite the drowsiness.

11 The right LL power is 2/5, which is true hemiparesis. Our patient's injury is left-sided, which indicates initial hemiparesis should be on the right side (contralateral). This marked unilateral hemiparesis is present in both right UL and LL.

12 Reflex testing can be important in EDH. Areflexia would indicate an LMN picture whilst hyperreflexia would point more towards a UMN issue. Asymmetrical reflexes may warrant use of the National Institutes of Health Stroke Scale (NIHSS) to assess for stroke. A growing EDH will often share common features with an UMN disease process, such as hypertonia, hyperreflexia and positive Babinski sign.

13 The CN exam in a suspected ICH such as in EDH must assess brainstem function and integrity of the optic nerve. While testing CN II, pupil size and reactivity to light must be measured. Unequal pupils may indicate brainstem pathology or raise suspicion of head trauma with subsequent haemorrhage.

14 Visual field assessment is crucial in EDH examination as it maps out important deficits. Characteristically, minor EDH may not initially present with visual field defects. As the haematoma grows, visual field deficits will appear due to compression of key nerves within the cavernous sinus.

15 CN III (oculomotor) nerve testing is paramount since part of the nerve resides in the cavernous sinus. Compression of this nerve can result in ptosis, eye muscle weakness and a fixed dilated pupil, ipsilateral to the side of the haemorrhage.

16 CN IV (trochlear nerve) and CN VI (abducens nerve) can be tested together. Shining a light into the pupil to elicit a direct and consensual response in both pupils and swinging the light from pupil to pupil to engage the 'swinging reflex' are important components. Compression of these nerves within the cavernous sinus as the extradural space fills up with more blood will produce impairment of the direct

and consensual eye response, swinging light reflex and accommodation.

17 Corneal reflex is expected to be present in EDH due to preservation of the afferent division of CN V and efferent division of CN VII.

18 LL neurological exam, particularly gait, is important to test. Any type of ICH will have far-reaching effects in the brain. With mild to moderate EDH, the patient will demonstrate an unsteady gait.

Investigations

NB. Due to the patient's high ICP and drowsiness (GCS 8), these investigations must be performed concurrently with resuscitation. Priority goes to protecting airway and investigations must not obstruct resus measures or delay treatment.

- A non-contrast CT brain reveals a **left-sided temporoparietal skull fracture, with an underlying hyperdense, sharply demarcated bi-convex EDH with mild midline shift** [1].

- FBE reports a mildly normal **WCC, microcytic hypochromic anaemia (Hb 110g/L) and normal platelets** [2].
- **UEC results are normal** [3].
- An ECG is in **sinus rhythm and unremarkable** [4].
- **Coagulation studies (i.e. clotting profile – prothrombin time (PT), activated partial thromboplastin time (aPTT), thrombin and INR) return normal results** [5].

1 An urgent non-contrast CT brain (CTB) is the gold standard investigation to confirm EDH. As soon as the patient presents to the ED and there is any suspicion of an EDH, a non-contrast CTB takes precedence over other investigations and less important parts of the history and exam. The shape of an EDH on a CTB is bi-convex or lentiform (lemon-shaped). It is generally sharply demarcated and appears hyperdense due to the haemorrhaging arterial blood. The more acute the bleed is, the less hyperdense it will appear on CT. If an EDH is sufficiently large, it can cause a midline shift as demonstrated by our CTB.

2 Often with EDH, active haemorrhage over a few hours can lead to anaemia. This has important implications for surgery. With a falling Hb and an impending major surgery, it is imperative to order a group and hold and cross-match units of the patient's blood group.

3 UEC is important in the setting of a surgical emergency. First, it identifies any electrolyte abnormalities that most

often need correction prior to surgery. Secondly, it assesses renal function and fitness for IV contrast in the setting of imaging (such as CT), as well as serving as a prognosticator for postoperative recovery.

4 An ECG is a simple and non-invasive investigation to assess electrical rhythm and informs preoperative cardiac risks. It is important to establish sinus rhythm and rule out atrial fibrillation or arrhythmias in the setting of a haemorrhage, to glean whether clotting medications or anticoagulation will be required postoperatively.

5 With any haemorrhage, it is imperative to conduct coagulation studies and observe the different durations of the clotting markers to ascertain any prolonged clotting times. These studies will inform anticoagulation and clotting medication guidelines immediately in the days leading up to the surgery.

Management

Immediate

Stabilise the patient [1] and monitor urine output. Keep the patient **fasted** [2]. Obtain IV access and check fluid status. **Seek urgent advice** [3] from the

neurosurgery team. Administer **IV mannitol** [4]. **Commence prophylactic IV antibiotics** [5]. Alert **airway anaesthetist and prepare intubation and resuscitation kit on standby due to ongoing drowsiness** [6].

Short-term

Perform an **urgent craniotomy and haematoma evacuation** [7]. Following the procedure, transfer the patient to the **ICU for monitoring** [8]. Review the patient's **surgical site** [9] and perform regular **neurological examinations** [10]. **Perform serial GCS exams to monitor neurological improvement** [11]. **Auscultate the lungs** [12] and **examine the lower limbs** [13]. The patient may require **dietitian review** [14]. They **may be discharged** [15] if vital signs remain stable with consciousness maintained (GCS >13), they can tolerate oral intake, have opened their bowels, neurological deficits and drowsiness have resolved, they are cleared by allied health and neurosurgery and are **back to a satisfactory level of function** [16].

Long-term

It is imperative for the patient to **follow up with the neurosurgery outpatient clinic** [17] for monitoring of postoperative complications.

---

1 Ensure the patient remains haemodynamically stable prior to operative treatment. In particular, BP and heart rate (HR) are important to stabilise as they are prognosticators for postoperative recovery. Since this is an acute situation, stabilisation may not be achieved, and surgery may be required. Systematic evaluation and resuscitation using priciples of advanced life support should be commenced to prevent further deterioration.

2 Keeping the patient fasted is crucial in their preoperative management. It allows the patient to have bowel rest, as well as reducing the risk of aspiration in the setting of anaesthesia. Ideally, patients should be fasted off solid foods for 6 hours, and clear fluids for 2 hours prior to induction of anaesthesia. This may not always be possible in the acute setting.

3 EDH warrants urgent neurosurgical evaluation. The type of management hinges on the patient's state. The decision to perform craniotomy with haematoma evacuation is based on the patient's GCS, neurological examination with key pupillary signs and neuro-radiological findings. Current practice dictates surgery be performed within 2 hours of loss of consciousness in patients with neurological deterioration following head trauma. Surgery is otherwise recommended for comatose patients due to acute EDH, onset of neurologic deterioration and signs of brain herniation. Our patient clearly demonstrated acute neurologic deterioration. Furthermore, our patient has a GCS of 8 (severe TBI) with marked unilateral hemiplegia and pupillary signs (dilated fixed left pupil) supplemented by a clear-cut CTB demonstrating EDH. Without life-saving surgery, the patient will die.

4 Commence IV mannitol to reduce the swelling around the brain from the haemorrhage and to reduce the ICP. This will help facilitate a smoother surgery.

5 Prophylactic IV antibiotics will be administered to prevent secondary meningitis from the skull fracture.

6 With a GCS of 8, ongoing drowsiness and irregular breathing, oxygen saturation should be closely monitored. The brainstem and its breathing centres are becoming compressed. An arterial blood gas (ABG) should be obtained to monitor for hypoxia and respiratory acidosis. Intubation will most likely be required to prevent impending respiratory failure.

7 Urgent craniotomy with haematoma evacuation by a neurosurgeon is the gold standard approach and management in this specific case. The ruptured MMA and any other affected vessels must be identified and ligated. This should ideally stabilise BP, HR and breathing. It should also resolve some of the neurologic deficits. Generally, patients have good prognosis and positive outcomes postoperatively for an EDH, even with large ones.

8 Patients must be monitored postoperatively for any immediate complications of surgery in the ICU. These include signs of shock (septic or hypovolaemic), infection, reaction to anaesthesia, DVT and PE, urinary retention or renal failure and new neurologic deficits.

9 Review the surgical site to ensure proper closure, as well as the amount of ooze and any signs of infection from the wound. Following a craniotomy, wound review can often occur quite early. Particularly after neurosurgery, risk factors for wound dehiscence include coughing, sneezing and straining with bowel movements.

10 Perform a modified neurological exam 24 hours after surgery. Once the patient is awake with independent breathing, perform daily neurological exams and compare findings to the initial neurological exam that was performed on presentation.

11 Serial GCS exams will help monitor for improvement in conscious state and inform timeline towards discharge.

12 Listen for any crepitations. The presence of crackles in the lung may indicate either an infective process or atelectasis.

13 Recent surgery and subsequent immobilisation in bed postoperatively are major risk factors for the development of DVT. Inspect the calves for unilateral swelling and erythema. Palpate the calves to ensure they are not tender. If clinically suspicious, order a Doppler ultrasound of the affected leg to diagnose, and then start the patient on anticoagulation.

14 If the patient is unable to breathe independently or maintain a GCS >13, dietitian review is required with a view towards other routes of nutrition. Only introduce oral intake after demonstration of independent breathing, improved GCS and bowel sounds on examination.

15 Complex neurosurgical cases on the background of an acute presentation normally take 1–2 weeks before discharge. Because of their large EDH and severe presentation that involved midline shift and brainstem compression, the patient will remain in ICU for a prolonged period until they can maintain consciousness and breathe independently. Discharge home will depend on cognitive and physical functionality, the ability to maintain a GCS >13 and social factors.

16 The patient should ideally be able to function at the level that they were able to prior to becoming ill. However, often this does not happen after a major neurosurgery on the background of an acute bleed. As a result, allied health – physiotherapy and occupational therapy – must perform further assessment of fitness for discharge home at a functional level. Marginal post-op improvements may warrant a transfer to a community rehabilitation centre for further physical therapy. This will be done once blood tests and vital signs are stabilised. At the rehab centre, physiotherapists and occupational therapists can work on gait and strength. Importantly, neurosurgery must also clear the patient for discharge.

17 Follow-up with the neurosurgeon is required to assess for postoperative complications such as incidental damage to any of the cranial nerves or other neural structures.

CASE 35: Hydrocephalus

History

- A **2-month-old** [1] female baby with **no known past medical history** [2] presents to the ED with **marked head enlargement** [3] and **lack of interest in feeding** [4], worsening over the **last 36 hours** [5].
- The parents also report symptoms of **generalised irritability** [6], **upper limb tremors** [7], **vomiting** [8] and **eyes that appear to consistently gaze downwards** [9].
- Additionally, they document recent failure of the baby to either **smile responsively** [10] or **vocalise to their commands** [11].
- Upon further questioning, a history of **premature birth** [12] was elicited, with the baby born at 34 weeks due to premature rupture of membranes.

[1] Hydrocephalus is a surgical condition that can occur at any age. It is broadly classified into either congenital or acquired subtypes, and accounts for around 1% of all paediatric hospital admissions worldwide.

[2] Past medical history is important in determining fitness for any investigative or surgical procedure, particularly with regard to any genetic disorders amongst infants. Additionally, it is also important for assessing risk of hydrocephalus, which often manifests in conjunction with congenital conditions such as Dandy–Walker syndrome and Arnold–Chiari malformations.

[3] The accumulation of CSF within the CNS causes the anterior and posterior fontanelles to bulge. As a result, this manifests as marked enlargement of the patient's head as one of the initial cardinal features. The head circumference is enlarged rapidly, and in most cases, surpasses the 97th percentile.

[4] As hydrocephalus progresses, torpor sets in, and infants often show lack of interest in their surroundings. This can include reduced feeding, as well as responsiveness to visual and audiological stimuli around them. As the hydrocephalus worsens, midbrain and brainstem dysfunction may result in lethargy and drowsiness.

[5] The progression of hydrocephalus typically occurs over a matter of hours to days. A timeline of <48 hours prior to first presentation at hospital is in keeping with current epidemiological data on this condition.

[6] The feature of generalised irritability is variable in infants with hydrocephalus. Most infants exhibit irritability for a variety of reasons, but this feature is often seen in conjunction with this condition.

[7] The increased pressure on the CNS causes bodily movements to become gradually weaker, with a prominent manifestation being generalised tremors of the upper limb.

[8] Symptoms of elevated ICP within the posterior fossa as a result of the raised levels of CSF include nausea and vomiting.

[9] Focal neurological deficits are a manifestation of increased ICP, with a prominent manifestation being the aptly called 'sunset eyes' (upper eyelids become retracted and eyes are turned downwards). This occurs as a result of raised pressure on the mesencephalic tegmentum, along with concurrent compression of the quadrigeminal plate, which causes vertical gaze palsy. In severe cases, vision may also be reduced due to compression of the optic nerve root.

[10] Infants and children who live with undiagnosed hydrocephalus for long periods of time can often exhibit developmental delays. In more acute cases, milestones that have already been met may show regression, highlighting the accelerated need to diagnose this condition. A thorough developmental history will need to be obtained from the parents or carers, to assess infant milestone progression.

[11] In a similar vein to social developmental milestones, infants may exhibit regression in language milestones as a result of increased ICP too. This can include failure to respond to audiological cues, or lack of imitation of speech sounds.

[12] Although rare, hydrocephalus can typically present as a delayed consequence of prematurity. Increased ICP typically manifests within the first 5 days after birth of a premature baby, but can occur up to 2 months after birth. Consequently, thorough maternal/parental history regarding circumstances of birth must be obtained.

Examination

- The infant appears **restless and uncomfortable** [1] , but there are no signs of **acute respiratory distress** [2] .
- Her central capillary refill time is <2 seconds, with **no pallor of the palmar creases** [3] .
- Vital signs reveal a **pulse rate of 110bpm** [4] , BP of **125/80mmHg** [5] and a **temperature of 38.3°C** [6] .
- The conjunctivae are not **pale** [7] , but it is noted **that the eyes exhibit a marked downward gaze, and the patient does not follow any finger movements** [8] .

- She is tracking well on the height and weight charts, at the 50th percentile for both variables, but is on the **97th percentile for head circumference** [9] .
- On abdominal examination, there is **no sign of any organomegaly** [10] , and **no visible tufts of hair on the lower back** [11] .
- There is no evidence of **ambiguous genitalia** [12] , and the anus is patent. Femoral pulses are strong and bilaterally palpable.

[1] General inspection of the patient can, at times, guide the clinician's level of concern for the acuity of the patient's pathology. In this particular context, those with hydrocephalus typically exhibit signs of irritability and/or obstreperousness, mechanisms which are both related to the increased ICP.

[2] Acute respiratory distress may indicate a sign of hypoxia and necessitates oxygenation if applicable. It can often be seen as a result of obstreperousness secondary to raised ICP. Infants requiring oxygenation will need to be managed urgently, due to risk of irreversible hypoxic brain injury otherwise.

[3] Causes of pallor in children include hypovolaemia (due to either blood loss or dehydration) or anaemia. Severe systemic pallor might necessitate immediate rhesus-negative blood transfusion.

[4] Changes in normal heart rate might be indicative of pyrexia, particularly if the patient is tachycardic. It is important to note that the normal HR of infants is significantly higher than their adult counterparts, but an isolated raised HR might prompt further physical examination of the cardiovascular and respiratory systems.

[5] In the setting of severe infection, patients may present with hypotension. The most important thing to determine in a patient with hypotension is if the patient is in shock. If so, fluid resuscitation and identifying the cause of shock is imperative. Other features that are highly suggestive of shock include abnormal mental state, tachycardia, oliguria, tachypnoea, metabolic acidosis and hyperlactataemia.

[6] Checking the patient's temperature is integral to determining their immediate wellbeing and subsequent prognosis. In particular, pyrexia might often hide underlying infection, necessitating urgent investigative procedures. One of the classic signs of meningitis, an important differential, is high grade fever, a symptom that is not predominantly seen in patients presenting with hydrocephalus.

[7] Conjunctival pallor has been documented to appear more frequently in patients with severe anaemia, and hence may be more sensitive than other signs. However, viewing this clinical sign in conjunction with 'sunset eyes', as seen in hydrocephalus, is difficult, and must therefore be approached with caution, to avoid further distress to the patient.

[8] As described earlier, the patient's 'sunset eyes' are visible. The patient also exhibits failure to follow any of the clinician's finger movements as a result of this.

[9] Isolated increase in head circumference parameters is visible due to hydrocephalus. Typically, this is above the 95th percentile. Young infants may also develop frontal bossing, an abnormal skull contour in which the forehead becomes prominent. Scalp veins could appear dilated as well.

[10] Abdominal distension or organomegaly may be associated with other GI pathologies in which infants exhibit restlessness, such as intussusception, and must therefore be ruled out. A thorough abdominal examination is also essential to determine evidence of any previous invasive procedures or surgeries, both of which have a risk of post-procedure infection.

[11] Tufts of hair on the lower back are most seen in spina bifida, a pathology commonly seen in conjunction with hydrocephalus, with approximately 90% of people born with spina bifida also having hydrocephalus. The spine should also be carefully examined for stigmata suggestive of an acquired Chiari II malformation associated with spinal dysraphism, such as a pit located above the gluteal crease.

[12] Ambiguous genitalia could be indicative of an underlying genetic disorder, which could be a cause of underlying neurological issues. Common genetic conditions include Turner syndrome (in females), Patau syndrome and Edwards syndrome, which can manifest with neurological complications.

Investigations

- FBE reports **mild anaemia** [1] with **normal leucocyte count** [2].
- **UEC results are normal** [3].
- **CRP is within normal limits** [4].
- Other blood parameters including LFT results are normal. A **urine dipstick is conducted** [5] and revealed to be normal as well.
- X-ray shows **no consolidation of the lung fields** [6], or any **intra-abdominal pathology** [7].
- Abdominal ultrasound shows **no concentric echogenic and hypoechogenic bands** [8].
- A lumbar puncture was carried out, revealing no changes to the **glucose or protein levels of the CSF** [9].
- A T2-weighted MRI is performed, confirming the diagnosis of **communicating hydrocephalus** [10].

1 Mild anaemia can often be seen as a result of hypovolaemia due to the infant not consuming fluids as a result of irritability. Often, this does not necessitate immediate intervention, but the need for fluid replacement must be kept in the back of the treating clinician's mind.

2 Infection is a common cause of raised leucocyte count. Possible differentials to hydrocephalus include meningitis or SIRS, which would raise the WCC.

3 UEC is important to determine any electrolyte anomalies as a result of prolonged vomiting secondary to raised ICP. It also assesses renal function and in turn, the patient's fitness for any procedural intervention or therapeutic options, such as shunt insertion.

4 C-reactive protein is one of many acute phase reactants that accompany inflammatory states. In meningitis, an important differential within the paediatric population, infection and inflammation take place, both of which elevate the CRP.

5 A urine dipstick and MC&S is often done as part of a full septic screen, particularly in the acutely ill infant. Conditions such as UTIs can often be seen within the early months of life, particularly due to congenital anomalies such as hydronephrosis or vesicoureteric reflux, and would merit further investigation with a renal tract ultrasound.

6 Consolidation of the lung fields is seen in either typical or atypical pneumonia, and chest X-rays are often done as part of a full septic work-up.

7 Abdominal X-rays are done in conjunction with chest X-rays and are helpful in ruling out intra-abdominal pathologies such as necrotising enterocolitis, which could also cause an acutely ill and febrile infant.

8 Ultrasounds of the abdomen are particularly sensitive for determining the presence of intussusception, which could provide an explanation for the infant's irritability and obstreperousness. As a bedside investigation, it is particularly useful within the emergency setting as well.

9 Lumbar punctures are both diagnostic and therapeutic for communicating (non-obstructive) hydrocephalus. For most cases of hydrocephalus, however, lumbar puncture is not necessary in the initial diagnostic evaluation. In particular, lumbar punctures are contraindicated if the patient has evidence of a space-occupying lesion such as an intracranial tumour or a brain abscess, because of the risk of cerebral herniation. Lumbar punctures are also essential to confirm a diagnosis of viral or bacterial meningitis, analysed through the CSF parameters.

10 Compared to other imaging modalities, MRI provides superior visualisation of pathologic processes in the CSF, including flow dynamics. In particular, T2-weighted imaging provides information regarding the CSF spaces and cisterns. Ultrasonography may be carried out if this imaging modality is not available, providing good information about the ventricular system, but should not be used as the anterior fontanelle closes (which occurs around the age of 18 months).

Management

Immediate

Monitor **vital signs** [1] and **urine output** [2]. Keep the patient **fasted** [3]. Obtain IV access and **consider usage of either diuretics** [4] or **fluid** [5]. **Seek advice** [6] from the neurosurgical team.

Short-term

Consider the need for and timing of intervention, given the **severity of symptoms and neuroimaging findings** [7]. Patients with acute rapidly progressive hydrocephalus require **urgent surgical intervention** [8].

For patients with **signs of herniation** [9] or marked deterioration, or those who are too unstable to undergo surgery, management often consists of placement of a **temporary external ventricular drain (EVD) or diuretic therapy** [10]. Following either of these procedures, the patient must be kept within hospital for **close monitoring** [11]. Perform regular **examinations** [12]. The patient may be discharged if **vital signs remain stable** [13].

Long-term

The patient is typically called back to hospital 10–14 days postoperatively for **suture removal** [14] at the neurosurgery outpatient clinic. Follow the patient up in an **outpatient neurosurgical (and if appropriate, paediatric developmental) clinic** [15] if necessary, for continuing wound management and monitoring for postoperative complications.

[1] Ensure the patient is haemodynamically stable prior to any procedural intervention. Temperature, BP and HR are all particularly important in the infant, due to their tendency to quickly fluctuate in an acutely ill young patient.

[2] Urine output is an indicator of fluid balance. In particular, due to nausea and emesis caused by increased ICP, it is possible that fluid levels within the acutely ill patient will fluctuate wildly, and thus fluid outputs and inputs must be closely monitored.

[3] Keeping the patient fasted is crucial in their preoperative management. It allows the patient to have bowel rest, as well as reducing the risk of aspiration in the setting of anaesthesia. Ideally, patients should be fasted off solid foods for 6 hours, and clear fluids for 2 hours prior to induction of anaesthesia.

[4] In those with acute rapidly progressive hydrocephalus, the use of diuretics may be considered in order to decrease CSF production. However, in newborn infants with post-haemorrhagic hydrocephalus, treatment with diuretics is generally not effective and is associated with complications, including electrolyte imbalances, ototoxicity and renal calcifications.

[5] The administration of fluid is dependent on UEC levels that may differ significantly from baseline parameters as a result of severe emesis. Patients are nil by mouth prior to surgery and so maintenance fluids are essential in keeping the patient adequately hydrated. IV fluid management is based around four principles – resuscitation, maintenance, replacement (of any fluid losses, such as from the GI tract) and redistribution (e.g. third spacing). Within the paediatric population, the 4–2–1 rule may be employed for fluid maintenance: 4ml/kg/hr for the first 10kg, 2ml/kg/hr for the second 10kg, and 1ml/kg/hr for every kg above 20, with the same rule being usable to calculate preoperative maintenance requirements.

[6] Hydrocephalus falls under the neurosurgeon's domain, and care should be directed by their advice. Often, pathway of care will shift from the ED team to either the paediatric team or the neurosurgical team, depending on the availability of the latter within the hospital.

[7] The need for and timing of procedural intervention in infants with hydrocephalus is determined by the severity of their symptoms, as well as findings documented on imaging. Asymptomatic patients who do not possess any symptoms suggestive of elevated ICP, such as papilloedema or bulging fontanelles, may be managed with watchful waiting. In a similar vein, those who are achieving expected developmental milestones, and do not have severe ventriculomegaly or obvious obstruction of the CSF pathway on neuroimaging, can also be managed without procedural intervention.

[8] Patients with acutely progressive hydrocephalus require either a CSF shunt or endoscopic third ventriculostomy. In those too unstable for surgical intervention, management can consist of placing a temporary external ventricular drain (EVD) or diuretic therapy. An EVD is a small catheter inserted through the skull, usually into the lateral ventricle, allowing for drainage of CSF.

[9] Brain herniation is the potentially lethal side-effect of markedly raised ICP and occurs when part of the brain is squeezed across structures within the skull. The brain may shift across structures including the falx cerebri, the tentorium cerebelli or even the foramen magnum. In particular, hydrocephalus may cause tonsillar herniation, which refers to the downward movement of the cerebellar tonsils through the foramen magnum, possibly causing compression of the upper cervical spinal cord or lower brainstem. Signs of brain herniation include decorticate posturing, lowered levels of consciousness, dilated pupils unresponsive to light, and vomiting due to compression of the area postrema.

[10] Insertion of an EVD may also be diagnostic, as connecting the drain to a transducer allows for measurement of ICP. Diuretics such as furosemide or acetazolamide may be used to decrease CSF production, but are considered less effective than EVD. Note that in newborn infants with post-haemorrhagic hydrocephalus, treatment with diuretics is generally not effective. Electrolyte disturbances, particularly with the usage of furosemide, must be considered and closely monitored as well.

[11] Patients must be monitored post-treatment for any immediate complications. For EVDs, this includes catheter occlusion and infection. Acute deterioration in those with life-threatening presentations of hydrocephalus, such as those showing signs of herniation, must also be

immediately managed. Infections are typically seen in the first postoperative month, and typically develop via colonisation by skin flora within the shunt itself. *Staphylococci* are predominant pathogens. Whilst shunt infections are often asymptomatic, patients may present with evidence of soft tissue infection with swelling, erythema, tenderness or purulent drainage. Principles of management therefore involve removal of the device, external drainage, parenteral antibiotics, and shunt replacement once the CSF is sterile. Should device removal not be feasible, IV antibiotics may be considered.

12 A thorough physical examination of the patient postoperatively is a must. A neurological examination will help assess severity of the condition, as well as determine if the patient has improved from their initial presentation. Monitor for postoperative complications, including infection and VTE.

13 Following treatment for hydrocephalus with a shunt, patients are discharged home with sutures/staples still in place. If vital signs are stable, patients may even be able to shower/bathe within 24 hours post surgery.

14 Appropriate surgical site care and plans for suture removal must be discussed with the patient (and/or carer) and the treating team prior to discharge from the hospital. Red flags that might necessitate a hastened second visit to hospital include developing symptoms of a severe headache not relieved by medication/rest, onset of worsening visual/speech problems or the development of heat/pain, or increased swelling around the incision site.

15 The need for ongoing follow-up depends on the severity of the illness, the complexity of the procedure and the patient's risk for postoperative complications. Some patients are fit and well enough to be managed by their GP, whilst some will require several follow-up visits with the neurosurgeons to ensure adequate recovery and resolution of any lingering symptoms. Paediatric patients must also be assessed by the hospital's developmental medicine team, to ensure that all social, adaptive, language and gross motor milestones are being met.

CASE 36: Lumbar myelopathy/radiculopathy

History

- A **45-year-old** [1] **male** [2] **lorry driver** [3] presents with **2 days** [4] of **severe lower back pain** [5] and **difficulty walking** [6], on the background of **chronic back pain** [7].
- The pain is **sharp** [8], originates from the **central** [9] lower back and **radiates** [10] down the back of his left thigh into his calf, stopping at the ankle.
- The patient denies any alleviating factors such as positioning. He reports **difficulty sitting, walking, and sleeping because of the pain** [11].
- He also feels **numbness and heaviness** [12] in his left leg.
- The patient denies **bowel** [13] or **bladder** [14] dysfunction.
- He reports a history of back pain over the last 25 years, initially more **prominent after standing for a long time** [15] and which is relieved by taking **paracetamol** [16].

- Six weeks ago, he experienced **sudden severe lower back pain** [17] whilst **lifting a heavy box** [18].
- The pain was not relieved by **bed rest** [19], **medications** [20] or **physical therapy** [21].
- He has presented to the ED twice in the past week. The prescribed analgesics provided minimal relief. He also reports his GP prescribing an **epidural corticosteroid injection** [22], with relief only lasting 2 weeks.
- He takes no other regular medications, and in particular, no **immunosuppressants or steroids** [23].
- The patient has no personal or family **history of cancer** [24], fever, unexplained weight loss or night sweats, nor intravenous drug use (IVDU) [25].
- He denies **abdominal pain** [26].
- The patient reports **smoking** [27] 10 cigarettes per day for the past 20 years.

[1] Intervertebral disc herniation is one of the most common causes of lumbosacral radiculopathy. Disc herniation occurs in all age groups, especially in young and middle-aged patients.

[2] Occupational posture that includes repetitive lifting, bending or twisting puts extra strain on the back. Prolonged sitting and vibratory loading also put more pressure on the discs. As such, a person's occupation may put them at higher risk of developing lumbosacral radiculopathy.

[3] Disc herniation is more common in males than in females at a ratio of 3:1. Similarly, lumbar spine stenosis is also more prevalent in males. This contrasts with degenerative spondylolisthesis which has been reported to be as much as 8 times more common in females. The reason is thought to relate to hormone-induced ligamentous laxity.

[4] Back pain that lasts <4 weeks is defined as acute, for 4–12 weeks as subacute and >12 weeks as chronic.

[5] Advancing disabling low back pain is an indication for surgery in patients with lumbar radiculopathy.

[6] Difficulty walking can be due to weakness or pain and needs to be investigated further in examination.

[7] A previous history of low back pain is a well-established risk factor for lumbar radiculopathy.

[8] Intervertebral discs are located between vertebrae. Their primary function is to provide cushioning and distribute the compressive load of the torso. The discs are composed of a central nucleus pulposus that is rich in proteoglycans, surrounded by a ring-structured annulus fibrosus composed of organised lamellar collagen. With age, the annulus fibrosus weakens, and sudden change in position can lead to bulging out of the central nucleus pulposus, resulting in nerve root compression.

[9] Sharp pain is characteristic of neuropathic pain. Other phrases that are commonly used including stabbing, throbbing, burning or electric shock-like.

[10] Axial lower back pain may be discogenic or mechanical. Musculoskeletal causes of pain tend to be localised.

[11] Nerve root dysfunction causes radiculopathy. This manifests as pain and paraesthesia following a dermatomal distribution, and muscle weakness following a myotomal distribution with or without diminished deep tendon reflex. Radiculopathy is a result of both nerve root compression and resultant inflammation of the affected nerve. The

compression can occur anywhere along the course of the nerve root.

12 Substantial functional impairment warrants further investigation. Prolonged sitting causes higher pressure and compressive forces on discs. It may also imply that sustained lumbar flexion causes mechanical deformation and aggravates the pain. Pain that is worse with bending forwards is a common clinical finding in disc herniation. Musculoskeletal pain, however, is typically worsened with repeated movements and improved with sitting through the effect of resting. If the complaint involves morning stiffness that is relieved by activities, then it is suggestive of an inflammatory condition such as ankylosing spondylitis or OA of the facet joint.

13 Bowel dysfunction can manifest as either constipation or incontinence. Sometimes changes in bowel habits are not apparent in the history. In all patients presenting with back pain, cauda equina syndrome (CES) needs to be excluded. CES is most frequently seen in patients with lumbar disc herniation. It is associated with bilateral leg pain, saddle anaesthesia and bowel/bladder dysfunction. CES is a surgical emergency where surgical decompression is preferably performed within 12 hours, and no later than 24 hours. Delayed decompression will result in increased risk of sexual dysfunction, urinary dysfunction or permanent neural damage. This is further discussed in *Case 31*.

14 The bladder relies on both parasympathetic and sympathetic plexus innervation for sphincter control. CES is associated with disruption of bladder contraction and sensation, and hence manifests as urinary retention followed by overflow incontinence.

15 In cases of neurogenic claudication caused by spinal stenosis, lumbar flexion increases the space of the central canal and alleviates symptoms. Therefore patients find it less painful when leaning over, going upstairs or sleeping in the foetal position, while extension decreases foraminal dimensions, therefore positions such as walking and standing straight exacerbate the symptoms.

16 Paracetamol is usually the first-line treatment in patients with non-specific back pain.

17 Acute disc herniation usually has an abrupt onset and is intense. Clinically, chronic radiculopathy more often involves intermittent neurogenic claudication in the region of buttock, hip or posterior thigh. Acute disc herniation on the background of chronic back pain from degenerative lumbar stenosis is common. Intervertebral disc herniation produces symptoms by direct compression of nerve roots in an already narrowed foramen.

18 Improper lifting technique may increase the chance of tearing the outer annulus, causing herniation of the nucleus pulposus, thereby compressing the adjacent nerve root.

19 It is widely accepted that the majority of patients improve with bed rest, then gradual mobilisation to normal activities as tolerated. Herniated discs will regress over time in >90% of patients, through spontaneous reabsorption by macrophage phagocytosis.

20 Medications for disc herniation range from simple analgesia to muscle relaxants and short-term opioids.

21 Physical therapies include physiotherapy, superficial heat, massage, acupuncture, traction and chiropractic manipulation. They have been shown to provide symptomatic relief in patients with lumbar disc herniation with radiculopathy. Physiotherapy aims to strengthen the supporting musculature to improve postural mechanics.

22 Spinal injections, including epidural steroid injections, facet joint injection or transforaminal injections, form the second-line treatment. They are indicated if an aetiology involves local compression of a nerve root or for non-surgical candidates of spinal canal stenosis. They are also indicated when the patient fails to respond to conservative treatment. Injections typically involve anti-inflammatories such as corticosteroids and an anaesthetic agent such as lignocaine, usually under contrast-enhanced fluoroscopy or CT guidance. They work by mechanically relieving the compression on the nerve root, as well as the anti-inflammatory effects against local inflammatory mediators. Injections serve as both diagnostic and therapeutic tools in cases where the aetiology is indeterminate. They usually provide short-term relief that lasts for 2–4 weeks. Epidural steroids should be used with caution in diabetic and osteoporotic patients. They are contraindicated in pregnant women and patients with active peptic ulcer disease or coagulopathy.

23 Consider malignancy as a differential if there is a history of cancer with new onset of lower back pain or with the presence of constitutional symptoms such as unexplained weight loss, anorexia and low grade fever. The pain is usually unremitting, worse with recumbency and interferes with sleeping. Primary tumours are rare, most of them are benign, slow growing, solitary, intradural mass. Metastatic tumours tend to be extradural and multifocal. Common primary cancers that metastasise to the lumbosacral spine include leukaemia, lymphoma, melanoma, breast and lung, and tumours in the pelvic region, such as colon and prostate.

24 Back pain associated with fever should raise suspicion for an infectious cause such as discitis or epidural abscess. Look for systemic unwellness, history of IVDU or use of immunosuppressants or steroids. Septic discitis needs urgent neurosurgical referral because of the potential to cause rapid destruction to adjacent vertebrae. Similarly, epidural abscess needs urgent surgical debridement or initiation of a course of antibiotics.

25 Saddle anaesthesia results from the irritation of S3, S4 and S5 which provides sensation to inner thigh, perineum and rectum area.

26 Abdominal organs may refer pain to the lumbar region. Therefore, conditions such as pancreatitis, abdominal aortic aneurysm, nephrolithiasis, pyelonephritis and pelvic inflammatory disease (PID) may manifest as back pain, but would not be consistent with the history of pain radiating down the lower limbs.

27 Smoking accelerates disc degeneration by causing vasoconstriction and ischaemia, and malnutrition of the disc. It also disturbs normal annular cell metabolism.

Examination

- The patient appears to be distressed with pain. **Vital signs are unremarkable** [1].
- He is **178cm tall and weighs 120kg** [2].
- In standing, the patient demonstrates **scoliosis** [3], but there appears to be no **muscle atrophy** [4].
- The patient walks with a left-sided antalgic gait and is able to **walk on his heels** [5] but **is unable to walk on his toes** [6].
- **Lumbar range of motion in all directions is restricted by pain** [7].
- There is paraspinal **tenderness over L5–S1 region with deep palpation** [8].
- His lower extremity muscle **tone** [9] is normal.
- Motor examination is unremarkable apart from **left-sided mild weakness of ankle plantarflexion and reduced ankle reflex** [10].
- **Babinski sign** [11] is negative.
- His **sensation to pinprick is diminished** [12] from the back of his left thigh, down the knee and along the lateral aspect of the foot to the fifth toe, but is **intact over the buttocks, posterosuperior thighs and perineal region** [13].
- With the patient lying supine, lifting his left leg straight up with an extended knee **reproduces pain and paraesthesia at an angle of 40°** [14].
- The left leg is then lowered 5° and the foot is dorsiflexed, once **again reproducing symptoms** [15].
- However, **passive flexion of the right hip** [16] fails to reproduce the symptoms.
- The patient is able to **stand on one leg without tilting his pelvis** [17].
- His **anal tone** [18] is normal on PR examination.

1 This confirms the absence of fever, making an infectious cause less likely.

2 Obesity is a risk factor for lower back pain and lumbar spinal spondylosis. Being obese also adds more stress on the discs, thus is a risk factor for disc herniation.

3 Scoliosis is a finding associated with muscle spasm. Other causes include cerebral palsy and muscular dystrophy.

4 Muscle atrophy is a result of weakness and underuse of muscles, whether that be due to pain or inability. It is more characteristic of pathologies of insidious onset such as spinal canal stenosis.

5 An inability to walk on one's heels demonstrates ankle dorsiflexion weakness, which may be due to L5 nerve root compression.

6 Walking on one's toes requires ankle plantarflexion. Inability to do so may reflect S1 radiculopathy.

7 Reduced range of motion can be a result of paraspinal muscle spasm or pain. As mentioned previously, pain exacerbated by forward flexion is more likely to be disc herniation, and pain that worsens with extension is more likely to be spinal stenosis.

8 Pain elicited by deep palpation may indicate spinal fracture or local infection. Muscle spasm may also be present.

9 Hypertonia is seen in UMN lesions, and hypotonia in LMN lesions.

10 S1 radiculopathy is associated with ankle plantarflexion weakness. It echoes with the previous finding of inability to walk on toes. Diminished Achilles tendon reflex is also seen in S1 radiculopathy.

11 Babinski sign is positive in UMN disease, for example in the spinal cord or in the brain cortex. Absence of Babinski sign does not differentiate normal from LMN lesions.

12 The sensory disturbance follows the dermatomal distribution of the S1 nerve root. In isolated sensory disturbance affecting the medial lower leg, consider saphenous neuropathy as a differential.

13 This is confirming the absence of saddle paraesthesia, a manifestation of CES.

14 The straight leg test (SLT) is a provocative test that demonstrates L4–S1 nerve root lesions due to disc herniation. When the symptoms are reproducible between 30° and 70°, it is thought to be positive. Supine SLT has a higher sensitivity than seated SLT for radiculopathy due to disc herniation.

15 This is known as Lasegue's sign, and is also a sign of nerve root irritation.

16 This is known as crossed straight leg test. It is not as sensitive, but more specific than the SLT for disc herniation.

17 Trendelenburg gait is seen in L5 nerve lesions, where there is gluteus medius weakness that fails to stabilise the hip joint when standing on one foot.

18 Loss of sphincter tone is a sign of CES.

Investigations

- **FBE is within normal limits** [1] .
- **CRP and ESR are not elevated** [2] .
- An **erect lumbar spine X-ray** [3] shows **straightening of the lumbar lordosis** [4] with **no malalignment** [5] .
- There is mild **disc space narrowing** [6] at **L4–5 and L5–S1** [7] .
- No other **focal bony lesion** [8] is observed.
- **MRI of the lumbar spine** [9] shows that at the level of L5–S1, there is diffuse **central** [10] **disc bulging** [11] with loss of disc height and **degenerative end-plate changes** [12] .

- There is a more focal **posterior** [13] **protrusion** [14] that is impinging on the left S1 nerve root.
- In combination with **facet joint hypertrophy** [15] and **thickening of the ligamentum flavum** [16] , this results in mild to moderate **central canal narrowing** [17] with almost **no CSF space** [18] surrounding the nerve root at this level.
- The **neural exit foramina** [19] are also mildly narrowed. The rest of the spine looks normal.
- No **bone oedema** [20] or **synovial cysts** [21] are identified.

1 An absence of leucocytosis is reassuring for excluding infectious causes.

2 CRP and ESR are indicators for an acute inflammatory process, occurring in conditions such as ankylosing spondylitis and malignancy.

3 Plain radiograph of lumbar spine is generally required for preoperative assessment of alignment. It provides no information on soft tissue elements. However, it is useful in excluding other pathologies such as vertebral compression fracture, degenerative spondylosis or metastatic spinal disease. It is not indicated in patients with non-specific back pain because of the relatively high exposure to ionising radiation and potential false positive findings, and resultant anxiety. Dynamic X-rays are taken with lumbar flexion and extension for segmental instability, if there is suspicion of spondylolisthesis.

4 Loss of lordosis means loss of the normal lumbar curve in the sagittal plane. It is due to loss of disc height.

5 Malalignment is obvious in displaced fractures and dislocations. Presence of overt malalignment implies further stenosis and nerve impingement.

6 Disc space narrowing is a main feature of lumbar disc degeneration. It is primarily due to reduction of water content in the nucleus pulposus with age.

7 L4–5 and L5–S1 are the two most common segments involved in degenerative changes and disc herniation, with nearly 90% of lumbar disc prolapse occurring at these levels. Isthmic spondylolisthesis is also mostly seen at L5/S1.

Degenerative spondylolisthesis and lumbar spine stenosis are more common at L4/5.

8 Focal bony lesions can be benign or malignant, sclerotic or lucent.

9 In patients with a history and physical examination consistent with lumbar disc herniation with radiculopathy, MRI without contrast is the most appropriate diagnostic test with high sensitivity and specificity. CT myelogram may be performed if MRI is contraindicated or if the result is inconclusive. In addition, MRI is also appropriate in patients with back pain radiating to the legs that lasts more than 1 month and who do not respond to conservative management. MRI is also appropriate if suspecting infection, tumour, trauma or with the presence of CES. MRI is superior to CT in rates of diagnosis. MRI can also demonstrate additional pathological changes such as stenosis and spondylolisthesis.

10 Central prolapse is generally associated with central back pain without radiculopathy. Massive central disc herniation may involve compression of the cauda equina, leading to bowel and bladder dysfunction.

11 Bulging means the disc materials extending out between 50% and 100% of the disc circumference. It is not considered as herniation. When the disc materials bulge out <50% of the disc circumference, it is considered as herniation. Between 25% and 50% is 'broad-based', and <25%, 'focal'.

12 End-plate changes often occur in conjunction with degenerative disc disease. It represents a continuum of degenerative changes starting from end-plate oedema and ending with end-plate sclerosis.

13 Posterolateral herniation is most common because the posterior longitudinal ligament is the weakest at this area. It typically causes symptoms at a lower level; for example, L4/5 disc herniation will compress L5 nerve root. In contrast, foraminal herniation, also known as lateral herniation, of L4/5 disc will cause symptoms in the L4 distribution.

14 Protrusion indicates an intact annulus fibrosus. Other types of herniation include extrusion and sequestered fragmentation. Extrusion is a herniation where there is a perforated annulus fibrosus, but the part herniated into epidural space remains continuous with disc space. A sequestered fragment refers to the condition where the herniated section loses its continuity with the disc space.

15 Loss of intervertebral disc height causes uneven distribution of pressure on the vertebrae and facet joints, leading to facet joint hypertrophy, osteophyte formation and ligamentum flavum hypertrophy. These changes result in stenosis at different locations including the central canal, lateral recesses, foramina or outside the foramina, presenting with various manifestations.

16 Ligamentum flavum hypertrophy is a result of cumulative mechanical stress along the dorsal aspect of the spine. It causes central spinal canal stenosis, compressing the exiting nerve root, leading to symptoms following the distribution of the lower level nerve root.

17 Central canal narrowing is a result of impingement on nerve roots.

18 CSF appears bright and spinal cord appears dark on T2 weighted images, therefore effacement of CSF indicates compression.

19 Foraminal stenosis describes narrowing between the medial and lateral border of the pedicle. It is usually a result of a combination of significant loss of disc height and foraminal disc protrusion or osteophytosis.

20 Bone oedema indicates recent fracture. Underlying tumour or pathological fracture need to be excluded.

21 MRI is reliable in differentiating disc herniation from synovial cysts. Synovial cysts arise from the synovial lining of the posterolateral synovial joint capsules, most commonly located at L4/5. Symptomatic synovial cysts result from compression of adjacent neural structures. Symptoms may resemble those of disc herniation. Plain radiographs do not regularly pick up synovial cysts. On MRI, they appear to be well circumscribed extradural smooth masses that are located in close proximity to facet joints. CT can better characterise its contents such as calcification, inflammation and blood.

Management

Immediate

Provide **analgesia** [1] to relieve symptoms.

Short-term

After **discussing management options** [2] with the patient, perform a **laminotomy and microdiscectomy** [3]. After the operation, **assess the patient's outcome** [4]. Ensure appropriate VTE prophylaxis. Order a postoperative CT to assess the positions of the screws and cage implants. Once the patient is well, **advise the patient on restrictions** [5] and discharge them home. Instruct them to stop **smoking** [6] for at least 12 months.

Long-term

Ensure the patient follows up with his GP for **wound care** [7]. Provide a customised lumbar brace. Review the patient in the neurosurgery outpatient clinic in 6 weeks to monitor for long-term complications such as a **recurrent herniation** [8].

1 Simple analgesia such as paracetamol and NSAIDs should be offered first, followed by opioids. If pain is still uncontrollable, discuss with the pain specialty team for advice around IV analgesia or other options.

2 Patients are candidates for spinal surgery if they experience symptoms that are persistent and incapacitating for >6 weeks despite non-operative management, there are progressive and significant neurological deficits, or if CES is present. The decision for surgery involves both the patient's preference and clinical judgement. Earlier surgery (within 6–12 months) for patients with symptomatic lumbar disc herniation is associated with faster recovery and better long-term outcomes. In patients with severe symptoms, surgical intervention is superior to non-operative management, whereas in patients with less severe symptoms, relief from surgery compared to no surgery appears to be equivalent in both short and long term. Positive predictors of good surgical outcomes include positive SLT, main complaint of leg pain, correlation of imaging results and clinical examinations, being married.

3 The type of surgical approach is tailored to specific conditions. Recent advances in surgical approach include a microdiscectomy and minimally invasive procedures that do not involve as much acceleration of degenerative changes, as opposed to aggressive removal of lumbar disc, thus reducing the incidence of chronic lower back pain resulting from degenerative disc disease or facet arthropathy. If the major cause of radiculopathy is spinal stenosis then a laminectomy needs to be considered.

4 Failure to relieve symptoms during the immediate postoperative period may be due to operating at the wrong level, insufficient decompression, missed segmental instability or incomplete removal of disc fragment.

5 Advise the patient to avoid prolonged sitting, bending, twisting, stretching or lifting objects that are heavier than 2kg. He cannot drive until cleared by occupational therapist assessment. The time frame to return to work varies with individuals depending on rate of recovery, residual neurology and clearance by allied health professionals.

6 Smoking leads to worse outcomes by impairing recovery.

7 Be especially alert for any erythema, oedema, purulent discharge or excessive pain.

8 Recurrent herniation is defined as herniation that occurs at the same level on the ipsilateral or contralateral side after 6 months post operation. Risk factors for recurrent herniation include young, male, smoker, occupational lifting and large annular defects. This can be managed by repeat surgery, which shows similar success to primary surgery. Otherwise, in the setting of no clear surgical goal (i.e. no clear evidence of mechanical compression of nerve roots), non-surgical treatment such as a corticosteroid injection or neuropathic analgesia would be appropriate.

CASE 37: Pituitary apoplexy

History

- A **50-year-old** [1] **male** [2] presents with **a sudden onset severe retro-orbital headache** [3] accompanied by **visual field impairment, specifically double vision** [4] over the past 2 hours.
- He also notes **nausea, vomiting** [5], **neck stiffness and photophobia** [6].
- His partner noted a **decrease in the level of consciousness that is worsening over the past 2 hours** [7].

- He **does not smoke** [8], and drinks alcohol socially.
- The patient admits to **HTN** [9], which was diagnosed 3 years ago and is well controlled by captopril.
- He denies any **recent coryzal symptoms** [10].
- He also denies **loss of weight** [11], **fever** [12] **and falls** [13].
- There is **nil personal or family history of strokes** [14] **and no recorded history of aneurysms** [15].

[1] Pituitary apoplexy is a rare neurosurgical condition that is normally present with a pituitary tumour, with a target age of onset of approximately 50 years old. It is important to note that a wide age range is reported. The age of the patient has significance as this is a life-threatening condition that requires urgent neurosurgical intervention and the peri- and postoperative outcomes in an older patient may differ from those of a younger patient.

[2] Pituitary apoplexy is inextricably linked to the presence of pituitary tumours, most of which are non-functioning. As a result, the incidence of pituitary apoplexy is higher among males than females, perhaps due to the presence of amenorrhoea which will lead to earlier detection. A small increase in the risk of haemorrhage into the tumour is correlated with large tumours (i.e. macroadenomas ranging in size from 18–24mm).

[3] A sudden onset severe headache (due to haemorrhage into the adenoma) is the most commonly reported symptom of pituitary apoplexy. The type and location of headache is often localised to behind the eyes or around the temples. This is consistent with the specific anatomy affected in pituitary apoplexy, where a sudden haemorrhage into the gland exerts pressure on the optic chiasm.

[4] Commonly, the pituitary macroadenoma is situated within the pituitary gland. With a sudden haemorrhage into the gland, pressure is exerted on the optic chiasm causing visual field loss in the outer halves of both eyes, which is the classic presentation of bitemporal hemianopia. The cavernous sinus, which houses several important nerves that govern eye movement, can also be affected by the bleed since it is adjacent to the pituitary gland. Compression of the sixth cranial nerve within the cavernous sinus leads to horizontal diplopia.

[5] Episodes of nausea and vomiting are quite common in pituitary apoplexy due to the raised ICP from the pooling of the blood. This rise in pressure will activate the chemoreceptor trigger zone in the vomiting centre of the medulla.

[6] Neck stiffness and photophobia are also common symptoms of pituitary apoplexy. They usually accompany the sudden headache. These signs of meningism arise due to blood irritating and inflaming the meninges. It is important to ask further questions at this point to identify any other potential causes of meningism (e.g. bacterial meningitis, viral encephalitis).

[7] Decreasing level of consciousness or drowsiness, as often noted by a loved one, is a worrying prognostic indicator.

[8] A thorough social and drug and alcohol history is necessary in order to elicit other precipitants for this episode, comorbidities and risks that might dampen postoperative outcomes. Smoking is considered a strong risk factor for strokes, HTN and cranial haemorrhages secondary to strokes and aneurysms. It is associated with an increased risk of peri-operative respiratory, cardiac and wound-related complications. Also ask about any previous exposure to general anaesthetic, and any allergies.

[9] Hypertension has been linked to pituitary apoplexy as an associated risk factor. Uncontrolled BP is also a major risk factor for strokes and SAHs. As a result, it is prudent to delve into a patient's past medical history and if significant conditions are elicited, medication compliance must be explored.

10 It is important to ask the patient about recent coryzal or flu-like symptoms, to rule out communicable diseases. This will allow the treatment team to gauge if there were any precipitating factors that may have led to the decompensation of the pituitary macroadenoma into pituitary apoplexy.

11 If the patient has experienced unintentional weight loss over a short period of time leading up to this decompensating event of sudden headache and raised pressure, urgent exploration is required to rule out a malignant cerebral tumour.

12 Recent febrile episodes within the setting of headache with drowsiness must be questioned to ease clinical suspicion of various differentials such as meningitis, communicable diseases, other infective processes (e.g. TB) and constitutional symptoms of malignancy.

13 A patient in this age group presenting to the ED with fluctuations in alertness warrants an abbreviated falls history. The falls history will help the clinician understand if a fall led to head trauma and subsequent bleed. It is also important as repeated falls and trauma to the head can cause a benign pituitary macroadenoma to haemorrhage.

14 Due to the overlapping symptoms of haemorrhagic strokes and pituitary apoplexy along with the course of the carotid artery in the cavernous sinus, previous and family history of strokes must be inquired about, to achieve clinical distinction between these syndromes.

15 Lastly, a burst aneurysm shares a strikingly similar clinical presentation to pituitary apoplexies due to common underlying mechanisms of sudden haemorrhages and raised pressure.

Examination

- The patient appears **drowsy, but can be roused and is alert to time, person and place** [1] .
- **GCS fluctuates between 12 and 13** [2] .
- There is **no pallor of the palmar creases** [3] .
- Vital signs are unremarkable, and the **patient is afebrile** [4] .
- Heart sounds are dual with no murmurs. Auscultation reveals vesicular breathing sounds and equal air entry with no apnoeic episodes. **Normal tone is noted (nil rigidity or hypotonia)** [5] .
- On motor examination, power is normal in all limbs except for a slight **weakness in right elbow flexion and finger extension** [6] .
- **Reflexes are symmetrical and not brisk** [7] .
- **Rapid alternating movements were slowed bilaterally** [8] .
- **Sensory exam is unremarkable – normal light touch and pin prick sensation throughout all UL dermatomes with normal proprioception** [9] .
- **Neck exam reveals marked rigidity and stiffness** [10] across all planes of movement (flexion, extension and rotation).
- Cranial nerve exam demonstrates **pupils are equal and reactive to light** [11] .
- Testing of visual acuity using a **Snellen chart reveals 6/25 bilaterally** [12] .
- Visual field and confrontational field testing demonstrate **bitemporal hemianopia** [13] .
- There is **normal pupil constriction and upper eyelid movement** [14] .
- In response to light, **the pupils constrict adequately, with intact swinging light reflex and normal accommodation** [15] .
- However, testing eye movement demonstrated **horizontal diplopia** [16] .
- Lower limb exam reveals that the patient is **mildly unsteady whilst walking on toes** and **during tandem gait** [17] . Otherwise gait is normal with nil spastic ataxic gait. The remainder of the exam is unremarkable.

1 A drowsy patient with fluctuating levels of consciousness on the background of sudden severe headache points towards possible neurologic deficits due to an underlying haemorrhage.

2 With declining levels of consciousness, the GCS is crucial as it helps define the degree of TBI. Our patient within the setting of pituitary apoplexy may have trouble opening eyes spontaneously with mild confusion, which may also impair his ability to obey commands, leading to a fluctuating score of 12–13.

3 Pallor indicates anaemia. Anaemia can lead to reduced oxygen delivery, and most importantly reduced end-organ oxygen utilisation. Anaemia in itself may cause respiratory distress, but it is also a negative prognosticator for postoperative recovery. Anaemia can also present due to intracranial haemorrhages.

4 Fever is a characteristic feature of most infections and with a patient that presents to ED with signs of meningism in the context of headache and falling GCS, meningitis must be considered. If suspicion for bacterial meningitis is high, a lumbar puncture should be ordered.

5 Increased tone would point to a UMN picture, whilst rigidity would indicate spinal pathology or a movement disorder rife with parkinsonian features. These signs are not generally present in pituitary apoplexy or ICH.

6 Muscle power is important to test within all planes of movement, to glean the degree or severity of haemorrhage. Due to the relatively close proximity of the cavernous sinus to the pituitary gland, haemorrhage can sometimes compress the carotid artery which courses through the sinus. Compression of the artery can lead to hemiplegia.

7 Reflex testing can be important in pituitary apoplexy. Areflexia would indicate an LMN picture whilst hyperreflexia would point more towards a UMN issue. Asymmetrical reflexes may warrant a NIHSS to assess for stroke. Within pituitary apoplexy, a severe bleed may result in areflexia.

8 Coordination testing is crucial in assessing for stroke-like symptomology. However, a sufficiently large haemorrhage can impair coordination and slow rapid alternating movements (dysdiadochokinesia).

9 Generally, a sensory exam will be normal in pituitary apoplexy. However, it is worth testing pain, temperature and proprioception to assess for any stroke symptoms or spinal cord pathology.

10 A neck exam testing all planes of movement is crucial in a patient presenting with drowsiness, sudden headache and signs of meningism (e.g. neck stiffness and photophobia). These symptoms overlap with ICH and meningitis.

11 The CN exam in a suspected ICH, such as in pituitary apoplexy, must assess brainstem function and integrity of the optic nerve. While testing CN II, pupil size and reactivity to light must be measured. Normal pupil size ranges from approximately 2–5 mm and are generally equal bilaterally.

Unequal pupils may indicate brainstem pathology or raise suspicion of head trauma with subsequent haemorrhage.

12 Visual acuity (VA) must be tested using a Snellen chart positioned at 90° horizontally and 6 metres away from the patient, with correction if the patient uses visual aids. In pituitary apoplexy, due to pressure from the haemorrhage compressing the optic chiasm and different sections of the optic nerve, VA decreases with corresponding visual field defects.

13 Characteristically, pituitary apoplexy presents with visual field loss impacting the outer halves of each eye. In other words, the bleed commonly compresses the optic chiasm leading to a characteristic bitemporal hemianopia.

14 CN III (oculomotor) nerve testing is paramount since part of the nerve resides in the cavernous sinus, adjacent to the pituitary gland. Compression of this nerve can result in eye muscle weakness and a dilated pupil.

15 CN IV (trochlear nerve) and CN VI (abducens nerve) can be tested together. Shining a light into the pupil to elicit a direct and consensual response in both pupils and swinging the light from pupil to pupil to engage the 'swinging reflex' are important components.

16 Our case is consistent with abducens nerve compression, as evidenced by the patient complaining of horizontal diplopia (rather than diagonal) while following the pen. This indicates some degree of cavernous sinus compression from the bleed and therefore must alert the clinician to make an urgent referral to neurosurgery.

17 A lower limb neurological exam, particularly gait, is important to perform. Any type of ICH will have far-reaching effects in the brain. The cerebellum can be affected, leading to disturbances in gait. Sometimes with pituitary apoplexy, the patient can become unsteady while demonstrating heel–toe gait, walking on toes and tandem gait.

Investigations

- FBE reports a mildly increased **WCC, microcytic anaemia and mildly decreased platelets** [1].
- **UEC results are normal** [2].
- **Coagulation studies return normal results** [3].
- **Blood glucose levels including random blood glucose and HbA1c are within normal limits** [4].
- **Thyroid function tests** [5] are normal.
- The results of the **hormonal panel** [6] – which include growth hormone (GH) IGF-1, prolactin

luteinising hormone (LH) IGF-1, follicle-stimulating hormone (FSH) and testosterone – are normal.
- **24-hour urinary free cortisol and a 48-hour low dose dexamethasone suppression test** [7] are also normal.
- **A T1-weighted sagittal MRI of the pituitary gland** [8] without contrast reveals a **hyperintense signal within the gland** [8].

1 Infection and inflammation are common causes of an elevated WCC. In this patient with an acute and serious condition such as pituitary apoplexy, active bleeding is

bound to cause inflammation in the surrounding arteries of the brain, resulting in a slightly elevated WCC. Often with pituitary apoplexy, active haemorrhage over a few hours can lead to microcytic anaemia. It has been noted that pituitary apoplexy can also result in mild thrombocytopenia, due to haemorrhage.

2 The precipitant for this particular patient's apoplexy must be identified. If hypopituitarism or another hormonal disorder is the culprit, there would be corresponding disturbances in the serum sodium. For example, low sodium is present in adrenocorticotrophic hormone deficiency whilst the other end of the spectrum paints a more diabetes insipidus picture.

3 With any haemorrhage, it is imperative to conduct coagulation studies and observe the different durations of the clotting markers to ascertain any prolonged clotting times. These studies will inform anticoagulation and clotting medication guidelines immediately in the days leading up to the surgery, especially in patients who take anticoagulants.

4 It is imperative to quickly screen BSLs in our patient due to their acute presentation, age group and drowsiness, to rule out hypoglycaemia. Acutely elevated or depressed BSLs within the setting of an acute bleed may also indicate a hormonal issue secondary to an adrenal gland disorder.

5 TFTs are an important preliminary panel of tests to assess the health of the thyroid. Normal thyroid function tests may protect the thyroid from unnecessary further scans and reinforces our initial history point of a non-functioning macroadenoma being the central cause of this pituitary apoplexy.

6 Perhaps the most important panel of blood tests for pituitary apoplexy is the hormonal panel. This panel contains a myriad of important tests that can gauge the health of an individual's pituitary and adrenal gland. We investigate these markers to either pinpoint or exclude hypopituitarism, functioning and malignant micro-/macroadenomas of the pituitary, and adrenal gland insufficiency as aetiologies. Combining this panel's normal results with radiological evidence of a pituitary macroadenoma, we can confidently pinpoint the haemorrhaging of non-functioning macroadenoma as the cause.

7 24-hour urinary free cortisol supplemented with a low dexamethasone suppression test are quality investigations to rule out Cushing's disease and adrenal disorders. Arranging these tests can be complex and should not delay treatment, especially in emergency neurosurgery.

8 The gold standard radiological investigation for pituitary apoplexy is a T1-weighted non-contrast sagittal MRI of the pituitary gland. MRI in this case is more sensitive and specific than CT and provides greater image optimisation of the haemorrhaging gland. It provides clarity to the clinician in terms of measuring the size of the adenoma and visualising its exact location and proximity to the gland. Furthermore, a T1 weighting and sagittal cut allows some insight into the surrounding structures (e.g. nerves within the cavernous sinus) that might be compressed. Other views of MRI are also required to confirm the complications and damage to surrounding areas by the haemorrhage. If unclear, contrast may be utilised to visualise specific arteries. Our MRI displays a hyperintense signal in the gland indicating a haemorrhage and pinpoints approximately a 22mm macroadenoma as the culprit.

Management

Immediate

Monitor **vital signs** [1] and urine output. Keep the patient **fasted** [2]. Obtain IV access and commence **fluid resuscitation** [3]. **Seek urgent advice** [4] from the neurosurgery team. If fluid bolus does not stabilise BP, commence **IM hydrocortisone administration** [5]. If cortisol levels are depleted, **commence cortisol replacement** [6]. **Commence IV dexamethasone** [7]. **Alert the anaesthetics team and prepare an airway kit on standby due to ongoing drowsiness** [8].

Short-term

Perform an **urgent transsphenoidal pituitary resection** [9]. Following the procedure, keep the patient in hospital for **monitoring** [10]. Review the patient's surgical site [11] and perform a complete **neurological examination** [12]. **Auscultate the lungs** [13] and **examine the lower limbs** [14]. The patient may be discharged if **vital signs remain stable** [15], **visual deficits and drowsiness have resolved** [16], the patient is **cleared by allied health/neurosurgery/endocrinology** [17] and is back to a satisfactory level of function.

Long-term

Follow the patient up in an **outpatient endocrinology clinic** [18] for continuing assessment and monitoring for postoperative complications, resurgence of symptoms and improvement. It is imperative for the patient to **follow up with neurosurgery** [19] for monitoring of post-op complications.

1 Ensure the patient remains haemodynamically stable prior to operative treatment. In particular, BP and HR are important to stabilise as they are prognosticators for postoperative recovery.

2 Keeping the patient fasted is crucial in the preoperative management of the patient. It allows the patient to have bowel rest, as well as reducing the risk of aspiration in the setting of anaesthesia. Ideally, patients should be fasted off solid foods for 6 hours, and clear fluids for 2 hours prior to induction of anaesthesia. This may not always be possible in the acute setting.

3 IV fluid is integral in fluid resuscitation and stabilisation of circulation. In the setting of acute haemorrhage and hypotension, shock may ensue. Patients are nil by mouth prior to surgery and so maintenance fluids are essential in keeping the patient adequately hydrated.

4 Pituitary apoplexy warrants urgent neurosurgical evaluation. The type of management hinges on the patient's state. Persistent and worsening visual deficits with ongoing drowsiness and hypotension on the background of a confirmed haemorrhaging pituitary macroadenoma on MRI warrant urgent transsphenoidal surgery to arrest the bleeding and decompress the pituitary gland and surrounding structures. Medical or expectant management can be pursued if the patient is not a surgical candidate and there are minor and improving visual and neurologic deficits supplemented by radiologic evidence of small adenoma with a minor bleed. This patient's condition warrants urgent transsphenoidal surgery.

5 Hypotension in pituitary apoplexy due to haemorrhage generally stabilises after a fluid bolus. If the hypotension is refractory to fluid resuscitation, intramuscular (IM) hydrocortisone can be administered to restore BP, as the cause of hypotension may be related to a cortisol deficiency.

6 It is important to measure serum and urinary cortisol levels in pituitary apoplexy in order to identify a cause for the bleed and hypotension. However, if a fluid bolus and hydrocortisone does not stabilise BP prior to surgery, it is imperative to keep an eye on cortisol levels. If cortisol levels are depleted, cortisol replacement must be commenced immediately.

7 IV dexamethasone is worthwhile for swelling reduction around the haemorrhage area within the brain. This aims to decrease the ICP, facilitating a smoother surgery with fewer complications.

8 With a GCS of 12–13 and intermittent drowsiness, an airway specialist with intubation and resuscitation kit must be alerted and placed on standby.

9 Urgent transsphenoidal surgery by a neurosurgeon to decompress the pituitary gland and optic chiasm is the gold standard approach and management in this specific case. Surgical instruments are passed through the nose with an approach towards the sphenoid bone. This enables access to the pituitary gland. The goals of surgery are to arrest the haemorrhage, decompress any structures (especially the pituitary gland) and clean out any major debris. This should ideally stabilise BP, improve VA, improve any remaining visual defects and gait whilst alleviating ongoing neurologic deficits. These goals can be achieved if surgery is performed within one week of onset of symptoms.

10 Patients must be monitored postoperatively for any immediate complications of surgery. These include signs of shock (septic or hypovolaemic), infection, reaction to anaesthesia, DVT and PE, urinary retention or renal failure, and new vision impairments and neurologic deficits.

11 Review the surgical site to ensure proper closure, as well as the amount of ooze and any signs of infection from the wound. Particularly after neurosurgery, risk factors for wound dehiscence include coughing, sneezing and straining with bowel movements.

12 Perform a complete neurological exam 24 hours after surgery and compare findings to initial neurological exam that was performed on presentation. There should be marked improvements in vision and peripheral neurology (if present). Once the patient is able to mobilise, gait should also be examined for any ataxia.

13 Listen for any crepitations. The presence of crackles in the lung may indicate either an infective process or atelectasis.

14 Recent surgery and subsequent immobilisation in bed postoperatively are major risk factors for the development of DVT. Inspect the calves for unilateral swelling and erythema. Palpate the calves to ensure they are not tender. If clinically suspicious, order a Doppler ultrasound of the affected leg to diagnose, and then start the patient on anticoagulation.

15 If the patient remains afebrile, is haemodynamically stable and looks well, they may be candidates for discharge. Complex neurosurgical cases on the background of an acute presentation normally take 1–2 weeks before discharge. The extended duration is to monitor for complications, any recurrence of symptoms and to ensure vision impairments have resolved/markedly improved.

16 Serial cranial nerve exams are imperative to test for improvements after surgery and tease out any unresolved visual field deficits.

17 The patient should ideally be able to function at the level that they were able to prior to becoming ill. However, often this does not happen after a major neurosurgery on the background of an acute bleed. As a result, allied health – physiotherapy and occupational therapy – must perform further assessment on fitness for discharge home at a functional level. If the patient is not cleared from an allied health point of view, they will have to be transferred to a community rehabilitation centre for further therapy. At the rehab centre, physiotherapists and occupational therapists can work on gait, depth perception and alternative ways to manage ADLs in this new setting of neurologic impairments.

18 Follow-up with an endocrinologist after surgery for pituitary apoplexy is crucial to monitor for long-term issues and conduct more investigations to identify any disorders with the patient's adrenal and pituitary gland that could have predisposed them to this apoplexy.

19 Lastly, follow-up with neurosurgery is required to assess for postoperative complications such as incidental damage to any of the cranial nerves. The follow-up MRI scans will also guide the surgeon to visualise any remaining tumour tissue, which can be managed via gamma knife radiation therapy, medications or further surgery.

CASE 38: Subarachnoid haemorrhage

History

- A **42-year-old** [1] **female** [2] with a **recent history of migraines** [3] and **long-standing history of hypertension** [4] presents to the ED with a 3-day history of **worsening headache** [5] .
- Simple analgesics and NSAIDs were taken by the patient as required over this time, with **little to no relief** [6] .
- The morning prior to presenting to hospital, the patient awoke with **terrible pain localised to the occiput region** [7] of her head and documents **some radiation of this pain to forehead** [8] .

- She also documented, in conjunction with the development of this severe headache, **newfound photophobia, phonophobia, nausea and vomiting** [9] , going on to describe the headache as a **"10/10 in pain" and unlike anything she has ever experienced** [10] .
- The patient does not have any **peripheral neuropathies** [11] and is **otherwise well** [12] .
- She is of **normal body habitus** [13] and **denies urinary symptoms** [14] .

[1] Subarachnoid haemorrhage (SAH) is a neurosurgical condition defined as spontaneous bleeding into the subarachnoid space. Although most commonly caused by trauma, other causes of SAH include spontaneous ruptured aneurysms, the presence of arteriovenous malformations (AVMs) or coagulopathies.

[2] As previously mentioned, most subarachnoid haemorrhages are due to the rupture of intracranial aneurysms. Consequently, there is some overlap of risk factors between aneurysm formation and subarachnoid haemorrhage development, with females slightly more likely to develop aneurysms compared to males. Other risk factors for the development of SAH that must be considered amongst women include pregnancy/parturition in patients with pre-existing AVMs or eclampsia, or usage of the combined oral contraceptive pill.

[3] The presence of a previous history of migraines is not meant to be indicative of one's risk of developing SAH. However, migraines may often be mistaken for the latter, and therefore careful consideration must be taken whilst obtaining the patient's history to ensure that both pathologies are appropriately differentiated. Unlike SAH, migraine headaches are usually one-sided and associated with a throbbing, pulsatile quality, and last for a shorter period of time. Often, moving into a quiet room can alleviate symptoms of a migraine, but this is not seen amongst those with SAH.

[4] Hypertension is a major risk factor for the development of SAH.

[5] Sentinel headaches, colloquially known as 'warning' headaches, are reported to occur in 30–50% of all

subarachnoid haemorrhages. Due to minor leaks resulting in loss of blood from the berry aneurysmal sac, sentinel headaches are associated with sudden focal or generalised pain within the head that may be severe in quality.

[6] Simple analgesics and NSAIDs, whilst indicated for migraines, typically have little to no effect on relieving the pain caused by an SAH. Non-relief from such medications is meant to steer a clinician's differential diagnosis towards the latter.

[7] One of the hallmarks of SAH is the development of a so-called pathognomonic 'thunderclap' headache, often described as the 'worst headache ever experienced by the patient'. Such a headache typically only lasts for a few seconds and after exertion but is one of the most sensitive signs of SAH.

[8] Thunderclap headaches, due to the severity of the quality of pain, are often reported by patients as radiating to other parts of their head, including the forehead. Conversely, note that migraines are typically unilateral and consequently do not exhibit this radiation in pain.

[9] Often as a direct result of the excruciating pain of the thunderclap headache, patients will present in conjunction with several other symptoms, including nausea/vomiting, photophobia and phonophobia. Other symptoms to take note of when garnering a patient history include decreased consciousness, as a result of cerebral ischaemia or raised ICP or ocular haemorrhaging, seen as a result of compression of the central retinal vein.

[10] Thunderclap headaches are rated by patients as a 10/10 in pain, and as such should be taken very seriously by

the treating physician. As previously mentioned, patients document this pain as the 'worst headache they have ever experienced', which typically occurs after some degree of exertion (such as walking up a flight of stairs).

11 Focal deficits, including cranial nerve palsies (particularly those of the oculomotor and trochlear nerves) are seen due to raised ICP. Consequently, hemiparesis within the patient is quite common, and preservation of motor function must be carefully elucidated whilst taking a history from them.

12 It is important to learn what the patient's baseline functioning is like prior to presentation. Often, conditions that can cause raised ICP, such as space-occupying lesions or hydrocephalus, present with a myriad of constitutional symptoms beforehand. Additionally, while rare in developed countries, pathologies such as neurocysticercosis can present with focal neurological deficits such as aphasia or weakness and must be carefully elucidated in the history as well. A

past history of genetic conditions such as Arnold–Chiari malformations must also be carefully documented, to exclude certain differentials such as hydrocephalus, which may present with similar focal neurological deficits.

13 A condition that may present in a similar manner to SAH is idiopathic intracranial hypertension (also known as benign intracranial hypertension). The incidence of this condition is significantly lower than that of the former but is primarily seen in between the 3rd and 4th decades of life, mainly in women. Benign intracranial hypertension is typically seen amongst obese females and associated with ophthalmologic symptoms such as narrowed visual fields, blurred vision and diplopia. Unlike in SAH, consciousness is always preserved.

14 Autosomal dominant polycystic kidney disease (ADPKD) is typically associated with berry aneurysms, and therefore a careful renal/genitourinary history must be conducted to exclude symptoms of haematuria.

Examination

- On general observation, the patient is of **normal body habitus** [1].
- The patient appears **uncomfortable but conscious** [2], and there are no signs of respiratory distress.
- Vital signs are stable, and the patient is **afebrile** [3].
- Heart sounds are dual with **no murmurs** [4].
- There is no sign of **tar staining** [5] around the fingernails.
- The conjunctivae are **markedly injected** [6], and **eye movements appear reduced** [7], particularly abduction and inferior movements of both eyes.

- Abdominal examination is otherwise normal, with **no masses palpable in the lumbar flanks** [8].
- The patient is **unable to move her neck around** [9], and it is documented that when the thigh is flexed at the hip and knee at 90° angles, **subsequent extension at the knee is resisted and painful** [10].
- Additionally, when the neck is flexed by the clinician, the **patient's hips and knees flex simultaneously** [11].

1 Documenting the patient's body habitus is important in discerning whether or not benign intracranial hypertension is a cause for their symptoms, which is typically seen amongst obese females between the ages of 30 and 40 years. It should be noted that this pathology is a diagnosis of exclusion and is typically much more uncommon when compared to the incidence of SAH, which is an emergency, and must therefore be carefully considered by the treating clinician.

2 The patient may exhibit signs of meningism, and as such may appear to be quite uncomfortable whilst at rest. Utilising the Hunt and Hess scale for grading the severity of SAH, confusion/lethargy is typically seen in Grade 3 or above, indicating a heightened mortality rate of >30%, and as such must be carefully managed. Patients with a high grade SAH quite often present in a state of coma; however, in order that this coma can be reversible, urgent treatment and monitoring are warranted.

3 Subarachnoid haemorrhages typically are not associated with concurrent fever. However, meningitis, which often presents with some of the same cardinal signs as subarachnoid haemorrhaging, including meningism, presents with raised temperature, and as such must be ruled out as an infective cause.

4 Particularly in older patients, the mid-systolic murmur of aortic stenosis which can be seen in conjunction with hypertension, may be audible. Murmurs may also be present in those with connective tissue diseases such as Ehlers–Danlos or Marfan syndrome, as both these conditions may predispose to the formation of intracranial aneurysms, which in turn may precipitate an SAH.

5 Smoking is a major cause of developing HTN, and long-term smoking history is one of the biggest modifiable risk factors for the development of SAH. Signs of smoking may often be seen through tar staining visible around the fingernails.

6 An injected conjunctiva might be visible amongst patients as a direct result of ocular haemorrhaging, which in turn can occur due to raised ICP. This raised pressure compresses the central retinal vein, which can cause haemorrhaging within the eyes in up to 40% of all patients. Known as Terson's syndrome, this is associated with a five-fold increase in mortality.

7 Eye movements may also become reduced as a direct result of subarachnoid haemorrhaging. This is due to haemorrhaging resulting in focal deficits, particularly affecting cranial nerves III and IV, which may disrupt normal eye movement. Oculomotor nerve abnormalities may indicate bleeding from the posterior communicating artery. Interruption of the oculomotor nerve also affects the parasympathetic function of the eye and may manifest as a lack of accommodation reflex.

8 An abdominal examination in the setting of SAH is not imperative, but necessary to rule out the presence of any concurrent genetic conditions, such as ADPKD. The abdominal examination may also be utilised to ensure there is no femoral-femoral pulse delay, given that aortic coarctation distal to the subclavian artery is seen in some cases of subarachnoid haemorrhaging.

9 Meningism is seen in conjunction with SAH. This is due to irritant blood spreading down into the 4th ventricle, and further down into the spinal cord, which can cause neck and back pain.

10 Kernig's sign is one of the physically demonstrable symptoms of meningism. Severe resistance of the hamstrings to move, as a result of meningeal irritation, causes an inability to straighten the leg when the hip is flexed to 90°. Kernig's sign takes around 6–12 hours to develop following the haemorrhage occurring.

11 Brudzinski's sign is another physically demonstrable symptom of meningism. With the patient in a supine position, the clinician keeps one hand behind the patient's head and their other hand on the patient's chest to prevent movement of the latter. Reflex flexion of the patient's hips and knees after passive flexion of the neck constitutes a positive Brudzinski's sign.

Investigations

- FBE reports a normal **WCC** [1].
- UEC results are normal apart from **marginally reduced sodium levels** [2].
- **CRP** [3] is normal.
- A **urine dipstick is normal** [4].
- A bedside ECG reveals **left ventricular hypertrophy** [5].
- An abdominal ultrasound reveals **no cysts on the kidneys** [6].

- A non-contrast CT scan of the brain reveals **hyperdense material seen filling the subarachnoid space** [7].
- A **lumbar puncture** [8] is also performed, revealing a **xanthochromic sample** [9].
- A **cerebral angiography is also performed, determining the source of the haemorrhage** [10] to be the anterior cerebral artery.

1 Infection and inflammation are common causes of an elevated WCC. Given that meningitis (either bacterial or viral) often presents with similar cardinal symptoms to those of SAH, including meningism and resisted limb movements, it is important to sway one's level of suspicion from one diagnosis to another by a simple blood test.

2 Urea, electrolyte and creatinine levels are a simple way to assess any electrolyte anomalies that require correction prior to procedural intervention. In the case of SAH, hyponatraemia may be quite common, with prevalence rates of 30–55%. This occurs due to either syndrome of inappropriate antidiuretic hormone secretion (SIADH) or cerebral salt wasting syndrome, and may potentially cause cerebrovascular spasm. Clinically significant hyponatremia among neurosurgical patients, which needs treatment, has been defined as a serum sodium level of <131mEq/L.

3 C-reactive protein is one of many acute phase reactants that accompanies inflammatory states. Acute phase reactants are proteins that increase or decrease by at least 25% during inflammatory states. In meningitis, infection and inflammation take place, both of which elevate the CRP. However, CRP levels typically are not as raised in the setting of subarachnoid haemorrhaging.

4 A urine dipstick test is particularly useful for ensuring there is no haematuria, which may be an underlying marker of polycystic kidney disease (PCKD). Haematuria is seen in up to two-thirds of all people with PCKD.

5 The risk factors of developing an SAH typically intersect with those of developing intracranial aneurysms, and as such, all patients must be thoroughly investigated from a cardiovascular point of view. A bedside ECG is a simple test to determine the presence of any left ventricular hypertrophy, which often occurs in the setting of long-standing HTN. Other changes in ECGs associated with SAH include QT prolongation and deep T waves.

6 ADPKD can typically be diagnosed with imaging of the lumbar flanks. This includes CT scans, MRIs or an ultrasound of the same area. In the setting of SAH, a quick and easy bedside test that may be performed by the emergency clinician is an ultrasound, allowing for quick visualisation of the kidneys.

7 The imaging modality of choice for investigating SAH is a non-contrast CT of the brain. However, CT is only useful within the first six hours of onset of symptoms, as its sensitivity diminishes thereafter. Often colloquially termed a 'star sign', SAH are visible on CT as hyperdense material (i.e. blood) filling the subarachnoid space. CT of the brain is also useful to determine the presence of acute hydrocephalus, intraventricular haemorrhages, intracerebral haemorrhages or large aneurysms.

8 A lumbar puncture may be performed by the treating clinician if the CT scan is negative but the patient's history still remains very suggestive of SAH. Given the invasive nature of this procedure, however, several contraindications exist, including infected skin over the puncture site and space-occupying lesions present on the lumbar vertebrae.

9 However, a lumbar puncture may only be done 12 hours after the patient's onset of symptoms, to allow breakdown of red blood cells (RBCs) so that a positive sample is xanthrochromic, due to bilirubin breakdown. Only this would allow for truly differentiating a puncture sample due to subarachnoid haemorrhaging versus a 'bloody tap'.

10 Following confirmation of an SAH, the origin of bleeding will need to be determined. If bleeding is likely to have originated from an aneurysmal leak, the choice of determining site of bleeding is between cerebral angiography and CT angiography. Four vessel cerebral angiography (in which dye is injected into the two carotid and two vertebral arteries) is considered the gold standard for determining the origin of aneurysms and demonstrates the source of haemorrhaging in >80% of all cases. Catheter angiography can also be therapeutic, as it allows for the possibility of coiling an aneurysm.

Management

Immediate

Admit the patient to **ICU** [1] and monitor **vital signs** [2]. Keep the patient **fasted** [3]. Obtain IV access and **administer antibiotics** [4] and **fluid** [5]. Elevate the **bed to 30° and provide oxygenation** [6]. **Seek advice** [7] from the neurosurgery team. Continue to re-examine the patient's **CNS, including their GCS** [8], and chart regular **BP measurements** [9].

Short-term

Commence the patient on **a calcium channel blocker** [10], either per os (PO) or through IV. The patient may be started on **levetiracetam** [11] as seizure prophylaxis. Surgery for SAH may be done through either open measures (**surgical clipping** [12]) or **endovascular coiling** [13]. Following the procedure, keep the patient in hospital for **monitoring** [14]. Following procedural intervention, review the **patient's surgical site** [15] and perform a **CNS neurological examination** [16]. **Auscultate the lungs** [17]. The patient may be discharged if **vital signs remain stable** [18].

Long-term

The patient may be commenced on **long-term antihypertensive therapy** [19] if not already begun. **Smoking cessation** [20] measures may be followed up with their GP. Follow the patient up in an outpatient clinic for continuing wound management and monitoring for postoperative complications.

1 Management of SAH involves general measures to stabilise the person while also using specific investigations and treatments. Thus, the patient would best be suited to monitoring by the ICU.

2 Vital signs of the patient must be closely monitored prior to any procedural intervention. The treating clinician must ensure the patient remains haemodynamically stable prior to operative treatment. In particular, BP and HR are important to stabilise as they are prognosticators for postoperative recovery.

3 Keeping the patient fasted is crucial in their preoperative management. It allows the patient to have bowel rest, as well as reducing the risk of aspiration in the setting of anaesthesia. Ideally, patients should be fasted off solid foods for 6 hours, and clear fluids for 2 hours prior to induction of anaesthesia.

4 Prophylactic antibiotics are important in preventing wound infection and intracerebral abscess formation.

5 IV fluid is integral in fluid resuscitation and stabilisation of circulation. Patients are nil by mouth prior to surgery and so maintenance fluids are essential in keeping the patient adequately hydrated.

6 The initial approach to raised ICP of any cause is head of the bed elevation (between 30° and 45°) to optimise cerebral venous drainage and normoventilation. Additionally, the impact of acute brain injury and delayed neurological deficits due to cerebral vasospasm (CVS) are major determinants of outcomes after SAH.

7 SAHs fall under the neurosurgeon's domain, and care should be directed by their advice.

8 The CNS must be closely monitored by the treating team, to check for progression of any symptoms which may indicate a worsened outcome. In a similar vein, the patient's GCS must also be recorded at regular intervals.

9 The charting of BP measurements at regular intervals is important to assess the risk of further aneurysmal leakage.

10 Calcium channel blockers such as nimodipine may be commenced in any patient to ensure systolic blood pressure remains <160mmHg. Nimodipine works to reduce CVS, which in turn reduces morbidity from cerebral ischaemia. In patients with malignant hypertension, labetalol may also be provided, but this does not have a protective effect on vasospasm.

11 Oral or IV dosages of levetiracetam may be provided to the patient as a method of seizure prophylaxis.

12 The choice between an endovascular modality of treatment or open craniotomy for surgical clipping depends on a multitude of factors, including the patient's suitability for the procedure and subsequent postoperative repair, and the treating surgeon's ability and experience. Microsurgical clipping is typically more definitive, with >80% of all aneurysms being completely obliterated. Additionally, there is less risk of rebleeding from the aneurysmal sac in the long term, so this modality of treatment might be more suitable for younger patients to ensure non-recurrence.

13 Endovascular coiling is a newer procedural intervention and allows for a minimally invasive method of treating SAH. Since there is no need for craniotomies, patients have a faster recovery time, and this method of treatment may be extended to those who might have been unsuitable for open surgery, such as the elderly. However, there is a higher chance of a second procedural intervention being required due to increased risk of rebleeding, and only 60% of aneurysms are completely obliterated.

14 Patients must be monitored postoperatively for any immediate complications of surgery. These include signs of shock, infection, reaction to anaesthesia, DVT and PE, urinary retention or renal failure, and postoperative ileus.

15 Wound infection post craniotomies is uncommon but must nevertheless be carefully checked for. If this does occur, it is associated with significant morbidity and requires complex treatment that often involves the removal of the bone flap and long-term antibiotic therapy.

16 A thorough physical examination of the patient postoperatively is a must. A neurological examination will help assess severity of the condition, as well as determine if the patient has improved from their initial presentation.

17 Postoperative fevers must be closely monitored by the treating team. Listen for any crepitations. The presence of atelectasis or pneumonia within the postoperative patient is typically seen after 1–3 days.

18 Following treatment for SAH either endovascularly or through microsurgical clipping, the vital signs are closely monitored within a hospital setting. If treated endovascularly, the patient may be able to be discharged home within 48 hours, at the discretion of the neurosurgical and intensive care teams.

19 If the causative factor of the aneurysmal leak is due to HTN, the patient may be commenced on BP-lowering agents by their GP, if not already on them. This can include either one or a combination of the following: ACE inhibitors/angiotensin receptor blockers, beta blockers or calcium channel blockers.

20 If the patient has a long history of smoking, cessation strategies may be explored by their GP. These can include attending social support or community-based resources, utilising pharmacological modes of treatment or nicotine replacement therapy.

CASE 39: Subdural haematoma

History

- A **65-year-old** [1] **male** [2] is brought in to the ED by ambulance after an **unwitnessed fall** [3] from a **presumed standing height** [4].
- The man has a long-standing history of poorly controlled **T2DM** [5] and **hypertension** [6] but is **unable to provide an explanation as to how he fell** [7].
- When questioned further, the patient says he played rugby extensively in his youth but reports that he does not play **contact sports** [8] any more.
- He denies **peripheral neuropathy** [9] and is **otherwise well** [10], and reports **living by himself** [11] with no problems for the last several years.
- The patient denies any **loss of weight** [12] and abstains from **drinking alcohol** [13] and **smoking** [14].

[1] Whilst subdural haematomas are typically caused due to acceleration–deceleration changes, and thus may be prevalent within any age demographic, the elderly are primarily at risk of developing this condition. This is because age-related brain atrophy makes bridging veins between cortex and venous sinuses vulnerable, allowing for accumulating haematoma between dura and arachnoid mater.

[2] Overall, subdural haematomas are more common in men than in women, with a ratio of approximately 3:1.

[3] Falls are the most common cause of injury in elderly adults. Unwitnessed falls pose a dilemma to the initial treating clinician, given that there is no unbiased third party available for corroborating the patient's history. Additionally, it would be difficult to conduct a thorough falls history with the patient in question, in order to appropriately determine its cause. In patients who have had an unwitnessed fall and are unable to provide a thorough history, it is essential to determine if this is due to a language barrier or altered mental status, as the latter might significantly change their management plan.

[4] The height from which the patient has fallen also plays a major role in guiding their management. Typically, the severity of injury increases with the height of the fall, but it is important to also take into consideration the manner in which the patient's body impacted on the surface.

[5] Diabetes is a major risk factor for falling. This is predominantly due to reduced balance performance, which occurs as a direct result of several diabetes-related complications, including peripheral neuropathies, sarcopenia and cerebrovascular accidents. Additionally, even amongst those with well-controlled T2DM, the risk of postural hypotension developed due to polypharmacy and autonomic dysfunction might heighten their risk of having a falls-related injury.

[6] Risk factors for developing subdural haematomas include concurrent antiplatelet or anticoagulant use, in addition to advanced age. Consequently, vasculopaths with a long-standing history of poorly controlled HTN are at higher risk of having a fall and thus developing subdural haematomas.

[7] History plays an important role when performing an assessment of the patient who has fallen. It is important to determine the circumstances before the fall, such as if the patient had any presyncopal symptoms, their general health and their usual modes of mobilisation (i.e. do they walk independently or require a stick/roller/wheelchair, etc.). The context of what occurred during the fall is also essential, such as determining if the fall was witnessed by a third party, whether there was any tongue biting (particularly amongst younger patients to diagnose epilepsy) or loss of voluntary bladder control (to imply a potential seizure). Following the fall occurring, it is important to determine how long the patient was lying there prior to being found/presenting to hospital, as the longer the patient lies down on a floor, the greater their risk of developing subsequent rhabdomyolysis.

[8] High impact contact sports, such as rugby, boxing and wrestling, are associated with a much higher risk of subsequent development of subdural haematomas. This is because repeated head impact may potentiate a severe structural brain injury, with both parenchymal and diffuse axonal injury being associated with subdural haematomas.

[9] Peripheral neuropathy, a common complication of uncontrolled diabetes mellitus, is defined as a disorder of one's autonomic and somatic nervous system. Those with peripheral neuropathy, which is typically seen in diabetics over the age of 60, are at an even higher risk of falling because numbness, decreased sensitivity to touch and muscle weakness can have significant adverse effects on their balance.

10 It is important to determine what the cause of a fall is in any presenting patient. Some of the most common aetiologies include disorders of the inner ear (labyrinthitis), a previous history of repeated falls and poor vision. Genetic conditions may predispose a person to developing autonomic neuropathy, which in turn can precipitate postural hypotension and thus subsequent falls. These include Shy–Drager syndrome and idiopathic orthostatic hypotension.

11 In patients who have been self-sufficient by themselves for a long period of time, a sudden fall without any explanation is a cause for concern. It is important to ascertain the patient's home circumstances when trying to determine the cause of their fall.

12 Space-occupying lesions, particularly within the supratentorial compartments of the brain, can impact cerebral blood flow, and thus cause the patient to lose consciousness and consequently suffer a fall. Often seen within the context of malignancy, a detailed history of the so-called 'B symptoms' must be obtained, by asking the patient about any prolonged fevers, drenching sweats at night time, and unintentional loss of weight.

13 Prolonged alcohol consumption can cause a hypoglycaemic state that may result in patients 'blacking out' and suffering a fall, which can precipitate a subdural haematoma. As such, a thorough alcohol history must be obtained, including the quantity, quality and frequency of drinks they consume. A long-term alcohol consumption history may also manifest as postural hypotension.

14 Long-term smoking histories can have a two-fold effect on increasing a person's risk of developing a subdural haematoma. Primarily, smokers often have a higher than average BP, which in turn can decrease cerebral blood flow and thus cause unconsciousness and subsequent falls. Additionally, there is significantly raised brain atrophy in smokers compared to non-smokers, which as previously mentioned increases the risk of lacerating bridging veins between the cortex and venous sinuses.

Examination

- Upon general observation, the patient is of **normal body habitus** [1].
- The patient appears **uncomfortable but conscious** [2].
- The patient does not appear **nauseous** [3].
- The patient's capillary refill time is **<2 seconds** [4].
- There is **no pallor of the palmar creases** [5].
- BP is raised at **146/96mmHg** [6].
- Pulse is **110bpm** [7] and regular.
- Heart sounds are dual with **no murmurs** [8].
- There is no sign of **tar staining** [9] around the fingernails.
- Peripheral neurological examination reveals **motor function grossly intact, with power being 5/5 for all movements** [10] assessed.
- **Babinski reflex** [11] is normal bilaterally.
- **CNS examination** [12] is also normal, with all cranial nerves appearing intact and functional.
- There is no **anisocoria** [13] visible.
- Gait is examined, revealing an **antalgic and unsteady gait** [14].
- It is noted that when conducting the history, the patient appears to display some **intellectual slowing** [15], and takes on average 2–3 seconds before answering each question posed.

1 Documenting the patient's body habitus is important in discerning whether or not malignancies are an indirect cause for their subdural haematoma. Typically, patients with malignancies present with a markedly cachectic appearance. In a similar vein, those who are markedly obese might have an increased risk of developing cerebrovascular accidents and must be carefully assessed as well.

2 Clinical progression for subdural haematomas can be separated into three distinct periods, including the initial traumatic event, the latency period and the final clinical presentation period. In the context of subdural haematomas, the patient may have fluctuating levels of consciousness, and as such may appear to be quite uncomfortable whilst at rest. Additionally, due to increased ICP secondary to bleeding, there may be marked irritability and personality changes visible within the patient.

3 Symptoms of elevated ICP secondary to haematoma within the posterior fossa include nausea and vomiting.

4 An adequate capillary refill time indicates the patient is perfusing well and thus would likely have preserved end-organ perfusion. In addition, it suggests the patient is adequately hydrated. Other signs of adequate hydration are warm peripheries, normal skin turgor, moist mucous membranes and normal urine output.

5 Both acute and chronic subdural haematomas can cause anaemia. Palmar pallor can indicate anaemia, as does conjunctival pallor.

6 Ensuring that there are no significant fluctuations in BP in the patient can aid in reducing the risk of vasospasm and thereby consequent cerebral ischaemia.

7 Tachycardia can be attributed to multiple aetiologies. Infection, anxiety, anaemia and arrhythmia are important causes to further investigate. Be sure to check the patient's other vital signs, including temperature, and feel the pulse for regularity.

8 Particularly in older patients, the mid-systolic murmur of aortic stenosis which can be seen in conjunction with HTN, may be audible. In severe cases, a flow murmur indicating anaemia may also be heard.

9 Smoking is a major cause of developing HTN, and long-term smoking history is one of the biggest modifiable risk factors for the eventual development of cerebral ischaemia. Signs of smoking may often be seen as tar staining visible around the fingernails.

10 After presenting with a recent falls history, peripheral neurological function must be closely assessed. Thorough check of all myotomes for muscle power and dermatomes for preserved sensation is imperative to ensure that nerve function is preserved.

11 The presence of a downgoing plantar reflex indicates that there is no UMN lesion present. Other signs of UMN lesions include hyperreflexia and hypertonia, both of which are assessed as part of the peripheral neurological examination.

12 In conjunction with a peripheral neurological examination, the CNS must be also examined following any head trauma. This includes examining all twelve cranial nerves, as well as conducting an ophthalmic and otoscopic inspection.

13 In severe cases of subdural haematomas, as the size of the bleed continues to increase and subsequent mass effect on the brain increases, pupillary changes often appear, with the most common documented change being unequal pupil sizes.

14 Gait examinations are performed as part of a routine peripheral nervous system inspection. However, within the context of a fall, suspicion of spinal fractures would delay a gait examination, as the patient must remain lying flat.

15 Apparent intellectual slowing after a TBI in the elderly must be carefully assessed. It must be noted that amongst patients from non-English speaking backgrounds, it is entirely possible that their delayed response to questions posed by the medical team might be due to a language barrier and not have an organic cause. Within the context of subdural haematomas, however, intellectual slowing, aphasia or slurred speech can all occur as a direct result of bleeding within the brain.

Investigations

- FBE reports a normal **WCC** [1].
- **UEC** [2], **CRP** [3] and LFT results are normal.
- A **urine dipstick is normal** [4].
- A bedside electrocardiogram is also performed, revealing **left ventricular hypertrophy** [5].
- A **colour flow duplex ultrasound scan** [6] of both carotids is performed, revealing no stenosis of the arteries.

- A non-contrast CT scan of the brain reveals **hyperdense material within the frontoparietal convexity** [7].
- Concurrent **CT of the patient's cervical spine** [8] is performed, revealing no fracture.

1 Infection and inflammation are common causes of an elevated WCC. Space-occupying lesions secondary to bacterial collections may result in raised ICP, and as such may manifest with similar symptoms to those of subdural haematomas, including confusion and dizziness.

2 UECs are important in the setting of a surgical emergency. First, they identify any electrolyte abnormalities that most often need correction prior to surgery. Secondly, they assess renal function and fitness for IV contrast in the setting of imaging, as well as serving as a prognosticator for postoperative recovery.

3 Infection and inflammation are common causes of an elevated WCC. In this patient, the presence of a space-occupying lesion such as an abscess may explain these findings.

4 In an elderly patient presenting with confusion, it is essential to perform aspects of a septic screen to rule out delirium. A urine dipstick is a quick non-invasive test to rule out the presence of nitrites within the urine, which can be indicative of a UTI.

5 A baseline electrocardiogram may be performed to quickly assess the patient's cardiovascular wellbeing, and thus fitness for any operative procedure. Acute spontaneous subdural haematoma is defined as neurological end-damage occurring due to systolic BP levels being >180mmHg, which in addition to examination, can be visible on an ECG as left ventricular hypertrophy when long-standing.

6 Transient ischaemic attacks (TIAs) can cause temporary loss of consciousness and may be one of the reasons for the patient to have a sudden, unexpected fall. Carotid artery stenosis, due to age-related atherosclerosis, is the primary cause of TIAs. Carotid artery stenosis is typically diagnosed by a bilateral duplex ultrasound scan of the neck, which is a non-invasive test with high sensitivity and specificity.

7 The gold standard investigation for a suspected subdural haematoma is a non-contrast CT scan of the brain. On a CT scan, subdural haematomas are classically crescent-shaped, with a concave surface away from the skull, colloquially referred to as the 'blue banana' sign (blue indicating the source of bleeding being from the veins, and 'banana' indicating the shape of the haematoma itself). Whilst 85% of all subdural haematomas are unilateral and commonly occur within either the frontoparietal convexity or middle cranial fossa, subdural haematomas may be bilateral, particularly in infants.

8 Within the context of any fall/trauma, imaging of the affected area needs to be performed to rule out fractures/other injuries. In this context, a CT scan of the cervical spine is performed to rule out any cervical injury. X-rays of the upper or lower limbs may also be performed on an ad hoc basis, depending on the patient's history.

Management

Immediate

Admit the patient to hospital and monitor **vital signs** [1] . Keep the patient **fasted** [2] . Obtain IV access and **administer fluid** [3] . Elevate the **bed to 30° and provide oxygenation** [4] . **Seek advice** [5] from the neurosurgery team. Continue to re-examine the patient's **CNS, including their GCS** [6] , and ensure **mental state examinations** [7] are performed.

Short-term

Analyse the **size of the subdural haematoma** [8] as measured on CT imaging. Surgery for larger subdural haematomas may be done through an **open craniotomy** [9] . On discussion with the neurological team, the patient may be started on **levetiracetam** [10] as seizure prophylaxis. Following the procedure, keep the patient in hospital for **monitoring** [11] . Following procedural intervention, review the **patient's surgical site** [12] and perform a **CNS neurological examination** [13] . **Auscultate the lungs** [14] . The patient may be discharged if **vital signs remain stable** [15] .

Long-term

Follow the patient up with **allied health** [16] , as well as in the neurosurgery outpatient clinic, for continuing wound management and monitoring for postoperative complications.

1 Vital signs of the patient must be closely monitored prior to any procedural intervention. In particular, BP and HR are important to stabilise as they are prognosticators for postoperative recovery.

2 Keeping the patient fasted is crucial in their preoperative management. It allows the patient to have bowel rest, as well as reducing the risk of aspiration in the setting of anaesthesia. Ideally, patients should be fasted off solid foods for 6 hours, and clear fluids for 2 hours prior to induction of anaesthesia.

3 Intravenous fluid is integral in fluid resuscitation and stabilisation of circulation. Due to anorexia, the patient may not have had much oral intake prior to presenting to hospital. Patients are nil by mouth prior to surgery and so maintenance fluids are essential in keeping the patient adequately hydrated.

4 The initial approach to raised ICP of any cause is head of bed elevation (between 30° and 45°) to optimise cerebral venous drainage and normoventilation.

5 Evacuation of large subdural haematomas falls under the neurosurgeon's domain, and care should be directed by their advice.

6 The CNS must be closely monitored by the treating team, to check for progression of any symptoms which may indicate a worsened outcome. In a similar vein, the patient's GCS must also be recorded at regular intervals.

7 Only about 20–30% of all subdural haematoma patients retain long-term brain function. Consequently, cognitive function must be regularly assessed to ensure that there are no drastic fluctuations in their score.

8 The size of the subdural haematoma as depicted on imaging will guide the proposed management of this condition. Small subdural haematomas can be managed by careful monitoring, as the blood clot is eventually resorbed naturally. Others may also be managed through a minimally invasive approach, wherein a small catheter may be inserted into the skull to suck out the haematoma.

9 Large haematomas require a craniotomy. In this procedure, the dura mater is exposed, and the offending clot is removed through suction, with the site of bleeding being controlled through evacuation of any remaining haematomas. The lacerated vessels must also be repaired.

10 Oral dosages of levetiracetam may be provided to the patient as a method of seizure prophylaxis. There is little evidence for this at present.

11 Patients must be monitored postoperatively for any immediate complications of surgery. These include signs of shock (septic or hypovolaemic), infection, reaction to anaesthesia, DVT and PE, urinary retention or renal failure, and postoperative ileus.

12 Wound infection post-craniotomy is uncommon but must nevertheless be carefully checked for. If this does occur, it is associated with significant morbidity and requires complex treatment that often involves the removal of the bone flap and long-term antibiotic therapy.

13 A thorough physical examination of the patient postoperatively is a must. A neurological examination will help assess severity of the condition, as well as determine if the patient has improved from their initial presentation.

14 Postoperative fevers must be closely monitored by the treating team. Listen for any crepitations. The presence of crackles in the lung may indicate either an infective process or atelectasis.

15 Following open surgery for subdural haematomas, vital signs are closely monitored within a hospital setting. If treated endovascularly, the patient may be able to be discharged home within 48 hours, at the discretion of the neurosurgical and intensive care teams.

16 If a subdural haematoma is due to a fall, the patient will need to be assessed by members of an allied health team to develop strategies to minimise risks of repeated falls. Physiotherapists play a major role in ensuring patients can return to their regular function as soon as possible after their accident, and typically liaise closely with the patient's GP as well. In a similar vein, if the patient's fall occurred at home, an occupational therapist may be able to pay them a visit to assess the safety of their own home with regard to the usage of stairs, fitting grab handles on their bathtub, etc. This functions to ensure that there is no subsequent fall that may occur within the same setting.

CASE 40: Traumatic spinal cord injury

History

- A **30-year-old** [1] **female** [2] presents to ED **brought in by ambulance** [3] after a **high speed motor vehicle accident** [4].
- The woman had fallen asleep when driving home following a **late-night party** [5], and is **unable to provide an explanation as to how she crashed** [6].

- When interviewed at hospital, her words are **slurred** [7], but she is able to provide an accurate history nonetheless.
- The woman does not document a significant past medical history apart from **multiple binges of alcohol** [8] each week and is currently **otherwise well** [9].

[1] Although cervical spine trauma is more common following high velocity mechanisms of injury, falls and low velocity mechanisms may also result in this pathology. High speed acceleration–deceleration injuries can occur within any age demographic. Blunt trauma is the leading cause of death in patients under the age of 45 years, with both blunt and penetrating trauma causing more deaths in children/adolescents than all other conditions combined.

[2] Typically, trauma injuries occur far more commonly amongst males, with some studies reporting a gender ratio variance of up to 2:1. However, younger females must also be considered at high risk of being involved within a trauma setting, particularly in the context of drugs and/or alcohol.

[3] Given the nature of this particular accident, the patient must be thoroughly handed over to the hospital treating team by the first responders, including whether thorough spinal immobilisation was achieved during the patient's transport. Spinal injuries may include, but are not limited to, complete/incomplete transection, cord oedema or spinal shock.

[4] Within the context of a motor vehicle accident, there are several things to be concerned of when deliberating on a patient's history. These include events occurring right before the crash (what speed was the patient travelling at, were they drunk/inebriated otherwise?), the crash itself (did the vehicle roll over, were there any external structures such as poles or glass that further injured the patient upon contact?) and immediately after the crash (who called the emergency services, was the patient conscious?, etc.).

[5] Within the context of any party, it is important to document whether or not any illicit substances were consumed, as well as obtain a parallel history from one of the woman's friends at the party if possible. This serves a two-fold purpose, as it not only ensures that the woman's immediate wellbeing is maintained, but also ensures that a thorough forensic history is documented, if the patient's accident involved multiple other vehicles, and if police involvement is required.

[6] Often, motor vehicle accidents occurring as a direct result of alcohol or any other drug can result in compromised history taking, as the patient may not remember their most recent actions. Within this context, obtaining a subsequent history from a third party would be ideal in order to ensure no vital information, such as the nature of the patient's accident, or any other relevant past medical history, is missed by the treating team. Important aspects that attempts must be made to obtain within a history taking include the mechanism of action of injury, i.e. was the victim's seatbelt being worn/was there a suspicion of head strike/was there any consequent loss of consciousness?

[7] Slurred speech or confusion after a high speed accident, such as within this context, should prompt the suspicion that the accident occurred due to substance abuse, which could have compromised the driver's decision-making skills. However, patients with intracranial injury may also present in this manner; thus a level of suspicion must remain, and further investigation must be considered.

[8] Considering the past history of increased alcohol consumption on a fairly regular basis, immediate management strategies must be commenced to address potential withdrawal, as well as electrolyte deficiency occurring within the patient, which are discussed in further detail below.

[9] Given the acute nature of this particular injury, the immediate wellbeing of the patient must be appropriately addressed prior to proceeding with basic management, including placing them within a cervical spine collar. Every patient with one or more of the following symptoms requires placement within a C-spine collar: midline tenderness, any focal neurological symptoms/signs, history of intoxication, or sustained loss of consciousness.

Examination

- On general observation, the patient appears **uncomfortable but conscious** [1] , with a **marked laceration on her forehead** [2] .
- A **primary survey** [3] reveals that the **patient's airway is patent** [4] , and she has maintained normal ability to breathe and speak, with no evidence of any **facial fractures** [5] .
- There is some **tachypnoea** [6] , but a respiratory examination reveals a **midline trachea** [7] and **bilateral air entry with no presence of any consolidation** [8] within either of the lungs.
- The patient's capillary refill time is **<2 seconds** [9] .
- There is **no pallor of the palmar creases** [10] , and BP is slightly lowered at **108/72mmHg** [11] .
- Pulse is **110bpm** [12] and regular.

- Heart sounds are dual with **no murmurs** [13] .
- The patient has a current **GCS** [14] of 15.
- An **abdominal examination** [15] is performed and revealed to be normal.
- However, a peripheral neurological examination reveals that there is **weakness of all upper and lower limb movements, rated as 2–3/5, with intact sensation** [16] .
- **CNS examination** [17] is normal, with all cranial nerves appearing intact and functional.
- **A musculoskeletal examination** [18] of the spine is performed as well.
- There appears to be no sign of **abnormal sacral sensation bilaterally or decreased anal tone** [19] .

[1] Within the context of any trauma setting, general inspection of the patient can, at times, guide the clinician's level of concern for the acuity of the patient's pathology. However, note that spinal injury cannot be excluded until further testing.

[2] Lacerations are commonly managed within an ED setting. The goals of laceration management include achieving haemostasis and optimising cosmetic outcome without increasing the risk of infection.

[3] Within the setting of the ED, the primary survey is designed to assess and treat any life-threatening injuries quickly. Utilising the 'ABCDE' model, the survey serves to assess **A**irways, **B**reathing, **C**irculation and any **D**isabilities observed within the patient. Adequate **E**xposure is required to ensure that no injuries are missed.

[4] Every trauma patient must be assumed to have a cervical spine injury on presentation until proven otherwise and must therefore be immobilised with a collar on presentation. Commonly, patients are collared by ambulance staff prior to arrival at hospital. Signs of airway obstruction include agitation, confusion, respiratory distress, and in very severe cases, central cyanosis.

[5] Whilst assessing the patient's airway, it is important to assess the presence of any facial fractures or skin burns, as this may affect how the patient should be intubated or provided with supplemental oxygen.

[6] Tachypnoea in a patient may indicate hypoxia, SIRS or anxiety. It is not a diagnosis in itself; however, it should prompt the clinician to urgently determine the cause for respiratory distress and treat appropriately.

[7] The presence of a deviated trachea can indicate a potential PTX or massive pleural effusion, and must therefore be immediately investigated and addressed.

[8] Presence of decreased air entry within the lungs in the setting of trauma can be indicative of an intrathoracic injury causing haemo-/pneumothorax. If air entry is not heard upon auscultation, closely monitor the patient's vitals to ensure they do not become hypoxic.

[9] An adequate capillary refill time indicates the patient is perfusing well and thus would likely have preserved end-organ perfusion. In addition, it suggests the patient is adequately hydrated. Other signs of adequate hydration are warm peripheries, normal skin turgor, moist mucous membranes and normal urine output.

[10] Within the context of trauma, internal bleeding due to serious injury is a possibility, and sustained unmanaged bleeding can result in lowered haemoglobin levels. Palmar pallor can indicate anaemia, as does conjunctival pallor, which could result in reduced oxygen delivery and thus subsequent impaired end-organ oxygen preservation.

[11] Ensuring that there are no significant fluctuations in BP within the patient can aid in reducing the risk of vasospasm and thereby consequent cerebral ischaemia. Given the age of this particular patient, BP is reduced but within normal ranges, but could also be related to her high levels of alcohol consumption.

[12] Tachycardia can be attributed to multiple aetiologies. Infection, anxiety, anaemia and arrhythmia are important causes to further investigate. Be sure to check the patient's other vital signs, including temperature, and feel the pulse for regularity.

13 A cardiac assessment is performed as part of a routine post-trauma screen to ensure the patient is perfusing well.

14 Typically used amongst trauma patients with decreased levels of consciousness, the Glasgow Coma Scale is a good indicator of severity of injury and neurosurgical prognosis. The scoring needs to be repeated often to provide a dynamic idea of the patient's wellbeing; any patient with deteriorating GCS requires immediate attention by their treating team.

15 Palpating the abdomen can help determine the presence of blunt abdominal injury. Ensuring that there is no ecchymosis or tenderness present post-accident will guide further investigation and management.

16 A thorough check of all myotomes for muscle power and dermatomes for preserved sensation is imperative to ensure that nerve function is preserved. Patency of the spinothalamic and dorsal column medial lemniscus, in addition to the other efferent pathways of the body, must also be closely assessed when there is a heightened risk of neck or suspected spine injury. Within this particular context, there is decreased motor function of all myotomes assessable (i.e. C5 and below). Given sensation is preserved, these findings are suggestive of a sensory incomplete Grade 'B' spinal cord injury, as defined by the American Spinal Injury Association (ASIA) Impairment Scale.

17 In conjunction with a peripheral neurological examination, the CNS must be also examined following any head trauma. This includes examining all twelve cranial nerves, as well as conducting an ophthalmic and otoscopic inspection.

18 A thorough examination of the spine must be performed, assessing spinal tenderness, muscle spasm, bony deformities, and spinous process malalignment. This is through the following method: the patient must be maintained within a neutral position, and then have their C-spine palpated; after which they must have a log roll performed, then have their thoracic and lumbar regions palpated.

19 Cauda equina syndrome is an emergency that can occur with any spinal cord injury below T10 vertebrae. Signs and symptoms that must be closely assessed by the treating team to rule out its presence include patient incontinence, presence of anterior thigh pain, quadriceps weakness, abnormal sacral sensation, decreased rectal tone and variable reflexes.

Investigations

- FBE reveals an elevated **WCC** [1].
- **UEC** [2] and **LFT** [3] results are normal.
- A **urine dipstick is normal** [4].
- A **toxicology screen** [5] is also performed, with negative results.
- An **arterial blood gas** [6], along with **blood cross-matching and clotting profiles** [7], is performed and recorded.
- With regard to imaging, an X-ray **trauma series** [8] reveals no obvious chest or pelvic injury.
- A **CT panscan** [9] is ordered, which of note shows **perched facet joints at C4–C5 with mild spinal canal narrowing** [10].
- An **MRI** [11] is ordered by the treating neurosurgical team as well.

1 Infection and inflammation are common causes of an elevated WCC. In the setting of trauma, the WBC count may also elevate, making it an unreliable marker of infection.

2 UECs are important in the setting of a surgical emergency. First, they identify any electrolyte abnormalities that most often need correction prior to surgery. Secondly, they assess renal function and fitness for IV contrast in the setting of imaging. In the setting of major trauma, it is important to weigh the risks and benefits of contrast imaging, between missing potential life-threatening injuries by refraining from IV contrast against the potential of contrast-induced nephropathy.

3 LFTs are typically done as a baseline investigative measure. Given the context of potential alcohol abuse within this scenario, the presence of deranged liver function may in turn guide the patient's treatment options (for instance, certain medications which are hepatically metabolised may be less efficacious in this demographic).

4 A urine dipstick is a non-invasive method of ruling out haematuria, the presence of which can in turn indicate potential lumbar flank trauma.

5 As part of any screening process within an emergency setting, a toxicology screen is performed. The goal of emergency toxicology is to provide clinically useful toxicology test results to support the needs of the poisoned or potentially inebriated patients in the ED.

6 An arterial blood gas assesses the presence of any metabolic or respiratory acidaemia or alkalaemia. Lactate is also a useful marker that may indicate ischaemia. The ABG also assesses oxygen saturation to determine whether or not the patient is exhibiting any respiratory failure post-accident.

7 In cases of severe blood loss post-trauma, blood cross-matching and clotting profiles must be assessed.

8 For any patient presenting to the ED following a motor vehicle accident, X-rays are no longer the gold standard of imaging for diagnosing injury. A trauma series of X-rays are initially performed as they are accessible and can usually occur in concurrence with treatment. Usually, a CXR and pelvis X-ray are performed, with the option of imaging any other limbs if suspicious of injury.

9 Instead, a CT panscan (from head to pelvis) may be performed to allow the treating clinician to get a better idea of the patient's internal injuries, if any, and thus proceed therapeutically from there.

10 A perched facet joint is a type of subluxation of the facet joint of a vertebral body. It is a radiological finding of a vertebral body's inferior articular process sitting on the superior articular process of the vertebra below. Unilateral perched facet joints can occur as a result of flexion-rotation injuries, whereas bilateral perched facet joints are more commonly seen in hyperflexion injuries. This is a concerning radiological finding and is considered an unstable C-spine injury, as any further subluxation of the vertebra may lead to a 'jumped' facet, where the affected vertebra may be locked in a distracted position and cause significant cord injury. In correlation with the patient's examination findings of an ASIA B spinal cord injury, this is a neurosurgical emergency that will require surgical decompression within 24 hours.

11 Within this particular scenario, since spinal cord injury is suspected, treating neurosurgeons order an MRI as well. The MRI is done within 24 hours of any surgery performed, to let the treating neurosurgeon team know if the surgical approach will be anterior or posterior. Additionally, MRI would also allow for close visualisation of soft tissue pathology, which can affect treatment. For example, if an intervertebral disc is protruded posteriorly into spinal cord, the surgeon would first need to perform a discectomy to prevent further obstruction of spinal cord, prior to performing reduction and fixation.

Management

Immediate

Admit the patient to **ICU** [1] and monitor **vital signs** [2]. **Intubate** [3] the patient if necessary. Obtain IV access and **administer fluid** [4]. **Seek advice** [5] from the neurosurgery team. Continue to perform neurological observations, **including GCS** [6]. On discussion with the neurosurgical team, consider the patient being commenced on **seizure prophylaxis** [7].

Short-term

Consider commencing the patient on **high dose steroids** [8]. **Surgery** [9] is performed to posteriorly decompress and stabilise the spine at C4/C5.

Following the procedure, keep the patient in ICU for close neurological **monitoring** [10]. Following procedural intervention, review the **patient's surgical site** [11] and perform a **CNS neurological examination** [12]. **Auscultate the lungs** [13]. The patient may be discharged if **vital signs remain stable** [14].

Long-term

Transfer the patient to a **spinal rehabilitation centre** [15] and continue to follow the patient up in the neurosurgery outpatient clinic for continuing wound management and monitoring for postoperative complications.

1 Management of any accident or trauma involves general measures to stabilise the person while also using specific investigations and treatments. Thus, the patient would best be suited to initial monitoring by the ICU.

2 Vital signs must be closely monitored prior to any procedural intervention. The treating clinician must ensure the patient remains haemodynamically stable prior to operative treatment. In particular, BP and HR are important to stabilise as they are prognosticators for postoperative recovery. BP dropping below systolic values of 90mmHg can result in spinal cord ischaemia, and thus must be carefully monitored.

3 Within the context of this particular case, intubation is not needed as the patient is breathing normally and saturating well. However, for any trauma case involving a high cervical spine injury, neurogenic shock is a possible complication, which can eventuate into respiratory depression requiring supplemental oxygenation and/or intubation.

4 IV fluid is integral in fluid resuscitation and stabilisation of circulation. Patients are nil by mouth prior to surgery and so maintenance fluids are essential in keeping the patient adequately hydrated. IV fluid management is based around four principles: resuscitation, maintenance, replacement (of any fluid losses, such as from the GI tract) and redistribution.

5 Management of suspected spinal cord injury falls under the neurosurgeon's domain, and care should be directed by their advice.

6 The CNS must be closely monitored by the treating team, to check for progression of any symptoms, which may indicate a worsened outcome. In a similar vein, the patient's GCS must also be recorded at regular intervals.

7 Anti-epileptics such as levetiracetam are occasionally administered as a method of seizure prophylaxis. Currently, there is limited evidence to its efficacy, but it is a growing practice in most major trauma centres.

8 A high dose of methylprednisolone or dexamethasone may be provided. Corticosteroids have been touted as limiting further spinal swelling and secondary injury. However, due to concurrent risks of developing GI bleeding and infection, their efficacy is dubious and large-scale evidence is currently lacking.

9 Surgery may often be required for a multitude of reasons, such as to relieve excess pressure on the cord, stabilise the spine or evacuate anything external compressing the cord itself, such as lodged objects, bone fragments or blood. When needed, surgical intervention within 24 hours of injury has the best outcomes. Depending on the treating surgeon's discretion, a more conservative approach may be chosen, involving bed rest, cervical collars, motion restriction devices, and optionally traction.

10 Patients must be monitored postoperatively for any immediate complications of surgery. These include signs of shock (septic or hypovolaemic), infection, reaction to anaesthesia, DVT and PE, urinary retention or renal failure, and postoperative ileus.

11 Wound infection after neurosurgery must be carefully checked. If this does occur, it is associated with significant morbidity and requires complex treatment that often involves long-term antibiotic therapy.

12 A thorough physical examination of the patient postoperatively is a must. A neurological examination will help assess severity of the condition, as well as determine if the patient has improved from their initial presentation.

13 Postoperative fevers must be closely monitored by the treating team. Listen for any crepitations. The presence of crackles in the lung may indicate either an infective process or atelectasis.

14 Following trauma-related injuries or accidents, the vital signs are closely monitored within a hospital setting. If stable, the patient may be able to be discharged at the discretion of the neurosurgical and intensive care teams.

15 Spinal cord injury patients often require extended follow-up within rehabilitation centres. Typically, the inpatient rehabilitation phase lasts 8–12 weeks and then the outpatient rehabilitation phase lasts a further 3–12 months, followed by yearly medical and functional evaluation. An MDT is involved, including occupational therapists, psychologists and physiotherapists to develop a plan of discharge that is appropriate for the person's condition.

CASE 41: Ankle injury

History

- **A 42-year-old female** [1] is brought into the ED after **slipping** [2] on a path.
- She reported feeling her **right ankle** [3] **twist** [4] and turn **under** [5], and both feeling and hearing a crack accompanied by immediate pain.
- She attempted to **walk** [6] but was unable to bear weight due to pain and her ankle feeling **unstable** [7], leading to her friends bringing her to the hospital.
- The patient denies any alcohol consumption that **evening** [8] and is a **non-smoker** [9].

- She reports **pain** [10] of 4/10 when it is still, increasing to 9/10 when she tries to move it, and it is most painful in the areas of the lateral and medial malleoli, with no radiation. It feels swollen, and she cannot move the joint normally but feels this is related to pain. She has not been able to walk since the accident.
- She has no **paraesthesias** [11] in the ankle or foot and she has had **no previous injuries or surgeries** [12] to her ankle.

[1] Rates of ankle fractures are similar in women and men, but the distribution varies based on age, with females having a higher rate between the ages of 50 and 70, and males having a higher rate as young adults. In spite of its greater prevalence in women who are in the peri- and postmenopausal age group, bone mineral density (BMD) does not appear to be a major risk factor.

[2] Ankle fractures are typically low energy fractures involving rotational forces.

[3] Ankle fractures are the most common fracture of the lower limb, and account for 10% of all fractures seen in the trauma setting. An ankle fracture is defined as one involving a fracture of any of the malleoli (lateral, medial or posterior), that may or may not include disruption of the syndesmosis. If there is involvement of the tibial articular surface, it is termed a pilon fracture which is considered to be a separate injury.

[4] Ankle fractures typically involve rotational force, leading to the talus rotating in the mortise causing malleolar fractures. Different fracture patterns are produced depending on whether the foot is everted or inverted.

[5] Bimalleolar fractures tend to result from eversion and are very unstable fractures requiring either an above-knee plaster to control rotation (by having the knee in flexion) or internal fixation.

[6] Depending on the extent of the injury, patients may still be able to walk in for an assessment.

[7] The ankle maintains stability through the formation of a ring (or ankle mortise) comprising the medial and lateral malleoli around the talus, as well as the ligaments of the ankle.

[8] In any situation involving an injury or trauma, it is important to determine if the individual may be intoxicated or have used recreational drugs. This is because pain can be masked by these substances, meaning that a patient may have injuries that are not reported and therefore not discovered, or report minor pain for what is actually a significant injury. Therefore, ruling out intoxication of any description is an important component of the history and examination.

[9] Cigarette smoking and elevated BMI are associated with ankle fractures.

[10] It is important to check how much pain a patient is in, and then address it. At a minimum this patient is going to need imaging, which will require moving her leg and ankle. She is also likely to need a cast. Providing analgesia early can make this a more pleasant experience for the patient, as well as making it easier for the radiology technician to get the patient into the right position/s for imaging.

[11] It is important to take a history using a systemic approach. A common format that is used is pain, areas of tenderness, radiation, associated joint swelling, limitations in joint movements, altered sensation and previous episodes.

[12] It is always important to know whether there has been previous trauma or surgery to a joint. Also ask about other problems present before the injury, such as swelling, clicking, locking or giving way (locking or giving way can indicate underlying meniscal issues).

Examination

- The patient is lying on a bed, appears comfortable, and has her right lower leg resting on a pillow. Her **observations** [1] are all within normal parameters, and she is afebrile.
- Heart sounds are dual with nil added, and lung fields are clear **bilaterally** [2].
- When compared to her left side, her right ankle appears **swollen** [3] with no obvious **deformity** [4], and **bruising** [5] is beginning to appear.
- There is no **broken or abraded skin** [6], no increased **pallor** [7] of the foot when compared to her left foot, and the capillary refill time in her toes is less than 2 seconds with normal sensation and pulses intact.
- She has no **evidence of trauma** [8] to her knee or foot, with no tenderness to palpation, and normal range of movement in her toes and knee, although she is reluctant to move as it impacts on her ankle.
- She is acutely tender to touch over both the **lateral and medial malleoli** [9], with no tenderness over the **midfoot** [10].

[1] Respiratory rate (RR) is a sensitive indication of patient deterioration but is often overlooked. HR can be elevated in patients due to multiple causes, including pathological (infection, anaemia, arrhythmia) and benign (anxiety). Hypotension can indicate severe infection or dehydration. It is important to determine if a hypotensive patient is in shock (look for other symptoms such as tachycardia, tachypnoea, hyperlactataemia, metabolic acidosis and oliguria). In cases of shock, fluid resuscitation and identification of the cause are imperative.

[2] A basic examination is necessary in all patients to ensure no other conditions are missed and is important in the preoperative patient as part of determining fitness for surgery.

[3] The examination covers 'look, feel, move', and always starts with the normal side to allow a comparison. Examine the unaffected side first for a comparison point, and have the patient suitably undressed for the examination. If the patient is too uncomfortable, consider giving some oral analgesia, wait 10–15 mins, and re-examine. Give the patient reassurance that you won't suddenly move their joint without warning.

[4] Obvious deformity may indicate a displaced fracture dislocation, which is an orthopaedic emergency. The degree of displacement may be somewhat masked by swelling, leading to greater displacement than that expected. The fracture needs to be reduced (with adequate analgesia +/– sedation), placed in a below-knee backslab, and then imaged to ensure adequate reduction. Neurovascular status must be checked both before and after reduction.

[5] The 'look' part of the examination typically covers the following points:
- swelling (effusion, synovitis), bony deformity, skin tenting
- colour changes: bruising, erythema, pallor, signs of neurovascular compromise
- skin involvement: abrasions, skin breaks
- scars: traumatic, surgical, infective
- muscle wasting around the joint and/or in the limb: can be an indication of pre-existing pathology that may have led to the injury.

[6] Broken skin creates increased complexity in areas that are subsequently covered by a cast, so always needs to be noted. Breaks in the skin over the fracture site are regarded as an open fracture and need to be managed early to minimise infection risk. They require immediate antibiotics, a washout as soon as possible in the ED and the fracture reduced. Before dressing the wound with gauze soaked in saline, take photos of the wound to prevent repeated exposure, as other doctors can then refer to the photo rather than undressing the wound. Give a tetanus shot if the wound is dirty or if you cannot be certain that the patient has had one within the past 5 years, and commence antibiotics.

[7] Check for pulses and capillary refill downstream of the injury. Blood supply can be disrupted by the fracture rupturing blood vessels, or by swelling leading to compression (including compartment syndrome). Look for a pale extremity with delayed capillary refill. If in any doubt, seek urgent advice from a senior.

[8] In any trauma situation, it is important to ascertain whether there may be any other injuries, especially as strong pain can distract from other injuries that may also need attention. The joints above and below the injury must always be checked. In ankle injury it is important to examine for tenderness over: proximal fibula, lateral malleolus and ligaments, medial malleolus and ligaments, navicular bone, calcaneus, Achilles tendon and base of the 5th metatarsal.

[9] Check for medial tenderness, which may be either malleolar or ligamentous. A medial ligamentous injury with no fracture may still destabilise the ankle, leading to talar shift.

[10] In this patient, this would be an indication for foot X-ray.

Investigations

- Take baseline bloods of **FBC** [1] and **UECs** [2] .
- **AP and lateral** [3] ankle **X-rays** [4] are **taken** [5] .
- The X-ray shows no dislocation or evidence of **talar shift** [6] , but **multiple** [7] **fractures** [8] of the ankle joint.
- A **CT** [9] is ordered which shows **tri-malleolar** [10] fracture with a comminuted fracture of the fibula extending above the **syndesmosis** [11] , the fracture pattern deemed to be **Lauge-Hansen classification** [12] SER Stage 4.
- There are no indications of **pathological fracture** [13] , and the soft tissues appear **normal** [14] with **effusions** [15] noted.

[1] FBCs are important as a baseline, as anaemia can lead to reduced oxygen delivery and therefore reduced end-organ oxygen utilisation. It also negatively impacts postoperative recovery and healing. Although we would not expect this patient to be anaemic, knowing her status before any potential surgery is useful. As this is a low blood loss surgery, she is not on any blood thinners, and she has no pre-existing conditions, a group and hold and coagulation studies may not be necessary.

[2] UECs are important in case of potential surgery, as it identifies any electrolyte disturbances that may need correction prior to surgery. It is also important in medication choice, as well as dose.

[3] The decision to order X-rays can be made by referring to the Ottawa Ankle Rules. According to the Ottawa Ankle Rules, ankle X-rays are indicated if the patient has any pain in the malleolar zone PLUS any of the following:
- bone tenderness at the posterior edge or tip of the lateral malleolus OR
- bone tenderness at the posterior edge or tip of the medial malleolus OR
- an inability to bear weight both immediately AND in the ED for four steps.

This set of rules is 99.7% sensitive and reduces unnecessary radiographs by as much as 40%. However, this cannot be used if the patient is uncooperative, intoxicated, has other distracting injuries, has gross swelling or has diminished sensation in their legs.

[4] The request form should include details about the history and examination findings, especially history regarding previous surgeries and injuries.

[5] Ankle injuries may extend to the foot. A foot X-ray is necessary if there is pain in the midfoot PLUS any of the following:
- inability to bear weight both immediately after the accident AND in the ED
- bone tenderness over the navicular bone
- bone tenderness at the base of the 5th metatarsal.

[6] Talar shift is defined as lateral displacement of the talus relative to the tibia. It typically requires surgical management. This is identified by checking the joint space for uniformity.

For this reason, the ankle must be in full dorsiflexion when being imaged, as in plantarflexion the talus (which narrows towards the posterior aspect) can appear translated within the mortise. A gap of >4mm between the talus and the medial malleolus in mortise view (AP X-ray with ankle in 15° of internal rotation) is indicative of talar shift.

[7] 60–70% of ankle fractures involve one malleolus; 15–20% are bimalleolar, and 7–12% are trimalleolar.

[8] Stable injuries can be managed conservatively with a below-knee cast, with the foot in neutral (90°). This includes fractures involving only the lateral malleolus (Weber A or B) with no talar displacement in the mortise.

[9] Complex ankle fractures require a CT scan for adequate surgical planning. This is particularly the case when there is a displaced posterior malleolus fragment, or if it is unclear on plain radiograph whether there is any displacement.

[10] Ankle fractures can be described anatomically:
- isolated lateral malleolar fracture
- isolated medial malleolar fracture
- bimalleolar fracture – fractures of the medial and lateral malleoli
- trimalleolar fracture – fractures of the medial, lateral and posterior malleoli; the posterior malleolus refers to the posterior tibia.

Diagnostically, the major consideration is stability of the fracture. Stable fractures can receive conservative management with a short leg cast, whereas unstable fractures require surgery.

Fracture	Stability
Isolated medial malleolus	Usually stable
Isolated lateral malleolus	Usually stable
Posterior malleolus	Usually unstable due to typically being associated with other malleolar fractures
Bimalleolar	Mostly unstable
Trimalleolar	Always unstable

11 This is a Weber C fracture. Weber classification is used to classify lateral malleolar fractures. They are graded according to where the fracture is relative to the syndesmosis (the ligament complex in the ankle joint joining the tibia to the fibula). More proximal injuries have a greater risk of ankle instability.

Weber classification of ankle fractures			
	Weber A	**Weber B**	**Weber C**
Level of fracture	Below level of syndesmosis of lateral malleolus	At level of syndesmosis of lateral malleolus	Above level of syndesmosis of lateral malleolus
Syndesmosis	Intact	May be partially torn	Usually injured, with widening of distal tibiofibular articulation surface

12 The Lauge-Hansen classification (*see Table opposite*) is another classification system, instead based on the mechanism of injury and ankle position at time of injury. This is more widely used in orthopaedic practice and has more detail than the Weber classification.

13 A pathological fracture is one that is due to a disease rather than an injury. They can be an incidental finding on X-ray, and include causes such as osteoporosis, cancer, osteomalacia and osteomyelitis. These would include cystic changes or areas of lucency. If a pathological fracture is identified, further imaging needs to be performed to check the whole lower leg for further lesions, as this may alter management.

14 Increased soft tissue lucency in the area of a fracture strongly suggests an open fracture as it indicates the presence of gas.

15 Effusions secondary to trauma are a result of microvascular leakage (from ruptured vessels) being greater than the clearance rate of synovial fluid, leading to a collection of fluid.

Lauge-Hansen classification			
Supination		**Pronation** Associated with syndesmosis instability	
SA Supination – adduction	**SER** Supination – external rotation	**PA** Pronation – abduction	**PER** Pronation – external rotation
10–20% of all ankle fractures	40–75% of all ankle fractures	5–20% of all ankle fractures	7–19% of all ankle fractures
Stage 1 Low avulsion lateral malleolus fracture or lateral ligament injury	Anterior talofibular ligament tear	Transverse medial malleolus fracture (or deltoid ligament tear)	Transverse medial malleolus fracture (or deltoid ligament tear)
Stage 2 Vertical shear fracture of medial malleolus	Spiral oblique distal fibula fracture at ankle mortise level	Anterior talofibular ligament or posterior talofibular ligament tear	Anterior talofibular ligament tear
Stage 3	Posterior malleolus fracture or posterior talofibular ligament tear	Transverse fibular fracture at or above ankle mortise – typically fibula fracture has butterfly segment (comminuted)	Spiral oblique fibula fracture above ankle mortise
Stage 4	Transverse medial malleolus fracture or deltoid ligament tear		Posterior malleolus or posterior talofibular ligament tear

Management

Immediate

Provide **analgesia if required** [1] and if **necessary** [2], perform a **closed fracture reduction** [3] in order to bring the fracture into **anatomical alignment** [4]. Manage any open fractures promptly.
Immobilise the fracture [5] and elevate the ankle to reduce swelling. Monitor **vital signs** [6] and order an **ECG** [7].
Keep the patient fasted until the **orthopaedics team** [8] confirms when the patient will be undergoing surgery. Once a surgical time is determined, insert a **cannula** [9], take **bloods** [10], commence **fluids** [11] and ensure patient is kept **fasted** [12].

Short-term

Surgical approach: open reduction, internal fixation **(ORIF)** [13]. Specific approach is dependent on injury. **Prophylactic antibiotics** [14] will be given in theatre. Postoperatively, elevate the limb to prevent ongoing swelling. Continue to monitor for **compartment syndrome** [15] and any **postoperative complications** [16]. Provide mobility aids on discharge and ensure adequate pain relief.

Long-term

Remain non-weight-bearing as per surgeon instructions (typically 6 weeks). Instruct the patient to remove the CAM (controlled ankle motion) boot daily to check **stitches** [17] and perform range of motion (ROM) exercises. At around 2 weeks, arrange for follow-up to remove stitches and review the wound. Follow the patient up again at 6 weeks with a repeat X-ray to assess for fracture healing. Commence weight bearing at this stage and engage physiotherapy to restore full functionality. Physiotherapy is centred on restoration of ankle mobility, strength, ability to bear weight, and balance. Home exercises, education and advice are provided by the physiotherapist prior to discharge. Instruct the patient not to drive until proper braking response time can be achieved, approximately 9 weeks postoperatively. ORIF is **successful** [18] 90% of the time, but the recovery is long. It is expected to take 2 years to reach maximal functionality.

---

[1] Pain relief makes examinations easier to perform. Musculoskeletal pain is often managed best with NSAIDs and non-opioids. Dose may need to be adjusted for patients at risk of renal dysfunction or those with pre-existing kidney injury. Consult guidelines on dosages for specific medications.

[2] If a closed reduction is necessary, analgesia will be required. There are a few options:
- Intravenous regional anaesthesia (Biers block): most common form of analgesia used; provides safe and effective regional analgesia. Limb is exsanguinated, the limb isolated from the central circulation by use of a tourniquet, and local anaesthetic is injected intravenously.
- Haematoma block: not suitable for open fractures. Lignocaine is injected into the fracture cavity and around the adjacent periosteum.
- Procedural sedation and analgesia: results in depressed level of consciousness, allowing the patient to maintain their own airway and oxygenation during painful procedure.
- Regional blocks: anaesthetic is injected near nerves to anaesthetise a specific part of the body by blocking those nerves; the name of the block relates to the nerve being blocked, e.g. brachial plexus block, femoral nerve block.

- General anaesthetic in theatre: deeper sedation requiring airway protection and an anaesthetist.

[3] After you have ensured there is adequate analgesia, apply traction using one person to apply traction to the foot in dorsiflexion while an assistant provides counter-traction at the knee. You may feel the fracture relocate with a 'clunk'. Try to be gentle in order not to further damage the soft tissues.

[4] A displaced ankle fracture must be reduced as an emergency, even if surgery is planned for the near future. Reductions reduce pressure on the soft tissues, decrease swelling and lower the risk of neurovascular compromise or skin breakdown. X-rays must always be repeated afterwards to confirm adequate reduction, and neurovascular examination repeated. Typically fracture dislocations are unstable and require fixation in theatre.

[5] Apply a backslab for fractures that are reduced or undisplaced or minimally displaced. Confirm good positioning through X-ray. This reduces pain by decreasing movement of the fracture. For non-operative fractures this is all that will be necessary, and the backslab is then replaced with a full cast after approximately a week, when swelling has decreased. For operative fractures it stabilises the joint prior to surgery – which may be delayed in order to allow swelling

to decrease. Backslabs are casts that are left open on one side in order to allow for swelling without constriction, which could otherwise lead to compartment syndrome.

6 Ensure the patient remains haemodynamically stable.

7 This may identify arrhythmias or MI and is otherwise important as a baseline prior to surgery.

8 The orthopaedic surgical team will typically consent the patient, as well as giving instructions on any specifics they want to be addressed, e.g. type of fluid, any antibiotics to be commenced prior to surgery, analgesia in addition to that already given.

9 For surgery insert at least a size 20 cannula. This will be suitable for most fluids, in a patient who is not expected to need a transfusion or rapid infusion. For planned surgeries the cannula is typically inserted by the anaesthetist prior to induction.

10 Routine bloods include FBE, UEC and LFTs. Correct any abnormalities such as anaemia, dehydration and coagulopathy. Group and hold and coagulation studies are not generally necessary, as this is a low blood loss injury and surgery.

11 IV fluids are used for fluid resuscitation and to maintain haemodynamic stability. As the patient will be nil by mouth until surgery, it is important that they receive fluids so they do not become dehydrated, as this could affect both their haemodynamic stability and kidney function. Hypovolaemia in the peri-operative period leads to low cardiac output with resultant decreased tissue perfusion, and severe hypovolaemia can result in shock and multi-organ failure. Peri-operative hypervolaemia is typically due to retention of fluids given during surgery, and can increase morbidity and mortality, and lengthen time spent in the ICU. Signs of fluid overload include elevated JVP, peripheral oedema and crackles in lung bases.

12 Patients should be fasted prior to surgery to lower the risk of aspiration of stomach contents. The general guidelines are 6 hours for food, and 2 hours for clear fluids. Patients can have a general anaesthetic in the unfasted state using RSI to reduce the risk of aspiration; however, this is better avoided and is generally reserved for emergency situations.

13 ORIF is indicated for open fractures, malleolar non-union, talar displacement, displaced medial or lateral malleolar fracture, bimalleolar fracture and posterior malleolar fracture with a large step-off.

14 Prophylactic antibiotics are important to prevent wound and bone infection. The most commonly used first-line antibiotic in orthopaedic surgery for closed long bone fractures is cefazolin.

15 Although a rare complication, compartment syndrome can lead to permanent injury, so early identification is crucial. It can either be due to swelling or bleeding into a closed space (either tissue fascia or casting for the fracture) impeding blood flow to and from the affected tissues. The classical 5 Ps to look out for are: pain, pallor, paraesthesia, pulselessness and paralysis. Early compartment syndrome tends to present solely with pain out of keeping with the injury and can be elicited on passive stretch.

16 Patients are monitored postoperatively for surgical complications, including infection, shock (septic or hypovolaemic), anaesthetic reaction, DVT and PE.

17 This is to ensure that there is no infection starting. Signs to look for are erythema, exudate, swelling.

18 This is improved by patients being compliant with their rehabilitation, which typically involves exercises that can be performed at home which are designed to restore full ROM and functionality.

CASE 42: Anterior cruciate ligament injury

History

- A **40-year-old** [1] **female** [2] presents to the ED complaining of left **knee instability and pain** [3] .
- She had been riding a bike when she needed to suddenly brake to **avoid a collision** [4] .
- With her left leg in extension and her foot planted hard on the pedal, she **twisted her upper body** [5] to come off the **bike** [6] .
- This resulted in a "popping" sensation in her left knee accompanied by **instant pain** [7] .
- After initially falling to the ground, she tried to stand and found her left knee was **unstable** [8] , described as "moving" when she tried to walk and leading to increased pain.
- She also reports her knee seems **swollen** [9] and she feels as though she **cannot straighten it** [10] .
- No other **injuries** [11] were reported including no head-strike or loss of consciousness.
- She has no previous history of **knee injuries or surgery** [12] .

[1] Along with other parts of the body that show age-related changes, the anterior cruciate ligament (ACL) may develop chronic degenerative changes by the age of 40 such as less organised fibres, fibres showing signs of deterioration, reduced numbers of stem cells and decreased cellular activity.

[2] Depending on the source referenced, females are anywhere from 2–10 times more likely than men to tear their ACL. This is thought to be due to numerous factors that place increased stress on the knee, including: differences in stress dispersion due to wider female pelvis; more typically flat-footed landing technique; more reliance on quadriceps to decelerate or change speed; and more upright posture when running. Additionally, hormonal variations may alter ligament laxity, which is an additional risk factor for younger athletes, either male or female.

[3] The most commonly injured ligament in the knee is the ACL.

[4] ACL injuries are most commonly associated with sporting activities that involve twisting, pivoting, sudden decelerations, and jumping – not generally with bike riding. This underscores the importance of understanding the mechanism of injury, and not subconsciously ruling out an ACL rupture due to the activity involved at the time of the trauma. They can also occur in high-energy trauma situations, such as MVAs, where a direct blow to the knee causes forced valgus deformity or hyperextension of the knee.

[5] ACL injury is classically a non-contact pivoting injury. The mechanism typically involves the knee being externally rotated, in 10–30° of flexion, and in a valgus position. This most often arises from: landing from a jump; a sudden change in direction with the foot firmly planted; or a non-contact deceleration (which can include a sudden directional

change). It is a relatively common knee injury, especially in sports that involve a degree of pivoting: netball, soccer, basketball, football, downhill skiing. Non-contact injuries are most common (70%), although contact injuries can occur.

[6] Risk factors for ACL injury can include non-anatomical factors, such as a high level of friction between the sporting surface and shoes so that the foot is somewhat held in place. In this instance, the foot is planted hard on the pedal, and the twisting to come off the bike has resulted in the foot remaining in a forward position, with the 'twist' going through the knee joint.

[7] The classic ACL presentation often describes feeling – or even hearing – a 'pop', accompanied by pain deep in the knee, and immediate swelling – often an acute haemarthrosis (blood within a joint).

[8] ACL provides 85% of the stability to the knee, preventing excessive anterior movement of the tibia off the femur, and providing rotational stability by preventing excessive tibial medial and lateral rotation. Instability is a key characteristic of ACL injury.

[9] The ACL receives its main blood supply from the blood vessels originating from the middle geniculate artery. The forces involved in an ACL rupture also damage branches of the middle geniculate artery, leading to haemarthrosis. Swelling to the knee is usually immediate, and quite pronounced, but can also be delayed and quite minimal.

[10] If the swelling is extensive, it can lead to a decreased range of movement, particularly difficulty in fully extending the knee.

11 In any trauma situation, it is important to ascertain whether there may be any other injuries. Strong pain can distract from other injuries that may also need attention.

12 It is always important to know whether there has been previous trauma in a joint. Of note, patients who have already had an ACL injury with ACL reconstruction surgery are up to six times more likely to have another ACL injury in the 24 months after their repair than someone who has never had an ACL tear. Also ask about other knee problems present before the injury, such as swelling, clicking, locking or giving way (locking or giving way can indicate underlying meniscal issues).

Examination

- The patient comes slowly and gingerly into the ED, walking without **actively extending her knee** [1] before getting onto a bed.
- Although she grimaces while getting onto the bed, once settled there she does not appear to be in significant pain, and has her leg slightly bent and **externally rotated at the hip** [2]. She reports she is able to move it but does not want to as it is painful.
- Her **HR is 115bpm and regular** [3], BP 130/80mmHg, RR 20 breaths per minute, temperature 36.7°C.
- She is slightly overweight, but not **obese** [4].
- The capillary refill time in her toes is <2 seconds, and sensation is normal throughout her **dermatomes** [5].
- Her knee appears to be **swollen and feels firm** [6]. There is no indication of scarring to the knee – either surgical or traumatic.

- **Palpation** [7] of the knee is uncomfortable, with some **tenderness of the patella** [8] but no tenderness on the **medial side of the joint** [9].
- Her medial collateral ligament appears to be **intact on examination** [10], as is the **lateral collateral ligament (LCL)** [11].
- You are concerned she may have an **ACL partial** [12] or complete tear, so commence performing the **appropriate tests** [13].
- The **anterior drawer test** [14] is not convincingly positive, but the **Lachman test** [15] is positive with anterior translation >10mm.
- You do not perform a **pivot test** [16].

1 Patients may adopt a quadriceps avoidance gait, which avoids subluxation of the joint by not actively extending the knee.

2 Movement in the acute phase is very painful and keeping the joint still in a semi-flexed position can provide some relief.

3 Heart rate can be elevated for multiple reasons, including non-pathological ones such as stress and pain. A regular heart rate is reassuring, but an ECG will rule out most cardiac concerns.

4 Physical diagnosis is more difficult in larger patients. Obesity is an additional risk factor for pre-existing joint damage, especially in the knee.

5 If there has been significant hyperextension with knee dislocation, the peroneal nerve or popliteal neurovascular bundle may be damaged.

6 Rapid onset tense swelling in a knee may indicate an acute haemarthrosis. Swelling that develops over a period of days is more likely to be a reactive effusion.

7 Palpate all the structures around the knee (bony landmarks, joint lines, ligament insertions) looking for tenderness, swelling, warmth and crepitus.

8 According to the Ottawa knee rules, in those aged between 18 and 55 years, X-rays are indicated if any of the following are present:
- isolated bony tenderness of the patella
- bony tenderness over the fibula head
- inability to flex the knee to 90°
- inability to bear weight (taking at least 4 steps) both immediately after the injury and at the time of the examination.

Have a lower threshold for obtaining an X-ray if the patient is <18, >55, intoxicated, has pre-existing bone disease (e.g. osteoporosis, RA), is re-presenting to the ED with the same injury and has not previously had an X-ray.

9 Tenderness in this location may indicate injury to the cartilage. There may also be a meniscal injury (present in >50% of ACL ruptures), and/or a medial meniscus tear. If there is ACL, MCL (medial collateral ligament) and meniscal tear, it is termed O'Donohue's triad. This is more likely to occur with contact injuries.

10 MCL injuries often occur in association with ACL tears. MCL injuries associated with ACL injury create an increased risk of developing stiffness in the knee, thus need to be considered in the management. If the MCL is injured, this tends to be addressed before reconstructing the ACL, by bracing it for approximately 6 weeks in conjunction with comprehensive rehabilitation.

11 The LCL is one of the structures that provide stability to the posterolateral corner of the knee (along with the popliteus muscle and tendon). If there is instability in this area, it can increase the likelihood of failure of ACL reconstruction. To assess the collateral ligaments, straighten the leg and apply a gentle valgus stress to the knee joint by moving the lower leg laterally. Examine for laxity or pain in the MCL. Then apply varus stress by moving the lower leg medially. Repeat these movements with the knee flexed to 20° (this relaxes the cruciate ligaments). Compare both sides.

12 Partial ACL tears are difficult to diagnose solely on physical examination.

13 Up to 90% of ACL tears can be diagnosed based on history and clinical examination findings. If you are concerned about patellar tendon rupture, ask the patient to do a straight leg raise. If they are able to perform this against resistance, it virtually excludes both transverse patellar fractures and patellar tendon rupture. If pain prevents them from doing this, get them to sit with the affected leg dangling free, and kick forwards. As with all tests, perform the test on the unaffected side first for a comparison point, and have the patient suitably undressed for the examination. If the patient is too uncomfortable, consider giving some oral analgesia, wait 10–15 mins, and re-examine. Give the patient reassurance that you won't suddenly pull or move their leg without warning. As much as possible, get the patient to relax their quadriceps and hamstring muscles.

14 Anterior drawer test:
- Patient: relaxed supine position, knees to approximately 90°. If unable to flex this far, assess with slight flexion of approximately 10°.
- Examiner: sitting on the patient's feet, place your hands around the upper tibia of the leg being tested with your thumbs on the supero-anterior aspect of the tibia. Pull anteriorly on the proximal tibia.
- Positivity of the test depends both on the end feel, and the amount of translation.
- Note that this test is fairly accurate, but a number of studies have shown it to be less accurate than the pivot shift test and the Lachman test. This is because hamstring spasm may prevent excessive anterior translation, giving a false negative anterior drawer test.

	Positive	Negative
End feel	Soft feel indicating secondary structures are stopping continued anterior translation of the tibia	Hard or firm end feel indicating intact ACL
Translation	Excessive anterior translation	Abrupt stop

15 Lachman test – this is the most sensitive test for ACL injury:
- Patient: relaxed supine position, knee being tested flexed to about 15°.
- Examiner: one hand holds and stabilises the distal femur, other hand grasps proximal tibia firmly. Pull anteriorly on the proximal tibia while holding the femur in a stable position.
- Although quite accurate, the Lachman test should not be the sole criterion to assess ACL integrity. A posterior cruciate ligament (PCL) tear may give a false positive Lachman result due to posterior subluxation.

	Positive	Negative
End feel	Soft feel indicating secondary structures are stopping continued anterior translation of the tibia	Hard or firm end feel indicating intact ACL
Translation	May be excessive anterior translation >10mm translation indicates Grade III A/B strain (see chart for grades)	Abrupt stop For Grades I to IIB sprain, can be 3–10mm translation (see chart for grades)

16 Pivot shift test:
- Although this is one of the most accurate tests for assessing knee instability, it can be difficult for the patient to relax enough to perform the test, as this position reproduces the patient's instability by mimicking the actual event. It is therefore easier to perform under anaesthesia. The pivot shift test assesses the ACL primarily, but also the LCL and posterior capsule.
- Patient: relaxed, supine position, knee being tested fully extended.
- Examiner: one hand cupping under the heel of the foot, palm of the other hand on the lateral aspect of the proximal tibia placing your 5th finger near the fibular head, lift leg so hip is flexed to approximately 30°. While holding the lower leg in internal rotation, slowly flex the knee while concurrently applying moderate valgus and internal rotation pressure to the proximal tibia.

	Positive	Negative
At 30° of flexion	Proximal tibia subluxes anteriorly on distal femur and returns into place with a "clunk" upon knee extension; reduces at 20–30° of flexion	No subluxation

Investigations

- A knee X-ray is ordered, which is grossly normal, with no sign of **Segond fracture** [1] or deep sulcus/lateral femoral **notch sign** [2].
- A multi-planar/multi-sequence **MRI** [3] is ordered, and the report reads:
  - "The extensor tendons are intact, and the patella is in normal **position** [4].
  - A large **joint effusion** [5] is identified in the suprapatellar recess extending into the posterior compartment.
  - No **chondromalacia** [6] identified.
  - Both **menisci** [7] show normal configuration and signal intensity without any obvious frank tear.
  - The ACL appears swollen and oedematous particularly involving its **mid and proximal segments** [8] although it appears to retain its normal orientation, suggesting high grade **partial tear** [9].
  - The posterior cruciate ligament is intact. The medial and lateral collateral complex appears **intact** [10].
  - Bone marrow oedema identified in the adjoining surfaces of the lateral femoral and posterior aspects of the lateral tibial condyle suggesting **bony contusion** [11] from previous anterior translation at time of injury.
  - Conclusion: high grade **partial tear of the ACL** [12]. No meniscal tear seen. Bony contusion in the lateral femoral and tibial condyles suggesting anterior translation at the time of injury."
- An **arthroscopy** [13] is not ordered.

[1] X-rays are usually of normal appearance, as ligaments are not visualised. If an avulsion fracture of the anterolateral ligament is present (Segond fracture), this is a positive sign of an ACL tear. Segond fractures are associated with an ACL tear in 75–100% of cases. As the tibial plateau is critical to weight bearing, this can impact on recovery and delay rehabilitation.

[2] The notch sign is a depression on the lateral femoral condyle at the junction between the weight-bearing articular surface of the tibia, and the patellar articular surface of the femoral condyle. It is considered to be an indirect sign of an ACL tear, and results from an osteochondral impaction fracture.

[3] MRI is the imaging modality of choice, as data seems to indicate that CT scans – while good at confirming an intact ACL – are less reliable in assessing torn ACLs. Some studies have reported MRI accuracy of 95% in identifying ACL tears, with less accuracy for proximal, partial or chronic tears. The presence of other major ligamentous injuries also reduces the accuracy.

[4] A key role of the MRI is to identify other coexisting knee injuries, especially tears of the other ligaments, and damage to the menisci.

[5] Effusions secondary to trauma are a result of microvascular leakage (from ruptured vessels) being greater than the clearance rate of synovial fluid, leading to a collection of fluid.

[6] Chondromalacia patellae (runner's knee) refers to deterioration and softening of the cartilage on the under-surface of the patella.

[7] Lateral meniscal tears are present in 54% of acute ACL tears.

[8] Approximately 70% of tears are in the mid-segment of the ACL, with 7–20% located proximally, and 3–10% distally at the tibial attachment.

[9] Signs on MRI indicating an ACL tear include primary signs (those that directly involve the ACL, e.g. swelling, discontinuity of ACL) and secondary signs (bony contusion, Segond fracture, etc).

[10] Patients who have an ACL injury and an additional LCL or PCL injury often experience debilitating instability that requires aggressive surgical management. An unrepaired LCL tear increases the risk of early ACL graft failure. LCL tears optimally are repaired within 1–3 weeks of the initial injury.

[11] This refers to a type of bone injury or bruise known as a 'kissing' bone bruise. It is common in ACL rupture, and indicates hyperextension during the process of injury. If both bone bruises are present, the probability of an ACL tear is very high, with only slightly lower probability if only one bruise is present. If the menisci and MCL are also injured, this increases the likelihood of bone contusion. Although undetectable on X-ray, these contusions can be discerned on MRI, and are thought to result from haemorrhage, oedema and microtrabecular fractures. Extensive bony and cartilage injury can negatively affect rehabilitation. If severe, delaying weight bearing may be a consideration. Bone bruises can remain visible on MRI for 12–14 weeks after the initial injury.

[12] Partial ACL tears are common, accounting for up to 43% of all ACL tears. Tears involving 50–75% of the ACL have a

high probability of progressing to a complete tear, and <50% of patients with unrepaired partial tears are able to return to their pre-injury activity level. The ACL generally does not heal from tears, and this is thought to be partly because of

its relatively avascular central core, although a tear involving <25% of the ACL has a reasonable prognosis.

13 Arthroscopy gives an absolute diagnosis but is seldom used due to its cost and invasive nature.

Management

Immediate

Provide conservative analgesia, strongly considering anti-inflammatory agents.

Short-term

Stabilise the knee with strapping or using a brace, whilst **awaiting surgery** [1] . Apply basic MICE principles to **reduce swelling** [2] . Refer to **physiotherapy** [3] for strengthening of the quadriceps and hamstrings.

Long-term

A key goal of ACL injury management is ensuring return of stability to the joint. Treatment choice is

dependent on numerous factors including the **degree of injury** [4] , **patient activity level** [5] , **degree of instability** [6] , patient expectations and their willingness to engage in intensive postoperative physical therapy. Consider the indications for **conservative** [7] and **operative** [8] management. Review the risks and benefits of performing a **patellar tendon autograft** [9] against a **hamstring tendon autograft** [10] . In the immediate period after surgery, ice therapy should be liberally used. Allow for **early weight bearing** [11] and encourage **full passive extension** [12] . Educate the patient on knee **precautions** [13] and aim for a guided **return to sports** [14] .

1 Surgery is typically delayed for weeks or months, to allow time for swelling to subside. Delays to surgery of greater than one year have been associated with increases in further injury, such as medial meniscal tears.

2 It is important for swelling to have subsided before undergoing ACL reconstruction. If the patient is not going to have a reconstruction, then reducing swelling becomes important in restoring ROM, enabling them to mobilise and engage in physiotherapy. Although RICE is still used for immediate first aid, for short-term treatment it has now been replaced by MICE. So advise the patient to Move the joint gently, Ice it intermittently; use bandaging to apply Compression; and Elevate the limb. The knee should be pain-free with full extension prior to surgery, as surgery on stiff, tight knees leads to complications and the patient may never regain full ROM.

3 This also helps to reduce the amount of effusion and improves strength, both of which are important in preparing for surgery. This mainly focuses on strengthening of the quadriceps and hamstrings.

4 ACL injuries are classified as grade I, II or III sprain. A grade III sprain is sometimes also referred to as an anterior cruciate deficient knee, as there is a complete tear of the ACL. A torn ACL is not considered to be something that will spontaneously heal.

	Grade I sprain	Grade II sprain	Grade III sprain
Ligament fibres	Stretched but no tear	Partial/ incomplete tear with haemorrhage	Completely torn (ruptured); ligament is in two parts Haemarthrosis within 1–2 hrs
Tenderness and swelling	Some tenderness and swelling	Some tenderness, moderate swelling with some loss of function	Tenderness with limited pain Anywhere from some to a lot of swelling
Stability	No instability, does not 'give out' during activity	Knee may feel unstable or give out during activity	Knee feels unstable or subluxates at certain times; rotational instability present

	Grade I sprain	Grade II sprain	Grade III sprain
Examination	No increased laxity Firm end feel	Increased movement with anterior drawer test but still a firm end point Painful with increased pain on Lachman and anterior drawer stress tests	Positive pivot shift test No end point evident
Translation	3–5mm translation	5–10mm translation Firm endpoint: grade IIA No endpoint: grade IIB	>10mm translation Firm endpoint: grade IIIA No endpoint: grade IIIB

5 This strongly impacts the decision on whether or not to repair. For example, a patient who is a professional footballer is much more likely to require a repair than a similar patient who works in an office and rides their bike for exercise. Activities that involve twisting motions of the knee (netball, dancing, football, skiing) are much more likely to require an intact ACL to resume activity.

6 Clinical evaluation is key to ruling in or out knee instability, which then strongly influences the decision on whether or not to proceed to surgery.

7 Conservative management may be considered in elderly patients, less active athletes, or those able to achieve stability that is sufficient for the activities in which they engage. Furthermore, those who are poor candidates for reconstruction arthroscopy may qualify for non-operative management. ACL-deficient knees are more likely to develop issues associated with reduced stability, such as chondral injuries, complex meniscal tears, arthritis, knee instability leading to decreased activity which may manifest as poor knee-related quality of life. The use of functional braces or protective equipment in patients who are ACL-deficient is controversial, with no clear evidence of benefit. The ACL provides stability to the knee by resisting anterior translation, and secondarily resisting varus and valgus forces. There can be a loss of proprioception when the ACL is injured, as it contains sensory mechanoreceptors that can provide information to the CNS on knee tension. The resulting loss of proprioception can be clinically significant.

8 ACL graft reconstruction provides stability to the ACL-deficient knee, thus preventing re-injury from repeated subluxations, and increasing the range of activities in which the patient can engage. Operative intervention is usually delayed at least 3 weeks after injury to prevent the development of arthrofibrosis (build-up of scar tissue within the knee) as a complication. Surgical repair usually involves intra-articular reconstruction of the ACL. This has a success rate of up to 95% in restoring activity and stability. If MCL injury is present, allow it to heal (regain stability) before performing ACL reconstruction, because varus/valgus instability may jeopardise the graft. If a meniscal tear is present, this is often repaired at the same time as the ACL reconstruction, as it has been observed to increase meniscal healing rate.

9 In a patellar tendon autograft reconstruction, the central portion of the patellar tendon is then removed to form the ACL graft, and the graft ends are attached to plugs of bone from the patient's patella and tibia. These plugs of bones help to anchor the new ACL. Its advantage is that patients have a high rate of return to play, and low rates of failure. However, it comes with the risk of postoperative knee pain, patellar fracture and potential for patellar tendon tear.

10 The new ACL may also be taken from the semitendinosus tendon, sometimes with the gracilis tendon added to make a stronger graft. The tendons are folded and braided together, before being placed in a similar method to that used for patellar tendon autograft. Its advantages are that the procedure allows for a smaller incision, and has less risk of peri-operative and anterior knee pain. However, the strength of the hamstring graft may be less than the patellar graft, with less peak flexion strength at 3 years.

11 Early weight bearing has been shown to reduce patellofemoral pain.

12 Ensuring full passive extension of the knee is particularly important if there has been an associated patellar dislocation or MCL injury.

13 Excessive and repetitive activity can lead to a loosening of the graft, which can then lead to a higher long-term likelihood of failure.

14 Follow-up should be regular, with close monitoring by the surgeon and physical therapist. Return to sport may take 6–9 months.

CASE 43: Colles' fracture

History

- A **64-year-old** [1] **right-hand dominant** [2] **female** [3] presents to the ED after **tripping on her rug at home** [4], putting out her hands to catch herself and landing on her **hands and knees** [5].
- She felt a **cracking sensation** [6] in her right wrist, accompanied by immediate pain. When she looked at her wrist it appeared misshapen, so she called an ambulance. She has no pain other than her wrist.

- She denies any **symptoms prior to the fall** [7], had no head-strike and no **loss of consciousness** [8], and has been otherwise well with **no previous injuries or problems with her wrist** [9].
- She has no significant **medical history** [10], is not on any **medications** [11], completed menopause at the age of 44 and did not use **HRT** [12], and is a **smoker** [13].
- She **lives alone** [14] and is **retired** [15].

[1] Wrist fractures are the most common fracture of the upper limbs in older adults, with wrist fractures being more common in women aged <75 years, and hip fractures more common in women >75. Distal radius fractures are also common in those aged 20–30 due to high energy injuries. In those >60 it is typically a low energy injury.

[2] In all upper limb injuries, it is important to determine handedness, as this influences decisions regarding management as well as suitability for discharge. Wrist fractures can lead to functional decline due to impacts on ability to carry out ADLs.

[3] Colles' fractures are more common in women due to postmenopausal osteoporosis and an increased risk of falls.

[4] Falls risk increases as people age, with 30% of people >65 and 50% of those >80 experiencing at least one fall per year. Falls are associated with increased morbidity and mortality, so ascertaining the type of fall is important as this will impact the decision on suitability for discharge.

[5] Always be aware of distracting injuries. As the patient landed on her knees it is important to examine them.

[6] A cracking sound or sensation is a common sign of a bone fracture.

[7] It is important to take a detailed history for all falls to ensure serious causes are not missed. This includes fall height, surface of impact, positioning, events before, during and after the fall, associated incontinence, and history of previous falls. In wrist injuries, fracture type is influenced by whether the hand was in flexion (Smith's fracture) or extension (Colles' fracture). If there were witnesses, obtaining a collateral history can be helpful.

[8] In all falls, ask about head-strike and loss of consciousness. Any head-strike or loss of consciousness requires a neurological examination. Head-strike also requires a cervical spine examination.

[9] It is always important to know whether there has been previous trauma or surgery to a joint. A Colles' fracture carries a risk of carpal tunnel syndrome.

[10] A provisional diagnosis of osteoporosis can be made based on non-traumatic fracture from standing height. Osteoporosis is the most common form of bone disease and is characterised by low bone density which makes these patients more susceptible to low trauma fractures. As the association between Colles' fracture and osteoporosis is so strong, a Colles' fracture in the elderly should prompt further investigation for osteoporosis, as this elevates the risk for hip fracture.

[11] Risk factors for Colles' fracture are mostly related to osteoporosis and include female gender, early menopause, smoking or alcohol excess and prolonged steroid use. Earlier menopause is associated with greater risk of developing osteoporosis, as oestrogen inhibits bone resorption. No previous oestrogen use is a risk factor for wrist fractures in women. Prolonged steroid use reduces the ability of the body to absorb calcium, and increased osteoclast activity, which can lead to bone loss with resultant osteoporosis.

[12] Hormone replacement therapy (HRT) reduces women's risk of osteoporosis. It is sometimes used as a treatment for osteoporosis, although is not recommended as the first-line treatment except for younger postmenopausal women (those <60).

[13] Smoking is a known risk factor for osteoporosis, with studies showing a clear relationship between smoking and

decreased BMD. Although the exact mechanisms are unclear, smoking is associated with earlier menopause in women, and nicotine has been shown to have an inhibitory effect on osteoblast production. Fracture healing is also negatively impacted by smoking, and it also increases the risks associated with surgery and anaesthesia.

14 Social history becomes important in determining the suitability for discharge of patients. Factors such as ability to care for themselves, ability and availability of others to care for them at home, or the availability of services impact on the decision as to whether a patient can be discharged or not. Allied health services' input should be sought early if there are concerns.

15 It is important to know if a patient is working, and what kind of work they do, as this helps to determine management including what degree of fracture alignment and reduction will be satisfactory. Someone working on a computer may require different management to someone who does heavier work.

Examination

- The patient appears comfortable and is holding her arm across her lower chest. Her wrist has an obvious deformity, with evident **dorsal angulation just proximal to the wrist accompanied by diffuse swelling** [1] especially when compared to her other wrist.
- There is no evidence of **broken skin** [2].
- On **examination** [3], she had no tenderness in her right **shoulder, elbow or metacarpophalangeal joints (MCPJs)** [4], and was able to move these **joints normally** [5] within the confines of her **wrist tenderness** [6].
- Her hand is **neurovascularly intact** [7] with no evidence of compromise to the **median nerve** [8] and no **snuffbox tenderness** [9].
- There are no notable injuries to her **knees** [10].
- Her observations are within normal parameters, and she is **afebrile** [11].
- Heart sounds are **dual with nil added** [12], and lung fields are clear bilaterally.

1 This is the classic 'dinner fork' or 'bayonet'-like deformity associated with Colles' fracture. This is due to backward angulation and displacement when viewed in pronation (the fingers are the prongs). Always ensure you compare both sides.

2 This is especially important in areas where the bone is close to the skin, including areas such as the wrist and ankle. Any break in the skin over a fracture needs to be treated as an open fracture, as it has increased risks of infection. This means it needs to be washed out within 24 hours and the fracture reduced. Early administration of IV antibiotics is crucial and is associated with improved mortality. Give a tetanus shot if the wound is dirty or if you cannot be certain that the patient has had one within the past 5 years.

3 As with all tests, perform the test on the unaffected side first for a comparison point, and have the patient suitably undressed for the examination. If the patient is too uncomfortable, consider giving some oral analgesia, wait 10–15 mins, and re-examine.

4 In any trauma situation, it is important to ascertain whether there may be any other injuries, especially as strong pain can distract from other injuries that may also need attention.

5 Always examine the joint above and below to ensure there are no other injuries that are being missed, including any other joints that may be affected. A fall onto outstretched hand (FOOSH) can also result in injury to the elbow, shoulder and clavicle.

6 It is important to take into consideration patients' pain when performing an examination. A patient with a Colles' fracture will not be able to perform full range of movement of their shoulder and elbow, as to do so would cause too much pain in the wrist. However, they should be able to perform limited movements to an extent that you can reasonably rule out an acute injury.

7 Stable Colles' fractures are minimally comminuted, whereas unstable fractures are distinctly comminuted, often with accompanying radial and/or ulnar styloid avulsions. These avulsions can potentially cause compression neuropathies, with the median nerve particularly at risk. Check for pulses and capillary refill downstream of the injury. Blood supply can be disrupted by the fracture rupturing blood vessels, or by swelling leading to compression which may occur in the carpal tunnel but can also include compartment syndrome of the forearm. Look for a pale extremity with delayed capillary refill. If in any doubt, seek urgent advice from a senior. A quick neurovascular examination of the upper limb is as follows:
- Median nerve:
  - motor: thumb abduction
  - sensory: sensation on radial surface of distal 2nd digit

- Anterior interosseous nerve: ask to make the OK sign – if distal interphalangeal joint (IPJ) of 2nd digit and IPJ of thumb extend, this suggests anterior interosseous nerve involvement
- Ulnar nerve:
  - motor: thumb adduction (Froment's sign)
  - sensory: ulnar surface of distal 5th digit
- Radial nerve:
  - motor: extension of IPJ of thumb
  - sensory: dorsal surface of 1st webspace.

8 Median nerve neurapraxia is a potential complication of a Colles' fracture due to direct damage to the nerve from the fracture, compression due to swelling or compartment syndrome. The median nerve passes through the carpal tunnel, and compression or damage can give symptoms similar to carpal tunnel syndrome, including numbness and tingling in the thumb and first three fingers of the hand, mostly on the palmar surface. Median nerve symptoms should resolve after reduction.

9 Scaphoid and ligamentous wrist injuries may also be present, as a fall onto an outstretched hand with the hands in dorsiflexion transmits forces through the proximal row of the carpus and along the long axis of the radius – mainly through the scaphoid and lunate.

10 If possible, observe the patient walking into the ED to observe their gait. She is reporting no pain in her knees on her history; however, still do a 'look, feel, move' of the knees.

11 RR is a sensitive indication of patient deterioration but is often overlooked. HR can be elevated in patients due to multiple causes, including pathological (infection, anaemia, arrhythmia) and benign (anxiety). Hypotension can indicate severe infection or dehydration. It is important to determine if a hypotensive patient is in shock: look for other symptoms such as tachycardia, tachypnoea, hyperlactataemia, metabolic acidosis and oliguria. In cases of shock, fluid resuscitation and identification of the cause are imperative.

12 This is a typical way of reporting that first and second heart sounds have been heard, with no other sounds such as murmurs. Murmurs may indicate structural heart defects or valvular heart disease. In patients who require surgery, murmurs would need to be investigated to determine fitness for general anaesthetic, and to ascertain increased risk of complications in the peri-operative period.

Investigations

- **FBE** [1] and **UECs** [2] are normal.
- AP and lateral X-rays of her wrist are ordered. They show an **extra-articular fracture** [3] of the distal radius, being dorsally angulated and displaced, involving both the radiocarpal and radioulnar joints, with an associated avulsion fracture of the **distal ulna** [4].
- **Bone density appears normal** [5] with no indication of **pathological fracture** [6].
- There is **soft tissue swelling** [7] that appears to be related to the fracture, but no other **soft tissue abnormality** [8].
- She is diagnosed with a **Colles' fracture** [9] **type II** [10].

1 FBE is an important baseline test, as anaemia can lead to reduced oxygen delivery and therefore reduced end-organ oxygen utilisation. It also negatively impacts postoperative recovery and healing. Although we would not expect this patient to be anaemic, knowing her status before any potential surgery is useful. As this is a low blood loss surgery, she is not on any blood thinners, and she has no pre-existing conditions, a group and hold and coagulation studies are not necessary.

2 UECs are important in case of potential surgery, as it identifies any electrolyte disturbances that may need correction prior to surgery. It also is important in medication choice, as well as dose.

3 The pattern of fracture tends to differ based on age. In children, distal radius fractures may have an epiphyseal slip due to an open epiphysis (similar to slipped capital femoral epiphysis in the hip). It is described as a Salter I or II fracture. In the young adult population, a higher energy force is required to cause the fracture, hence it tends to be comminuted, with intra-articular extension. In the elderly, weak forces combined with a weaker bony cortex tend to manifest as extra-articular fractures.

4 Colles' fractures classically have a transverse fracture of the distal radius, located around 2.5cm proximal to the radio-carpal joint, with dorsal displacement and angulation, along with radial tilt. It may also involve comminution at the fracture site, radial shortening, radial angulation, loss of ulnar inclination and associated avulsion fracture of the ulnar styloid process.

5 Plain X-rays are not a sensitive test for osteoporosis, as >30–50% bone loss is required before it will be apparent. Therefore, a report stating that there is no apparent decrease in BMD still requires further investigation. Early indications of osteoporosis on X-ray are decreased cortical thickness and loss of bony trabeculae.

6 A pathological fracture is one that is due to a disease rather than an injury. They can be an incidental finding on X-ray, and include causes such as osteoporosis, cancer, osteomalacia and osteomyelitis. These would include cystic changes or areas of lucency. If a pathological fracture is identified, further imaging needs to be performed to check the whole lower arm for further lesions, as this may alter management.

7 Effusions secondary to trauma are a result of microvascular leakage being greater than the clearance rate of synovial fluid, leading to a collection of fluid.

8 Increased soft tissue lucency in the area of a fracture strongly suggests an open fracture as it indicates the presence of gas.

9 Colles' fracture is a term typically used to describe a fracture at the distal end of the radius, at the cortico-cancellous junction.

10 Wrist fractures can be classified by a number of systems using different parameters. This is the most common one:

Frykman classification		
Fracture classification	**Location**	**Additional fractures**
Type I	Transverse metaphyseal fracture (includes both Colles' and Smith's fractures as angulation is not a feature)	Nil
Type II	Same as type I	Ulnar styloid fracture
Type III	Involvement of the radiocarpal joint (includes Barton, reverse Barton and chauffeur fractures)	Nil
Type IV	Same as type III	Ulnar styloid fracture
Type V	Transverse fracture involving distal radio-ulnar joint	Nil
Type VI	Same as type V	Ulnar styloid fracture
Type VII	Comminuted fracture involving both radiocarpal and radio-ulnar joints	Nil
Type VIII	Same as type VII	Ulnar styloid fracture

Management

Immediate

Provide **analgesia** [1]. Based on the patient's case and fracture pattern on X-ray, consider the indications for **backslab** [2], **closed reduction** [3] and **operative fixation** [4]. **Insert an IV cannula** [5] and **commence fluids** [6]. Keep the patient **fasted** [7] whilst awaiting **orthopaedics consultation** [8].

Short-term

It is decided that operative fixation is most appropriate for this patient. **Prophylactic antibiotics** [9] are given in theatre. An **ORIF** [10] is performed; however, **alternative techniques** [11] were considered. Monitor the patient postoperatively for any **signs of complication** [12]. The patient may be discharged once vital signs are stable. Provide adequate analgesia.

Long-term

Follow the patient up in the orthopaedics outpatient clinic. Monitor for **long-term complications** [13]. Refer the patient for a **BMD scan** [14]. Engage allied health to continue rehabilitation for **ROM exercises** [15], and subsequently **strengthening** [16]. Advise the patient that recovery time is **dependent on numerous factors** [17], and it may take up to 2 years for healing to occur. **Residual ache or stiffness** [18] is likely to be present until this point.

1 Pain relief makes examinations easier to perform. Musculoskeletal pain is often managed best with NSAIDs and non-opioids. If necessary, opioids can be prescribed but with caution due to their addictive nature. Dose may need to be adjusted for patients at risk of renal dysfunction or those with pre-existing kidney injury. Consult guidelines on dosages for specific medications.

2 Undisplaced fractures can generally be managed in a backslab immediately. Early casting can assist in pain reduction, by stabilising the joint. They can also be utilised to immobilise the joint whilst deciding on definitive management. The positioning of the hand and wrist is similar to that used in rugby to hold the ball in preparation for the kick. Alternatively, instruct the patient to hold out their forearm (supporting their wrist with their other hand or getting someone else to do it), and with their radius upward let the hand and wrist fall into a relaxed position (similar to a handshake position). Backslabs are left open on one side to allow for swelling without constriction, which could lead to compartment syndrome. Confirm good positioning through repeat X-ray.

3 Closed reduction is indicated in mildly angulated/displaced fractures. Prior to performing closed reduction, analgesia must be provided. This may be in the form of regional anaesthesia or procedural sedation. After you have ensured there is adequate analgesia, apply traction using one person to apply traction to the hand while an assistant provides counter-traction at the elbow. You may feel the fracture relocate with a 'clunk'. A fracture is always accompanied by soft tissue injury. Careful handling and gentle reduction can help to preserve the blood supply to the soft tissue and bone, thereby assisting fracture healing.

4 Surgery or manipulation under general anaesthetic is indicated in significantly angulated, deformed and comminuted fractures. Patients with symptoms of nerve compression and/or compound fractures require urgent manipulation under anaesthesia (MUA). Timing of surgery is not as important if the nerves are not compromised and it is not a compound fracture. MUA is also required for fractures that show a loss of normal forward radial tilt on lateral X-ray.

5 For surgery insert at least a size 20 cannula. This will be suitable for most fluids, in a patient who is not expected to need a transfusion or rapid infusion. For planned surgeries the cannula is typically inserted by the anaesthetist prior to induction.

6 IV fluids are used for fluid resuscitation and to maintain haemodynamic stability. As the patient will be nil by mouth until surgery, it is important that they receive fluids so they don't become dehydrated, as this could affect both their haemodynamic stability and kidney function. All fluids should be charted, so that it is clear how much and what has been given, as both hypo- and hypervolaemia can create problems. Peri-operative hypovolaemia leads to low cardiac output with resultant decreased tissue perfusion, and severe hypovolaemia can result in shock and multi-organ failure. Peri-operative hypervolaemia is typically due to retention of fluids given during surgery, and can increase morbidity and mortality, and lengthen time spent in the ICU. Signs of fluid overload include elevated JVP, peripheral oedema and crackles in lung bases.

7 Patients should be fasted prior to surgery to lower the risk of aspiration of stomach contents. The general guidelines are 6 hours for food and 2 hours for clear fluids. Patients can have a general anaesthetic in the unfasted state using RSI to reduce the risk of aspiration; however, this is better avoided and is generally reserved for emergency situations.

8 The orthopaedic surgical team will typically consent the patient, as well as giving instructions on any specifics they want to be addressed, e.g. type of fluid, any antibiotics to be commenced prior to surgery, analgesia in addition to that already given.

9 Prophylactic antibiotics are important to prevent wound and bone infection. The most commonly used first-line antibiotic in orthopaedic surgery for closed long bone fractures is cefazolin.

10 ORIF is performed using a volar plate or dorsal plate, fixed with screws. This can be combined with percutaneous pinning and external fixation. If the fracture is complex and comminuted, bone grafting may be required.

11 External fixations need to be managed cautiously as they are prone to distal radio-ulnar joint contracture due to being held in a pronated position. Percutaneous pinning involves K-wires being placed into the fracture dorsally and used to reduce the fracture until they are driven into the proximal radius. As mentioned above, these techniques may be used as an aid for internal fixation or used solely as the definitive management of the fracture.

12 Monitor for postoperative complications such as pneumonia, surgical site infection and UTI. In addition, assess the neurovascular status of the arm regularly to ensure there are no signs of compartment syndrome.

13 Delayed union refers to a failure of union in 1.5x the expected time. Non-union refers to a failure of union in 2x the expected time. This can be related to either excess mobility at the fracture site (hypertrophic non-union) or poor blood supply (atrophic non-union). A potential complication, Sudeck's atrophy/osteodystrophy is a complex disorder involving pain, abnormal blood flow, sensory abnormalities, sweating and trophic changes in superficial or deep tissues.

14 The most common type of BMD scan is the dual energy X-ray absorptiometry (DEXA) scan. It provides a T-score comparing the patient's BMD to that of a 30-year-old of the same sex and race. Diagnosis is based on degree of BMD:
- Normal BMD: T-score of +1.0 to −1.0
- Osteopenia referring: T-score of −1 to −2.5
- Osteoporosis: T-score lower than −2.5.

Treatments are aimed to increase BMD to reduce fracture risk (most common in pelvis, hip and wrist). Conservative treatment includes increasing calcium and vitamin D levels and engaging in weight-bearing exercise. Smoking cessation and low alcohol intake are also important. The most commonly prescribed medications are bisphosphonates, although other treatments can also be used including selective oestrogen receptor modulators.

15 Commence with passive ROM, progressing to active ROM. Focus on wrist flexion and extension within the limits imposed by patient pain. Adding further ROM exercises assists in limiting scar tissue and adhesion formation. Attention needs to also be paid to the joints above and below the fracture site (fingers, elbow, shoulder).

16 Later on, once the patient is cleared to load-bear, strengthening exercises are performed along with ROM exercises to attain increased flexibility.

17 Recovery depends on the degree of bone displacement, the number of bone fragments, presence of intra-articular fracture, and the patient's age, gender and medical history.

18 This may be permanent and is particularly true for high energy injuries, where the patient is over the age of 50, and those who have some osteoarthritis. The stiffness is typically minor and not sufficient to negatively affect function.

CASE 44: Monoarticular arthropathy

History

- A **55-year-old** [1] **male** [2] with a history of **gout** [3], **hypertension** [4] and **T2DM** [5] presents with a **tender and swollen** [6] left **knee** [7] which **began yesterday at midday** [8] and has **worsened over the last 24 hours** [9].
- He has recurrent gout in his left knee with a **recent acute attack** [10], but states this **feels different** [11] to previous gout flares.
- He has associated **fevers and malaise** [12].

- He denies any **trauma** [13] and has no **respiratory** [14] or **genitourinary** [15] symptoms.
- His regular medications are **hydrochlorothiazide** [16], **metformin/dapagliflozin** [17] and **atorvastatin** [18], and he takes **ibuprofen** [19] for acute gout flares.
- He is married and has had **no new sexual partners** [20], works as a **gardener** [21], has **occasional alcohol** [22], is a **non-smoker** [23] and has never been an **IVDU** [24].

1 Increasing age is a risk factor for gout and septic arthritis. Gout is very uncommon in younger people and if present, tends to reflect a genetic or renal issue rather than lifestyle factors. In septic arthritis, incidence and likelihood of poorer outcomes increases with age, and the likely causative pathogen is different for different age groups, with *N. gonorrhoeae* being important to consider in sexually active young adults.

2 Men are more likely than women to develop gout, primarily because hyperuricaemia occurs earlier in men (immediately after adolescence) whereas in women it tends to occur after menopause (oestrogenic compounds enhance the clearance of uric acid through the kidneys). Gender is not a risk factor for septic arthritis. Rheumatoid arthritis and SLE (important differential diagnoses) are more likely in women.

3 Gout is a chronic disease and typically presents with multiple acute flares with periods of intercritical gout in between. Urate-lowering medications in patients with recurrent gout reduce the likelihood of progression to chronic tophaceous gout.

4 Patients with hypertension should specifically be asked if they take loop and thiazide diuretics, which are risk factors for gout. The presence of hypertension should also raise suspicion for impaired renal function, which can be a cause and consequence of hyperuricaemia.

5 Diabetes is a risk factor for septic arthritis and cardiovascular disease. There are peri-operative implications including impaired healing, increased infection risk, labile BGLs due to fasting and considerations for timing of ceasing oral hypoglycaemic agents. The presence of diabetes should prompt consideration about cardiovascular disease, renal disease and autonomic dysfunction in surgical patients.

6 Differentials for swollen, tender joints are broad, ranging from OA, autoimmune arthritis, crystal deposition disorders, trauma and septic arthritis. Septic arthritis is a time-critical diagnosis and should be at the top of your differential list because of the consequences of delayed diagnosis.

7 The causes of a monoarticular arthritis are different to polyarticular arthritis, with gout and septic arthritis being important differentials to consider. Knees are the joints most affected by septic arthritis (50% of septic joints), followed by hips, shoulder, elbow, ankle and sternoclavicular (IVDU). Gout typically affects the lower extremities, particularly the first MTP joint or knee.

8 Acute onset over hours–days suggests an inflammatory process such as gout, septic arthritis or trauma. Onset over weeks to months is typical of an inflammatory arthritis such as rheumatoid arthritis or psoriatic arthritis, whereas OA has gradual onset over years. Gout flares are twice as likely to occur overnight or early in the morning as during the daytime.

9 In septic arthritis, joint damage can occur within 8 hours of symptom onset, therefore early diagnosis and treatment are essential to minimise risk of serious complications.

10 Multiple attacks of gout in the knee suggests this could be another gout flare; however, previous joint arthritis (e.g. gout) makes it easier for bacteria to seed the joint.

11 Distinguishing between an acute gout flare and septic arthritis is very difficult as they have near-identical presentations. It can be easy to put this presentation down to another gout flare, but always try to keep septic arthritis in mind because gout can predispose a patient to septic arthritis and, occasionally, they can also present concurrently.

12 Systemic symptoms such as fever, malaise and weight loss raise the suspicion of infection. However, patients with gout can present with fever and malaise while patients with septic arthritis may not have any systemic symptoms.

13 Trauma to a joint can present with pain, swelling and inflammation, and a history of trauma should prompt imaging to assess for fracture or joint injury. Patients who have a history of loss of consciousness, confusion or recent alcohol or drug intoxication may not have any recollection of a fall and it may not be possible with these patients to exclude a traumatic cause based on history alone.

14 Septic arthritis has three mechanisms of infection: trauma with direct inoculation into the joint, extension of infection from adjacent tissue such as osteomyelitis, or, most commonly, via haematogenous seeding of the synovial membrane. A lower respiratory tract infection may be a source for bacteraemia and haematogenous seeding.

15 Urinary tract infections may likewise provide a source for haematogenous seeding of the joint. If a patient has a UTI and suspected septic arthritis, empirical antibiotic therapy should include cover for Gram-negative bacteria. The patient should also be asked about genital discharge, which may indicate gonorrhoea, a common pathogen for septic arthritis.

16 Urate is secreted and reabsorbed in the proximal tubules, with most of the secreted urate being reabsorbed. Loop and thiazide diuretics reduce urate excretion directly, by enhancing the reabsorption of urate and indirectly, by inducing a volume-depleted effect which reduces urate secretion into the tubule. The net effect is to induce or exacerbate hyperuricaemia and precipitate attacks of gout. Loop diuretics increase the relative risk of gout by approximately 80%.

17 In a potentially septic patient, or during the peri-operative period, metformin should be withheld to mitigate the risk of lactic acidosis. Withholding sodium-glucose co-transporter-2 (SGLT2) inhibitors should also be considered due to the potential for hypovolaemia and acute renal injury. UTI is a common adverse effect of SGLT2 inhibitors, therefore a urine MC&S should be performed to determine if there is bacteriuria and a possible source of seeding if the joint is septic.

18 This patient presents with multiple features of metabolic syndrome. Gout is often considered a 'benign' disease; however, it can be considered as part of the metabolic syndrome. Counselling about lifestyle changes is not only helpful for the management of gout but will also reduce the risk factors associated with metabolic disease.

19 This patient has numerous risk factors for renal injury: gout, use of dapagliflozin and use of NSAIDs. Poor renal function is a risk factor for gout and has implications for treatment options. Ask the patient about recent NSAID use and doses.

20 It is important to ask patients about sexual partners to determine likelihood of gonococcal arthritis, which accounts for 20% of septic arthritis and is the most common cause in sexually active younger adults and adolescents. Gonococcal infection most often manifests as a dermatitis-arthritis with tenosynovitis, vesiculopustular skin lesions and polyarthralgia without purulent arthritis (60% of cases) or as purulent arthritis without skin lesions (40%).

21 Certain occupations put patients at increased risk of OA and subsequent joint damage which can predispose to septic arthritis. This patient should be asked about minor penetrating trauma (e.g. kneeling on plant thorns) which could be an infection source and a low threshold should be maintained for potential foreign bodies in the joint which may not be detected on imaging studies. The patient's occupation also has implications with regard to prognosis if the joint is septic, as he is at high risk of losing joint function and it would have a significant impact on quality of life. Early referral to social work is recommended.

22 Alcohol consumption is a risk factor for gout. The consumption of beer and spirits (but not wine) is a risk factor for developing the first episode of gout, whereas consumption of beer, wine and spirits is a risk factor for recurrent gout flares with a significant dose–response relationship. Patients at risk of gout should be counselled about reduction of alcohol intake. Heavy alcohol consumption can also lead to hepatic insufficiency, which is a risk factor for septic arthritis and has implications for the use of medications and therapy.

23 Smoking status is an important consideration for surgical candidates. Current smokers should be offered nicotine replacement therapy in the peri-operative period to reduce surgical risks and improve wound healing.

24 Intravenous injection is an important risk factor for septic arthritis. People who inject drugs have a different range of possible pathogens and require more broad-spectrum empirical antibiotic therapy. The outcomes in these patients are generally worse, with a higher likelihood of repeat surgeries, longer hospital stays and higher mortality. Clinicians should also have a low threshold for suspecting infective endocarditis, as septic arthritis may be the presenting manifestation of infective endocarditis.

Examination

- The patient looks **comfortable and alert** [1] with a **large body habitus** [2] .
- He is **febrile at 38.5°C** [3] but otherwise **haemodynamically stable** [4] .
- **Mucous membranes** [5] look dry.
- Heart sounds are dual with **no murmurs** [6] .
- The skin is normal with **no rashes** [7] , **visible plaques or nail changes** [8] , and the **conjunctiva** [9] are clear.
- Other joints are **normal** [10] with no **nodules** [11] .
- The knee is **erythematous, swollen and hot to touch** [12] , and there are no **wounds or scars** [13] .
- **Active and passive range of movement** [14] is limited due to pain.

[1] A patient who looks unwell or has altered mentation should raise suspicion for sepsis and warrant urgent investigations and treatment.

[2] Obesity is a risk factor for gout. Other modifiable risk factors include hypertension, hyperlipidaemia, cardiovascular disease, diabetes mellitus, chronic kidney disease, dietary factors, alcohol and medications altering urate balance.

[3] Fever is present in 75% of patients with septic arthritis, usually below 39°C with no associated chills. Although patients with gout flares can be febrile, septic arthritis must be considered as a potential cause of this patient's presentation and he will require joint aspiration to confirm the diagnosis.

[4] The vitals do not suggest the patient is septic. Signs of life-threatening organ dysfunction in adults are confusion, tachypnoea, hypoxaemia, hypotension, lactataemia or oliguria.

[5] The patient is dehydrated, likely due to inadequate oral intake. Replace fluids to minimise possible complications such as acute kidney injury (AKI) or rapid deterioration if he becomes septic.

[6] Listen carefully for added sounds that may indicate infective endocarditis, or other cardiovascular pathologies which should prompt further investigation. If murmurs are detected, request an ECG and refer for an echocardiogram. If infective endocarditis is suspected, collect three sets of blood cultures, commence on appropriate empiric antibiotic therapy, and request both TTE and TOE.

[7] Extra-articular symptoms, such as skin rashes, might suggest systemic inflammatory arthritis, such as SLE, or systemic infection, such as disseminated gonorrhoea or disseminated intravascular coagulation (DIC) in a septic patient. Also look for mottled skin and assess peripheral perfusion, which may be early signs of organ dysfunction in a septic patient.

[8] Skin plaques, particularly on the extensor surfaces of the joints, onycholysis and pitting nails are typical presentations of psoriasis. Psoriatic arthritis is a seronegative inflammatory arthritis which affects up to 30% of people with psoriasis and can present as an acute monoarthropathy.

[9] Scleritis, episcleritis and uveitis may be present with systemic inflammatory arthritis.

[10] Look for swelling, erythema, skin changes, deformity and muscle wasting. Feel the joints for warmth, tenderness and swelling. Assess movement of joints, looking at passive and active movement, stability of joint and crepitus.

[11] Nodules may be due to OA or RA, or may be tophi from chronic undertreated gout.

[12] Compare the affected joint with the unaffected joint, particularly if signs are subtle. Tap the patella to assess for large joint effusions and the bulge sign for small effusions. Effusion is usually the result of synovitis but may also be blood (haemarthrosis) or pus. Use the back of your hand to compare temperatures. The combination of swelling, erythema and warm joint supports an inflammatory/infective process rather than OA.

[13] Look for small wounds which may be caused by penetrating injury (e.g. plant thorns, injections). Previous surgery, particularly joint replacement, could be an infection source and change how the condition is managed.

[14] Reduced range of active motion could be due to a joint issue or the tissues adjacent to the joint (tendons, ligaments, muscles, bursae). Reduced range of passive motion is supportive of an intra-articular process.

Investigations

- **Urinalysis** [1] is unremarkable.
- **ECG** [2] shows normal sinus rhythm.
- FBE shows a significantly **elevated WCC** [3].
- UECs show moderately **elevated creatinine** [4].
- **ESR and CRP** [5] are significantly elevated.
- **LFTs** [6] are normal.
- **Serum uric acid** [7] is elevated.

- Two sets of **blood cultures** [8] are taken.
- Plain X-ray of knee shows **joint effusion** [9].
- A **large volume (5ml) of purulent synovial fluid is aspirated** [10] from the knee, with initial analysis showing **elevated WCC (75 000 cells/mm³)** [11], **Gram-positive cocci in clumps** [12], **monosodium urate crystals** [13] and the **culture** [14] is pending.

1 Positive urinalysis with leucocytes and nitrites suggests a UTI may be a source of haematogenous spread of bacteria in septic arthritis and guides empirical antibiotic therapy. Urine samples that are positive should always be sent for MC&S. First void urine should be collected if gonococcal infection is suspected. Catheterisation is a risk factor for septic arthritis.

2 A routine ECG may be helpful for patients with cardiovascular risk factors who are likely to have surgery. An ECG in this patient is not entirely indicated.

3 Infection and inflammation are responsible for elevated WCC. A low or normal WCC in immunosuppressed patients may occur.

4 Elevated creatinine may be acute or chronic. Review previous UEC results to determine the chronicity of renal dysfunction. Withhold nephrotoxic medications and give IV hydration judiciously if the patient is not fluid-overloaded. Be mindful that giving IV hydration to patients with chronic kidney disease can cause fluid overload. There are multiple possible causes for reduced kidney function in this patient – dehydration, early sign of organ dysfunction due to sepsis or as a consequence of gout. Renal complications from chronic hyperuricaemia include uric acid nephrolithiasis and chronic urate nephropathy, which can cause chronic kidney disease.

5 CRP and ESR are acute phase reactants which elevate during inflammation and infection. A CRP >100mg/L is strongly suggestive of a bacterial infection (80% likelihood). CRP tends to be more useful than ESR in septic arthritis because it rises and falls rapidly, making it a good marker to assess response to therapy. ESR and CRP are elevated in most inflammatory arthritis, therefore normal levels suggest a non-infectious/inflammatory cause such as stress fracture or OA.

6 Patients with chronic liver disease are more likely to be immunodeficient and at increased risk of septic arthritis or clotting deficiencies and haemarthrosis (consider testing coagulation profile). Acute changes in LFTs could be an early sign of organ dysfunction due to sepsis, particularly elevated serum bilirubin.

7 Hyperuricaemia is necessary but not sufficient to precipitate gout attacks. It is also not uncommon to have normal to low serum urate levels during an acute flare (up to 40% of attacks).

8 50% of people with septic arthritis have positive blood cultures. Take blood cultures prior to initiating antibiotic therapy.

9 Imaging is of secondary importance to aspiration of the knee, which should not be delayed. The role of imaging is to assess for fracture or dislocation if trauma was a factor, to provide further information if the diagnosis is unclear, or if aspiration is unsuccessful. In septic arthritis imaging may show joint space widening, peri-articular osteopenia or adjacent osteomyelitis. Ultrasound and CT may be useful to guide joint aspiration.

10 The decision on whether to aspirate a hot, swollen in a patient with known gout can be difficult. It is recommended that all patients who present with a short history of a hot, swollen, tender joint with a restriction of movement should be considered to have septic arthritis until proven otherwise. Additional factors in this patient further support the decision to aspirate (the patient is febrile, the symptoms feel different to other gout attacks, he has other risk factors for septic arthritis and his occupation requires a well-functioning knee, therefore delaying the diagnosis and treatment of septic arthritis would have a significant impact on his occupation). Joint aspiration is the gold standard investigation which must be done prior to commencing antibiotics, to confirm the diagnosis and guide therapy. The only exception to commencing antibiotics prior to aspiration is if the patient is septic, in which case IV antibiotics should be commenced within 1 hour of presentation (blood cultures should be taken at a minimum though). Aspiration can be performed on patients who are anticoagulated, although testing INR in warfarinised patients to exclude supratherapeutic INR would be prudent, as illness is a risk factor for high INR. Joint fluid should appear clear – a turbid or frankly purulent sample is strongly suggestive of infection.

11 A WCC >50 000 cells/mm³ is considered diagnostic of septic arthritis; however, patients can have lower counts, particularly if they are immunosuppressed. A higher WCC correlates with a higher likelihood of septic arthritis. Septic arthritis should be presumed in patients with joint replacement and a WCC >1100 cells/mm³. WCC can also be raised in acute gout flares or inflammatory arthritis.

12 Clumps of Gram-positive cocci are suggestive of *Staphylococcus aureus* infection and empirical antibiotics should be tailored towards this finding. Sensitivity for Gram stain is only 30–50% (crystal arthropathy can cause both false positive and false negative Gram stain results), therefore antibiotics should not be withheld. While waiting for culture results, Gram stain is useful to guide initial therapy (Gram-negative bacilli suggest *E. coli* or *P. aeruginosa*, Gram-positive cocci suggest *S. aureus*, *S. epidermidis*, *S. pneumoniae*, Gram-positive diplococci suggest *N. gonorrhoeae*).

13 Monosodium urate crystals confirm the presence of gout. Septic arthritis occurs concurrently with gout in 5% of cases.

14 All specimens must be sent for culture to confirm the pathogen and determine antibiotic sensitivities. Polymicrobial septic arthritis is very uncommon and usually due to a penetrating injury.

Management

Immediate

Monitor **vitals** [1] and commence **empirical IV antibiotics** [2] and **IV hydration** [3]. Refer to the **orthopaedics team** [4] to guide further management.

Short-term

Adjust antibiotics according to **joint aspirate and blood cultures** [5]. The patient is taken for **knee arthroscopy with washout** [6]. Repeat **FBC, CRP** [7] and **UEC** [8] daily. **Cease hydrochlorothiazide** [9]. Arrange

a **central IV catheter** [10]. Arrange **allied health** [11] review. Patient can be **discharged** once he is **clinically improved** [12], deemed safe for discharge by allied health and on **oral antibiotics** [13].

Long-term

The patient is discharged to a **rehabilitation centre** [14] prior to returning home. He is commenced on **urate-lowering medication** [15] and followed up in the outpatient clinic. Due to significant joint damage a **prosthetic joint** [16] is recommended.

1 Observe patient for trends in vitals (increasing respiratory rate or decreasing systolic blood pressure (SBP) which could indicate deterioration, onset of sepsis or complications such as PE.

2 Do not wait for culture results to decide on choice of antibiotic, because joint destruction can occur within hours. The choice of antibiotic should cover the likely pathogens, with the most common being *S. aureus*. IV flucloxacillin is most appropriate to treat this patient, although vancomycin should be used for patients with an increased risk of MRSA. In young patients, *N. gonorrhoeae* should be covered and people who inject drugs should have broad-spectrum antibiotics to cover Gram-negative bacteria and MRSA. Make reference to hospital or local antibiotic guidelines to determine an appropriate empirical regimen.

3 Fluid resuscitation should be carefully managed to avoid complications. This patient has dry mucous membranes and elevated creatinine, therefore a 500ml bolus should be appropriate (a young, healthy patient can tolerate a 1L bolus), followed by maintenance and replacement fluids. Monitor fluid balance to ensure appropriate hydration and observe for signs of fluid overload (crackles in lung bases, elevated JVP, peripheral oedema), particularly in a patient who has risk factors for chronic kidney disease.

4 The patient will require admission to hospital with orthopaedics input, as he may require arthroscopy or surgical debridement and, in the longer term, possible joint replacement if severe damage has occurred.

5 Negative culture results from joint aspirates do not exclude septic arthritis, as false negatives can occur with crystal arthropathy, inflammatory arthritis, haemarthrosis, if antibiotics were administered prior to sample collection, or if the joint is seeded with pathogens which are difficult to culture. Nucleic acid amplification testing may be useful in these situations. Viral arthritis and fungal arthritis will also be culture negative. Viral arthritis is more likely to present with polyarticular arthritis and fungal arthritis in immunocompromised patients. Bacteraemia should prompt investigation of source of haematological seeding and will also determine duration of antibiotic therapy, with a minimum 4 weeks for *S. aureus* bacteraemia.

6 All operative options involve some form of drainage and/or washout as septic arthritis is, in essence, an abscess. Needle aspiration is the simplest and easiest treatment but may not be adequate for severe infections or joints which are difficult to access. Arthroscopy allows better washout and insertion of a percutaneous drain. Surgical drainage may be required if adequate drainage is not achieved, a foreign body is suspected (penetrating trauma), or if there is persistent effusion for 7 days or more despite aspiration and/or arthroscopy. Patients may require several aspirations/arthroscopies if they have severe infection; the synovial fluid should be analysed each time to monitor response to treatment (expect WCC to decrease and fluid to be sterile).

7 CRP is an acute phase reactant which rises and falls quickly in response to infection and resolution; monitor WCC and CRP to assess response to treatment. If they do not fall, consider other sources of infection or inflammation, or the presence of other pathogens which may not be sensitive to antibiotics.

8 Monitor creatinine to determine if there is resolution of AKI or if there is a chronic renal injury. Surgical patients often require monitoring and replacement of electrolytes (particularly potassium and magnesium) due to fasting and shifts between intracellular and extracellular fluid. Consider replacing these electrolytes if they are at the low end of normal range.

9 Hydrochlorothiazide and other loop diuretics decrease the excretion of uric acid. Changing to an alternative antihypertensive agent such as an ACE inhibitor may be better for the patient in the long term.

10 Follow local guidelines for duration of antibiotics; however, for confirmed *S. aureus* joint infection, a minimum of 2 weeks IV therapy and a total duration of 4 weeks IV + oral antibiotic therapy is recommended. A central venous catheter or PICC has a lower risk of infection compared to a peripherally inserted venous cannula; however, there is no recommended time frame to replace these central lines, and the risk of infection increases over time. Regardless of the type of cannula, the site should be reviewed daily for signs of complications (infection or DVT being most common).

11 Physiotherapy will play a key role in assessing joint mobility, identifying issues which may require long-term solutions and arranging equipment to expedite discharge home if required. This patient will also require social work to assist with issues relating to work and possible loss of income. Occupational therapy may be required if there is permanent loss of function that requires interventions to maintain independence and quality of life. A dietitian can discuss dietary and lifestyle changes to reduce recurrence of gout.

12 Knee effusion and erythema should be reduced and pain brought under control. Monitor FBE and CRP for objective evidence of improvement.

13 Some patients may be discharged home on IV antibiotics provided suitable services are available and in place (i.e. hospital in the home or similar).

14 Only 40% of patients with septic arthritis are discharged home; the majority require some form of rehabilitation. Factors such as age and comorbidities such as diabetes and heart failure have a greater likelihood of longer admission or inpatient rehabilitation.

15 Hyperuricaemia carries an increased risk of recurrent gout flares, formation of tophi and development of CKD, but is also indirectly associated with an increased risk of cardiovascular disease (likely due to lifestyle factors). Therefore adequately treating hyperuricaemia has multiple benefits beyond simply minimising the risk of gout attacks. Long-term treatment for gout is two-pronged; non-pharmacologic lifestyle modifications (including diet changes and review of medications which affect urate excretion) and pharmacologic urate-lowering medications. Allopurinol is the first-line agent for treating hyperuricaemia; however, it should not be started during an acute flare-up as it can precipitate acute gout attacks. Ensure appropriate prophylaxis with colchicine or NSAIDs is given when starting allopurinol and educate the patient about risk of acute attacks when commencing allopurinol.

16 Up to one-third of patients may have poor outcomes (amputation, arthrodesis, prosthetic surgery or severe functional deterioration). The prognosis depends on age, pre-existing joint disease, organism virulence (*S. aureus* being the most destructive), duration of infection prior to initiating treatment and whether the patient is an IVDU. In-hospital mortality from septic arthritis is 3–5%.

CASE 45: Neck of femur fracture

History

- A **75-year-old** [1] **male** [2] is brought in to the ED by ambulance after **tripping on a rug on his way to the toilet** [3] .
- **He landed on his right side on wooden flooring** [4] , had **immediate right hip pain** [5] but **denies any other pain** [6] .
- After falling, he was **unable to get up** [7] .
- He denies **incontinence** [8] or **urgency** [9] .
- There were **no preceding symptoms** [10] and he has had **no previous falls** [11] .
- He has **no history of trauma or surgery to his hip** [12] , no significant **past medical history** [13] , and

is not on any regular **medications** [14] , particularly **anticoagulants** [15] .
- A **social history** [16] reveals he **lives alone** [17] , with regular family visits.
- He is independent of all his **pADLs** [18] and **dADLs** [19] .
- He appears well-nourished and **cooks his own meals** [20] .
- He has **never smoked, and only drinks occasionally** [21] .
- He is uncertain **when the fall happened** [22] and seems mildly **confused** [23] .
- He has a score of 21 on **MMSE** [24] .

[1] A neck of femur fracture (NOF) is a common orthopaedic presentation, most typically as low energy injuries in elderly patients. When they occur in younger patients, significant forces are usually involved (e.g. road traffic collision or fall from height), meaning a higher likelihood of other significant injuries which may need attention first. Falls occur in approximately one-third of elderly people who live independently (per year), and in 10% of these falls a hip fracture is the result (with 90% of these in those over the age of 70). More than 10% of those who experience a hip fracture will be unable to return to their previous home, with most of the remainder experiencing ongoing disability or pain.

[2] Hip fractures are more prevalent in women, with postmenopausal women being twice as likely to have a hip fracture as their premenopausal counterparts.

[3] It is important to ascertain whether the patient simply slipped and fell, or if something led to the fall, especially if there are potentially modifiable risks.

[4] It is important to get a thorough history of the mechanism of injury to ensure the injury matches the mechanism. In a fracture sustained with minimal trauma (e.g. stepping off a pavement), it would raise the suspicion of a pathological fracture, as would previous history of hip pain or cancer.

[5] Fractures are painful, so initiate analgesia early. NOF may also present with pain in the hip, groin and/or knee.

[6] A fall can result in more than one injury, commonly of the ipsilateral wrist or proximal humerus. Head strike is common and must be ruled out. If there is a head strike,

the cervical spine needs to be examined for possible injury. Details such as fall height, surface fallen onto, and positioning can help to identify other potential injuries of which the patient may not be aware. If there were witnesses, getting a collateral history can be helpful.

[7] Reduced mobility with a sudden inability to bear weight are common in an NOF; however, patients may still be able to walk (albeit with difficulty).

[8] Incontinence, particularly urge incontinence, is a risk factor for falls, as patients may trip while rushing to the toilet.

[9] Urgency may be a sign of urge incontinence and/or UTI. It is important to have a low level of suspicion for UTIs in the elderly, as they are more susceptible and don't always present with classic symptoms. UTIs are also a potential cause of delirium, which may be mistaken for dementia. Women are more susceptible to UTIs than men.

[10] A detailed history of the circumstances surrounding all falls is imperative, to ensure serious causes are not missed. Questions should include what happened before the fall (including symptoms such as dizziness, chest pain or palpitations), during the fall (incontinence or tongue biting may indicate seizure activity) and after the fall, including if they were able to resume normal activities afterwards.

[11] Previous falls are a strong predictor of the likelihood of future falls.

[12] It is important to know about previous trauma or surgery to a joint.

13 Past medical history may allude to conditions that increase fracture risk and/or falls risk. Conditions that increase fracture risk include previous cancer (potential for pathological fracture), osteopenia or osteoporosis, endocrine disorders, reduced activity, low body weight and cigarette smoking. Conditions that increase falls risk include previous stroke, incontinence, Parkinson's disease, fear of falling, decreased mobility, impaired balance and gait, visual impairment, polypharmacy (especially antidepressants, psychoactive medications, benzodiazepines and antipsychotics), reduced muscle strength and poor reaction times.

14 Medications are among the most common risk factors for falls in the elderly, as well as one of the easiest to modify. Medications that increase drowsiness or worsen confusion make patients less sure-footed. Medications that lower BP can lead to or worsen postural hypotension. Diabetes medications can cause hypoglycaemia.

15 Anticoagulants are problematic in falls due to increased haemorrhage risk leading to significant blood loss, including internally from a pelvic fracture into the pelvic cavity, or into the brain secondary to head strike. Other medications (e.g. steroids) can reduce BMD.

16 A thorough social history is imperative, as treatment is aimed at restoring patients to their previous functional level. Secondly, it influences decisions regarding discharge. Patients who live alone may need to remain in hospital longer and have services provided for their return home.

17 Living arrangements impact on decisions regarding discharge. In the elderly and impaired it is also important to identify sinister causes of injuries, including neglect and abuse. Consider non-accidental injury if the history of the incident does not fit with the injury.

18 Personal activities of daily living (pADLs) are everyday personal care activities. These are necessary for independent living and caring for oneself. These include: bathing, dressing, grooming, mouth care, toileting, transferring to/from bed/chair, walking, climbing stairs and eating.

19 Domestic activities of daily living (dADLs) are activities related to independent living and include shopping, managing medications, doing housework, using the phone, doing laundry, cooking, driving or using public transportation.

20 Calcium and vitamin D are important for healthy bones. Nutrition can be an issue in the elderly due to various factors including decreased vision and mobility making shopping and food preparation difficult, and ill-fitting dentures affecting ability to eat.

21 Alcohol and tobacco negatively affect bone mass, resulting in a higher risk of fracture. Alcohol use also leads to an increased falls risk.

22 Long lie is defined as a prolonged period of time spent on the floor (>1 hour) due to an inability to get up. It is an indicator of social isolation, weakness and illness, and is associated with high rates of morbidity and mortality. It can lead to muscle injury due to tissue compression, resulting in rhabdomyolysis potentially causing renal failure, and death.

23 Sudden behavioural changes in elderly patients may be due to delirium. There are two types: hyperactive and hypoactive delirium. Signs of hyperactive delirium include agitation, hallucinations and restlessness. Hypoactive delirium is more difficult to detect, as patients present more withdrawn or drowsy. It is associated with a higher mortality. Patients may also present with aspects of both hyper- and hypoactive delirium. Delirium typically has an acute onset and a fluctuating course of disturbance in attention, level of arousal, and other aspects of mental status. Approximately 70% of delirium is not identified in the ED. If not identified, it leads to increased mortality (approximately double) and longer hospital stays.

24 The Mini Mental State Examination comprises 30 questions to assess for cognitive impairment. It is especially important in elderly patients who may be suffering from delirium and/or dementia.

Examination

- The patient appears **uncomfortable** [1], and his right leg is **abducted and externally rotated** [2].
- On comparison with his left leg it appears **visibly shorter** [3].
- Examination reveals no **broken skin** [4], some **ecchymosis, and swelling in the right inguinal area** [5].
- Pain is exacerbated by **palpation of the greater trochanter** [6].
- He has normal **sensation to his lower limb, and pulses are intact** [7].
- He has **no abdominal pain, nausea or vomiting** [8].
- His **observations are within normal parameters** [9], and he is **afebrile** [10] with normal **central capillary refill time** [11].
- **Heart sounds are dual with nil added** [12], and lung fields are **clear bilaterally** [13].
- His **calves are soft and non-tender** [14].
- His right wrist, elbow and knee are **non-tender** [15].

1 This injury is acutely painful and requires analgesia promptly.

2 An abducted, externally rotated leg is the classic positioning for a NOF.

3 Leg shortening is due to the pull of the short external rotators.

4 Broken skin over a fracture is regarded as an open fracture, which has a higher risk of infection requiring a washout as soon as possible and fracture reduction. Before dressing the wound with gauze soaked in saline, take photos to prevent repeated exposure, as other doctors can then refer to the photo rather than undressing the wound. Give a tetanus shot if the wound is dirty or you cannot be certain the patient has had one within the past 5 years, and commence antibiotics urgently. In elderly patients the skin is often fragile, so note all broken skin/skin tears even if nowhere near the potential fracture, and treat accordingly.

5 Physical findings on examination include:
- limited range of motion of the hip (especially internal rotation)
- shortened injured leg, with external rotation and abduction
- pain elicited by attempted passive hip motion
- antalgic gait (if patient is able to bear weight); may be unable to stand on the affected leg
- ecchymosis (bruising): not always present
- tenderness to palpation of the inguinal area over the femoral neck +/– swelling.

6 A classic finding of a NOF is exacerbation of pain on hip rotation, and on palpation of the greater trochanter. Avoid vigorous examination if you suspect a fracture, as it is incredibly painful and you also run the risk of displacing the fracture.

7 Although neurovascular compromise is rare after a NOF, it is still essential to perform a full neurovascular examination, so that any deficits can be addressed urgently.

8 He has potentially had a long lie, putting him at risk of rhabdomyolysis. The classic triad of rhabdomyolysis symptoms are muscular pain in the shoulders, thighs or lower back, muscle weakness and myoglobinuria (red/brown urine) with decreased urine output. However, up to 50% of patients with rhabdomyolysis have no muscle-related symptoms. Other signs include abdominal pain, nausea and vomiting, fever, tachycardia and confusion.

9 RR is a sensitive indication of patient deterioration but is often overlooked. HR can be elevated in patients due to multiple causes, including pathological (infection, anaemia, arrhythmia) and benign (anxiety.) Hypotension can indicate severe infection or dehydration. It is important to determine if a hypotensive patient is in shock (look for other symptoms such as tachycardia, tachypnoea, hyperlactataemia, metabolic acidosis and oliguria). In cases of shock, fluid resuscitation and identification of the cause are imperative.

10 Older patients do not always mount a fever in response to infection, even in serious infection. Thus, absence of fever should not be taken as an absence of infection.

11 Normal central capillary refill time suggests the patient is euvolaemic, making major blood loss and dehydration less likely.

12 Murmurs may indicate structural heart defects or valvular heart disease. In patients requiring surgery, murmurs need investigation to determine fitness for general anaesthetic, and ascertain increased complications risk in the peri-operative period.

13 A chest infection can be a cause of delirium in the elderly, so must be ruled out. Atypical pneumonia may not cause lung consolidation, leading to lung fields sounding clear. If pneumonia is a concern and there is a likelihood of atypical pneumonia (e.g. immunosuppressed patients), a CXR should be ordered.

14 DVT may present as tight, tender calves, erythema and measuring >3cm greater in circumference than the normal calf.

15 In all traumas it is important to assess for other injuries, especially as strong pain can distract from other injuries.

Investigations
- FBE shows no **anaemia** [1] and no raised **WCC** [2].
- **UECs** [3], LFTs and **creatine kinase (CK)** [4] are normal.
- **Group and hold and coagulation studies** [5] are also ordered.
- A catheter is inserted, with approximately **1L entering the bag** [6].
- A **urine dipstick test is normal** [7] and the sample is sent to the laboratory for **urinalysis and MC&S** [8].
- A **CXR** [9] is clear.

- AP pelvis **X-ray** [10] shows a **single fracture line** [11] running between the greater and lesser trochanters of the right femur in the **intertrochanteric line** [12].
- There are no other fractures, making this a **2-part fracture** [13].
- **Shenton's line** [14] is discontinuous, with shortening of the femur.
- **Soft tissue swelling** [15] is noted with no signs of **pathology** [16].
- **ECG** [17] is normal.

1 Pre-operative anaemia in an NOF is a risk factor for peri-operative death. Some of this anaemia is likely to be due to blood loss associated with the initial trauma, making it even more important to have a baseline haemoglobin before surgery. Anaemia can lead to reduced oxygen delivery and end-organ oxygen utilisation. It negatively impacts postoperative recovery and healing. In severe dehydration, haemoglobin and haematocrit appear higher than the actual level.

2 This is an indication of infection and inflammation. This result decreases the likelihood of an infective source for this patient's delirium. However, it could also indicate an inadequate immune system response to infection, so urinalysis and a CXR should still be ordered to look for a source.

3 UECs are important in case of potential surgery, as they identify electrolyte disturbances that may need correction prior to surgery, and factor into medication choice and dose.

4 Elevated CK indicates rhabdomyolysis, with positive results typically at least 5 x the upper limit of normal. It begins rising as early as 2 hours after muscle injury, peaking in 24–72 hours. Serum aminotransferases are also commonly elevated. Myoglobinuria is only observed in 50% of cases.

5 NOF can result in significant blood loss, some of which occurs prior to surgery. A baseline coagulation profile can be useful, and a group and hold prior to surgery ensures a better transfusion match as it can take a few hours to process.

6 Urinary retention is a potential cause of delirium, as are faecal impaction/constipation, infection, medications and other causes. Relieving urinary retention may lead to the resolution of an episode of delirium if it is the sole cause. Normal bladder capacity is 400–600ml.

7 Blood, protein, nitrites and leucocytes on urine dipstick are all indicators of a UTI. Even in the presence of a UTI, urine dipstick may not be positive. If suspicion is strong, consider sending the urine sample for microscopy, culture and sensitivities.

8 Urine MC&S identifies the causative organism and the antibiotic susceptibilities and resistance. This is valuable if empiric antibiotic therapy is not working.

9 In elderly patients with possible delirium, a CXR is often ordered to exclude pneumonia.

10 It is useful to assess both hips for more informed preoperative planning. Additionally, it helps to rule out other differential diagnoses such as pelvic fractures (especially those of the pubic ramus) and fractures of the femoral head, femoral diaphysis and acetabulum. If pathological fracture is suspected, include full-length femoral X-rays.

11 If X-ray is equivocal in spite of a high clinical suspicion for fracture, obtain more imaging. The gold standard is an MRI; however, in practice a CT tends to be ordered as they are fast to perform and quickly available.

12 Fracture line runs in the intertrochanteric region (outside of the joint capsule) making it an extracapsular fracture. The femoral head receives its blood supply in a retrograde fashion (distally to proximally from femoral neck to femoral head), mostly through the medial circumflex artery which lies directly along the intracapsular femoral neck. An extracapsular fracture does not usually interfere with this artery, whereas an intracapsular fracture typically does, resulting in loss of blood supply and avascular necrosis of the femoral head. Therefore, although extracapsular fractures are typically managed with either an intramedullary nail or a dynamic hip screw, intracapsular fractures generally require either a half (hemiarthroplasty) or total hip replacement. Intracapsular NOFs follow the Garden classification.

Intracapsular neck of femur fracture – Garden classification			
Garden 1	**Garden 2**	**Garden 3**	**Garden 4**
Incomplete femoral neck fracture	Complete femoral neck fracture	Complete femoral neck fracture	Complete femoral neck fracture
Undisplaced	Undisplaced	Partially displaced	Fully displaced
Often impacted and likely to unite with bedrest, but as prolonged bedrest is associated with complications, typically stabilised with screws through the neck into the femoral head		Unlikely to unite, high risk of avascular necrosis Elderly: hemiarthroplasty often recommended Patients with pre-existing joint disease and who are still active with a reasonable life expectancy are offered total hip replacement Younger patients: reduction and screws to preserve their femoral head as long as possible	

13 Although there is no formal classification system for extracapsular hip fractures, identifying how many parts there are to the fracture gives an indication of stability and surgical difficulty.

Intertrochanteric (extracapsular) neck of femur fracture		
2-part	**3-part**	**4-part**
Fracture through intertrochanteric line	Fracture through intertrochanteric line	Fracture through intertrochanteric line
	Fracture of lesser trochanter (can be single fragment or comminuted)	Fracture of lesser trochanter (can be single fragment or comminuted)

Intertrochanteric (extracapsular) neck of femur fracture		
2-part	3-part	4-part
		Fracture of greater trochanter (can be single fragment or comminuted)

14 Shenton's line is a line drawn along the medial aspect of the femoral neck and inferior border of the superior public ramus. Disruption of this line indicates a NOF.

15 Effusions secondary to trauma result from microvascular leakage (from ruptured vessels) exceeding the clearance rate of synovial fluid, resulting in fluid collection.

16 A pathological fracture is one due to disease rather than injury. They can be an incidental X-ray finding and include causes such as osteoporosis, cancer, osteomalacia and osteomyelitis. If a pathological fracture is identified, further imaging needs to be performed to check the whole femur for further lesions, as this may alter management.

17 Arrhythmias can be another cause of falls, so should be ruled out.

Management

Immediate

Provide **analgesia** [1] and a **femoral nerve block** [2] if possible. Obtain IV access, take **bloods** [3], commence **fluids** [4] and keep the patient **nil by mouth** [5]. Monitor vital signs and **urine output** [6] through insertion of a **urinary catheter** [7]. Order an **ECG** [8] and screen for **cognitive impairment** [9]. The **orthopaedic team** [10] will assess for **fitness for surgery** [11], including anaesthetic assessment for **fitness for anaesthesia** [12]. Identify other medical conditions and discuss early with the medical team to prevent surgical delays, including obtaining **MDT input** [13].

Short-term

Surgery is typically within **36–48 hours** [14], with **various surgical options** [15]. Prophylactic **antibiotics** [16] are given in theatre. Postoperatively, monitor **vitals** [17]. **Encourage mobility** [18] as soon as possible. Administer **VTE prophylaxis** [19]. Engage **allied health** [20] for physical rehabilitation and discharge planning.

Long-term

Continue **rehabilitation** [21] until the patient reaches the limit of their personal recovery. Follow the patient up in the orthopaedic outpatient clinic with a repeat X-ray to monitor progress of fracture healing.

1 Pain relief makes examinations easier to perform. Musculoskeletal pain may be managed with NSAIDs and non-opioids, with dose adjustments for patients at risk of renal dysfunction or with pre-existing kidney injury. Consider opioids, weighing up their risk of sedation and potential dependence against their quick analgesic effect.

2 NOFs are very painful, so typically a block is given. This is performed with aseptic technique, typically using guided ultrasound to identify structures (nerve, artery, vein). Local anaesthetic is used to numb the skin, before using a needle to pierce the skin and approach the nerve. Perineural infiltration of long-acting local anaesthetic is given. It is important to ensure the ropivacaine is not injected into a blood vessel, which can lead to local anaesthetic toxicity; thus aspiration to ensure no blood comes back is essential before first injecting and should be repeated every 5ml. This provides analgesia for an average of 16 hours.

3 Group and hold, FBC, U&E, LFTs, coagulation and bone profile. Correct any abnormalities such as anaemia, dehydration and coagulopathy.

4 Intravenous fluids are used for fluid resuscitation and to maintain haemodynamic stability. As this patient will be nil by mouth it is important they receive fluids so they do not become dehydrated, as this could affect both their haemodynamic stability and kidney function. Hypovolaemia in the peri-operative period leads to low cardiac output with resultant decreased tissue perfusion, and severe hypovolaemia can result in shock and multi-organ failure. Peri-operative hypervolaemia is typically due to retention of fluids given during surgery, and increases morbidity and mortality, and time spent in the ICU. Signs of fluid overload include elevated JVP, peripheral oedema and crackles in lung bases.

5 Patients are fasted prior to surgery to lower the risk of aspiration. The general guidelines are 6 hours for food, and 2 hours for clear fluids. Patients can have a general anaesthetic in the unfasted state using RSI to reduce the risk of aspiration in emergency situations.

6 Urine output is an important indicator of fluid balance and renal function. Reduced renal function secondary to hypovolaemia can lead to acute kidney injury if not addressed early.

7 This patient will not be able to mobilise for some time, plus catheterisation makes urinary output easier to measure.

8 Baseline ECG may identify arrhythmias or MI – both potential causes of falls.

9 Cognitive screening may identify delirium or underlying cognitive impairment. This is important as these findings will have implications on consent for medical treatment. Consent via an appointed medical treatment decision-maker or next of kin may be required.

10 The orthopaedic surgical team typically consents the patient, as well as gives instructions on any specifics they want to be addressed prior to surgery.

11 One tool often used is the Nottingham Hip Fracture Score, which calculates 30-day mortality after hip fracture surgery. It asks questions on: age, gender, abbreviated mental test score, Hb on admission, residence, comorbidities and active malignancy in the last 20 years (excluding SCC and basal cell carcinoma (BCC)). This generates a predicted mortality rate as a percentage.

12 Although uncommon, some patients may be too unfit for surgery in which case their fracture may need to be managed with bed rest and traction. Surgery for an NOF has a 10% postoperative mortality, as these patients are often already frail. Discussion with anaesthetics is always required, to ensure the patient is fit for anaesthesia.

13 Mortality is often related to patients having multiple comorbidities. MDT involvement with specialist ortho-geriatrician input helps reduce the mortality rate.

14 This is a very painful fracture, and these patients are typically elderly and already frail. As such, prolonged time in bed waiting for surgery leads to rapid deconditioning, making eventual rehabilitation more difficult. Not delaying surgery results in earlier mobilisation and a decrease in morbidity and mortality. Extracapsular NOFs carry a high mortality rate of up to 30% at one year, with predictors of mortality including: significant comorbid conditions, abnormal ECG preoperatively, decreased pre-injury cognitive function, decreased mobility prior to fracture, and being older than 85 years.

15 There are several operative options:
- Dynamic hip screw: for stable fractures; a large lag screw is placed through a plate into the head of the femur. The plate runs down the lateral side of the femur and is attached with bone screws. The lag screw slides down the barrel of the plate as the patient mobilises, which compresses the fracture, thus stabilising it. If there is rotational instability of the femoral head, an additional hip screw can be inserted to prevent rotation. This enables full weight bearing immediately. This is the most common surgical management of extracapsular fractures.
- Intramedullary nail (Gamma locking nail): used for stable and unstable fractures. This is preferred for reverse oblique fractures (where the fracture runs from below the greater trochanter to above the lesser trochanter) and subtrochanteric fractures (fracture extends below the lesser trochanter). The intramedullary nail is placed through the greater trochanter directly into the bone marrow and is held in place with a distal fixation screw through the femur. A lag screw is then placed through this nail, entering the femoral head and neck. The intramedullary nail allows for impaction and compression of the fracture site, enabling early weight bearing. It is called a gamma locking nail because the combination of the lag screw and the intramedullary nail forms a Y shape, resembling the Greek letter γ (gamma). These implants are more expensive than a dynamic hip screw.
- Cannulated hip screws: can be used for non-displaced intracapsular fractures; involves the use of three parallel screws in an inverted triangle formation.
- Hip hemiarthroplasty: for displaced subcapital fractures; half of the hip joint (femoral head and neck) is replaced with a prosthetic implant which extends into the proximal femur.

16 Prophylactic antibiotics are important to prevent wound and bone infection. The most commonly used first-line antibiotic in orthopaedic surgery for closed long bone fractures is cefazolin.

17 Prolonged bed rest increases the risk of complications such as atelectasis, pneumonia, pressure injuries, thromboembolism and deconditioning, which in turn lead to increased morbidity and mortality.

18 The recommendation is for progressive weight bearing as tolerated soon after surgery, leading to full weight bearing, based on patient's general physical status. Partial weight bearing may last for 8–10 weeks depending on degree of fracture healing. Full weight bearing should be achievable after 3 months.

19 This includes medications such as low molecular weight heparin (LMWH) or warfarin, and mechanical methods such as thromboembolism deterrent (TED)/compression stockings, and intermittent pneumatic compression.

20 In hospital, physiotherapists will work with the patient and provide them with instructions on safe mobility on discharge. This includes ROM exercises for the hip, knee and ankle, and strengthening exercises typically 6 weeks post-surgery (dependent on surgeon instructions). Balance and proprioception rehabilitation are also required, as both decrease rapidly with inactivity. Regular exercise can maintain muscle mass, slow down bone loss, and improve balance and coordination, thereby reducing the risk of a subsequent fall and fracture. Progressive resistance exercise programmes have been demonstrated to achieve improvements to physical performance and quality of life that are both significant and maintained over time. Occupational therapists help prevent further falls by optimising the home environment. This includes a living environment assessment (lighting, trip hazards such as loose rugs, necessity for handrails in toilet and bathroom, etc.) as well as an assessment of ability to perform ADLs.

21 This is dependent on multiple factors, including patient age and condition, severity of fracture, and type of surgery used. Rehabilitation may be undertaken in a rehabilitation facility or in the patient's home, depending on their age and condition. Physical therapy can help a patient to recover their strength and mobility and may take up to 3 months. A large number of patients living in the community do not regain the functional level they had prior to their injury.

CASE 46: Neck trauma

History

- An **inebriated** [1] **19-year-old male** [2] with **no known past medical history** [3] presents with **worsening neck pain** [4] after **diving head first into a sand bar** [5] at the beach **30 minutes earlier** [6].
- He **denies loss of consciousness** [7] and although **initially painless** [8], he now complains of **worsening right-sided neck pain** [9].

- He has **no other injuries** [10].
- He denies any **limb weakness or sensory changes** [11], **dizziness** [12], **visual disturbances, headache, nausea or confusion** [13].
- He **smokes occasionally** [14] and **binge drinks most weekends** [15].

[1] Alcohol is a risk factor in 25% of all spinal cord injuries. When a suspected spinal injury does occur, alcohol depresses the CNS, which masks pain and neurological deficits, making it difficult to diagnose or exclude an injury. The threshold for suspecting spinal injuries in inebriated patients should be very low, and a spinal injury should not be excluded through physical assessment alone, until they are sober.

[2] Vertebral fractures are most common in young men (through trauma) and older women (due to osteoporosis). In general, young men are at high risk of traumatic injuries, particularly motor vehicle accidents.

[3] Past medical history is important to determine suitability for surgery, the likelihood of complications and to interpret findings during your examination. Medical conditions such as osteoporosis, cervical spondylosis and spinal arthropathies including rheumatoid arthritis and ankylosing spondylitis increase the risk of spinal injuries.

[4] Neck pain in the setting of this mechanism of injury should immediately raise suspicion of a cervical spine injury and the patient should be immobilised with a C-spine collar.

[5] The mechanism of injury provides crucial information to identify which injuries need to be considered. In this case, axial loading on the cervical spine increases the likelihood of a vertebral fracture, whereas head strike against a sand bar (as opposed to a hard surface such as a submerged rock) makes an intracranial bleed less likely.

[6] Primary spinal cord injuries refer to the immediate effect of the trauma on the cord. Secondary injuries are delayed progressive changes which evolve over hours and may be due to hypoxia, oedema, inflammation or other chemical changes. Although this patient did not initially have any neurological changes, secondary injury processes can still be occurring.

[7] LOC occurs when there is a significant insult to the brain. The absence of LOC is reassuring, particularly in the setting of a low-speed head strike against a soft surface like sand, but does not exclude an intracranial injury.

[8] Immediate neck pain at the time of injury is more consistent with vertebral injury, whereas delayed pain, even by a couple of minutes, is more suggestive of a muscular injury such as whiplash. Although this information is reassuring, it's important to look at the whole clinical picture in this patient by completing the history and examination before making any decisions about how to proceed.

[9] Unilateral delayed pain is more in keeping with a soft tissue injury to the paravertebral muscles.

[10] Distracting injuries (such as a long bone fracture or intra-abdominal injury) can mask more subtle signs of a spinal injury. Evidence of a distracting injury is therefore a contraindication to using clinical examination to 'clear' cervical injuries.

[11] Neurological deficits would be expected if there was injury to the spinal cord, nerve roots or peripheral nerves. While the lack of neurological deficits is reassuring, the patient's inebriated state may hide more subtle findings.

[12] Neurogenic shock is a form of shock that results from a severe injury to the CNS and can present with bradycardia, hypotension, warm and flushed skin and possible respiratory arrest.

[13] Intracranial injury can affect the cranial nerves, causing visual disturbances, vertigo, hearing disturbances, etc. Mass effect from intracranial bleed may cause similar symptoms as well as headache, confusion and nausea. Dissection of the carotid or vertebral arteries may cause stroke-like symptoms.

[14] Smoking is associated with an increased risk of peri-operative respiratory, cardiac and wound-related

complications. Consider prescribing nicotine replacement therapy while patients are admitted, to reduce surgical risks, and counsel about smoking cessation prior to discharge.

15 Binge drinking is a high risk activity for traumatic injuries in this age group. In heavy drinkers, consider the risk of alcohol withdrawal or liver dysfunction.

Examination

- The patient appears **alert** [1] , **comfortable** [2] , is **talking in full sentences** [3] , **lying flat in bed** [4] and wearing a **well-fitting C-spine collar** [5] .
- He is **haemodynamically stable** [6] and has a brisk **central capillary refill time** [7] .
- The lungs are clear to auscultation with normal vesicular breath sounds from the **bases to the apices** [8] , heart sounds are dual with no added sounds and there are no **carotid bruits** [9] .
- The abdomen is **soft and non-tender** [10] .
- The chest wall, long bones and main joints are **non-tender on palpation and movement** [11] .
- There is **midline tenderness** [12] on palpation of the cervical spine at levels C7 to T2.

- There is **no further spinal tenderness on log roll** [13] and **anal tone and sensation** [14] is intact.
- **Cranial nerves II–XII** [15] are intact.
- **Sensation is reduced** [16] **bilaterally** [17] in the **C7–T1 dermatomes** [18] of the upper limbs.
- **Power is 4/5** [19] for **elbow and wrist extension, and finger extension, flexion, adduction and abduction** [20] .
- **Upper limb reflexes are ++ bilaterally** [21] .
- In the lower limbs, **sensation and power are reduced throughout** [22] .

1 The Glasgow Coma Scale is a useful tool to monitor and accurately assess patients' consciousness and changes over time. A quicker assessment tool is AVPU (Alert; responds to Voice; responds to Pain; Unresponsive) with the transition between V and P corresponding roughly to a GCS of 8 and consideration for intubating the patient. AVPU is useful when initially assessing patients or when GCS needs to be estimated quickly.

2 A comfortable patient suggests that any pain is well controlled or minimal, the patient is not anxious, and there is no respiratory distress. Initial impressions can guide a clinician's concern about the acuity of a patient.

3 The patient is unlikely to have any respiratory issues (such as pneumothorax (PTX)).

4 Patients with a potential spinal injury should stay in spinal precautions (lying flat in bed without flexing or rotating the spine) until they are cleared of an injury or if an injury is identified, it has been stabilised with a brace or fixation.

5 A poorly fitting C-spine collar provides insufficient stability to the spine and can result in neurological injury if a fracture is present. The collar should be adjusted and refitted. Between 3% and 25% of all spinal cord injuries are attributed to improper immobilisation and transport after the injury.

6 There is no evidence to suggest the patient is in spinal shock or has any other injuries such as PTX or internal organ laceration. In a haemodynamically unstable patient, the focus should be on ABC: airway, breathing and circulation. If the airway is at risk of compromise, the priority should be on protecting the airway with intubation rather than protecting the C-spine.

7 A brisk capillary refill time suggests the patient is not in shock or dehydrated, relevant in that he is inebriated and has been at the beach.

8 Auscultate while the patient is lying flat in bed, listening at the sides, the axilla and apices of the chest. Signs of a PTX include reduced or absent breath sounds or subcutaneous emphysema. A small PTX may not have any clinical signs. If a PTX is suspected, consider using an ultrasound to look for signs.

9 Bruits would suggest carotid artery dissection which would require further investigation, such as a CT angiogram of the neck and head.

10 Internal organ injury such as laceration to the spleen, liver or kidneys can occur in a trauma setting and lead to exsanguination. Abdominal or renal tenderness should raise the suspicion of these injuries and prompt further assessment and investigation.

11 A full but brief assessment of the shoulders, clavicles, chest wall, arms, pelvis and legs is important to identify any other injuries that may be masked by more painful injuries, but it also ensures the log roll can be performed safely to assess the spine without causing further damage if another injury is present.

12 Midline tenderness is concerning for a fracture or ligamentous injury which would result in an unstable spine, and this would necessitate radiographic imaging. A cervical spine can be cleared and the collar removed without imaging only if the patient is awake, alert AND has no neck pain, tenderness or neurologic deficits AND has no distracting injuries. The Canadian C-spine rule is a well validated tool to identify patients who do not require imaging to clear a cervical spine injury. This tool can be used for inebriated patients, provided they are alert and cooperative.

13 The entire spine must be carefully assessed to identify all potential vertebral injuries. In trauma settings, it is not uncommon to find multiple discontinuous vertebral fractures, particularly in high energy injuries.

14 Digital rectal examination assesses the S3–S5 dermatome. Reduced tone or sensation may be present if there is a spinal cord injury; however, it is not a reliable sign and can have false positives and false negatives, therefore any findings should be viewed in the context of the overall clinical picture.

15 Cranial nerve deficits can occur if there is intracranial injury.

16 A positive neurological finding such as reduced sensation strongly increases the likelihood that a spinal injury has occurred.

17 Bilateral neurological deficits suggest a segmental injury as opposed to an injury to peripheral nerves (i.e. brachial plexus injuries) or other rarer injuries such as Brown-Séquard syndrome, in which one side of the cord is affected resulting in symptoms on one side of the body.

18 Sensation is often preserved in dermatomes below the site of injury in incomplete spinal cord injuries because sensory tracts are more peripheral and less vulnerable than motor tracts.

19 The combination of sensory and motor deficits, which use different pathways in the spinal cord, is compelling evidence that a spinal cord injury has occurred. Reduced power indicates an incomplete spinal cord injury has occurred, and the focus should be to stabilise the spine and prevent a complete injury.

20 The innervation for these muscle groups originates from C7–T1 which corresponds to the dermatomes of reduced sensation and suggests a C7 injury has occurred.

21 In the acute setting, spinal shock may result in hyporeflexia and flaccid tone. If the injury is permanent, over days to weeks increased tone and hyperreflexia will usually predominate.

22 An injury at the cervical spine results in all neurological functions below this point being affected.

Investigations

- **FBE** [1] , **UECs** [2] and **LFTs** [3] are all normal, and **blood alcohol level is 0.19** [4] .
- **CT scan** [5] of the C-spine shows **anterior wedge fracture of C6** [6] , **burst fracture of C7** [7] and **spinous process fractures C6–T1** [8] .

- **MRI** [9] of the spine shows **no contusion** [10] , **mild spinal cord oedema** [11] , **intact posterior longitudinal ligament** [12] and **interspinous ligaments** [13] with **moderate interspinous oedema** [14] .

1 An acutely low haemoglobin, or a decreasing trend in a trauma patient, may indicate a haemorrhage and prompt further investigations to look for a bleed.

2 Assessing renal function and electrolytes is an important investigation in a trauma patient. It determines if the patient is suitable for surgery or IV contrast, it may indicate urinary retention in a spinal injury or renal laceration in a trauma patient, electrolyte imbalances may need to be corrected or investigated and some drugs may need to be adjusted or withheld.

3 Deranged LFTs may indicate hepatic laceration in a trauma patient.

4 Blood alcohol level (BAL) confirms if a patient is sober or inebriated. A BAL <0.05 in an apparently 'intoxicated' patient should raise suspicion of a head injury or other causes (delirium, electrolyte imbalance, illicit drugs, etc.).

5 Choice of imaging modality is dependent on several factors. Use the Canadian C-spine rule to decide if imaging is required at all. X-rays may be suitable in patients with a low likelihood of injury, but it is difficult to confidently exclude an injury based on X-ray. CT is the mode of choice for identifying bony injury; however, the higher radiation dose must be factored into your decision-making, particularly in younger patients. A CT should be requested if patients have neurological deficit, require concurrent CT of head or other region of body, have previous spinal surgery or have reduced GCS.

6 All spinal injuries should be referred to a spinal team for review of images, assessment and guidance about management. Management of spinal fractures differs depending on the type of fracture and other associated injuries. In general, anterior wedge fractures are stable and can be managed conservatively unless there is severe loss of height of the vertebral body (>50%) or there are multiple adjacent wedge fractures.

7 A burst fracture results from vertical compression on the vertebral body (the nucleus pulposus of the disc is pushed into the centre of the vertebral body, causing it to burst outwards). Bone fragments displaced posteriorly may impinge on the spinal cord. Burst fractures can be stable or unstable; however, unstable fractures may require surgery.

8 Isolated spinous process fractures are generally considered stable; however, in the context of this case with multiple fractures and neurology, there is a high suspicion the combination of injuries makes this an unstable injury.

9 MRI is the modality of choice to assess soft tissue including the spinal cord, discs and ligaments. MRI should be considered in patients if they have a normal CT and ongoing neurology or have a high suspicion for ligamentous injuries. The type and severity of injury to ligaments can determine whether or not an injury is stable and how they should ultimately be managed.

10 Spinal cord contusion can result in spinal cord injury. Other vascular injuries around the spinal cord can also result in injury. For example, extradural haematomas can compress the cord, whereas spinal cord infarction can occur due to injury to the anterior spinal artery which supplies the anterior two-thirds of the spinal tract. Early anticoagulation is contraindicated in patients with spinal cord injuries to minimise the risk of extradural haematomas; seek advice from a spinal team to determine timing for anticoagulation.

11 Spinal cord oedema can occur as a result of disc herniation or direct compression of bone, or as a result of secondary processes (ischaemia, hypoxia, inflammation, toxicity). Oedema develops within hours of injury, peaks between days 3–6 and recedes after day 9.

12 The posterior longitudinal ligament provides stability to the spinal column; disruption of this ligament would make it an unstable injury.

13 Injury to the interspinous ligaments is consistent with the spinous process fractures and the severity of the injury. Isolated injury to these ligaments is generally a stable injury.

14 Oedema would be expected, given the other injuries.

Management

Immediate

Monitor **vital signs** [1] and **urine output** [2] . Keep the patient **fasted** [3] . Obtain IV access and **administer fluid** [4] . Ensure adequate **analgesia** [5] and **keep patient in spinal precautions** [6] while **seeking advice** [7] from the spinal surgery team.

Short-term

The spine is **immobilised with a Long Miami J collar** [8] . **Erect X-ray** [9] after fitting brace shows adequate spinal alignment. Ensure patient is **anticoagulated** [10] while an inpatient. Arrange **allied health** [11] assessments, monitor **changes in neurology** [12] and ensure appropriate **pressure area**

care [13] is provided. Patient can be discharged home when they are **fit and well** [14] , and have **adequate home supports** [15] to manage daily activities, otherwise refer to a **specialist rehabilitation centre** [16] .

Long-term

Follow the patient up in an **outpatient clinic** [17] with X-rays prior. Patients with permanent loss of neurologic function (partial or complete) should have **ongoing multidisciplinary support** [18] to reduce complications including **cardiovascular** [19] , **urological** [20] , **respiratory** [21] and **psychological issues** [22] and other **allied health** [23] input. **Long-term anticoagulation** [24] should be considered.

1 Ensure the patient remains haemodynamically stable and monitor for signs of delayed spinal shock.

2 Urine output is a measure of renal function and fluid status. Reduced urine output may be a result of hypovolaemia and early identification and rectification can help prevent acute kidney injury. In the setting of a spinal cord injury, reduced urine output may also indicate urinary retention due to spinal cord injury, and a bladder scan should be requested.

3 Keeping a patient fasted prevents unnecessary delays if an urgent surgical intervention is required. In a patient who is inebriated, lying flat in spinal precautions and wearing a stiff

C-spine collar, keeping them fasted will also help minimise risk of aspiration and movement of the cervical spine from eating, and aid compliance with the spinal precautions.

4 IV fluid is integral in fluid resuscitation and stabilisation of circulation, particularly in the setting of alcohol intoxication and while the patient is being fasted. IV fluid management is based around four principles – resuscitation, maintenance, replacement (any fluid losses such as from the GI tract) and redistribution (e.g. third spacing). Ensure the patient is on a fluid chart in order to monitor fluid input and output. Replace the losses based on this chart, and also ensure that adequate maintenance fluid is being given.

5 The patient presented because of pain; ensure adequate analgesia is provided to keep them comfortable and improve compliance with spinal precautions.

6 Maintaining stability of spine will minimise further injury to spinal cord until definitive treatment has occurred.

7 Assessing and managing spinal injuries is a highly specialised area of medicine; contact the spinal team early for advice and management.

8 There are a variety of options to stabilise the spinal column, ranging from short and long collars, external halos and surgical fixation. This patient will always need to wear the collar, even while showering and sleeping, and requires one person to assist with removing the collar to change the pads. The collar may need to be worn for at least 6 weeks while bone repair takes place.

9 Erect X-ray ensures the collar has stabilised the spine in a load-bearing position and is an appropriate fit. The spinal team should review the X-ray and decide if the collar is adequately fitted before the patient can be cleared to mobilise.

10 Trauma promotes a physiological prothrombotic state, with spinal cord injury carrying the highest risk of VTE which can persist for months to years. In general, prophylactic anticoagulation can be started as soon as an extradural haematoma is excluded.

11 Patients with spinal cord injury can have a complex array of needs. Physiotherapy can assist in the short term with things like assessing mobility, assigning exercises and conducting chest physio to maximise respiratory effort and minimise chest infections. Occupational therapists assess functional deficits and help put in place strategies to address those deficits including in-home assessments and equipment needs. Social work helps with issues such as social security payments, sick leave, family issues, etc. Psychologists help patients deal with the psychological issues surrounding the trauma and injuries.

12 Neurological function may deteriorate as the consequences of secondary injuries (hypoxia, oedema, excito-toxicity, etc.) manifest around 8–12 hours post-injury.

13 People with spinal cord injury are at increased risk of pressure area injuries, particularly those with complete or severe injury. These complications can be avoided through appropriate care.

14 The patient should have adequate pain control, be haemodynamically stable and any other injuries or issues treated.

15 Home supports are dependent on the severity of injury and functional limitations. At a minimum, the patient should have someone to assist with removing the brace after showering, to replace the wet pads, and be capable of performing ADLs or have interventions in place to support them to meet these needs.

16 Specialist spinal injury centres are available in several key locations in the UK to provide ongoing care to people who are unable to safely be discharged home. Early referral to these centres is advised, particularly for patients with complete or severe cord injury, or those with significant barriers to discharge.

17 The spinal team will review fracture repair and decide if further interventions are required, such as internal surgical fixation for non-union of fractures. The duration and decision to remove the collar will be made during these outpatient appointments.

18 Spinal cord injuries are complex, involve multiple systems and have significant impacts on people's lives. People with spinal cord injuries are at risk of many complications beyond their neurological injury, and utilising a variety of specialists provides better outcomes for patients and reduced morbidity and mortality.

19 Spinal cord injuries above T6 are at risk of autonomic dysreflexia resulting in vasoconstriction and hypertension below the level of injury (due to uninhibited or exaggerated sympathetic stimuli) with insufficient compensatory bradycardia and vasodilation above the injury. Risk factors for coronary artery disease are higher in people with chronic spinal cord injury and incidence of coronary artery disease is 3–10 times higher.

20 Most patients with spinal cord injury require support to manage bladder dysfunction and avoid issues including retention, incontinence and infection.

21 Training respiratory muscles can help redress dyspnoea and loss of exercise tolerance resulting from ventilatory failure from cervical spine injuries. Chest physiotherapy and vaccination can help to minimise risk of chest infections from impaired cough and reduced ability to clear lung secretions.

22 Psychological issues are likely to persist beyond the acute time period following trauma. Permanent or complete neurological dysfunction can have a major impact on patients' mental health and ongoing function.

23 Continuing physiotherapy, social work, occupational therapy, wound care, orthotics, etc. may be required to support patients after discharge and long-term.

24 The risk of VTE persists after discharge and increases with more severe injuries. Prophylactic anticoagulation up to 3 months may be appropriate for some patients.

CASE 47: Open fracture

History

- **A 25-year-old** [1] **male** [2] **motorcycle rider** [3] with no previous medical history is **brought in by ambulance** [4] with an **open fracture** [5] of **lower left leg** [6] after hitting a **car at 60km/h (37mph)** [7].
- **Helmet and safety gear** [8] were being worn.
- There was no **head strike or loss of consciousness** [9].
- Paramedics report **significant blood loss** [10] from leg, and the patient was **normotensive (SBP 110mmHg) and tachycardic (115bpm)** [11] at the scene.

- **Pressure dressing** [12] was applied and **1L normal saline** [13] was given intravenously for BP support during transfer.
- The patient **denies spinal tenderness** [14] or **neurological deficit** [15].
- **Methoxyflurane** [16] was given by paramedics for pain relief.
- He **drinks alcohol socially** [17], was not **drinking** [18] before the accident, is a **non-smoker** [19] and denies **recreational drug use** [20].
- He last **ate or drank 3 hours ago** [21].

In an acute trauma setting, the typical sequential approach of history, examination, investigations and management does not occur because many of these events are happening concurrently. Although it may appear haphazard, the sequence of events is very logical and structured because the focus is on saving life, organs and limbs. This case is presented in the typical sequential structure of a medical case but differs from how an actual trauma setting would be managed. For example, a brief history may be handed over from the paramedics while someone is gaining IV access and collecting blood for tests and yet another team is assessing and potentially securing the airway. This is all overseen by a trauma 'lead' who has overall responsibility. X-rays may be accessible in the resus bay, with key imaging available before all injuries are identified. A comprehensive history might be obtained after many of the injuries and problems have been initially managed. So, when reading this case please keep these points in mind.

1 Open fractures are often the result of high energy trauma due to road traffic accidents, industrial or workplace accidents, or falls from height. Younger people are at greater risk of road traffic accidents, whereas falls are more likely to occur in older people. Older people are also more likely to have osteoporosis and are at risk of fracture with minimal force; however, these fractures are unlikely to be open.

2 The incidence of traumatic injuries, such as open fractures, is higher in men than women. Regarding tibial shaft fractures, men are likely to sustain these at a younger age while women tend to be older, presumably reflecting the high risk behaviours of young men and osteoporosis in older women.

3 Understanding the mechanism of injury allows the clinician to predict the likely set of injuries and their severity. Some presentations, such as motorcycle accidents, carry higher morbidity and mortality. Other high risk presentations include pedestrians hit by motor vehicles, falls from height greater than 6m and severe motor vehicle accidents. A motorcyclist presenting after a road traffic accident has a very different set of possible injuries compared with a driver or passenger in a car, or a pedestrian hit by a car.

4 The arrival method by which a patient presents to hospital often gives some insight into the acuity of their presentation. A patient self-presenting rather than being brought in by ambulance is likely to have less severe injuries.

5 Any open fracture is a severe injury. When assessing severe injuries to the extremities, a useful approach is to evaluate the four functional components of the limbs: bone, soft tissue, blood vessels and nerves. An open fracture carries an increased risk of osteomyelitis and potential limb amputation if the injury is very severe. The location of the injury is an important clue about the mechanism of injury and other possible injuries. For example, femoral fractures result from high energy impact (except with osteoporosis or bone lesions) and a high index of suspicion for pelvic fractures or abdominal-pelvic organ injury should be maintained.

Likewise, patients with fracture of the humerus may also have thoracic injuries.

6 Approximately 3% of long bone fractures are open, with the tibia being the most involved bone because of the lack of soft tissue over the shin. About 25% of tibia fractures are open, with 58% of open tibia fractures being the result of road traffic accidents.

7 It is important to obtain as much detail about the circumstances of the accident as possible. Questions to ask include how fast both drivers were travelling, the type of road and the speed limit, who hit whom and where on the vehicle/body they were hit, whether any other vehicles or obstacles were hit, whether they were able to extricate themselves from the vehicle and/or mobilise afterwards. The clearer the picture of the circumstances of the accident, the easier it is for the clinician to predict potential injuries and, importantly, not to miss any injuries.

8 A key aspect of the initial history should include any safety devices such as helmet, safety gear, any restraints used and what type (i.e. seat belt in a car vs. 5-point restraint in racing car) and whether any airbags deployed. A rider not wearing a helmet is at a very high risk of intracranial injury, even with low-speed incidents. Ask if there was any damage to the helmet, and if so, where on the helmet it was. Likewise, a rider not wearing appropriate clothing may have significant skin abrasions requiring review and management by the plastics or burns team.

9 Intracranial injury is one of the major concerns with motorcycle crashes. Lack of head strike or LOC in a helmeted rider is reassuring and there is a low likelihood of injury.

10 While estimating the volume of blood loss can be difficult, questions such as whether there were pulsing sprays of blood (arterial injury) or the number of gauze pads used can give an idea of the extent of bleeding. Patients with tibial fracture from significant trauma often have other injuries, with about 15% having an internal organ injury, therefore external blood loss may not represent the true volume of haemorrhage.

11 These vitals are consistent with class II (moderate) haemorrhage involving 15–30% blood loss which typically presents with tachycardia (100–120bpm), tachypnoea (RR 20–24 breaths per minute), skin which can be cool, clammy and pale with reduced capillary refill time. Systolic blood pressure is preserved in patients with moderate haemorrhage (or slightly reduced); however, reduced pulse pressure may be recorded (the diastolic BP is elevated). Class III haemorrhage (30–40% blood loss) and class IV haemorrhage (>40% blood loss) should be considered severe and are typified by hypotension, tachycardia >120bpm, tachypnoea and altered mental status. Haemodynamics are stable with class I haemorrhage (<15% blood loss). An easy way to remember the difference between each class of haemorrhage is to think of tennis scores (15, 30, 40).

12 Pressure is the first-line management of any bleed.

13 The use of IV fluids in trauma patients should be minimised and only used to resuscitate patients with a mean arterial pressure (MAP) <65mmHg until blood products are available and they can be transfused. Resuscitation with IV fluids causes dilution of platelets and clotting factors, and hypothermia, leading to impaired clotting. Permissive hypotension is a concept in which the goal of resuscitation is to maintain enough pressure to adequately perfuse organs rather than return them to a 'normal' pressure which can rupture fragile thrombi and lead to further blood loss. Excessive infusion of crystalloid fluids (ratio of crystalloid fluid to packed RBC more than 1.5:1) in patients with severe trauma is associated with poorer outcomes.

14 The risk of spinal injury in a motorcycle accident is very high and a low threshold should be maintained for suspecting this type of injury. Cervical spine injuries cannot be excluded on clinical assessment alone if there is a distracting injury (such as an open tibia fracture), therefore imaging of the cervical spine may be appropriate in this patient.

15 Neurological deficit may be a result of a spinal injury or damage to the peripheral nerves in the leg, and both should be considered in a patient complaining of this symptom.

16 Methoxyflurane is a rapid-acting, inhaled non-opioid analgesic with short duration, primarily given for pain relief following trauma. It is an anaesthetic agent which produces an analgesic effect when inhaled at low concentrations.

17 Patients with excessive alcohol consumption may be at risk of alcohol withdrawal and should be put on alcohol withdrawal precautions. These patients are also at risk of liver damage, which has implications for medications and anaesthetics.

18 Alcohol is a significant risk factor for traumatic injuries and has legal implications in road traffic accidents. Acute alcohol intoxication also has anaesthetic implications and is important to disclose in a peri-operative setting.

19 Smokers are at greater risk of surgical complications, ranging from increased VTE, MI, stroke, respiratory compromise, poor wound healing and wound infection. Prescribe nicotine replacement therapy to regular smokers while an inpatient in order to prevent withdrawal, and counsel patients about smoking cessation prior to discharge, requesting GP follow-up if the patient is agreeable.

20 Recreational drug use can have implications for haemodynamics (methamphetamines and cocaine are sympathetic stimulants), interact with anaesthetic agents or alter the efficacy of analgesics (opioid tolerance). Patients who regularly inject drugs are also much harder to cannulate and may require alternative approaches to gaining IV access, such as ultrasound or intraosseous.

21 Patients should be fasted at least 6 hours prior to surgery to reduce the risk of aspiration during anaesthetic induction. If emergency surgery is required and there is any doubt about timing of last meal, RSI and intubation is used; however, this carries increased risks and the surgery should be delayed if possible.

Examination

- **On primary survey** [1], the patient is **alert** [2], **talking in full sentences** [3] and in **visible distress from pain** [4].
- The chest wall is **non-tender with no deformities** [5], lung sounds are clear with equal air entry [6], RR is 22 breaths per minute [7], and oxygen saturations 99% [8] on air.
- Abdomen is soft and non-tender [9].
- BP is 115/85mmHg with HR 110bpm [10] and there is a 15cm soft tissue injury [11] with bone protruding antero-medially from the left lower leg [12] and no active haemorrhage [13].
- Dorsalis pedis and posterior tibial pulses [14] are palpable, ankle pressure index 1.05 [15], active flexion and extension of great toe [16] is preserved and sensation [17] is intact.
- The wound is contaminated with road gravel [18].

1 Open fractures are often high energy injuries; therefore, the focus should be on identifying other life-threatening injuries and managing these. The primary survey is a simplified but comprehensive initial approach to identifying problems in trauma patients which pose the most immediate threat to life. The primary survey is discussed in *Case 21*.

2 GCS is a commonly used tool to assess and communicate patients' cognitive state; however, in an urgent scenario, AVPU may be more appropriate. The transition between P and U corresponds approximately to a GCS of 7–8 and is an indicator to consider intubation. In a trauma setting, early intubation is recommended if there is any doubt about a patient's ability to protect their airway.

3 The ability to talk in full sentences demonstrates the patient is maintaining his own airway and is not in obvious respiratory distress.

4 This patient requires analgesia; however, short-acting agents such as fentanyl and midazolam are preferable to avoid adverse haemodynamic effects.

5 A tender chest may be due to a rib fracture and therefore underlying lung injury. Look for unequal inspiration, paradoxical movement (chest wall moves in on inspiration) or any other obvious deformity or injury. Palpate for crepitus and obvious deformity.

6 Auscultate the lungs at the axilla and apices. Tension pneumothorax will have reduced breath sounds on side of injury. Haemothorax may have crackles or reduced breath sounds.

7 Patients with long bone fractures are at risk of fat emboli and DVT which can lead to PE. An elevated respiratory rate could be due to PE but is also consistent with moderate haemorrhage or pain and does not necessarily imply pulmonary injury.

8 Impaired oxygen saturations are an objective sign of impaired ventilation and would warrant further investigation for potential PE.

9 Intra-abdominal injury can lead to rapid exsanguination if there is a severe bleed. Any tenderness in the abdomen should warrant a FAST ultrasound assessment to determine if there is any evidence of intra-abdominal injury.

10 This patient is normotensive, with slightly reduced pulse pressure and tachycardia <120bpm which are consistent with moderate haemorrhage and hypovolaemic shock.

11 When describing the size of a soft tissue wound, estimate the entire area of tissue affected, not just the skin break which may be small. One of the issues with an open fracture is the extent and severity of soft tissue injury which may be quite extensive beyond the open wound. Severe soft tissue injuries can lead to rhabdomyolysis.

12 Approximately one in four tibial shaft fractures is open, which is defined as any skin laceration and fracture which communicate with each other. Any soft tissue wound adjacent to a fracture should be considered an open fracture until proven otherwise. The Gustilo–Anderson system classifies open fractures according to the size of the wound, extent of soft tissue injury, bone injury and vascular injury, and degree of contamination, to determine the severity of the fracture. A higher grade of fracture is associated with increased risk of infection and likelihood of loss of limb.

13 Conduct a complete vascular assessment. Signs of arterial injury include active haemorrhage, expanding or pulsatile haematoma, bruit or thrill over wound, absent distal pulses, ischaemia at extremities (pallor, pain, paralysis, cool to touch). Arterial injury in a penetrating wound would require immediate surgery to explore and repair the vascular injury, particularly in this patient who is showing signs of hypovolaemic shock. In a closed wound, signs of arterial injury are not as reliable as open injuries, and if patients are haemodynamically stable a CT angiogram may be appropriate to investigate further. Venous injury can generally be managed with pressure.

14 A complete vascular assessment should begin by palpating pulses (femoral, popliteal, posterior tibial and dorsal pedis). Compare the injured to the uninjured limb. If pulses cannot be palpated (dorsalis pedis is notoriously difficult) and there are no signs of ischaemia, a Doppler ultrasound scan can be used to confirm blood flow is present.

15 Equivalent to the ankle brachial pressure index (also known as the injured extremity index), this index should be performed on all haemodynamically stable patients with severe limb injuries. A ratio >0.9 has a high negative predictive value for vascular injury and patients can be monitored with neurovascular observations to determine if there is any deterioration. If the ratio is <0.9, consult with vascular surgeons for further advice and investigations.

16 Flexion of the great toe is through the flexor hallucis longus which attaches proximally to the inferior two-thirds of the posterior surface of the fibula and interosseous membrane and is innervated by the tibial nerve. Extension of the great toe is through the extensor hallucis longus which attaches proximally to the anterior fibula and is innervated by the deep fibular nerve. Testing movement of the great toe provides a quick assessment of both tibial and fibular nerve function.

17 Sensation is provided by branches of the femoral nerve (saphenous), fibular and tibial nerves. Loss of dermatomal sensation may indicate a direct nerve injury (i.e. severed nerve) or indirect injury (i.e. compartment syndrome).

18 The wound requires washout and debridement to remove foreign bodies and prevent infection developing. Obvious contaminants can be physically removed or irrigated with sterile saline water; however, the patient will require theatre for fracture fixation and a more thorough inspection and debridement can be done at that time.

Investigations

- **VBG** [1] and **FBE shows Hb of 75g/L** [2] **and platelets 75 x 10⁹/L** [3] .
- **UECs** [4] are normal.
- **LFTs and lipase** [5] are normal.
- **Coagulation profile** [6] is normal.
- **Blood alcohol level** [7] is 0.0, **blood group and cross-match** [8] is sent.

- **ECG** [9] shows normal sinus rhythm.
- **X-rays** [10] show **midshaft** [11] **segmental comminuted** [12] fractures of the **tibia and fibula** [13] with **disrupted overlying soft tissue** [14] .
- The **knee and ankle** [15] are enlocated with no other fractures.

1 Most major EDs have access to venous blood gas machines which can provide crucial information in a matter of minutes. Of interest in this patient are haemoglobin and lactate levels, which would provide an indication of blood loss and impact of hypovolaemia on tissue perfusion.

2 A full blood count provides a more accurate measurement of haemoglobin; however, in the setting of acute haemorrhage, the haemoglobin may initially be normal. A haemoglobin <80g/L (or <100g/L in patients at risk of acute coronary syndrome) is a common threshold for transfusion (although if there is active bleeding, transfuse at higher levels).

3 Platelets can be rapidly lost or consumed during significant haemorrhage or diluted if there is excessive resuscitation with IV fluids. A platelet count <50 x 10⁹/L is a threshold for replacement with platelets.

4 Assessing renal function is important because these patients may have an acute kidney injury secondary to hypovolaemia, pre-existing kidney dysfunction or a physical injury due to the trauma. This information is crucial in the peri-operative period as it will impact on decisions about

medications, administration of contrast, threshold for blood transfusion or IV fluid resuscitation. Rhabdomyolysis is also a potential complication when large areas of soft tissue are injured, particularly if compartment syndrome is present and can cause acute tubular necrosis in the kidneys. If there is renal dysfunction, electrolyte abnormalities or dark urine, test CK to assess for rhabdomyolysis.

5 A routine set of trauma blood tests includes LFTs and lipase to assess injury to the liver or pancreas (along with UECs, this assesses the major abdominal organs). LFTs are also a useful test due to the role of the liver in metabolism of medications (with implications for drug interactions and dosages) as well as potential clotting disorders in liver failure.

6 Coagulation can be affected by consumption or loss of clotting factors and platelets, dilution of blood, medications (i.e. anticoagulants) or medical conditions (i.e. liver cirrhosis) and should be tested in all patients. An INR >2.0 or fibrinogen <3µmol/L are thresholds for transfusing fresh frozen plasma or cryoprecipitate, respectively.

7 There are ethical and legal considerations with testing blood alcohol levels in patients involved in road traffic accidents and you should understand your obligations about mandatory testing and reporting in your local jurisdiction. Test BAL if a patient is confused, if there is any doubt about intoxication and to determine level of risk or complications with anaesthesia.

8 A trauma patient who is actively bleeding and shows signs of hypovolaemic shock will require immediate blood transfusion which cannot wait for group and cross-match. However, all trauma patients with haemorrhage should have a blood group and cross-check as they may require further transfusions and it is best to use matched blood products as soon as possible to avoid depleting valuable reserves of O-negative blood.

9 The patient is tachycardic and hypotensive, most likely due to blood loss. However, it is good to have a baseline ECG to exclude cardiac abnormalities, particularly in the preoperative period. If a pulmonary embolism is considered possible, an ECG is essential with signs of a PE including sinus tachycardia (seen in 44% of patients), S1Q3T3 (classic finding in 20% of patients), right bundle branch block (18% of patients), right axis deviation (16% of patients), P pulmonale (9% of patients), atrial fibrillation/flutter (8% of patients);

however, the most common finding is non-specific ST and T wave changes (50% of patients). Patients with a higher cardiovascular risk profile should also have a baseline ECG before any surgery.

10 Plain film X-rays should be taken of the site of injury as well as the joint above and below. At least two projections (AP and lateral) are required. CT is usually required if there is any doubt of fracture or for surgical planning if required.

11 The midshaft and proximal tibia are thicker and tend to be associated with high energy forces, as opposed to the distal shafts which can fracture with lower energy impacts.

12 Transverse, comminuted and segmental fractures are associated with high energy forces. Spiral and oblique fractures tend to occur with low energy or rotational forces.

13 A concurrent fibula fracture often occurs with tibia fractures from high energy forces.

14 Increased lucency of the soft tissue overlying or adjacent to a fracture is strongly suggestive of an open fracture.

15 The joints above and below a fracture are imaged to exclude additional fractures or dislocations.

Management

Immediate

Insert **2 large-bore cannulas** [1] and **collect blood** [2] for testing and group and cross-match. **Transfuse 2 units of cross-matched blood** [3] and commence **IV antibiotics** [4] and **tetanus prophylaxis** [5]. The wound should be **irrigated and padded with gauze** [6], **stabilised with splint and bandaged** [7]. Monitor **vital signs** [8] and **urine output** [9]. Discuss with the **trauma or orthopaedics team** [10].

Short-term

The patient is transferred to a **definitive trauma centre** [11] and undergoes surgery to **clean the**

wound [12], apply **temporary external fixation** [13] and **repair soft tissue coverage** [14]. **The wound is assessed regularly** [15], and **neurovascular observations** [16] and routine **postoperative monitoring** [17] performed. **Early VTE prophylaxis** [18] should be commenced. **Definitive internal fixation** [19] is performed a few days later.

Long-term

Follow up in outpatient clinic 4–8 weeks [20] after discharge, with X-ray prior to appointment.

1 At least 16G cannulas or bigger are required to enable rapid transfusion if the patient begins to exsanguinate. If peripheral IV access cannot be obtained, intraosseous or central venous catheter under ultrasound guidance may be required.

2 Obtaining IV access and bloods occurs as soon as a patient arrives in the ED, even while paramedics are giving a history to the trauma lead. Ensure enough blood is collected to fill required tubes.

3 Although this patient has signs of moderate hypovolaemic shock, he does not meet the requirements for emergency transfusion (ongoing bleeding, symptomatic anaemia, SBP <90mmHg, tachycardia >120bpm) and can wait for cross-matched blood. Two units should be given to return the haemoglobin above 80×10^9/L. No other blood products are required to be transfused (fresh frozen plasma, platelets, cryoprecipitates) in this patient. Patients with signs of severe haemorrhage and ongoing bleeding should trigger the threshold for massive transfusion protocol and be given blood products to maintain adequate perfusion (guided by parameters including mean arterial pressure, heart rate, oxygen saturations, urine output, lactate and base deficit). The blood products should be given in equal amounts (1:1:1 ratio of red blood cells, plasma and platelets).

4 Administering IV antibiotics is one of the most important steps in managing open fractures which should commence as soon as possible and continue for 24–72 hours after wound closure. A delay in initiating antibiotics more than 3 hours after the injury leads to increased risk of infection. The type of antibiotic is determined by the type of wound and exposure to pathogens. Refer to local antibiotic guidelines for empiric therapy.

5 Tetanus prophylaxis should be administered if there is any doubt about vaccination history.

6 Irrigate with saline solution to remove gross debris and contamination. This should be a gentle clean so as not to dislodge blood clots. Definitive cleaning of the wound will occur in theatre, as open fractures require surgical exploration, debridement, irrigation and fixation. Gauze padding is applied to protect the wound and absorb wound seepage.

7 The aim of stabilisation is to reduce pain, minimise soft tissue trauma and prevent disruption of clots while awaiting definitive treatment.

8 Haemodynamic instability could indicate further haemorrhage or other issues such as fat embolism.

9 Consider inserting a urinary catheter to accurately record urine output which could drop if there is inadequate renal perfusion or kidney injury from rhabdomyolysis, or if IV contrast has been given for CT scan.

10 This injury requires specialist management; the trauma or orthopaedics team should be notified and involved in the patient's management as soon as possible.

11 Patients with serious trauma have significantly reduced morbidity and mortality if transferred to a designated trauma centre (10.4% compared with 13.8%, relative risk 0.75). With regard to open fracture, the most important predictor of infection is early transfer to a trauma centre (aside from early IV antibiotics).

12 In the absence of life-threatening injuries, surgery within 6 hours has no benefit compared with surgery within 6–24

hours (provided antibiotics are initiated early). The wound is explored, foreign materials and devitalised tissue debrided, and irrigated with copious saline. The injury should be classified according to the Gustilo–Anderson classification.

13 Definitive internal fixation is often delayed in open fractures until the wound is clean enough to minimise risk of osteomyelitis. Temporary external fixation stabilises the fracture to prevent further damage to surrounding tissue from bone movement, and can allow repair to soft tissues and vascular injury if required.

14 Repair and coverage of the soft tissue injury is required to allow healing and minimise development of infection, which would delay definitive fixation of the fracture.

15 The wound should be assessed for signs of infection daily and evaluated in theatre every 24–96 hrs, depending on the appearance of the wound at the previous assessment.

16 Compartment syndrome can still occur in the setting of an open fracture. Early signs of compartment syndrome include pain out of proportion to the injury, tense swollen compartments and pain with passive stretching. Rapid progression of symptoms over the course of a few hours is an important clue to the development of compartment syndrome. Motor deficits are a late sign and associated with irreversible damage to nerves and muscles. Compartment syndrome is a medical emergency and should be treated immediately by removing any compression (dressings, splints, casts, restrictive clothing) and definitively with a fasciotomy.

17 Patients must be monitored postoperatively for any immediate complications of surgery. These include signs of shock (septic or hypovolaemic), infection, reaction to anaesthesia, DVT and PE, urinary retention or renal failure.

18 Trauma creates a physiological hypercoagulable state in patients which increases the risk of VTE events beyond the inherent risk in other surgical patients. Anticoagulation with heparin or enoxaparin should be commenced as per the surgeon's preference; heparin may be more appropriate in patients who may need further urgent surgery.

19 Timing of definitive fixation is at the orthopaedic surgeon's discretion.

20 Follow-up is required to assess wounds, monitor for complications and assess union of the fracture.

CASE 48: Osteoarthritis and total hip replacement

History

- **A 70-year-old** [1] **male** [2] presents to the orthopaedic outpatient clinic after referral from his GP for a **total hip replacement** [3] due to **osteoarthritis** [4] .
- He has been experiencing ongoing pain in his left hip and knee for some **years** [5] .
- In his hip, he reports **pain** [6] of 7/10, mostly experienced in the **groin** [7] , exacerbated by rising from a chair, and **walking up stairs** [8] and which sometimes keeps him **awake at night** [9] .
- In his knee he reports **pain** [10] of 4/10 experienced generally **throughout the knee** [11].
- He experiences pain and stiffness particularly in the **morning** [12] .

- This is making it difficult for him to walk, with a negative effect on his ability to manage things around the home, and also to **socialise with friends** [13] , leading to him reporting he is feeling **"a bit down"** [14] .
- He reports rupturing his left anterior cruciate ligament 30 years previously, resulting in an ACL repair and **partial meniscectomy** [15] with good return of function, but is concerned he may also need a **knee replacement** [16] .
- He has a **BMI of 34** [17] but as part of **conservative management** [18] has lost 5kg over the past few years.
- He has no other **medical conditions** [19] .

1 It is estimated that approximately 85% of people over 70 years of age will have osteoarthritis (OA). It can affect any synovial joint, but it is most common in the knee, followed by hips and hands. Hip prostheses are designed to last 15–20 years, and therefore may never need revising in older patients. Knee replacements in those under 65 are generally avoided if possible.

2 OA has a higher incidence in women than men, especially in patients over 50.

3 90% of total hip replacements are due to end-stage osteoarthritis of the hip.

4 'Osteoarthritis' means inflammation of a joint. The most common kind is 'wear and tear' or primary OA. The articular cartilage begins to degrade, with thinning and sometimes cracking occurring over time. This can lead to pieces of cartilage coming loose and floating within the knee, which leads to further irritation of the joint. Over time, the cartilage can wear away completely, leading to bone rubbing on bone. More than 10% of men and 13% of women older than 60 will experience OA.
The other type is secondary OA, which affects joints that have been previously damaged through fractures, joint injury (chondral lesions), acquired or congenital deformities, avascular necrosis and diabetic neuropathy (Charcot joints).

5 OA typically has an insidious onset, affecting joints well before patients notice any symptoms, and then progressing from pain that resolves with rest, to pain that is ongoing and can be very debilitating.

6 The degree of pain can be useful as a comparison point for before and after surgery, to give an indication of degree of improvement.

7 Pain from OA of the hip is most often felt in the groin but can also be experienced in the lateral hip or deep in the buttock.

8 In knee OA, walking downhill is painful. In hip OA, walking uphill is painful.

9 This is a common complaint associated with severe OA, although other causes of night pain such as malignancy and infection need to be ruled out. Poor sleep can have a major impact on quality of life so should not be dismissed lightly. Pain at rest and pain that disturbs a patient's sleep are indication for a knee replacement.

10 OA in one joint can predispose patients to develop it in related joints, by causing them to alter their stance and gait to accommodate the initial joint affected. This then forces other joints out of alignment, predisposing those joints to OA also.

11 Knee OA presents with generalised pain throughout the knee, worse at night, and which can come on after exercise, standing for long periods, or lifting loads. Typically, no particular point of tenderness can be elicited on palpation. A Baker's cyst in the popliteal fossa may cause pain and tenderness at the back of the knee, but this is secondary to OA, and is not OA itself. If pain is elicited over the joint lines, it is more likely to be due to a meniscal tear. If the joint is unstable and the patient reports that it "gives way", a cruciate ligament rupture should be considered.

12 Symptoms of osteoarthritis include:
- deformity: including characteristics particular to OA such as Bouchard's nodes at the proximal interphalangeal joints (PIPJs), and Heberden's nodes at the distal interphalangeal joints
- pain: characteristically dull aching pain, most noticeable during or after movement; may keep patients awake at night and worsens throughout the day
- stiffness: most notable after awakening or a period of inactivity, improves throughout the day
- swelling: can be caused by soft tissue inflammation around the joint; Baker's cyst in the popliteal fossa is indicative of knee OA
- crepitus during movement: grinding or crunching sensation.

13 Even in those over 80 years old, joint replacements can transform patient lives, enabling a degree of mobility they may not have been able to achieve in many years. Severity of symptoms and effect on patients' lives help to determine the most appropriate treatment, including if and when surgery should be considered.

14 Quality of life as reported by patients is markedly lower in those with OA of the knee, when compared to age-matched norms, and it deteriorates in step with disease progression. Patients with knee OA have been reported as having twice the rate of depressive symptoms as those without knee OA.

15 Meniscectomy is a recognised risk factor for the development of OA and is no longer performed. Tibial plateau fractures are also associated with developing OA.

16 A total knee replacement involves implantation of a three-piece prosthesis to replace the femoral condyles and tibial plateau, with at least one polyethylene piece between the tibia and femur for shock absorption. The patella may also be replaced (typically in approximately 50% of cases secondary to implant failure, maltracking patella and osteolysis).

17 Risk factors for OA include increasing age, previous injury (e.g. ligament injury), family history of OA, being overweight and damage to the joint from other forms of arthritis.

18 Conservative management of OA includes simple analgesia, heat, minimal load exercise (such as swimming and cycling), weight loss, physiotherapy, mobility aids and local joint injections (corticosteroid or local anaesthetic).

19 Other significant medical conditions (particularly cardiac and respiratory conditions and illnesses) may preclude surgery.

Examination

- Observations are within normal parameters, and he is **afebrile** [1].
- **Heart sounds** [2] are dual with nil added, and lung fields are clear bilaterally.
- On **hip examination** [3], his gait is **antalgic** [4].
- **Passive flexion** [5] of the hip joint is painful, and there is a **leg length discrepancy** [6], with the left leg measuring 2cm less than the right. There is pain on palpation over the groin and greater trochanter on the left side.
- **Thomas test** [7] is positive to 30°, and there is a positive left **Trendelenburg sign** [8].
- On knee examination, the legs are well aligned with no **varus or valgus deformity** [9].
- There is some **crepitus** [10] on passive movement, and there is no palpable **Baker's cyst** [11]. The knee has preserved ROM.

1 RR is a sensitive indication of patient deterioration but is also often overlooked. HR can be elevated in patients due to multiple causes, including pathological (infection, anaemia, arrhythmia) and benign (anxiety). Hypotension can indicate severe infection or dehydration. It is important to determine if a hypotensive patient is in shock, in which case they may have other symptoms such as tachycardia, tachypnoea, hyperlactataemia, metabolic acidosis, and oliguria. In cases of shock, fluid resuscitation and identification of the cause of the shock are imperative.

2 Murmurs may indicate structural heart defects or valvular heart disease. In patients who require surgery, murmurs would need to be investigated to determine fitness for general anaesthetic, and to ascertain increased risk of complications in the peri-operative period.

3 As with all musculoskeletal examinations, perform the test on the unaffected side first for a comparison point, and have the patient suitably undressed for the examination.

4 Antalgic gaits develop as a way to mitigate pain whilst walking, typically with a shortened stance phase relative to the swing phase. Patients will often also use mobility aids.

5 Early OA presents with reduced ROM for abduction and rotation. More advanced OA adds difficulty with adduction, flexion and extension.

6 Reduced joint space and deterioration of joint ends can result in reduced true leg length (measured from anterior superior iliac spine to the tip of the medial malleolus).

7 The Thomas test assesses for fixed flexion deformity, which may be present in OA. The patient lies supine. The examiner places their hand under the patient's back to identify lumbar lordosis (which is a predictor of tight hip flexors). Ask the patient to flex the non-affected side, bringing their knee to their chest, then holding it in place. The leg on the table is the one being tested and should be able to remain on the table. If there is a contracture, it will raise off the table, and the angle between the thigh and table can then be measured to reveal the degree of fixed flexion deformity of the hip. Alternatively, the patient can raise their hips up together, then straighten their hips in turn.

8 In OA of the hip, a positive Trendelenburg sign can be an indication of pain inhibiting normal function of the abductor muscles. Ask the patient to stand on one leg for 30 seconds whilst keeping their upper body upright. If balance is an issue, support them or allow them to hold on to something. See if the pelvis stays level. Test their unaffected side first. The test is positive if the pelvis drops on the contralateral side whilst standing on the affected leg, or if they can only maintain a level pelvis by leaning their upper body to the affected side.

9 Varus deformity refers to excessive inward angulation towards the midline of the body. Varus knee or genu varum results in bow-leggedness. OA is commonly associated with varus knee, both as a cause and an effect. Valgus deformity is excessive outward angulation.

10 Crepitus in a joint is a popping or crackling sound (or sensation) that is indicative of OA.

11 Baker's cyst is also known as a popliteal cyst. It is a swelling in the popliteal fossa containing synovial fluid, often secondary to inflammation of the knee, which may be caused by OA, gout, haemophilia, psoriasis, other forms of arthritis (reactive, rheumatoid and septic), injury (e.g. cartilage tear) or lupus.

Investigations

- Weight-bearing **X-rays** [1] of the knees **(lateral and AP)** [2] show mild narrowing of the joint space of both knees which is worse on the left.
- The left knee shows a loss of joint space **medially** [3], accompanied by some osteophytic lipping, but no sclerosis.
- There is no varus deformity and the lateral compartment joint space is well preserved. This is **Grade 3 osteoarthritis** [4].
- Pelvic X-rays show that the sacrum and **sacroiliac joints appear normal** [5], right hip has mild narrowing of the joint space, but the left hip shows severe OA, with marked joint space narrowing, subchondral sclerosis and formation of multiple osteophytes. There is greater loss of joint space medially.
- None of the X-rays shows any visible fractures, and outside of the imaged joints there are no **focal areas of sclerosis or lucency** [6].

1 The request form should include details about the history and examination findings, especially history regarding previous surgeries and of injuries.

2 AP views are used to assess the medial compartment – the compartment most commonly affected by OA, potentially leading to a varus deformity of the knee wherein the distal leg is medially angulated relative to the knee. This view also shows the lateral compartment clearly. The lateral view is used to assess the patellofemoral compartment; also a skyline view provides a better assessment of this compartment. Skyline views are typically only performed if the patient has a lot of anterior knee pain.

3 OA that affects all knee compartments (medial femorotibial, patellofemoral, lateral femorotibial) and is severe is best treated by total knee replacement. OA in only one compartment (typically the medial femorotibial joint) can be treated with uni-compartmental knee replacement. This preserves the other compartment(s) and is most typically considered in young patients who then retain the option for a future total knee replacement.

4 OA has its own grading system - the Kellgren–Lawrence Grading System.

Kellgren–Lawrence Grading System					
	Grade 1	Grade 2	Grade 3	Grade 4	Grade 5
Joint space narrowing	Nil	Doubtful	Possible	Definite	Marked
Osteophytic lipping	Nil	Possible	Definite	Multiple osteophytes	Large osteophytes
Sclerosis	Nil	Nil	Nil	Present	Severe
Deformity of bone ends	Nil	Nil	Nil	Possible	Definite

5 Features of OA on X-ray are:
- loss of joint space: one of the earliest signs of osteoarthritis; non-specific as it is present in most types of arthritis, e.g. psoriatic and RA.
- subchondral sclerosis: joint surface appears sclerotic and more white.
- subchondral cysts within the sclerosis: also found in RA, gout, pseudogout and avascular necrosis. They are seen just under the joint cartilage, and typically are both numerous and small.
- osteophytes: small bony protuberances along joint margins. This finding helps to distinguish OA from other arthropathies, as it is specific to OA. These are typically best seen at the joint margin and are abnormal small bony growths.

6 A pathological fracture is one that is due to a disease rather than an injury. They can be an incidental finding on X-ray, and include causes such as osteoporosis, cancer, osteomalacia and osteomyelitis. These would include cystic changes or areas of lucency. If a pathological fracture is identified, further imaging needs to be performed to check the whole femur for further lesions, as this may alter management.

Management

Immediate

Provide the patient with information about his **surgery** [1] including risks, benefits and rehabilitation. Obtain **consent** [2] for **surgery** [3] and advise the patient to **fast** [4] prior to surgery.

Short-term

As this is a planned procedure, a cannula is inserted in theatre and **IV fluids** [5] commenced. **Prophylactic antibiotics** [6] will be given in theatre before the first incision, and extra precautions put in place to reduce the risk of **infection** [7]. The **surgery** [8] is performed by **exposing the hip area** [9] before removing the damaged joint and inserting the prosthesis. Following the procedure, commence the patient on **VTE** prophylaxis [10]. Provide **postoperative analgesia** [11]. Monitor **drain tube outputs** [12]. **Mobilise the patient** [13] after surgery with the aid of allied health. Stitches or staples from the wound are removed in approximately 10–14 days.

Long-term

Patients are given exercises to complete for the first month post-surgery. They are also shown how to safely shower, dress, toilet themselves and climb stairs, and **movements they need to avoid** [14]. Patients are advised **not to drive** [15] for 3 months after surgery. Monitor the patient for at least 1 year after the procedure. Look for signs of **infection** [16]. Patients should be made aware of the **risk factors** [17] and **strategies** [18] to mitigate this risk.

1 The primary goal is pain relief, with improvement in function and mobility being secondary aims. There are various surgical options, including:
- arthrodesis: surgical immobilisation of a joint by bone fusion
- arthroplasty: surgical reconstruction or replacement of part or all of the joint surface
- osteotomy: joint realignment by removal of bone to change alignment – used to correct hallux valgus, genu valgum, genu varus; not commonly performed in hips
- excision: joint removal without fusion.

2 The consent form should outline the indications for the surgery, the risks (both general and specific), and details of the anaesthetic. Risks of this surgery include: DVT and thromboembolism, wound infection, dislocation of the hip joint, the joint breaking (during or after surgery), nerve injury, urine retention and bladder infection, bowel blockage, loosening or wearing out of the joint, difference in leg length, bleeding into the wound, infection around the joint years later, failure of the joint, increased risks in smokers (of wound and chest infections, heart and lung complications and thrombosis) and death.

3 There are various forms of arthroplasty, the two most common hip arthroplasties being hemiarthroplasty (half the hip joint is replaced – i.e. the femoral head) and total arthroplasty (both the femoral head and socket are replaced).

4 Patients should be fasted prior to surgery to lower the risk of aspiration of stomach contents. The general guidelines are 6 hours for food, and 2 hours for clear fluids. Patients can have a general anaesthetic in the unfasted state using RSI to reduce the risk of aspiration; however, this is better avoided and is generally reserved for emergency situations.

5 IV fluids are used for fluid resuscitation and to maintain haemodynamic stability. All fluids are charted, so that it is clear how much and what has been given, as both hypo- and hypervolaemia can create problems. Hypovolaemia in the peri-operative period leads to low cardiac output with resultant decreased tissue perfusion, and severe hypovolaemia can result in shock and multi-organ failure. Peri-operative hypervolaemia is typically due to retention of fluids given during surgery, and can increase morbidity and mortality, and lengthen time spent in the ICU. Signs of fluid overload include elevated JVP, peripheral oedema and crackles in lung bases. In a normovolaemic patient not actively losing large amounts, 3L per day is considered standard, leading to the typical protocol of administering 1L over 8 hours. Hypovolaemia is typically managed with an initial bolus, followed by ongoing fluids.

6 Prophylactic antibiotics are important to prevent wound and bone infection. It takes approximately 10 minutes for IV antibiotics to adequately penetrate bone.

7 Due to the devastating effects of joint infection, orthopaedic surgeries involve extra precautions to reduce the risk, including surgeons in exhaust bodysuits to provide a barrier between the operating team and the patient. Laminar airflow ensures 300 or more air changes per hour.

8 First the joint is exposed before dislocating the femoral head and removing it at the neck. It is then replaced with a metal stem which is either cemented or "press fitted" into the hollow centre of the femur. A metal or ceramic ball is then placed on the upper part of the stem, and a spacer made of plastic, ceramic or metal is placed over this to provide a smooth gliding surface between the new ball and socket. For a hemiarthroplasty, this basically completes the surgery.

A hemiarthroplasty is typically used for either NOFs in older patients who don't have OA in the joint, or older patients who have primary arthritis with complete joint destruction. In a total hip arthroplasty, the acetabulum likewise has its damaged cartilage surface removed and is replaced with a metal socket that is fixed in place with screws, 'press-fit' or cement.

9 Different approaches can be used to access the hip joint, each having advantages and disadvantages. The common factors that guide the choice of operative approach include surgeon preference, risk of dislocation, and risk of damage to structures implicated in the approach.

10 Following surgery, especially arthroplasty, there is a significantly increased risk of VTE. Administration of LMWH such as enoxaparin halves the rate of DVT and lowers the rate of fatal PE by ~75%. LMWH is preferable to ordinary heparin. On discharge, new oral anticoagulant drugs are typically prescribed for a few weeks as they are easier to take (dabigatran, rivaroxaban, apixaban).

11 Analgesia is typically charted by the anaesthetist in theatre. Dosage may need to be adjusted for patients at risk of renal dysfunction or those with pre-existing kidney injury. Frequently, the patient is administered a nerve block prior to operation, most likely to be an epidural, which can provide effective analgesia for many hours. Postoperatively, a patient-controlled analgesia (PCA) device delivers a dose typically of opioids such as fentanyl or oxycodone into their IV when it is pressed. It has a pre-set dose and a lockout period so that patients cannot overdose. The epidural and PCA can be used for the first 24–48 hours, depending on patient pain.

12 A drain tube is inserted into the incision to drain blood and serous ooze and is removed 24–48 hours after surgery or once the drainage has stopped.

13 It is variable as to when patients are allowed to be fully weight-bearing, and this advice is given by the surgeons. Generally, patients are allowed to mobilise soon after surgery, given no immediate postoperative complications such as dislocation or intra-operative fracture.

14 The standard hip precautions consist of movements that need to be avoided for the first 3 months. These include flexing past 90°, bending down to pick things up off the floor, crossing legs at the knees or ankles, and lying on the operated hip. Patients are advised to sleep on their back for the first 6 weeks, using pillows between their legs to avoid rolling over.

15 Patients are advised not to drive due to the inhibited ability to apply strong force to brakes in a sudden braking situation (regardless of side). They should also avoid being a passenger in a car for the first 6 weeks.

16 One of the most feared complications of total hip replacement is prosthetic joint infection. Infective symptoms to look out for post arthroplasty include new pain, new loss of function, fever or wound inflammation. The most common causative organisms of prosthetic joint infections are staphylococcal skin commensals. Metalware infections are notoriously difficult to treat, as bacteria tend to create an antibiotic-impermeable biofilm over the metalware. Early treatment generally involves debridement and antibiotics; however, in the setting of chronic infection and sequelae, radical debridement with removal of all prosthetic material and involved soft tissue and bone is required. Antibiotic-impregnated cement may be placed into the joint space.

17 Risk factors for joint infection are obesity, diabetes, RA, age and steroid use.

18 Steps to avoid infection include taking antibiotics before any dental or medical procedure, as well as prompt medical treatment of all suspected UTIs.

CASE 49: Osteosarcoma

History

- A **17-year-old** [1] **Caucasian** [2] **male** [3] , with **no known medical history** [4] , presents with **3-month history** [5] of dull **left thigh pain** [6] .
- The pain was initially present **during physical activity** [7] , is now **worse at rest** [8] and with **recent swelling** [9] over the site.

- He denies any **precipitating trauma** [10] , **fever** [11] , **weight loss, sweats** [12] or any other **constitutional symptoms** [13].
- There is **no pain in any other limbs or joints** [14] .
- **Family history** [15] is unremarkable.
- He is very active and a promising **football player** [16] .

[1] Osteosarcoma is a rare cancer which has a bimodal age distribution, with peaks in the second decade and after 65 years of age. Although rare, osteosarcoma is the most common primary bone tumour in children and adolescents and the fifth most common cancer in adolescents aged 15–19 years. Primary bone tumours such as osteosarcoma and Ewing sarcoma are responsible for 6% of all childhood cancers.

[2] Sickle cell disease is an important differential to consider in a patient with limb pain. The prevalence of sickle cell trait is highest in people from the Mediterranean, India and Caribbean countries and of African descent. Leg pain in sickle cell patients can be due to vaso-occlusive disease, bone infarction or DVT.

[3] Males are more likely to develop osteosarcoma than females; however, females generally develop osteosarcoma earlier than males due to the relationship between onset of cancer and growth spurts, which usually happen earlier in girls.

[4] Some patients with osteosarcoma have a genetic predisposition, particularly with genes associated with retinoblastoma and Li–Fraumeni syndrome. In older adults, osteosarcoma is generally a secondary cancer due to previous radiation exposure, Paget disease and other benign bone lesions (e.g. fibrous dysplasia, chronic osteomyelitis).

[5] The time course of symptoms is important; swelling that has arisen within days is likely an inflammatory/infective type cause (i.e. an abscess), while symptoms that have been present for years and are not progressive are more likely to be benign lesions (i.e. fibroma, osteoma). The pattern of progressively worsening symptoms over the course of months is more suspicious for a malignant lesion.

[6] The differential list for thigh pain is very broad. Using a surgical sieve (such as VITAMINC) to consider possible causes can help broaden your list and reduce the likelihood of missing the more uncommon presentations such as

neoplasm. Neoplasm should be considered in patients (particularly if they are young) complaining of generalised hip, thigh or knee pain, especially if there are systemic symptoms (fever, night sweats, weight loss) or an absence of precipitating factors such as trauma or overuse. Other differentials to consider include haematoma, myositis ossificans (bone-like tissue growth in muscle after an injury), stress fracture, tendon avulsion injury, osteomyelitis, gout and non-malignant bone lesions.

[7] Osteosarcoma often starts with pain during activity which can be dismissed as muscular ache or injury from contact sports.

[8] A history of progressively worsening pain, which is worse at rest, is the typical pattern for osteosarcoma but can occur with other bone tumours or soft tissue sarcomas. Keep in mind, however, that the pain may only occur after exercise. Pain at night or at rest is likely due to growth of the lesion in bone, whereas pain with weight-bearing activities is typically due to an inflammatory process. The other important diagnosis to keep in mind with this type of pain is chronic osteomyelitis.

[9] Swelling localised to the site of chronic pain in a limb is a red flag for osteosarcoma or some other malignant process. Causes of swelling in a limb can be growth of tissue (i.e. a tumour) or influx of fluid (i.e. inflammation, haematoma, lymphoedema, pus). A rapidly growing mass over weeks or months is more concerning of a malignant process compared to a benign slow-growing mass. A mass which waxes and wanes in size suggests a ganglion cyst or vascular malformation.

[10] Acute pain and swelling after trauma to a limb would be indicative of a fracture. Chronic pain and swelling after trauma could be due to bone callus, osteomyelitis, a venous thrombotic event, or myositis ossificans.

11 Fever could be due to an infective or inflammatory process (i.e. osteomyelitis) or malignant process as in osteosarcoma.

12 The B symptoms of fever, unintentional weight loss and sweats are typically associated with a malignancy, classically lymphomas; however, they may also be due to infections (tuberculosis, HIV, malaria, etc.), endocrinopathy (hyperthyroidism, phaeochromocytoma, carcinoid syndrome) or other rarer causes (temporal arteritis). When present in a patient with osteosarcoma, B symptoms suggest the disease is in the late stages.

13 Chest pain or respiratory symptoms could be associated with sickle cell disease or an autoimmune condition. Osteomyelitis could be associated with malaise and fever.

14 Pain in other bones or joints could be due to metastatic spread of cancer to bone at multiple sites, or an autoimmune condition such as rheumatoid or juvenile arthritis, particularly if the pain is more arthralgic than bone pain.

15 Osteosarcoma has an association with some genetic conditions; therefore, family history can be of use. Family history may also be of some benefit in evaluating for other cancers which may arise in, or metastasise to the bone (breast cancer, multiple myeloma, etc.) or alternative diagnoses (i.e. sickle cell).

16 Chronic thigh pain in someone who is physically active could be due to an 'overuse' injury such as stress fracture or referred pain from the hip or knee (osteitis pubis, tendinopathy, OA). Patients who play contact sports may attribute pains to an injury and present later. The treatment of osteosarcoma, which includes any combination of radiation, chemotherapy, surgical resection and amputation, will also have implications for the patient's future sporting activities.

Examination

- The patient appears **well** [1] and **comfortable** [2].
- **Neurovascular exam** [3] of the limbs is normal.
- There is a palpable **mass** [4] above the left knee, which is **tender** [5], **deep** [6], **firm** [7], **non-mobile** [8] and **poorly circumscribed** [9] with no **erythema, warmth or changes of overlying skin** [10].
- **Full musculoskeletal** [11] assessment reveals no other masses or tenderness.
- The **heart sounds are normal, abdomen** [12] is soft and non-tender and **lungs** [13] are clear.

1 A sick-looking patient immediately raises concerns of someone who is systemically unwell and requires immediate management. A patient who is cachectic would have a severe chronic underlying disease (e.g. metastatic cancer, chronic osteomyelitis). Most patients with osteosarcoma present due to symptoms of pain or swelling and would not be experiencing the systemic effects that might be present with metastatic disease.

2 Discomfort can be due to pain or effects associated with other symptoms (e.g. breathlessness in sickle cell crisis, nausea due to infection). If a patient appears uncomfortable, identify the cause and manage accordingly.

3 Neurovascular signs such as limb weakness, altered sensation, reduced or absent reflexes, unequal pulses, pale peripheries, venous distension or oedema occur when there is injury or disruption to the nerves, arteries or veins, and might indicate mass effect from growing tumours or direct local invasion.

4 Patients presenting with lumps or bumps is very common, and it can be difficult to distinguish between benign and concerning masses.

5 A mass which is tender to palpation is a key examination finding for osteosarcoma. Soft tissue sarcomas are generally painless, only becoming painful due to mass effect and compression of adjacent tissues.

6 A superficial mass, particularly if it is over muscle bulk, is unlikely to be a bone tumour, which will feel like a deep mass (except when the bone itself is superficial, such as the anterior tibia). When palpating a mass, visualise the different tissues beneath your fingers, and consider where the mass is and how it might relate to each of the tissues (i.e. skin, adipose tissues, tendons, muscles, arteries, veins, lymphatics, nerves, cartilage, bones).

7 A soft or fluctuant mass is due to fluid or a soft tissue (such as adipose tissue) and could be a deep abscess, oedema, haematoma or, in the case of adipose tissue, a lipoma. Being a bone tumour, an osteosarcoma will be a firm/hard mass.

8 'Mobility' of masses refers to how tethered they are to adjacent tissues. Osteosarcoma will not be mobile as it is a growth of the bone tissue. Other sarcomas which are not adherent to the bone will be somewhat mobile but if adherent to adjacent tissues they are not technically 'mobile' (consider how an enlarged lymph node would feel different from a leiomyosarcoma in the quadriceps).

9 Try to palpate the edge of the mass and determine if you can find a boundary and how clear it is. A well-circumscribed margin is a reassuring sign, suggesting that whatever process is occurring is very localised and local invasion is absent or very limited. A tumour which has invaded adjacent tissue will not have a clear margin and it will be difficult to tell where it ends.

10 Erythema and warmth can be associated with a tumour, haematoma or infection. A rapidly enlarging, red, warm and tender mass is highly suggestive of an abscess or infection, particularly if there is an associated wound to the skin and constitutional symptoms.

11 Bones are the second most common site for metastasis of osteosarcoma (behind lungs). Pay particular attention to the spine, proximal femur and humerus, which are the most common sites for bone metastases.

12 A complete physical examination should be done to provide a comprehensive clinical picture of the patient. Bone is also a very common site of metastatic spread from other cancers (highly vascular and dynamic tissue with constant turnover). Patients with metastatic spread would be expected to have some clinical signs based on their primary cancer (e.g. lung cancer, bowel cancer, liver cancer).

13 The lungs are the most common site of metastasis of osteosarcoma, with 10–20% of patients presenting with pulmonary metastases.

Investigations

- **FBE** [1] and **UECs** [2] are normal.
- LFTs show markedly **elevated ALP** [3] ; **calcium and phosphate** [4] are normal.
- **Plain film X-ray** [5] shows **destructive lesions** [6] within the trabecula of the **distal femur** [7] with **periosteal growths** [8] .

- **MRI** [9] shows **extension of the tumour beyond the cortex** with **enhancement and oedema involving the adjacent soft tissues** [10] .
- **Chest CT** [11] and **radionuclide bone scan** [12] with **SPECT** [13] does not show any **metastatic lesions** [14] .

1 Lymphoma can occasionally arise as a bone lesion (primary lymphoma of bone), in which case a raised WCC would be expected. Osteomyelitis or another infective/inflammatory cause may also result in an elevated WBC count.

2 Renal function should be assessed to determine fitness for administration of medications, IV contrast (i.e. for CT scans) if required, and for future surgery. Additionally, patients with cancer are at increased risk of kidney injury through mechanisms such as tumour lysis syndrome and other processes not well understood. Renal failure is one of the core presenting problems for patients with multiple myeloma.

3 ALP is an enzyme derived from the liver, bones and placenta (detectable in 3rd trimester of pregnancy). An elevated ALP without a concomitant rise in GGT suggests a bone source (provided patient is not pregnant). ALP can also be fractionated to identify if it originates from liver or bone.

4 Calcium and phosphate levels can be affected by bone turnover and are regulated by parathyroid hormone. Test parathyroid hormone levels in patients with deranged calcium or phosphate. Elevated levels of calcium and phosphate can affect renal function, while small changes in calcium level can have significant neurological effects.

5 Plain film X-ray is the initial investigation choice. Characteristic findings of osteosarcoma include blastic and destructive lesions of the trabecular bone, periosteal reaction, indistinct margins or a soft tissue mass.

6 Osteosarcoma can present with both destructive and ossifying lesions.

7 The distal femur is the most common site for osteosarcoma. Areas of bone which have the greatest increase in bone length and size are the most frequent sites for osteosarcoma, particularly the metaphyseal regions of the distant femur, proximal tibia and proximal humerus.

8 Periosteal growths are extensions of bone tissue into the soft tissue and suggest a malignant process, particularly if the margins are indistinct.

9 MRI is an important step for staging and surgical planning. Macroscopically, osteosarcomas are bulky tumours which invade into the medullary cavity. The extent of medullary invasion is often more extensive than the bulky appearance would suggest, thus MRI can identify the extent of invasion and allow surgeons to plan their excision.

10 These features of local invasion beyond the bone tissue are a feature of a malignant process.

11 80% of osteosarcoma metastases are in the chest. CT is the best modality to assess the thorax for metastatic spread; however, any suspect lesions which are indeterminate should be biopsied for histologic confirmation to avoid false positive results.

12 Bone scan with technetium is the best imaging modality to assess the entire skeleton for additional lesions.

13 SPECT (single-photon emission computed tomography) is like a PET scan in that it can assess the whole body for areas of metabolic and functional activity (i.e. active tumours). It has a lower cost, is more widely available, uses different radioisotopes, but has poorer contrast and spatial resolution.

14 Metastatic spread at time of diagnosis is common and is the single greatest prognostic factor. Patients with no overt metastatic spread at diagnosis may often have small metastases that are not detectable. The incorporation of adjuvant chemotherapy has increased long-term survival significantly (from 16% to 70%), most likely due to the destruction of distant small metastases before they become detectable.

Management

Immediate

The patient is referred to an **orthopaedic surgeon specialising** [1] in sarcomas where the tumour is **biopsied** [2], and the diagnosis of a **high grade** [3] **intramedullary osteosarcoma** [4] is confirmed.

Short-term

The patient is commenced on **neo-adjuvant chemotherapy** [5] after which the tumour is **surgically resected** [6] with a **bone graft** [7] to repair the defect.

The patient is referred to **physiotherapy** [8], **social work** [9] and **psychology** [10] prior to discharge home.

Long-term

Histology of the tumour at time of resection shows **good response to neo-adjuvant chemotherapy** [11], and the patient is continued on the same chemotherapy regimen for 6 months. He is followed up with **regular plain film X-ray, MRI, CT chest and whole-body bone scan with SPECT** [12] for surveillance.

1 Referral to an experienced specialist orthopaedic surgeon can improve outcomes in terms of survival and limb-sparing surgery. The surgeon is the lead clinician with regard to investigation and treatment, but nearly always works as part of an MDT to provide the best care.

2 The biopsy approach is determined by the orthopaedic surgeon and may be an open incisional biopsy or radiologically guided needle biopsy. The planning for biopsy considers implications for further surgery and aims to minimise the risk of seeding the tumour into other tissues.

3 Tumour grading is essential to determine prognosis and the therapeutic approach (chemotherapy and timing of surgery).

4 Intramedullary is the most common type of osteosarcoma, accounting for 80–90% of tumours. It typically affects the metaphysis of long bones and is most common in adolescents and young adults.

5 Neo-adjuvant chemotherapy can reduce the extent of the tumour, leading to an increase in limb-salvage resections and survival. Good response to the regimen of chemotherapy agents also predicts the response to post-surgical adjuvant chemotherapy.

6 Resection of tumour can involve amputation or limb-salvage resection. Limb-salvage resection requires an appropriate anatomical approach to be possible and neo-adjuvant chemotherapy to shrink or control the growth of the tumour with adequate margins. There is no difference in overall or disease-free survival between limb-salvage surgery and amputation, provided there is appropriate patient selection.

7 The bone defect is repaired by a bone graft, which can be autologous (tissue from the same individual), allograft (donated from a cadaver or living donor) or synthetic.

8 Physiotherapy is essential to assist the patient to recover function after a bone resection. If an amputation is required, a prosthetist should be involved in the patient's rehabilitation.

9 The impact of chemotherapy and surgery can exacerbate life stressors (or be a life stressor in itself), therefore early referral to social work can help to identify and manage issues (financial, work, study, home supports, etc.).

10 A potentially life-ending illness can be a major psychological burden for patients and their families. Refer early to a psychologist and link patients in with support and advocacy groups (e.g. Teenage Cancer Trust).

11 One aspect of neo-adjuvant chemotherapy is that it acts as a trial of chemotherapy medication; thus, a good response before surgery means that it will continue to have a good response after surgery. It is also a predictor of better overall prognosis.

12 The timing and frequency of monitoring and surveillance is guided by NICE guidelines and aims to assess immediate and short-term response to treatment, as well as longer-term surveillance for recurrence or metastatic spread. The imaging modality should be the same as that used at diagnosis. The vast majority of recurrences happen within 10 years; however, these patients will require indefinite follow-up due to the risk of treatment-related toxicity.

CASE 50: Rotator cuff injury

History

- **A 60-year-old** [1] , **right-hand dominant** [2] female, with well-controlled **T2DM and hyperlipidaemia** [3] presents with **right-shoulder pain** [4] which is **well-localised** [5] and **non-radiating** [6] since a **fall 2 days ago** [7] where she tripped and landed on an **outstretched arm** [8] .
- She has associated **weakness** [9] in that shoulder.
- She denies any **head strike** [10] , **neck pain** [11] or **neurological deficits** [12] .
- She had **chronic pain in the right shoulder** [13] which was **treated with NSAIDs** [14] and **physiotherapy** [15] for the last 6 months and has not had any **previous surgery** [16] or **intra-articular injections** [17] . She is well otherwise.
- The patient is a **retired teacher who regularly swims and plays tennis** [18] .
- She is a **non-smoker** [19] and non-drinker.

[1] Increasing age is a risk factor for rotator cuff injuries and severity of the injury. 28% of patients over the age of 60 have a full thickness tear, increasing to 65% in those over the age of 70. Age is also relevant when deciding how to manage these injuries as older patients with multiple comorbidities may be better managed conservatively, whereas younger, healthier and more active patients would benefit more from definitive surgical repair.

[2] Handedness is important from both a pathophysiological perspective and in determining management and outcome. Overuse of the joint is a risk factor for rotator cuff injuries; therefore, these injuries are more likely to occur in the dominant arm. An injury to the patient's dominant arm has greater subsequent impact on their quality of life and may influence the decision about conservative vs. surgical treatment.

[3] Comorbidities such as diabetes mellitus, RA, hyperlipidaemia, obesity and Marfan or Ehlers–Danlos syndromes can contribute to tendon pathology and are important risk factors for joint injuries. Diabetes is also a risk factor for adhesive capsulitis. Patients with diabetes and hyperlipidaemia have a higher risk for cardiovascular disease, which can impact decisions around surgery and should be further investigated if surgery is indicated.

[4] There are many possible causes of shoulder pain which can involve any of the structures of the joint itself (bones, ligaments, glenoid labrum), peri-articular tissues (tendons, muscles, bursae) or referred pain from the cervical spine. Patients with rotator cuff tears can be asymptomatic or present with severe acute pain, classically over the lateral deltoid and worse with overhead activities. There is no clear correlation between degree of pain and extent of tear and the absence or presence of pain should not influence clinical decisions.

[5] Poorly localised pain often has an extrinsic cause (referred pain); consider thoracic (MI, PE or pneumonia) or abdominal pathology (gall bladder disease) in patients with localised shoulder pain and normal shoulder examination. Women and diabetics with acute coronary syndrome often present with atypical symptoms and tend to fare worse due to delay in diagnosis and treatment.

[6] Sharp pain radiating from neck into shoulder can be due to cervical nerve root impingement.

[7] Rotator cuff injuries can be chronic, acute or acute on chronic injuries. Trauma is a common cause of acute injuries. Patients who present with a fall, even clearly mechanical falls, should be further assessed to determine if there are any underlying risk factors that put them at increased risk of further falls.

[8] Obtain a detailed history of the circumstances of the fall, the height from which they fell, what they landed on. Ask the patient to demonstrate the position of the arm when they landed and where on the arm they landed (with their non-injured arm!) to understand the direction of the forces and the likely injuries.

[9] Weakness in the shoulder can be due to pain, injury to the tissues required for movement (tendons and muscles) or neurological injury (brachial plexus or cervical spine) and is therefore a non-specific symptom. Weakness in a full tear rotator cuff injury is a necessary part of the diagnosis.

[10] Any patient presenting with a fall should be asked about head strike, and if the fall was witnessed, seek confirmation from the witnesses.

[11] Cervical radiculopathy may present with neck pain, particularly if there are neurological signs such as weakness, reduced sensation or diminished tendon reflexes.

12 An injury to the nerves of the brachial plexus or cervical roots can present with neurapraxia distally to the injury. A full neurological and cervical spine examination is required to exclude neurological injury. Traumatic brachial plexus injuries generally occur due to stretch of the plexus from a downward force on the shoulder. The mechanism of injury in this patient does not correlate with a traumatic brachial plexus injury.

13 Rotator cuff injuries can be considered as a continuum of disease from impingement → tendinopathy → rotator cuff tear → rotator cuff arthropathy. Natural ageing and overuse of the joint can lead to degeneration of the tissues, weakness of the rotator cuff tendons, joint subluxation and impingement. Often a rotator cuff injury begins with impingement of the supraspinatus tendon then leading to a small tear of the supraspinatus which then further progresses to a full tear of any of the rotator cuff muscles.

14 Long-term regular use of NSAIDs is not advised due to the risk of GI ulcers, effect on renal function and cardiovascular events.

15 Conservative treatment of partial tears and injuries is often the most appropriate course of action, with physiotherapy being the primary treatment. The aim of

physiotherapy is to modify activity to prevent further injury, restore flexibility of the joint and strengthen the muscles to improve shoulder stability and function. Non-operative treatment has a variable success rate between 33% and 92%.

16 A surgical history can provide much useful information, particularly if there has been any surgery to the injured joint or other joints. Previous surgery is also useful to gain an understanding of anaesthetic risks (difficult airways, reactions to anaesthetic agents, etc.).

17 Glucocorticoid injections may be used to treat inflammatory shoulder pains such as inflammatory arthritis or bursitis, but can increase the risk of septic arthritis if the injection is intra-articular.

18 Some occupations and sports which require overhead activities are risk factors for rotator cuff and shoulder injuries and they generally present at a younger age and involve the glenoid labrum. Typical activities which produce a high frequency of rotator cuff injuries include swimming, tennis, throwing balls, golf, etc.

19 Smoking is associated with an increased risk for rotator cuff tear and has implications for surgery (hypercoagulability, poor wound healing, respiratory illness, etc.).

Examination

- The patient **appears comfortable** [1] with her arm in a sling.
- She is **haemodynamically stable and afebrile** [2].
- **Cardiopulmonary assessment** [3] is unremarkable, **brachial and radial pulses** [4] are equal, and **neurological assessment** [5] is unremarkable.
- On **examination of the shoulders** [6], there are no **abrasions, bruises, joint deformities** [7], **erythema, swelling** [8], **scars** [9] or **atrophy** [10] to the shoulder.

- On palpation, the **humeral greater tuberosity is tender** [11] and there is no **warmth or effusion** [12].
- **Active abduction is painless** [13] **and reduced to 20°** [14] **and external rotation reduced to 60°** [15].
- **Passive movement** [16] is not restricted.
- **'Empty can' test** [17], **'drop arm' test** [18] and **resistance against external rotation** [19] demonstrate weakness of the right shoulder.

1 Shoulder pain at rest may suggest fracture or shoulder dislocation in a trauma patient, or septic or inflammatory arthritis. Other possible causes of shoulder pain could be referred pain from diaphragmatic irritation (splenic injury, ruptured ectopic pregnancy, hepatobiliary disease), respiratory (upper lobe pneumonia, apical lung tumour, pulmonary embolus), cardiovascular (myocardial ischaemia) or neurological (cervical nerve root compression, brachial plexus lesion, spinal cord lesion, suprascapular nerve compression).

2 Vital signs outside normal parameters should trigger further assessment and investigations to ensure the patient is fit for surgery if required. Fever in a patient with a painful joint would raise suspicion of septic arthritis, particularly if the joint was inflamed, swollen or had recent surgery.

3 Auscultation of the lungs and heart can quickly screen for any major cardiovascular or respiratory issues that may relate to the current presentation (i.e. myocardial ischaemia or pneumonia) or which may impact surgical management.

4 Absent or reduced pulse to the affected arm could indicate a vascular injury to the axillary artery or thoracic outlet syndrome.

5 Assess power in all muscle groups and sensation in all dermatomes. Cervical root compression often affects C5–C6, which are responsible for shoulder abduction.

6 Shoulder exams, like all musculoskeletal exams, follows the same principles of adequate exposure, 'look, feel, move' and special tests.

7 Fully expose the joint and examine from all angles, comparing the injured side with the uninjured side.

Deformity or asymmetry would suggest underlying fracture or dislocation. Direct trauma onto the shoulder can result in acromioclavicular dislocation and would present with abrasions, bruising or deformity. Deformity of joints may also be due to chronic arthritis.

8 Erythema over the joint is due to underlying inflammation and suggests there may be active arthritis or infection.

9 Look for evidence of previous surgery or injuries.

10 Atrophic muscles indicate a chronic underlying pathology.

11 The supraspinatus distally attaches to the greater tubercle of the humerus and forms the superior aspect of the rotator cuff. Tenderness may be due to injury to this muscle or the joint underneath (labrum tear, fracture, ligamentous injury, etc.). To avoid missed injuries, palpate all bones and joints from the sternoclavicular joint around to the scapula.

12 A joint which is hot to touch should immediately raise suspicion of septic arthritis and would require joint aspiration. Swelling can be due to synovitis (joint feels boggy) or a joint effusion (swelling is fluctuant, and fluid can be pushed through the joint).

13 Weakness in range of movement that is painless is strongly suggestive of a complete rotator cuff tear or neurological injury.

14 Abduction of the shoulder tests the glenohumeral joint and deltoid/supraspinatus function to 90°, with elevation usually possible to 180° with the additional movement of the scapula. Often these two joints move together, so it can be difficult to distinguish between glenohumeral and scapula pathology if abduction is reduced. The 'empty can' test isolates the glenohumeral joint and can help confirm pathology limited to this joint. Initiation of abduction is provided by the deltoid, with the supraspinatus providing

additional power when the joint is partially abducted, therefore weakness at minimal abduction only suggests deltoid pathology. The inability to abduct more than 20°, particularly when the limitation is not due to pain, suggests a significant injury to the supraspinatus such as a complete tear.

15 External rotation of the shoulder is achieved through the infraspinatus and teres minor.

16 Reduced active movements of joints can be due to pathology with the joint itself (i.e. OA) or with the muscles and tendons acting on the joint or nerves innervating those muscles. In general, if active AND passive movement are reduced, the pathology is likely to be intra-articular, whereas if passive movement is preserved but active movement reduced, the pathology is likely to be muscular or neurological.

17 The 'empty can' test requires both shoulders to be abducted to 90°, flexed to 30° and arms supinated (thumbs pointing to ground as if emptying a can). Push down on both hands to test resistance (strength of abduction). This test isolates abduction of the glenohumeral joint from the scapula. Weakness suggests injury to the supraspinatus and this test would be positive if this tendon was injured (i.e. it has high sensitivity and negative predictive value).

18 The 'drop arm' test involves elevating the arm to 180° and then asking the patient to slowly lower the arm laterally. A positive result occurs when the patient is unable to maintain abduction and the arm drops to the side (usually when it reaches 90° abduction), which is strongly suggestive of supraspinatus tendon tear.

19 The elbows should be flexed at 90° and the patient externally rotates their arms against resistance. Weakness in one shoulder suggests infraspinatus pathology and would be positive if there was a tear in the tendon of this muscle. The involvement of more than two tendons in a rotator cuff tear is categorised as a 'massive' tear.

Investigations

- **FBE** [1] and **UECs** [2] are normal.
- **ECG** [3] shows normal sinus rhythm.
- Plain film **X-rays** [4] show no fracture or dislocation with **preserved joint space** [5].
- **Ultrasound** [6] shows a **complete tear of the supraspinatus tendon** [7] and **partial thickness tear** [8] of the infraspinatus tendon.
- The patient is sent for **MRI** [9], which confirms the ultrasound findings.

1 In an otherwise healthy person, a normal full blood count is expected. Elevated WCC would suggest underlying inflammation or infection. A GI bleed (from regular NSAID use) is often detected from a low haemoglobin in routine FBE.

2 This patient is diabetic and been taking regular NSAIDs so is at increased risk of kidney dysfunction. Testing renal

function will be beneficial in the setting of potentially nephrotoxic medications.

3 The patient has some cardiovascular risk factors, therefore an ECG is a straightforward investigation for ischaemic heart disease and for surgical decision-making.

4 The use of plain film X-rays should be the first-line imaging of the shoulder if there is a history of trauma, joint deformity or suspected OA. Otherwise, X-rays have very limited use in the investigation of other causes of shoulder pain. Views should include AP, AP in internal/external rotation, axillary and outlet.

5 Loss of joint space and/or presence of osteophytes would indicate the presence of OA.

6 Ultrasound can have up to 90% specificity and sensitivity when performed by an experienced radiologist, which is equivalent to an MRI. Other benefits of ultrasound are its low cost, ease of access, safety and ability to perform dynamic imaging, so it should be the second-line imaging after plain film X-ray. Ultrasound may be of limited value in assessing very small tears, very large tears or partial thickness tears.

7 A complete tear of the tendon is full thickness and full width, resulting in the muscle becoming detached from the insertion point. This finding correlates with the patient's inability to abduct the arm more than 20° and would require surgical repair.

8 A partial thickness tear often starts from the articular surface of the tendon, which has a poorer blood supply than the bursal surface (and is more susceptible to chronic injury), which then progresses towards the bursal surface. An equivocal finding on ultrasound may be due to the limitations of ultrasound or the radiologist and may require further imaging with MRI to confirm the degree of injury.

9 MRI should be requested if ultrasound is negative and there is ongoing pain, or if the ultrasound findings are equivocal and further detail is required. It is the imaging modality of choice for suspected rotator cuff injuries if an experienced sonographer is not available. MR arthrography is the gold standard imaging technique if MRI is normal, but rotator cuff injury is still suspected.

Management

Immediate

Provide adequate **analgesia** [1] and **contact the orthopaedics team** [2] for review. Do **not fast the patient** [3] unless advised otherwise by the orthopaedics team.

Short-term

The patient is **scheduled for theatre as an outpatient** [4]. **Physiotherapy** and **occupational therapy** [5] review the patient, and she is **discharged home from the ED** [6]. An uncomplicated **arthroscopic repair of the tendons** [7] is performed 2 weeks later.

Long-term

The patient is given an **abduction brace for 6 weeks** [8] and attends **regular physiotherapy** [9]. **At 6 months** [10] she is cleared to return to playing tennis and has no further issues.

[1] In most patients, regular paracetamol and NSAIDs should provide enough pain relief. Limit dose and duration of NSAIDs in patients at risk of renal dysfunction.

[2] This patient will require surgical repair, therefore early referral to orthopaedics is warranted.

[3] Most rotator cuff injuries do not require immediate surgery, and many can be managed conservatively with physical therapy only. Injuries which require immediate surgery are not urgent and may be delayed up to 6 weeks.

[4] Indications for immediate surgery (i.e. a trial of conservative management is not recommended) are acute full thickness tears with significant loss of function or acute on chronic tears in otherwise healthy adults. These injuries should be operated on within 3 weeks and no later than 6 weeks to prevent muscle atrophy which is associated with poorer surgical outcomes, particularly in older patients. These patients will be scheduled into a non-urgent theatre list.

[5] Physiotherapists can advise about exercises and stretches to minimise further injury and maximise joint mobility, as well as arrange braces or slings for comfort if required. Occupational therapists can assess the degree of functional impairment. Both teams can also assist with assessing falls risks and advising modifications to reduce future falls risks.

[6] There is no indication to admit this patient to hospital.

[7] Arthroscopic repair is recommended over open repair due to the lower complication rates, quicker recovery and better outcomes; many arthroscopies are performed as day cases.

[8] This is a brace which prevents the arm from abducting, with the aim to reduce strain on the repair and allow time for it to heal.

[9] Physiotherapists guide the rehabilitation programme and are integral in returning patients to work.

[10] Most patients can do light activities above shoulder height at 3 months, and more vigorous activities at 6 months. This time frame depends on the degree of injury, success of surgery and other variables. It can take up to 2 years for full strength and ROM to be regained.

CASE 51: Appendicitis

History

- A **10-year-old** [1] **male** [2] with **no significant past medical history** [3] presents with **constant** [4] **right lower quadrant abdominal pain** [5] worsening over the **past 48 hours** [6].
- The patient reports that the pain was initially **central before migrating to the right lower quadrant** [7].
- His parents report he has **not been interested in food** [8], had a **fever** [9] at home, has had a couple of **vomits** [10] and **loose stools** [11] and is complaining of **abdominal pain when passing urine** [12].
- The pain is aggravated by **movement and coughing** [13].
- He grew up in a **smoke-free** [14] home.
- His parents **deny any recent coryzal symptoms** [15].
- The patient has no known **allergies and takes no regular medications** [16].

[1] Appendicitis is one of the most common acute abdominal surgical conditions and is the most common reason for emergency abdominal surgery in children. It can present at any age but is most commonly seen between the ages of 10 to 19 years. In childhood 95% of cases are in children over the age of five. It is important to consider the age of the patient when considering differentials. In particular, gynaecological pathologies must be considered in post-menarchal females as a cause of the pain, and a gynaecological history should be taken as part of the initial history.

[2] The incidence of appendicitis is slightly lower in females compared to males, at a ratio of 1:1.3 male to female.

[3] In children, past medical history is important as it may indicate other potential differentials as a cause of the patient's pain. It also outlines the general health of the child and also identifies whether they have ever had any previous abdominal surgery, which is important to consider when proceeding to operative management as it may indicate altered anatomy or presence of adhesions.

[4] Constant abdominal pain suggests localised peritonitis, which is in keeping with a diagnosis of appendicitis. Intermittent abdominal pain would lower clinical suspicion of appendicitis as that would suggest the pain may be due to another cause. Cramping pain may occasionally also be present in appendicitis.

[5] Classically, abdominal pain will be present in the right lower abdominal quadrant. However, variation in anatomy may also cause atypical presentations of appendicitis-related pain. Flank or back pain may be present with a retrocaecal appendix. Suprapubic pain may be present with a pelvic appendix. If the appendix is long and the tip is inflamed the pain may occur on the left side or upper abdomen due to migration of the tip towards that area. It is important to consider that the appendix may lie in different positions for children with congenital abnormalities of intestinal position; examples include after repair of diaphragmatic hernias, gastroschisis or omphaloceles, or in cases of uncorrected malrotation.

[6] Appendicitis usually declares itself within a few days and migration of the pain to the lower right quadrant often occurs within the first 24 hours. Advanced presentations are more commonly seen in younger children, often due to non-specific or difficult-to-elicit symptoms. There is a strong correlation between likelihood of perforation and duration of symptoms.

[7] Pain usually begins as a dull, periumbilical pain before localising to the right lower quadrant once the parietal peritoneum becomes inflamed.

[8] Anorexia is almost always associated with acute appendicitis. However, in the paediatric population particularly, absence of anorexia is less specific at excluding appendicitis, as this symptom may be absent in up to 40% of children.

[9] Fevers generally present within 24–48 hours after symptom onset.

[10] 75% of patients with appendicitis will also experience nausea and vomiting. Often vomiting will only occur once or twice as a response to the appendiceal inflammation. Other causes of nausea and vomiting should also be considered, e.g. gastroenteritis or bowel obstruction. The onset of pain typically occurs before vomiting and is a sensitive indicator of appendicitis.

[11] Diarrhoea is a relatively common finding in paediatric appendicitis, but the presence of both diarrhoea and vomiting without other features suggestive of appendicitis may lend itself more towards a diagnosis of acute gastroenteritis, which is more common in this age group. Constipation is a late finding in appendicitis.

12 Abdominal dysuria – the presence of abdominal pain during micturition – is sometimes reported. This is due to the inflamed appendix irritating nearby urinary structures.

13 Pain is worse on movement and coughing as this further aggravates the peritoneal inflammation being caused by the appendix. A typical history from a child is finding the car ride to the hospital very uncomfortable when passing over bumps in the road.

14 Exposure to passive smoking is a weak risk factor for increased incidence of acute appendicitis.

15 An important differential for appendicitis in the younger patient is mesenteric adenitis. Also known as mesenteric lymphadenitis, it refers to inflammation and swelling of intra-abdominal lymph nodes that can cause similar pain to that of appendicitis. Most commonly this is caused by a viral URTI and will often have preceding or concurrent associated coryzal symptoms, including rhinorrhoea and pharyngitis, and other lymphadenopathy, particularly cervical. An abdominal ultrasound may reveal enlarged (>8mm in diameter) mesenteric lymph nodes and importantly, a normal appendix. Mesenteric adenitis is a self-limiting condition and management involves supportive care and good hydration. Symptoms generally resolve in 1–4 weeks.

16 It is important to elicit a complete medication history to minimise any drug interactions or to avoid causing adverse reactions during management.

Examination

- The patient appears **unwell** [1] and is **lying still** [2] in bed.
- His capillary refill time is <**2 seconds** [3] .
- Pulse is **120bpm** [4] and regular.
- Blood pressure is **105/60mmHg** [5] .
- Respiratory rate is **22 breaths per minute** [6] .
- Temperature **38.5°C** [7] .
- No cervical **lymphadenopathy** [8] is present.
- Heart sounds are dual with **no murmurs** [9] .
- Auscultation reveals vesicular breathing sounds and **equal air entry** [10] .
- The abdomen appears mildly **distended** [11] and there is no evidence of **surgical scars** [12] .
- There is mild **generalised abdominal tenderness** [13] with **maximal tenderness in the right lower quadrant** [14] .
- Pain is worsened with **percussion** [15] .
- There is no **involuntary guarding or rebound tenderness** [16] .
- There is **pain in the right lower quadrant during palpation of the left lower quadrant** [17] .
- **Bowel sounds are present** [18] .
- **Inguino-scrotal exam is normal** [19] .
- The patient has **difficulty walking and hopping on one foot** [20] .
- The **psoas sign and obturator sign** [21] are negative.

1 General inspection is an important guide for the examiner to give an indication of how unwell the patient might be. A child who appears alert and happy and is easily engaged with games or toys is less likely to be having an acute surgical pathology than a child who appears flat, uncomfortable and miserable.

2 Lying very still in bed can be an indicator of peritonitis. Children may lie in bed with one or both hips flexed and can at times be reasonably comfortable as long as they are not moved.

3 A capillary refill time of <2 seconds indicates that the child remains well hydrated. Children can be very quick to become dehydrated when they are unwell, particularly considering in appendicitis if they have increased outputs in the form of vomiting and diarrhoea, or decreased inputs as they are not eating and drinking. Other assessments of fluid status may include testing both central and peripheral capillary refill, mucous membranes, presence of sunken orbits and skin turgor, and assessment of haemodynamics and urine output.

4 For a 10-year-old child, a pulse rate of 120bpm is classified as a tachycardia. Pulse rate may be increased for a number of reasons, such as in response to fever, pain, dehydration or anxiety from being unwell and in hospital.

5 Acute hypotension would be represented by a SBP of <80mmHg in a 10-year-old child. This patient is maintaining their BP but it is important to continue regular monitoring as it could change rapidly if they became dehydrated or septic. Other signs suggestive of shock may include tachycardia, altered mental state, oliguria, tachypnoea, metabolic acidosis or a raised lactate.

6 22 breaths per minute is within the normal range for a 10-year-old, but some paediatric patients may develop tachypnoea as part of their presentation. This may be due to splinting, where the child tries to reduce their respiratory efforts in order to minimise movement of the anterior abdominal wall during respiration which can aggravate inflamed peritoneum, causing pain. They may breathe more quickly as a result. Tachypnoea could also be a sign of shock.

7 Fever is a characteristic feature of most infections, including appendicitis. Classically appendicitis is associated with a low grade fever (≤38.5°C).

8 The presence of tender cervical lymphadenopathy and a recent viral URTI may suggest that symptoms are more likely associated with mesenteric adenitis rather than acute appendicitis.

9 Occasionally a murmur may be audible during auscultation when the patient has not previously been known to have a murmur. Usually these are innocent murmurs and they are detectable during a febrile illness as the heart is beating harder and faster, causing increased turbulence in the blood flow and thus making the murmur louder. They will not be audible when re-auscultating once the patient has defervesced. It is important to liaise with the paediatric cardiology department if there are any concerns regarding the finding of a new or known murmur when preparing for surgery.

10 Occasionally abdominal pain may be an atypical presentation of lower lobar pneumonia. The patient may also have similar features to those of appendicitis, including fever and vomiting. Careful history and examination can help differentiate whether this may be an unusual presentation of pneumonia. A CXR may be useful to help evaluate this differential if a high index of suspicion for pneumonia is found.

11 Abdominal distension is commonly associated with increased intestinal gas. However, it may also be associated with bowel obstruction, inflammatory bowel disease, coeliac disease or lactose intolerance.

12 Previous abdominal surgery introduces increased operative risks, as there may be abdominal adhesions and distorted anatomy. This may lead to increased intraoperative blood loss, longer operative times, accidental damage to nearby structures and a higher chance of not being able to attempt laparoscopic surgery or needing to convert to open surgery intraoperatively.

13 Diffuse tenderness is found in approximately half of appendicitis presentations in children under 5 years of age. As children grow older, diffuse tenderness may become less likely and pain is maximal over the area where the overlying parietal peritoneum has become inflamed as localised peritonitis develops.

14 McBurney's point tenderness is described as maximum tenderness over the point that is one-third of the distance from the anterior superior iliac spine to the umbilicus. It will be a positive finding in approximately 82% of children from the age of 5 onwards. In younger children signs are often less specific and localised tenderness is present in only 38% of presentations.

15 Pain with percussion will be present in 79% of children over the age of 5.

16 Guarding is the involuntary contraction of abdominal wall muscles in an attempt to protect inflamed organs. It is a common manifestation of peritonitis and may be localised over the appendix in the right lower quadrant. Patients with a retrocaecal appendix may not show signs of guarding in the right lower quadrant due to not coming into contact with the parietal peritoneum. Rebound tenderness is a reliable sign of peritoneal irritation but it can be painful to test for in children who do have appendicitis and falsely positive in those that do not. It can be tested by palpation of the abdomen followed by a quick release, with the release of palpation also eliciting abdominal pain. Involuntary guarding and rebound tenderness are present more often with perforation.

17 Rovsing's sign refers to pain in the right lower quadrant upon palpation of the left lower quadrant. It is indicative of right-sided localised peritonitis and is a highly specific indicator of acute appendicitis.

18 The presence of bowel sounds indicates that the bowel is likely not obstructed. In some cases, there may be hypoactive bowel sounds over the right side of the abdomen compared to the left.

19 It is important to check for unknown hernias as part of the abdominal exam, as a hernia causing obstruction may mimic appendicitis with similar features of abdominal pain, diarrhoea, vomiting, anorexia and fever if the hernia has been incarcerated for some time. A scrotal exam looking for signs of testicular torsion is also important as torsion may sometimes present with abdominal rather than scrotal pain, particularly in younger patients where symptoms are often less specific. Features to look for when considering torsion include a high-riding testes, transverse lie, testicular swelling and absence of the cremasteric reflex.

20 In children >5 years with acute appendicitis, difficulty walking may be seen in up to 82%, and pain with coughing in 79%. Refusal to ambulate, or difficulty doing so, increases suspicion for appendicitis, including in children <5 years.

21 The psoas sign is associated with a retrocaecal appendix. It is tested by reproducing right lower quadrant pain with passive hip flexion. If the inflamed appendix is lying against the right psoas muscle, it will be irritated by the shortening of the muscle when drawing up the right knee with hip flexion. The obturator sign is associated with a pelvic appendix. If the inflamed appendix lies against the right obturator muscle, abdominal pain can be elicited by internal rotation of the right hip at 90° flexion.

Investigations

- **Urinalysis** [1] and a **BGL** [2] is normal.
- Full blood examination results show a normal **haemoglobin** [3], raised **WCC** [4] and mildly **elevated platelets** [5].
- **Urea, electrolytes and creatinine** [6] results are normal.

- **CRP** [7] is elevated.
- **Ultrasound** [8] of the abdomen reveals a **non-compressible, tubular structure in the right lower quadrant** [9] with a **diameter of 7mm** [10] with associated **wall thickening** [11].
- There is no **free fluid** [12] identified in the pelvis.

[1] A urine dipstick and further testing with microscopy and culture is a simple test to quickly exclude a UTI or renal colic as a cause of abdominal pain and vomiting. However, in the paediatric population, sterile pyuria can be present in up to 25% of patients with appendicitis, as is the presence of haematuria, albeit less commonly, in patients where ureter and bladder may be irritated by a nearby inflamed appendix. In post-menarchal females, a urine beta-hCG should also be performed to quickly exclude gynaecological pathologies as a cause for abdominal pain, such as ectopic pregnancy.

[2] Diabetic ketoacidosis is an important, non-surgical cause for abdominal pain that must not be missed. The child may have a history of polydipsia and polyuria leading up to their presentation and once insulin deficiency and ketoacidosis become significant, the patient will develop anorexia, vomiting and abdominal pain with associated hyperglycaemia, ketosis and metabolic acidosis.

[3] Prior to surgery, it is important to ensure adequate levels of haemoglobin in the blood and to consider transfusion pre- or intra-op if not. If an otherwise healthy child with no significant medical history has a low haemoglobin, this may also indicate an underlying condition as a cause, such as inflammatory bowel disease, that may need to be investigated further.

[4] Infection and inflammation are common causes of an elevated WCC; it may also be raised in response to vomiting.

[5] Platelets are an acute phase reactant and may be raised in settings of infection and inflammation such as this one. Acute phase reactants are proteins that increase or decrease by at least 25% during inflammatory states. Other notable acute phase reactants include CRP, fibrinogen, haptoglobin, ferritin, albumin and transferrin. However, it is not required to test for all these when considering a diagnosis of appendicitis.

[6] UECs are important in the setting of a surgical emergency. First, it identifies any electrolyte abnormalities that most often need correction prior to surgery. Secondly, it assesses renal function and serves as a prognosticator for postoperative recovery.

[7] C-reactive protein is another acute phase reactant. When both CRP and WCC are elevated, specificity for appendicitis is approximately 90%, although sensitivity remains at 40%.

[8] Imaging is not always required in the paediatric population. If appendicitis can be reliably confirmed on history, examination and pathology alone, then there is often no role for imaging. Imaging may be considered when the history and exam is equivocal for appendicitis or the need to confirm or exclude an alternative pathology is required. Plain films are usually of little value and are rarely performed. In some cases, they may be done to look for free air under the diaphragm in the setting of perforation or if bowel obstruction is a differential. MRI is an emerging modality for imaging for appendicitis, which offers the benefits of no radiation exposure; however, it has limited availability, is expensive, and younger children require a general anaesthetic in order to get complete images of adequate quality, something that poses its own risks.

[9] A non-compressible tubular structure in the right lower quadrant suggests an oedematous, inflamed appendix. In some cases, a normal appendix visualised on ultrasound may actually have early or tip appendicitis. In these cases, a serial examination and ultrasounds or further imaging modalities may be considered if clinical concern for appendicitis remains high.

[10] Dilation of the appendix >6mm is generally a reliable measurement to characterise appendicitis.

[11] Wall thickening of >2mm is another sign on imaging that suggests an inflamed appendix.

[12] Free fluid is suggestive of perforation of the appendix. Other findings on ultrasound may include thickening of the mesentery, localised tenderness to probe pressure, the presence of a calcified appendicolith or echogenic fat signifying inflammatory fat changes due to increased oedema and engorgement of lymphatics.

Management

Immediate

Take the patient's **weight** [1] . Establish IV access and commence **IV antibiotics** [2] and **fluids** [3] . Monitor the patient's **vital signs** [4] and **commence strict fluid balance monitoring** [5] . Ensure the patient has adequate **analgesia** [6] . Keep the patient **fasted** [7] . **Seek advice** [8] from the paediatric general surgery team.

Short-term

Perform an **emergency** [9] **appendicectomy** [10] . Following the procedure, keep the patient in hospital for monitoring [11] . The patient may be slowly graded up to a full **diet** [12] . Review the patient's **surgical site** [13] and perform daily **abdominal examinations** [14] . **Auscultate the lungs** [15] . The patient may be discharged if **vital signs remain stable** [16] and the **patient can tolerate oral intake** [17] .

Long-term

Follow the patient up in an **outpatient clinic** [18] postoperatively to ensure adequate wound closure and that the patient has been able to resume their normal activities, e.g. sport and school.

[1] Fluids and medications are dosed by weight in the paediatric population so it is important to get an accurate weight for safe prescribing.

[2] Follow local hospital protocol for antibiotic choices in appendicitis. Remember to consider if the patient has any drug allergies. Antibiotics are important in reducing the risk of intra-abdominal abscess formation.

[3] Intravenous fluid is integral in fluid resuscitation and stabilisation of circulation. In unwell patients, commence fluids at two-thirds of the patient's maintenance rate. In children the standard fluids used are 0.9% sodium chloride with 5% glucose +/− 20mmol of potassium chloride. If the patient is stable, fluids can be given at full maintenance rate while fasting. If the patient is dehydrated or shocked, 0.9% sodium chloride fluid boluses at 10–20ml/kg should be given initially, and this may be repeated if required.

[4] Ensure the patient remains haemodynamically stable prior to operative treatment.

[5] It is important to monitor fluid balance to ensure timely and accurate replacement of losses (i.e. diarrhoea, vomiting) and as part of ongoing fluid status assessment. Urine output is an important indicator of fluid status. If urine output declines this may indicate hypovolaemia or shock and should be rectified to prevent or lessen effects of acute renal failure.

[6] It is important to ensure the patient remains as comfortable as possible to help alleviate any anxiety associated with their situation.

[7] Keeping the patient fasted is crucial in their preoperative management. It allows the patient to have bowel rest, as well as reducing the risk of aspiration in the setting of anaesthesia. Ideally, patients should be fasted off solid foods for 6 hours, and clear fluids for 2 hours prior to induction of anaesthesia.

[8] Appendicitis should be referred to the general paediatric surgical team who generally see any paediatric patients up to the age of 16. They will usually come to assess the patient themselves and consent the patient for an appendicectomy. In rural areas the adult general surgical team may see children above a specific age, or the patient may need to be transferred to a service with an available paediatric surgical service.

[9] Evidence suggests that adverse outcomes are not increased for children with early appendicitis who receive prompt antibiotic administration and undergo appendicectomy within 24 hours of diagnosis. However, for children with advanced appendicitis without appendiceal mass or abscess, proceeding to emergency surgery is recommended to prevent progression to sepsis. Patients with development of appendiceal mass or abscess can be managed one of two ways. For patients who appear unwell, they should proceed to the same urgent management as for advanced appendicitis. For patients who appear well, and have generally presented late (>5–7 days from when they first became unwell), a well localised abscess or phlegmon may be treated non-operatively. These patients receive percutaneous drainage of their abscess or phlegmon and also receive IV antibiotics. After resolution, they are scheduled for an elective appendicectomy (called an interval appendicectomy) approximately 8–12 weeks later. The delay is to ensure the underlying appendicitis is definitively treated to avoid the morbidity associated with immediate appendicectomy.

[10] Appendicectomies can be performed laparoscopically or in an open approach. The laparoscopic approach is favoured for a lower rate of wound infections, less pain postoperatively, shorter duration of hospital stay and for cosmetic reasons. In some cases, the surgeon may decide an open approach (laparotomy) is preferred based on certain patient factors (i.e. any previous surgeries) or the procedure may need

to be converted to open intraoperatively if a change in circumstances arises.

11 In simple appendicitis, patients are monitored overnight to identify any immediate complications from surgery, such as shock, ongoing infection, reaction to anaesthesia or urinary retention. Patients with advanced appendicitis will often have an indwelling catheter, long-term cannula and sometimes a nasogastric tube inserted intraoperatively.

12 Many paediatric surgeons will start patients back on a regular diet immediately following laparoscopic appendicectomy for simple appendicitis. For more unwell children, diet will be upgraded more gradually, starting with clear fluids, although diet is often guided by the child themselves and parents are encouraged to feed their child if they are requesting something, even if it does not match their current diet level, as it may indicate they are ready to progress.

13 Daily review of the surgical site while the patient is in hospital is important in order to identify any early signs of wound dehiscence or infection so that they can be corrected. Generally, wounds are closed with absorbable sutures, so no stitches need to be removed in the future.

14 Palpate the abdomen daily to examine for clinical recovery of peritonitis and listen for bowel sounds. The absence of bowel sounds, or hypoactive bowel sounds, may indicate postoperative ileus.

15 Particularly for patients requiring a longer-term stay it is important to auscultate the lungs to identify any crepitations which may indicate atelectasis or developing infection. It is important to ensure postoperative analgesia is adequate so that patients will use their entire lung volume during respirations rather than being limited by abdominal pain.

16 If the patient remains afebrile, is haemodynamically stable and looks well and has completed their required course of antibiotics, they are generally well enough to be discharged home. For simple appendicitis cases this is usually the next day postoperatively; for advanced appendicitis this may be 5 days or longer.

17 The patient must be able to tolerate oral intake prior to discharging home. This is to ensure they continue to stay hydrated. Parenteral nutrition is indicated in previously healthy children who are unable to eat after one week, and in previously undernourished children after a few days.

18 Generally following up a patient 4–6 weeks postoperatively is sufficient, particularly if the patient had simple appendicitis with laparoscopic intervention and was able to be discharged home the following day. It is important to ensure that patients have been able to return to their normal activities and are still achieving developmental milestones as expected. For complex patients their follow-up might be brought forward for closer observation in the longer-term postoperative period.
Before discharge the patient should be advised of red flags to re-present to hospital, including recurrence of abdominal pain, fevers and vomiting. The development of a postoperative collection, particularly in cases of complex or perforated appendicitis, is an important differential to consider and should be investigated with an US. In these cases a further course of IV antibiotics may be required and if the collection is of a significant size, percutaneous drainage of the collection is also performed.

CASE 52: Hirschsprung disease

History

- A **3-day-old** [1] **male** [2] neonate is reviewed in the **postnatal ward** [3] due to **bilious vomiting** [4] over the past day and increasing **abdominal distension** [5].
- He was born at term via a normal vaginal delivery. He is exclusively breastfed and has been having **feeding difficulties** [6].
- He **did not pass meconium until 48 hours of life** [7].

- He has not had any **fevers** [8].
- The patient's mother reports her **antenatal testing** [9] was normal and she had normal **antenatal ultrasounds** [10].
- The neonate's **older sister has Hirschsprung disease** [11].
- The neonate passed his **newborn hearing screen** [12].

[1] Hirschsprung disease, also known as congenital aganglionic megacolon, is named eponymously after Danish physician Harald Hirschsprung who described the condition in 1888. It is a congenital disorder affecting bowel motility due to failure of the formation of the gut's myenteric and submucosal plexuses during embryonic development. The majority of affected patients are diagnosed during the neonatal period or in the first few months of life. In approximately 10% of cases, Hirschsprung disease is not diagnosed until after the first few years of life and very rarely in adolescence or adulthood.

[2] There is a slightly increased incidence of Hirschsprung disease in males compared to females. Overall, Hirschsprung disease affects one in every 4000 live births and accounts for one-fifth of all neonatal intestinal obstructions.

[3] Hirschsprung disease is not evident immediately from birth, so most babies will be cared for routinely on a postnatal ward unless any other comorbid conditions warrant a higher level of care from birth. Short-segment Hirschsprung disease affects the rectosigmoid colon and makes up 80% of cases. Short-segment Hirschsprung disease may not present until later in life, often with less specific symptoms such as chronic constipation or failure to thrive, which can delay time to diagnosis. Long-segment Hirschsprung disease extends proximally from the sigmoid colon and makes up a further 15% of cases. Total colonic aganglionosis is when the entire colon is affected, making up <5% of cases. Rarely, Hirschsprung disease may extend in to the small bowel.

[4] Vomiting is a non-specific symptom that can be attributable to many causes. In presentations of Hirschsprung disease bilious vomiting is a feature of distal bowel obstruction due to the functional obstruction caused by the non-innervated bowel. During embryonic development, neural crest cells, which are precursors to enteric ganglion

cells, fail to migrate from the neural crest to the developing colon between weeks 4–7 of gestation. This results in an aganglionic distal colon in the newborn which is incapable of relaxing and therefore allowing stool to adequately pass, resulting in a functional rather than mechanical obstruction. Other congenital conditions which cause mechanical obstruction and may also present with bilious vomiting include intestinal atresia and intestinal malrotation with volvulus. Sepsis is another important differential to rule out as a cause of vomiting in the neonate. Vomiting is also a feature of Hirschsprung-associated enterocolitis, an extreme complication of Hirschsprung disease that requires prompt identification and management due to the potential morbidity and mortality associated with it. It is thought to be due to stasis of stool in the bowel lumen, predisposing to bacterial proliferation and subsequent migration of bacteria into the adjacent bowel wall, which can rapidly result in septic shock if not addressed quickly. Hirschsprung-associated enterocolitis can sometimes be the first presentation of Hirschsprung disease.

[5] Abdominal distension is another classical finding in neonates with Hirschsprung disease. Neonates affected by intestinal atresia may also demonstrate abdominal distension. The more distal the atresia, often the greater the level of abdominal distension. Colonic atresia often presents later than a more proximal intestinal atresia and may present similarly to Hirschsprung disease. Sometimes both colonic atresia and Hirschsprung disease may occur together. A neonate with confirmed colonic atresia should also be investigated for Hirschsprung disease. Children who present with subacute features of Hirschsprung disease may report chronic abdominal distension. Abdominal distension is also a feature for infants presenting with Hirschsprung-associated enterocolitis.

6 Neonates with Hirschsprung disease may demonstrate poor feeding or feed intolerance. New feeding intolerance or anorexia in an infant or child with Hirschsprung disease, if combined with other features, should raise concern for possible Hirschsprung-associated enterocolitis.

7 Delayed passage of meconium is a key feature of the history that points towards a diagnosis of Hirschsprung disease. Most neonates will pass meconium within the first 24 hours of life. By 48 hours of life all neonates without any comorbid conditions will have successfully passed meconium. Up to 90% of neonates with Hirschsprung disease will have a history of delayed passage of meconium, with first passage occurring at >48 hours of life. However, a history of the neonate passing meconium within 48 hours does not exclude a diagnosis of Hirschsprung disease if other features or history are present. Neonates with an intestinal atresia will also have a history of not passing meconium, although this is often absolute rather than a delayed passage, depending on the location of the atresia. Meconium ileus due to cystic fibrosis can also cause delayed passage of meconium. Meconium plug syndrome is another cause of functional bowel obstruction in the neonate and is the most common cause of functional bowel obstructions in this age group. In this condition, thick inspissated meconium blocks or 'plugs' the distal colon or rectum. Contrast enema is often both diagnostic and curative. Neonates should stool normally following the enema but if stooling remains an issue they should be investigated for other potential causes, including Hirschsprung disease. Small left colon syndrome, an uncommon cause of delayed passage of meconium and most commonly seen in neonates of mothers who have gestational diabetes, is another cause of delayed passage of meconium due to transient dysmotility of the left side of the colon causing a functional obstruction.

8 Fever in a neonate is a medical emergency and requires urgent investigation and intervention. A febrile neonate requires a full septic work-up including a lumbar puncture to help identify the cause of the fevers. There should be no delay in administration of empirical antibiotics, although blood, urine and CSF cultures should ideally be collected prior. Difficulty in obtaining samples should not delay antibiotic administration and antibiotics should be commenced if obtaining the samples is taking longer than anticipated. If there is difficulty establishing IV access, then the first dose of antibiotics should be given IM while access is established. Fever is one of the presenting symptoms of Hirschsprung-associated enterocolitis.

9 Antenatal testing and screening are a routine part of antenatal care for an expectant mother to ensure a safe pregnancy and delivery for mother and baby, and to try to pre-empt and correct any issues early should they arise. Antenatal testing involves regular reviews with GPs, midwives and obstetrician gynaecologists. These reviews involve general physical check-ups, including assessment of height, weight and BP for the mother, as well as fundal height measurements for an estimation of the development of the foetus. Urine samples are taken to look for evidence of infection or pre-eclampsia. Glucose tolerance testing is performed to identify early evidence of gestational diabetes mellitus. Blood tests are performed, including for mother's blood group and antibodies, haemoglobin levels, vitamin D levels, and to identify the presence of or immunity to various infections that could be passed on to the foetus or neonate by vertical transmission. This includes rubella, varicella, CMV, parvovirus, herpes simplex virus, toxoplasmosis, hepatitis B and C, syphilis and HIV. The above collection of conditions may lead to infant morbidity and mortality through a variety of means including various neonatal infections, leading to sepsis, congenital abnormalities, rashes, intrauterine growth restriction and developmental delays. A swab of the vagina late in pregnancy assesses for the presence of Group B streptococcus. Group B streptococcus can be a cause of early-onset sepsis in the newborn, and a positive finding of Group B streptococcus on swab or urine microscopy and culture is an indication for maternal antibiotic coverage during labour to reduce the chances of infecting the newborn during delivery.

10 As part of routine antenatal testing the mother will be referred for antenatal ultrasound scans. A dating scan is the first antenatal ultrasound performed, usually done at 10–13 weeks' gestation in normal pregnancies to predict the current gestation of the pregnancy and delivery date by measuring the size of the developing foetus. Around 12 weeks' gestation, a nuchal translucency antenatal ultrasound is performed, although this is sometimes combined with the dating scan. This scan measures the size of the nuchal fold of the foetus which can provide an estimation of the likelihood of the foetus having a chromosomal abnormality. A blood test may also be performed around the time of the nuchal translucency scan known as combined first trimester screening and the results are interpreted together to estimate the risk of the foetus having a chromosomal abnormality including Down syndrome (trisomy 21). Neonates with Down syndrome have a higher likelihood of having Hirschsprung disease than the general population. Up to 16% of cases of Hirschsprung disease occur in neonates with Down syndrome. Hirschsprung disease is also seen as a feature of many other syndromes, the most well-known including Waardenburg syndrome and multiple endocrine neoplasia type 2 (MEN-2) and when occurring as part of a constellation of features it is referred to as syndromic Hirschsprung disease. An antenatal morphology scan is performed at around 20 weeks' gestation for review of foetal morphology and growth, amniotic fluid volume and blood flow in the foetus and placenta. Hirschsprung disease can be associated with congenital heart disease or renal tract anomalies which may be identified antenatally on ultrasound scans. Further antenatal ultrasounds may be performed later in pregnancy depending on the advice of the mother's care provider.

11 There is a familial link, with the chance of a particular family member having Hirschsprung disease being 3% if a relative has short-segment disease, increasing to 17% if the relative has long-segment disease. This risk increases further if the relative is a female sibling or if multiple family members have Hirschsprung disease. The aetiology of Hirschsprung disease, particularly when occurring outside of other syndromes, is complex and likely related to various genetic factors and inheritance patterns.

12 Newborn hearing screens are routinely done for all neonates in the first few weeks of life, often before they are discharged from hospital. Hearing impairments are present in 5% of patients with Hirschsprung disease.

Examination

- The neonate appears **lethargic and irritable** [1] .
- The **heart rate is 160bpm** [2] .
- The **respiratory rate is 50 breaths per minute with no work of breathing** [3] evident.
- **Oxygen saturation on air is 97%** [4] .
- The **temperature is 36.8°C** [5] .
- The neonate has **a capillary refill time of 3 seconds** [6] .
- **Heart sounds are dual and there are no murmurs** [7] .
- **Chest is clear** [8] to auscultation with no added sounds and good air entry throughout.

- Upon general inspection of the abdomen, there is no evidence of an abdominal wall defect. The **abdomen is distended** [9] .
- The abdomen is soft to palpation with **no guarding or rigidity** [10] and **no palpable masses** [11] .
- The patient's **nappy is dry** [12] .
- The **anus is patent and in a normal position** [13] .
- The patient does not have any **facial or form features associated with genetic or congenital anomalies** [14] .

1 Depending on duration and severity of symptoms, the neonate may appear well-looking or may present unwell. Lethargy could be a symptom of dehydration, particularly if the neonate has been feeding poorly and vomiting. The neonate may be irritable as they are hungry or in pain from abdominal distension or intestinal obstruction. In cases of Hirschsprung-associated enterocolitis the neonate may present shocked and obtunded.

2 Normal heart rate for a term neonate is 110–170bpm. The presence of a tachycardia may be a response to hypovolaemia, sepsis, pain or distress. Tachycardia is a feature of Hirschsprung-associated enterocolitis.

3 Normal respiratory rate for a term neonate is 30–60 breaths per minute. Respiratory compromise may be evident due to abdominal distension causing diaphragmatic elevation that is preventing adequate chest expansion. Respiratory changes may also be present in the setting of an aspiration pneumonia caused by the repeated bouts of vomiting.

4 In term neonates oxygen saturations should be ≥95%. If saturations are <95% further investigation is warranted, for example looking for signs of sepsis, an airway or respiratory pathology or a cardiac pathology.

5 A fever is not usually seen in an isolated presentation of Hirschsprung disease without associated enterocolitis. However, a fever may be present in other diagnoses such as sepsis due to another cause.

6 Neonates are particularly susceptible to rapid volume depletion, especially in the setting of poor oral intake and vomiting, so a careful fluid balance assessment should be

performed. Other signs to identify are evidence of oliguria or anuria, sunken fontanelles, poor skin turgor, dry mucous membranes and altered conscious level. In neonates, capillary refill time should be assessed centrally by pushing one finger onto the neonate's upper sternum for five seconds, then removing and counting the time taken for colour to return to the area after release. In newborns, capillary refill time should be <3 seconds.

7 A full assessment of the neonate should be performed. Cardiac examination may identify added sounds or murmurs suggestive of a congenital heart defect. In patients with syndromic Hirschsprung disease, up to 50% may have an associated cardiac defect. A neonate with non-syndromic Hirschsprung disease is unlikely to have any cardiac pathology.

8 Lung field auscultation may indicate signs of pneumonia, which may have developed due to aspiration following repeated vomiting.

9 Abdominal distension is a frequent finding in presentations of Hirschsprung disease as a result of the functional bowel obstruction.

10 The abdomen should be assessed for peritonism. The presence of peritonitis is associated with severe Hirschsprung-associated enterocolitis causing bowel perforation.

11 In older children, faeces may be palpable in the left lower quadrant. In severe cases, a faecolith may be palpable. Children with chronic constipation that has limited response to toileting and bowel plans should be considered for abdominal plain film at baseline as part of investigation for Hirschsprung disease. A rare complication of short-segment Hirschsprung disease that is most commonly seen in undiagnosed children is volvulus of a dilated section of faeces-filled bowel, usually affecting the sigmoid colon.

12 The neonate's nappy should be inspected to assess for any passed meconium, and as part of a fluid assessment to ensure urine is still being produced. Explosive, foul-smelling diarrhoea is associated with Hirschsprung-associated enterocolitis and rectal bleeding may also be present with severe cases.

13 Some neonates with Hirschsprung disease may also have anorectal malformations. Examination of the anus may reveal a tight anal sphincter or narrowed, empty rectum. Explosive passage of stool following digital rectal examination

(performed either with a digital rectal thermometer, anal dilator or the fifth finger) is another common finding in Hirschsprung disease. An explosive, foul-smelling passage of gas and stool following rectal examination supports a diagnosis of Hirschsprung-associated enterocolitis in the presence of other features. Bacterial overgrowth in the static stool causes the malodour.

14 A full top-to-toe assessment of the child should be completed, looking for physical indications of chromosomal anomalies or congenital malformations. External features that may be present in neonates with Down syndrome include small low-set ears, brachycephaly, epicanthal folds, a low nasal bridge with a short nose and small nostrils, a small down-turned mouth, single palmar creases and a wide space between the first and second toes.

Investigations

- An **abdominal plain film** [1] shows dilated bowel loops and no free air in the rectum.
- A **contrast enema** [2] reveals a dilated colon with a narrowed rectosigmoid colon distally.
- A **suction rectal biopsy** [3] is performed which shows an absence of ganglionic cells.
- The neonate had the **newborn screening test** [4] at 3 days of life.
- A **urinary tract ultrasound** [5] is normal.
- Consider **genetic testing** [6].

1 Abdominal X-rays are a good first-line investigation and while they are unable to diagnose Hirschsprung disease, they may demonstrate features of intestinal obstruction such as absence of or decreased rectal gas and dilated bowel loops proximal to the obstruction. Other causes of intestinal obstruction may be seen on abdominal plain film including the 'double bubble sign', which is a classical finding in duodenal atresia. Intestinal malrotation may also be identified. Dilated small bowel loops with air–fluid levels are suggestive of a jejunal or ileal atresia. Abdominal plain films are part of the work-up for Hirschsprung-associated enterocolitis.

2 Contrast enema is the next line in investigating for potential Hirschsprung disease and should be performed in all infants in whom Hirschsprung disease is suspected. No bowel preparation is required prior to a contrast enema. A contrast enema may reveal a transition zone which delineates the change between the aganglionic bowel segment, which appears narrowed though in some cases can appear to have a normal diameter, to the normal, functioning colon which appears dilated. This appearance on contrast enema is pathognomonic of Hirschsprung disease. However, if the contrast enema does not reveal this classical appearance or appears normal it is not sufficient to rule out Hirschsprung disease, particularly if other features of history and exam are consistent with this diagnosis. In some instances where Hirschsprung disease is suspected but the contrast enema was inconclusive, a repeat contrast enema is performed 24 hours later and if residual contrast from the first enema

is identified within the bowel lumen, this finding also suggests Hirschsprung disease. In patients with total colonic aganglionosis, the colon may appear normal on contrast enema but dilated loops of small bowel may be evident. The contrast enema has some limitations; a false-negative result may be obtained if the patient has had a DRE within the preceding couple of days, as this can temporarily dilate the rectum and obscure a potential transition zone. If an infant presents with suspected Hirschsprung-associated enterocolitis based on history but without formal diagnosis, a contrast enema should not be performed in the acute setting due to risk of bowel perforation.

3 Suction rectal biopsy is the gold standard investigation for diagnosing Hirschsprung disease. This can be done without anaesthesia at the bedside or in an outpatient setting. A special apparatus to perform the biopsy can usually be obtained from the hospital's sterilising centre and supply. Generally, 3 biopsies are taken to provide an adequate sample size of tissue for histological analysis. The first biopsy is taken at least 2cm above the dentate line, as this region contains physiological hypoganglionosis. Subsequent biopsies are taken proximal to the first biopsy, usually in increments of 1cm. The absence of ganglion cells confirms the diagnosis of Hirschsprung disease. Other findings on histological analysis include hypertrophic nerve fibres (although these may not become apparent unless the infant is >8 weeks of age) and increased acetylcholinesterase staining in the muscularis mucosae, which further support the diagnosis. If the suction rectal biopsy is inconclusive or insufficient tissue was obtained for analysis, it can be repeated, or alternatively full thickness biopsies can be obtained under general anaesthesia. The tissue sample obtained for rectal biopsy must contain muscularis mucosae in order to be a sufficient sample. A normal rectal biopsy, with adequate tissue samples, rules out a diagnosis of Hirschsprung disease.

4 The newborn screening test is performed on all newborns to identify and detect any chronic conditions early in life in order to provide early intervention and management to improve the infant's quality of life. They are usually performed between 24 and 48 hours of life and may be repeated in any neonates that have received blood products or were born at a low birth weight. Cystic fibrosis and congenital hypothyroidism are two of the many conditions screened for as part of the newborn screening test. Both of

these conditions are causes of delayed passage of meconium in the neonate.

5 Infants with Hirschsprung disease have a higher rate of other congenital anomalies, whether syndromic or non-syndromic. The most common of these is urinary tract anomalies, occurring in one-fifth of all patients with Hirschsprung disease and increasing to two-fifths in patients with syndromic Hirschsprung disease. The most common anomalies are hydronephrosis and renal hypoplasia.

6 If syndromic Hirschsprung disease is suspected, genetic testing such as karyotype analysis or microarray may be considered, usually with the support of a clinical geneticist. Genetic screening may extend to the patient's family members.

Management

Immediate

Transfer [1] the neonate to the special care nursery or neonatal ICU. Refer to the **paediatric surgical team** [2]. Insert a **nasogastric tube** [3]. Make the patient **nil by mouth** [4]. Consider if **IV access** [5] is required. **Monitor** [6] the patient's fluid status and vital signs. Organise for **urgent abdominal imaging** [7].

Short-term

Commence the patient on **bowel washouts** [8] and organise for a **suction rectal biopsy** [9]. Once

Hirschsprung disease has been confirmed, schedule the patient for elective **pull-through procedure** [10]. **Monitor** [11] the patient postoperatively.

Long-term

Patients should be followed up in the **paediatric surgical outpatient clinic** [12] and be monitored and managed for any complications of Hirschsprung disease.

1 A neonate with bilious vomiting and abdominal distension is a surgical emergency until proven otherwise. They should be transferred to a setting where they can receive specialised care and management.

2 Care of the neonate should be jointly managed between the neonatal team and the paediatric surgical team. The paediatric surgical team should receive an early referral to expedite investigations and management.

3 An NGT should be inserted, especially if the neonate has ongoing vomiting. It should be left on free drainage with regular aspirates to help provide decompression. The aspirates can also be reviewed and colour and consistency noted. NGTs are required for gastric decompression in Hirschsprung-associated enterocolitis.

4 The patient should cease feeds while the cause of the bilious vomiting and abdominal distension is investigated; if an acute surgical cause is identified they may require

immediate surgical intervention. This also helps to reduce the chance of the neonate developing an aspiration pneumonia from repeated vomiting.

5 IV access for fluid support should be considered in an unwell, flat or dehydrated neonate. If the neonate is stable and investigations are readily available, IV access may not be required, as feeds may be able to be recommenced in only a few hours if an acute surgical cause is excluded. An infant or child presenting with Hirschsprung-associated enterocolitis requires urgent IV access for fluid resuscitation and broad-spectrum antibiotic administration.

6 The neonate should be monitored for any change in their vital signs that may indicate a worsening in their condition and warrant a change in management.

7 Abdominal imaging should be organised urgently to identify any acute causes of neonatal bowel obstruction. In the acute setting, this would usually involve an abdominal plain film or an upper GI contrast study. An upper GI contrast study is important to identify a small bowel atresia or intestinal malrotation with volvulus as a cause of the neonate's symptoms. The development of volvulus is a surgical emergency as it leads to small bowel ischaemia, necrosis and intestinal perforation. A contrast enema can be performed once an acute surgical cause requiring urgent intervention has been excluded.

8 Most infants should begin having twice-daily bowel washouts for stool lavage and to provide bowel decompression. Parents can be taught how to perform bowel washouts and be supervised doing them in hospital before their baby is discharged so they can continue being administered at home. Washouts are normally done using a wide-bore catheter or rectal tube, large catheter-tipped syringe and saline warmed to body temperature. Bowel washouts, along with bowel rest and antibiotics, make up the management for Hirschsprung-associated enterocolitis. Neonates with total colonic aganglionosis may not have good results with bowel washouts, and surgery may be performed sooner in these cases.

9 Rectal suction biopsy should be performed to confirm the diagnosis of Hirschsprung disease.

10 Definitive treatment for Hirschsprung disease involves resection of the affected segment of bowel. This procedure does not need to be performed as an emergency, so affected infants can be discharged and return electively for their procedure. Some health services may require an infant to be above a certain body weight before being able to proceed with surgery. The surgery may be done anywhere between 1 week to 2–3 months of life. Usually performed laparoscopically or trans-anally, the aganglionic segment of bowel is resected and the normal bowel is pulled down closer to the anus, while preserving the function of the internal anal sphincter. Frozen sections should be taken intraoperatively to help guide the resection margins. Acute surgical resection in Hirschsprung-associated enterocolitis is only required if the patient is not responding to non-operative measures or there is evidence of bowel ischaemia or perforation. In these cases, a colostomy is formed with formal resection and pull-through done at a later date. Long-segment Hirschsprung disease or total colonic aganglionosis may also require the formation of a colostomy to decompress the dilated bowel, with a planned pull-through at a later time.

11 As with any surgical procedure, patients should be monitored in the postoperative period to ensure good wound healing, no evidence of anastomotic leak, no development of secondary infection and that they are tolerating feeds and able to pass stool.

12 Patients should be reviewed in paediatric surgical outpatient clinic to ensure they are gaining weight well and reaching developmental milestones as expected. The patient or their parents may report postoperative complications including constipation, diarrhoea or faecal incontinence. Postoperative Hirschsprung-associated enterocolitis can occur post pull-through. Recurrent Hirschsprung-associated enterocolitis in the postoperative patient raises suspicion for the presence of strictures or residual aganglionic segments. These patients may require a repeat pull-through procedure when well. Patients with total colonic aganglionosis are more likely to experience complications.

CASE 53: Hypospadias

History

- A 2-day-old **male** [1] neonate is reviewed on the postnatal ward due to concerns raised by the midwives of an abnormal **appearance of his genitalia** [2] on his **routine newborn assessment** [3].
- He was born at **term** [4] via a normal vaginal birth.
- He was a planned pregnancy and **conceived naturally** [5].

- His mother is **37 years old** [6], from a **Caucasian background** [7] and has **no significant medical history** [8].
- He had a normal **morphology ultrasound** [9] at **20 weeks' gestation** [10].
- Serial antenatal ultrasound scans demonstrated **intrauterine growth restriction** [11].
- The infant's **father was born with hypospadias** [12].
- Neither of the infant's parents are **smokers** [13].

1 Hypospadias is a congenital abnormality affecting only male infants where the urethral opening is abnormally positioned on the ventral side of the penis. It can present with varying degrees of severity and can also be associated with penile curvature, called chordee, and incomplete foreskin closure around the ventral aspect of the glans. It is one of the most common congenital anomalies affecting male infants, affecting approximately 1 in 250 live births.

2 An understanding of the normal penile anatomy of the newborn male is important to both understand the diagnosis and subsequent surgical correction of hypospadias. The normal penis in a newborn male born at term usually measures 2.5–3.5cm in length. The foreskin is circumferential and adherent to the glans penis, covering the coronal sulcus. Retraction of the foreskin is usually not possible until later childhood. The normally-positioned urethral meatus will usually be visible through the tip of the foreskin without needing retraction, positioned centrally on the glans penis. Internally, the male urethra traverses through the corpus spongiosum on the underside of the penis, while located superolaterally are the paired corpora cavernosa. These structures are enveloped by the tunica albuginea and Buck's fascia.

3 Routine newborn assessments are top-to-toe physical examinations performed to screen for any apparent congenital abnormalities or medical conditions that may require urgent or routine follow-up or intervention. They are typically performed in the first few hours following birth, again prior to discharge from hospital and once more in the community at 6 weeks of life, at this time typically with a GP.

4 Prematurity is a reported risk factor for hypospadias.

5 Conception via *in vitro* fertilisation is a reported risk factor for hypospadias.

6 Advanced maternal age, where a mother's age is >35 years, is a reported risk factor for hypospadias.

7 The incidence of hypospadias varies in different population groups, with the highest incidence reported to be in people from Caucasian backgrounds.

8 Maternal diabetes mellitus that is pre-existing, rather than gestational diabetes which develops during pregnancy, is a reported risk factor for hypospadias.

9 Morphology ultrasounds are typically performed at 20 weeks' gestation. They are a standard part of antenatal screening and are performed to look at foetal morphology in detail to identify any potential structural abnormalities. On the 20-week morphology scan, approximately 50–60% of foetal structural abnormities are able to be detected. This reduces to 30% when just considering foetal cardiac abnormalities. The views obtained in the scan can sometimes be affected by technical limitations such as foetal position *in utero*, increased maternal body habitus, or the presence of maternal abdominal scarring. Occasionally the morphology ultrasound may be repeated if inconclusive views are obtained of key foetal anatomy. Hypospadias is typically not detected on morphology ultrasound.

10 Hypospadias is thought to occur due to disruption to androgenic stimulation which is required for the differentiation and normal development of external male genitalia. The aetiology is likely multifactorial and affected by both environmental and genetic factors. While hypospadias may be seen as a part of some genetic syndromes, such as Denys–Drash syndrome or Opitz G/BBB syndrome, in most cases the cause of hypospadias is unknown. There are some risk factors that are thought to increase the likelihood of hypospadias occurring. Embryologically, the external genitalia begin to differentiate around the 7th to 8th week of gestation, formed from the genital tubercle, genital swellings and genital folds. The genital tubercle begins to elongate and eventually forms a phallus, the future penis. The genital swellings eventually form into scrotal swellings and subsequently the scrotum. The genital folds begin fusing at their medial edges, ultimately forming the penile urethra. In hypospadias, there is impaired fusion of the genital folds, ultimately affecting the eventual positioning of the urethral meatus and the development of the foreskin. The degree of fusion failure will determine how proximal the eventual urethral meatus is. Penile curvature, or chordee, is a normal part of the development of the external male genitalia and will usually resolve after fusion of the genital folds into the penile urethra. In hypospadias, chordee may still be evident but can also occur in cases where the urethral meatus is in the normal anatomical position, referred to as chordee without hypospadias.

11 Intrauterine growth restriction is a reported risk factor for hypospadias. There can be many causes of intrauterine growth restriction, but placental insufficiency as one cause has also been associated with hypospadias. The cause of intrauterine growth restriction should be determined if possible and measurement of weight, length and head circumference plotted on a growth chart to identify whether the growth restriction is symmetrical or asymmetrical. Symmetrical intrauterine growth restriction is when there is a global restriction of the head and body and can be associated with neurological consequences. Asymmetrical intrauterine growth restriction is characterised by a normal head size but restricted growth of the body.

12 Having a father who had hypospadias increases an infant's risk for also having hypospadias.

13 Exposure to tobacco smoke antenatally is a reported risk factor for hypospadias. Additionally, exposure to pesticides antenatally is reported as a risk factor for hypospadias.

Examination

- The infant is **alert and reactive** [1] to examination.
- His **observations are within normal range** [2] and he has **stable temperatures** [3].
- He has **no obvious dysmorphic features** [4].
- Palpation of the head reveals a **symmetrical-shaped head** [5] with palpable, **level anterior and posterior fontanelles** [6] with **no head swellings** [7].
- The **face is symmetrical** [8] and **eyes are of a normal shape and size** [9].
- **Red reflexes are present** [10] bilaterally.
- The **ears are well shaped with no additional structures** [11].
- The **nares are patent** [12].
- Inspection and palpation of the **mouth is normal** [13].
- There are **no swellings identified in the neck** [14].
- The **chest is symmetrical with good air entry and no work of breathing** [15].
- **Heart sounds are dual with no murmurs** [16] audible on auscultation.
- **Femoral pulses are palpable** [17] bilaterally.
- The **abdomen is soft and non-distended** [18] and the infant has a **three-vessel cord** [19].
- Inspection of the external genitalia reveals a **penis with a urethral meatus opening on the proximal aspect of the ventral glans penis and a foreskin that does not cover the ventral surface of the glans** [20].
- The **penis is curved by 20 degrees** [21].
- The **scrotum is symmetrical and both testes are palpable within the scrotum** [22].
- The **anus is patent** [23].
- There are **no abnormalities identified on examination of the spine** [24].
- The **upper and lower limbs are symmetrical** [25] and the **hips are stable** [26].
- During the examination the newborn **passes urine and he is noted to have a downward stream** [27].

1 As with assessment of patients of any age, a general 'end of the bed' assessment to identify whether the patient is well-appearing or unwell-appearing is included as part of the newborn examination. Reviewing infant alertness and motor activity also forms part of a neurological assessment, along with assessing tone and primitive reflexes.

2 Vital signs should be routinely reviewed as they can be an early indication of an unwell neonate; for example, they could indicate a developing sepsis, or could also help identify the presence of unseen congenital abnormalities, or changes in haemodynamics or saturations could be suggestive of cardiac pathology.

3 Both hyperthermia and hypothermia can be signs of infection and sepsis in a neonate.

4 The presence of obvious features on examination which do not fit with a normal newborn appearance, such a cleft palate, unusual head shape or limb abnormalities, could indicate the presence of a syndrome.

5 Head shape and suture lines should be palpated. During labour and birth, suture lines may become overlapping or overriding; this causes temporary head asymmetry but is a normal part of birth moulding. An asymmetric head shape that persists beyond a few days of life with persistent ridging of suture lines may indicate craniosynostosis, which is an abnormal early fusion of cranial sutures that requires neurosurgical referral. Wide sutures can indicate hydrocephalus causing raised ICP. Skull asymmetry may be seen in Opitz G/BBB syndrome.

6 The anterior fontanelle is formed by the junction of the coronal, sagittal and metopic sutures. The posterior fontanelle is formed by the junction of the sagittal and lambdoid sutures and is smaller than the anterior fontanelle. Bulging fontanelles can indicate raised ICP.

7 Palpation of the scalp should be performed to look for any head swellings, which may be suggestive of caput, cephalohaematoma or subgaleal haemorrhage.

8 Facial palsies may be evident following an instrumental delivery or prolonged labour and usually resolve within a few weeks. A persistent facial palsy suggests an underlying central cause.

9 Wide-set eyes, formally referred to as hypertelorism, is associated with many syndromes, most notably Apert syndrome, Patau syndrome or Opitz G/BBB syndrome. Epicanthal folds and upslanting palpebral fissures are often associated with Down syndrome. Downslanting palpebral fissures may also be seen in Apert syndrome or Treacher Collins syndrome. Short and narrow palpebral fissures may be seen in DiGeorge syndrome.

10 Red reflexes, assessed with an ophthalmoscope, should be present in all neonates and indicates a clear lens and normal underlying structures. A diminished red reflex, white reflex, asymmetrical reflexes, or the presence of dark spots in the red reflex should all be assessed further by a neonatal ophthalmologist.

11 The ears should be examined for their general shape, size and positioning on the head. The presence of any preauricular skin tags or pits should also be identified. Abnormalities of the external ear increase the likelihood of abnormalities of the middle or inner ear and may also be associated with hearing loss. Hearing assessments are performed on all infants prior to discharge from hospital. External ear abnormalities may also be seen as part of other congenital syndromes and are sometimes associated with renal malformations. Ear tags are sometimes seen in association with hypospadias.

12 Neonates are obligate nasal breathers so patency should be established. If there are concerns about patency then a feeding tube should be passed down the nares to exclude choanal atresia. A particularly wide or narrow nose may be associated with other congenital anomalies.

13 Cleft lip is evident on general inspection but cleft palate or a submucosal palate can be harder to identify and therefore thorough inspection and palpation of the palate should be performed. The presence of a bifid uvula may indicate the presence of a submucosal cleft palate.

14 The neck should be palpated for any masses, which could indicate the presence of branchial cleft cysts, thyroglossal duct cysts, haematomas or a cystic hygroma. Trauma to the sternocleidomastoid during delivery may result in torticollis. Excess skin on the nape of the neck may indicate some genetic syndromes such as Down syndrome. Clavicles should also be palpated for fractures from a traumatic birth such as shoulder dystocia. The congenital absence of the clavicle may be seen in some congenital syndromes.

15 Pectus excavatum or pectus carinatum may be visible, either as part of a syndrome or as an isolated finding. Widely spaced nipples may indicate a genetic syndrome such as Turner syndrome. Accessory nipples are common, occurring as frequently as 1 in 40 births.

16 Murmurs can be normal in the first 24 hours of life due to a patent ductus arteriosus, which later closes. A persistent murmur in a stable neonate should be evaluated with an echocardiogram. If there are concerns of cardiovascular compromise and the presence of a murmur, then urgent echocardiogram and transfer to a tertiary unit is warranted. Cardiac anomalies are sometimes associated with hypospadias.

17 Coarctation of the aorta may present with diminished femoral pulses.

18 Abdominal distension may indicate intestinal obstruction or an intestinal atresia or ascites. A scaphoid abdomen may indicate the presence of a congenital diaphragmatic hernia. An abdominal wall defect such as omphalocele or gastroschisis is evident at birth or diagnosed on antenatal scans. Umbilical hernias are common due to rectus diastasis in the newborn and most will resolve without intervention by 5 years of age. Persistent or particularly large umbilical hernias should be corrected surgically. It is normal to palpate the liver edge in a newborn just below the costal margin.

19 Umbilical cords typically contain three vessels – two arteries and a vein. The umbilical cord and placenta are examined after birth to identify how many vessels are present. The present of a two-vessel cord with only one artery and one vein is associated with a higher rate of congenital or chromosomal abnormalities. Two vessel cords are more common in twin gestations.

20 Hypospadias can vary in severity depending on where the urethral meatus opens on the ventral surface. The urethral opening may be glanular, subcoronal, distal penile, midshaft, proximal penile, penoscrotal, scrotal or perineal. Close inspection of the glans penis in cases of hypospadias may reveal a blind-ending urethral pit where the urethral meatus would normally open. 10% of cases of hypospadias are very mild, sometimes classified as forme fruste of hypospadias, where the urethral meatus may be located only 1–2mm from the usual meatal opening, there is no chordee and the foreskin still circumferentially covers the glans penis. Standard hypospadias, occurring in approximately 65% of cases, has a urethral opening anywhere along the penile length, failure of closure of the foreskin on the ventral surface causing a dorsal-hooded foreskin (also known as a dorsal hooded prepuce), a normal penile length and varying degrees of chordee. More commonly the urethral opening is more distal. Severe hypospadias, occurring in approximately 20% of cases, has a urethral meatus located on the scrotum or perineum and severe chordee. In cases of severe hypospadias, a disorder of sexual development should be considered.

21 Chordee or curvature of the penis caudally is normal until 15° of curvature. Up to 40° of curvature is classified as mild. up to 80° of curvature is classified as moderate and severe chordee is where the curvature of the penis is >80°.

22 The scrotum should be evaluated to see if both testes are descended into the scrotum or, if not present in the scrotum, whether they are palpable more proximally in the inguinal canal. Up to 5% of term neonates and 30% of preterm neonates will have an undescended testis, also called cryptorchidism. Testes should have fully descended by 6 months of age. 10% of infants with hypospadias will have cryptorchidism, particularly in those with a proximal hypospadias. In these cases where hypospadias is present and one or both testes are not palpable, a disorder of sexual

development should be considered. A bifid scrotum may also suggest the presence of a disorder of sexual development. Hydroceles are a common finding on scrotal examination which resolve spontaneously. The scrotum should also be assessed for the presence of any inguinal hernias.

23 Imperforate anus can be associated with hypospadias or as part of a VACTERL syndrome (for more information on VACTERL see *Case 55, History* Note 10). It may not always be apparent unless there is a delayed passage of meconium or features of distal intestinal obstruction.

24 The spine should be examined for any evidence of a neural tube defect, including looking for a sacral dimple, abnormal tuft of hair or skin discolouration, all of which may suggest an underlying abnormality.

25 The limbs should be inspected for any movement abnormalities or discrepancies in length. Hands and feet should be carefully inspected for any evidence of syndactyly or polydactyly. These can be an isolated finding or part of a syndromic presentation. Fraser syndrome is associated with cutaneous syndactyly as well as genitourinary anomalies. A single palmar crease can be a normal finding but is also associated with Down syndrome.

26 The hips should be examined to identify developmental dysplasia of the hip. The Ortolani and Barlow manoeuvres are performed to detect any evidence of hip instability.

27 A downward urinary stream may be noted in some neonates with hypospadias.

Investigations

- A thorough examination revealed no other congenital abnormalities, and thus **no further investigations were required** [1].

- Consider **blood tests** [2] and **imaging** [3].

1 Thorough examination should always be performed in the first instance to identify any other congenital anomalies or the presence of a suspected syndrome.

2 If neither testis is palpable, a heel-prick blood test for serum electrolytes should be performed as a screening tool for congenital adrenal hyperplasia. Congenital adrenal hyperplasia is a rare, autosomal recessive condition causing a deficiency in certain enzymes responsible for cortisol, aldosterone and androgen production. It is the latter case that affects virilisation of the foetus and thus causes genital ambiguity in the neonate. Hyperkalaemia and hyponatraemia are evident on examination of serum electrolytes. Sometimes hypoglycaemia will also be a present. Generally, neonates will remain metabolically stable until one week of life. An adrenal crisis can have a sudden onset and be life-threatening.

3 Renal tract imaging is not required in isolated cases of hypospadias as the external genitalia develop after the main stages of renal development, which occurs before 7 weeks' gestation. Moreover, the external genitalia and renal tract arise from different embryological structures. If the neonate developed a UTI, then renal imaging would be warranted. In cases of severe hypospadias or hypospadias with an absent testis unilaterally or bilaterally, the infant should be investigated for a disorder of sexual development. This would include a pelvic ultrasound to identify the presence of any internal genitalia and a karyotype to identify sex chromosomes.

Management

Immediate

If the neonate is stable and examination confirms an isolated hypospadias in an otherwise well neonate, then they are appropriate to remain on the **postnatal ward** [1] and be discharged home at the usual time post birth. The family should be counselled on the implications of hypospadias and the **treatment required** [2]. Advise the family to **not circumcise** [3] their child.

Short-term

Refer to a paediatric urologist [4] for initial assessment and planning.

Long-term

Correction of hypospadias [5] is performed surgically between 6 and 18 months of age. Often patients are able to be **discharged home the same day** [6] as their procedure. They should be commenced on a **prophylactic antibiotic** [7] to prevent UTIs. **Strenuous activities should be avoided** [8] for 4 weeks postoperatively. Educate the parents on signs of **surgical complications** [9]. **Postoperative reviews** [10] are continued until adolescence.

---

1 An otherwise well neonate who requires no further investigations and is able to successfully pass urine can remain on the postnatal ward with their parents.

2 Mild forms of hypospadias do not necessarily require any surgical intervention. Forme fruste of hypospadias generally does not require correction as there is no impairment of passage of urine and sexual function is preserved.

3 The child should not be circumcised as the foreskin tissue can be used as part of the reconstruction process. Additionally, traditional circumcision techniques could pose a risk for the child with hypospadias due to the altered anatomy.

4 Hypospadias correction is done electively and all cases of hypospadias that are not classified as mild should be assessed by a paediatric urologist. The goal of surgery is to achieve a penis with as close to normal appearance as the standard anatomy and that provides normal penile function.

5 There are various methods of hypospadias repair and their choice depends on severity of the hypospadias. They may be done as a one- or two-stage procedure, and if a two-stage procedure is required then at least 6 months is required between procedures to promote adequate wound healing and reduce the risk of infection. For a two-stage hypospadias repair, the first stage is started at 6 months of age to initially reduce penile curvature and begin steps to create a new urethral meatus. The second stage occurs 6 months later where the urethra is reconstructed.

6 A catheter may or may not be required, depending on the extent of reconstruction performed. It can generally be allowed to fall out at home when dressings are removed on day 2 or 3 postoperatively. Longer-term catheters following more complex repairs will be removed during a follow-up appointment postoperatively. Parents and carers should be educated on catheter hygiene and care. Simple analgesia should also be utilised to control pain postoperatively.

Bloody discharge from the penis is normal postoperatively and twice-daily bathing of the area is important to help with postoperative swelling.

7 The patient should be on prophylactic antibiotics until a few days post removal of their catheter. Trimethoprim or nitrofurantoin are most commonly used.

8 Although sometimes difficult, toddlers and young children who have undergone hypospadias repair should avoid strenuous activities or activities that involve straddling, such as bike riding, for 4 weeks post operatively.

9 Signs of a UTI include high fevers, irritability or vomiting. Signs of a local wound complication include erythema or offensive discharge from the penis, excessive bleeding from the penis, difficulty passing urine, change in urinary stream or wound dehiscence. If any of these complications occur then parents should bring their child immediately to the ED for assessment. Two urinary streams suggest the formation of a urethrocutaneous fistula, which can occur in up to 20% of patients post correction of hypospadias. A thin urinary stream or straining during urination suggests the formation of a urethral stricture. Ballooning on the ventral aspect of the penis on urination and dribbling post voiding suggest the formation of a urethral diverticulum from an outpouching of the reconstructed urethra. Subsequent operations to correct postoperative complications are also generally performed 6 months following the initial procedure, except in the case of a urethral diverticulum, where correction may occur sooner as it can predispose to UTIs.

10 In general, follow-ups should be organised for patients 6 weeks after their initial surgery, 12 months after their initial surgery, after completing toilet training and as an adolescent. At each of these reviews the development of any complications should be identified and penile function and cosmetic outcome should be reviewed.

CASE 54: Inguinal hernias

History

- An **8-month-old** [1] **male** [2] with **no significant past medical history** [3] is brought in to the ED by his parents after noticing a **right-sided groin lump** [4] during his last nappy change.
- His parents report that they had at times spotted a small bulge in their child's groin when he had been **crying or straining** [5] over the past few months but became concerned as this lump had not disappeared like the others did.

- He had been well earlier in the day, but has been **inconsolable** [6] for the past few hours and had two **vomits** [7] at home.
- He was born at **term** [8] after an unremarkable pregnancy.
- His parents report no significant **family history** [9].

[1] Inguinal hernias will occur in up to 5% of all newborns. Of this, up to one-third will be incarcerated, with this often being the first presentation of hernia. Indirect inguinal hernias are the most common type of hernia in children and occur when abdominal contents pass into the inguinal canal. The inguinal canal is formed anteriorly by the aponeurosis of the external oblique muscle and posteriorly by the transversus abdominis muscle and transversalis fascia. Invagination of the transversalis fascia forms the opening of the inguinal canal, also called the internal or deep inguinal ring, which is located anatomically at the midpoint of the inguinal ligament and superolaterally to the inferior epigastric vessels. The inguinal canal allows passage through the abdominal wall of the spermatic cord from abdomen into scrotum in males and of the round ligament into the labia majora in females. The canal ends just superior to the pubic tubercle with a triangular opening in the aponeurosis of the external oblique muscle, known as the external or superficial inguinal ring, and is bounded inferiorly by the inguinal ligament. In infants, the inguinal canal is short and traverses the abdominal wall perpendicularly rather than obliquely as it does in adults. This anatomical lie causes the external inguinal ring to sit almost directly over the internal ring, increasing the risk of developing indirect inguinal hernias. Femoral hernias, where abdominal contents pass inferiorly to the inguinal ligament through a weakness of the abdominal wall into the abdominal canal, are rare. Direct inguinal hernias, where abdominal contents pass through a weakness in the transversalis fascia medial to the inferior epigastric vessels, are also rare. When they do occur, it is usually following prior surgical correction of an indirect inguinal hernia. Direct inguinal hernias are more common in adults.

[2] Males are more likely to develop inguinal hernias than females with a male-to-female ratio of 4:1. In males, the incidence of developing an inguinal hernia is highest during the first month of life. This is why testing for inguinal hernias is completed as part of the baby check assessments. However, females rather than males are more likely to develop incarceration of an inguinal hernia when present.

[3] Inguinal hernias are more likely to occur in children who have conditions that increase intra-abdominal pressure; examples include ascites, respiratory disease, peritoneal dialysis, mechanical ventilation, connective tissue diseases, abnormalities of the genitourinary system such as hypospadias or ambiguous genitalia, and existing abdominal wall defects.

[4] Hernias are more likely to occur on the right side as opposed to the left. Embryologically, the testes descend with the processus vaginalis (an outward pouching of the peritoneum) through the inguinal canal between the 7th and 9th month of gestation into the scrotum. Once the testis has fully descended, the processus vaginalis will have obliterated by 2 years of age. The right testis descends later than the left testis and thus the obliteration of the processus vaginalis also occurs later, allowing more time for a hernia to develop. A similar process occurs in females; however, the ovaries do not descend into the inguinal canal and remain in the abdomen. Similar to males, an outpouching of peritoneum called the diverticulum of Nuck extends into the labia majora and obliterates by 7 months of age. When these outpouchings do not obliterate spontaneously as intended, they are referred to as a patent processus vaginalis and canal of Nuck in males and females, respectively. It is via these patent channels through the inguinal canal that abdominal contents can pass through and allow herniation of intra-abdominal contents, including bowel. If the channels are only narrowly patent, they may permit only the passage of peritoneal fluid, causing a hydrocele. Hydroceles may be visualised as a fluid-filled swelling in the hemiscrotum or labia majora, which can

fluctuate in size or be reducible with pressure as they are still communicating with the peritoneal cavity. They should be observed and surgically corrected if they persist beyond 2 years of age, as it indicates that the processus vaginalis has not obliterated. Pathological hydroceles may also be present with testicular torsion, epididymitis or scrotal trauma, as swelling and fluid develops around the infected or inflamed area. Bilateral hernias are seen in approximately 50% of infants who are born preterm, reducing to 10% in infants born at term.

5 Parents of children with an inguinal hernia may describe a history of an intermittent bulge noticed in the groin during periods of increased intra-abdominal pressure, such as when straining or crying. They are usually asymptomatic of this mass and it will spontaneously self-reduce, usually once intra-abdominal pressure returns to normal.

6 Due to their young age, infants demonstrate pain through irritability and crying and are unable to be consoled through usual methods.

7 Vomiting may be a feature of an incarcerated hernia if the hernia contains a loop of bowel, and indicates bowel obstruction.

8 Approximately 10% of all infants born prematurely will develop an inguinal hernia. The frequency of development of inguinal hernias is also increased in infants of low birth weights.

9 A child is more likely to develop an inguinal hernia if there is a family history of inguinal hernia.

Examination

- The infant is **crying and unsettled** [1] but **not unwell-looking** [2].
- **Heart rate is 170bpm** [3].
- BP, oxygen saturation and respiratory rate are within normal limits for age. **Temperature is 36.5°C** [4].
- There is **no abdominal distension** [5] and **no evidence of previous surgical scars** [6] on abdominal inspection.
- The **abdomen is soft to palpation and there is no guarding or rigidity** [7], although examination is

difficult due to abdominal wall musculature tensing while crying.
- A **firm, tender mass is palpable in the groin and extends into the right hemiscrotum** [8].
- The **skin overlying the lump is erythematous** [9].
- Both **testicles are palpable in the scrotum and are non-tender and in the correct position** [10].
- The lump **cannot be reduced** [11].

1 Incarcerated hernias are exceptionally painful as they are stuck in position and cannot be reduced. Infants express their discomfort through crying and irritability.

2 Given the usually rapid presentations to hospital, infants are often still well-appearing as they have not yet become dehydrated due to losses or poor oral intake, and have not developed sepsis due to tissue necrosis or bowel perforation secondary to hernia strangulation. Incarcerated hernias can become strangulated within 2 hours, where hernia contents suffer from arterial compromise due to worsening oedema from lymphatic and venous obstruction. The longer the strangulation persists, the more likely tissues will develop necrosis from ischaemia and potentially bowel perforation if bowel is involved.

3 Tachycardia may be present as a response to distress and pain. In late presentations, this may be a sign of shock.

4 Generally, a fever is not a feature of an incarcerated hernia; however, in a delayed presentation a patient may have a fever if necrosis and infection of tissue or peritonitis from perforation develops.

5 Abdominal distension may be a finding in bowel obstruction from an incarcerated or strangulated hernia.

6 Direct inguinal hernias may herniate through a weakness in the abdominal wall caused by previous surgical correction of an indirect inguinal hernia. Direct inguinal hernias can also become incarcerated and herniated.

7 General abdominal examination should be performed, looking for evidence of peritonitis caused by a necrotic, gangrenous tissue or bowel or due to bowel perforation. Abdominal examination can sometimes be difficult in children when they are scared, in pain or distressed. Ensuring the child has adequate analgesia is important to help ease their distress due to pain. Modifying the examination to make it less confronting, such as examining while the child is in their parent's or carer's arms or lap can also be useful. Sometimes serial examinations and distraction techniques may be needed for a proper assessment to be completed ,which can take some time.

8 Incarcerated hernias will present as a firm, discrete mass that is tender to palpation in the groin and may or may not extend into the scrotum or labia majora.

9 Surrounding oedema and erythema is usually present as congestion develops and lymphatic and venous flow is impaired.

10 The testes should be examined as part of the hernia assessment to exclude acute testicular pathology. The hernia may be palpable extending into the scrotum. The testes should be evaluated to ensure both are descended, are lying in the correct orientation and are non-tender, in order to exclude a testicular torsion as a cause of the pain and vomiting. The testicle of the ipsilateral side may appear dark blue as pressure on the spermatic cord causes venous congestion.

11 If the hernia cannot be reduced then it is deemed incarcerated, and if compromise of the vasculature has started to occur then it is called strangulated. During earlier presentations where just an intermittent inguinal mass has been noted and the patient remains asymptomatic, a differential to exclude is that of a retractile testis. The testis can move into the inguinal canal and present as an inguinal mass due to an amplified cremasteric reflex, and consequently the hemiscrotum of that side will be empty.

Investigations

- Physical examination of this patient is **diagnostic** [1] of incarcerated inguinal hernia.

- Consider the need for **bloods** [2] and **imaging** [3] such as ultrasound of the groin.

1 Usually, no investigations need to be completed before proceeding to management, as examination is enough to confirm the diagnosis.

2 For patients presenting unwell, with evidence of fluid depletion or hernia strangulation, completing a basic blood panel for FBC, UEC, VBG and blood group and hold may be useful as part of a baseline work-up and preparation for surgery.

3 In settings where patients present with an intermittent groin swelling, an ultrasound may be performed if diagnosis

cannot be confirmed on clinical examination. Ultrasounds have a 93% accuracy at diagnosing acute groin swellings. In females presenting with an incarcerated inguinal hernia, gentle reduction may be attempted and if unsuccessful, an ultrasound should then be obtained to exclude reproductive organs being herniated into the hernia sac. A large number of inguinal hernias in females will contain an ovary or Fallopian tube. If reproductive organs are not present then further attempts at manual reduction can be made.

Management

Immediate

Give **adequate analgesia** [1]. Keep patient **nil by mouth** [2]. Attempt emergency **manual reduction** [3] of an incarcerated inguinal hernia in the **ED** [4]. Refer to the **paediatric surgical team** [5].

Short-term

Once the incarcerated hernia has been successfully reduced the patient should be booked in for elective

surgical repair [6] of the hernia. Most hernia repairs can be done as a day-surgery; however, particularly young infants should remain for 24 hours of **apnoea monitoring** [7] postoperatively.

Long-term

Patients should be followed up in the **paediatric surgical outpatient clinic** [8] post discharge.

1 Incarcerated hernias are extremely painful, as is the process of manual reduction. Infants should therefore be given adequate pain relief, such as intranasal fentanyl, before any attempts at correcting the hernia are made.

2 Patients should be given nothing orally in preparation for surgical reduction, should manual reduction of the hernia fail.

3 Manual reduction should be attempted in the first instance unless the child is very unwell or has evidence of peritonitis, bowel obstruction or perforation. Manual reduction has a very high success rate, with 95% of attempts achieving successful reduction.

4 Manual reduction should be attempted by a senior emergency physician.

5 If manual reduction is unsuccessful the paediatric team should be urgently consulted. They will re-attempt manual reduction using procedural sedation, icing the area to help ease swelling and putting the infant in Trendelenburg position – supine with head down and legs elevated. Continuous pressure for several minutes may be required to induce a successful reduction.

6 Timing of repair may be hospital- and surgeon-dependent. Some may choose to surgically repair the inguinal hernia immediately after successful manual reduction. Others may admit the child for observation and repair the hernia within 24–48 hours following manual reduction, allowing oedematous and inflamed tissues to settle before surgery. Others may discharge the child home with warning signs to look out for should the incarcerated hernia re-occur, and bring the patient back for elective repair within 5 days in order to have the lowest chance of re-herniation and incarceration. For patients with a delayed presentation and demonstrating signs of possible bowel obstruction, perforation, peritonitis or necrosis, the paediatric surgical team should be consulted immediately for emergency surgical intervention. These patients will require antibiotics,

may require a laparotomy and may require bowel resection with anastomosis or stoma formation. They will have an extended inpatient stay.

7 Due to their young age and the effects of anaesthesia, young infants should be monitored postoperatively as they have an increased chance of apnoeic events.

8 Postoperatively patients may develop scrotal oedema, haematomas or hydroceles. They should be followed up in outpatient clinic to ensure resolution of these complications. Scrotal oedema usually resolves within 3 weeks, though haematomas and hydroceles may take up to 3 months to disappear. Additionally, patients who may have presented to their GP or ED with readily reducible inguinal hernias may be booked in to surgical outpatient clinic for evaluation by the paediatric surgical team and to organise an elective booking for repair. Once an inguinal hernia is diagnosed, repair should occur promptly but not as an emergency, to reduce the chance of the hernia becoming incarcerated while they are awaiting their procedure. Parents and carers should be carefully informed of the signs and symptoms to look for in incarcerated hernias and advised to present immediately to the ED if their child is displaying these features. Assessment of the testes should also be undertaken during clinic review to ensure they are symmetrical. In cases of prolonged, irreducible hernia there can be compression of the nearby testicular vessels and this may rarely lead to atrophy of the ipsilateral testis.

CASE 55: Intestinal malrotation with volvulus

History

- A **one-month-old infant** [1] is brought in by ambulance to the ED with repeated **bilious vomiting** [2] for the **past four hours** [3].
- The parents report the vomiting started **suddenly** [4] and the baby has been **inconsolable** [5] since it began.
- The baby has **not had any fevers** [6].
- They **passed meconium at birth** [7] and have stooled normally since.
- They were **born at term** [8] via a normal vaginal delivery.
- The patient's mother reports her **antenatal testing** [9] was normal and she had normal **antenatal ultrasounds** [10].

[1] Intestinal malrotation is a congenital disorder of embryonic intestinal development that can predispose to intestinal volvulus, an acute surgical emergency. The true incidence is unknown as it is possible for people to live their entire lives while remaining asymptomatic. Of those that develop symptoms, it is estimated to occur in one in every 6000 live births. Malrotation with symptomatic sequelae is most frequently seen in the first year of life, and frequently in the neonatal period, with up to 75% of cases being identified during this time period. However, intestinal malrotation will also present in older children and adolescents and may even not be diagnosed until adulthood.

[2] Vomiting is a feature of acute intestinal obstruction and is seen in over 90% of presentations of intestinal malrotation with volvulus. In most cases the vomiting is bilious but in some cases it is non-bilious. Other congenital conditions which cause mechanical or functional obstruction and may also present with bilious vomiting include intestinal atresia and Hirschsprung disease. Sepsis is another important differential to rule out as a cause of vomiting in the neonate.

[3] The time period to presentation in intestinal malrotation with volvulus is often rapid, due to the severity of the patient's symptoms.

[4] As a volvulus due to intestinal malrotation can happen acutely without any prior warning, symptom onset is sudden. Malrotation occurs during embryonic development due to interruption of the normal rotation of the embryonic gut between the fourth and tenth weeks. During normal development, the developing primary intestinal loop grows quicker than the embryonic cavity can accommodate for. The loop will move into the yolk stalk (which becomes the umbilicus in the foetus) with the axis of the loop being the origins of the superior mesenteric artery. At this point the primary intestinal loop rotates 90° anticlockwise. When the primary intestinal loop returns to the abdomen it rotates a further 180° and begins fixation to the retroperitoneum, with

the proximal bowel attaching early at the ligament of Treitz (also known as the suspensory ligament of the duodenum) in the area of the duodenojejunal flexure and the distal colon attaching more gradually. This process results in the formation of the normal wide-based mesentery from the ligament of Treitz to the ileocaecal valve. There are various forms of abnormal intestinal rotation. The two most common are non-rotation and malrotation. Non-rotation, where the normal rotation of the primary intestinal loop does not occur, results in an orientation where small bowel occupies the right side of the abdomen and the colon occupies the left side of the abdomen. In malrotation, the proximal aspect of the primary intestinal loop remains unrotated and the distal aspect only undergoes 90° of rotation. This results in a caecum that is fixated to the right, mid to upper, lateral wall of the abdomen by bands of peritoneum. These bands, known as Ladd bands, extrinsically compress the duodenum and are a rarer cause of duodenal obstruction in the neonate. Ultimately, malrotation leads to the eventual midgut being supported on a narrow mesentery, increasing the risk of volvulus and vascular comprise of the mesenteric blood vessels.

[5] Identification of pain can sometimes be difficult in infants and young children, who may not be able to vocalise their feelings or have difficulty in localising their pain. In these age groups the behaviour of the child is important to take into account when assessing pain. In infants, distress, inconsolable crying and irritability can all be features of acute pain. Older children with intestinal malrotation without volvulus may have non-specific abdominal pain that could be attributed to other causes such as food allergy, irritable bowel syndrome and functional abdominal pain. Other symptoms of intestinal malrotation without volvulus in the older child include failure to thrive, chronic diarrhoea and cyclical vomiting. Rarely, they may present with pancreatitis or biliary obstruction.

6 Intestinal malrotation and intestinal malrotation with volvulus do not have fevers as a presenting symptom. Fevers can develop in intestinal malrotation with volvulus associated with sepsis and bowel necrosis causing perforation and peritonitis.

7 A history of delayed passage of meconium may raise suspicion for Hirschsprung-associated enterocolitis. Hirschsprung disease is associated with a history of delayed passage of meconium longer than 48 hours, and Hirschsprung-associated enterocolitis can sometimes be the first presentation of the disease. Other prominent features of Hirschsprung-associated enterocolitis include fever, offensive diarrhoea and abdominal distension, as well as vomiting.

8 Prematurity is a strong risk factor for necrotising enterocolitis, which may present similarly to intestinal malrotation with volvulus, particularly in a neonate. For preterm and low birthweight neonates being monitored in a neonatal intensive care setting who develop new feed intolerance, haemodynamic instability and vomiting, both necrotising enterocolitis and intestinal malrotation with volvulus are important differentials and warrant urgent investigation.

9 Antenatal testing and screening are a routine part of antenatal care for an expectant mother to ensure a safe pregnancy and delivery for mother and baby, and to try to pre-empt and correct any issues early should they arise. Antenatal testing involves regular reviews with GPs, midwives and obstetrician gynaecologists with various blood tests, urine tests, vaginal swabs and testing for gestational diabetes mellitus being performed at various stages of the pregnancy.

10 As part of routine antenatal testing, the mother will be referred for antenatal ultrasound scans. An antenatal morphology scan is performed at around 20 weeks' gestation for review of foetal morphology and growth, amniotic fluid volume and blood flow in the foetus and placenta. Any unusual findings on antenatal ultrasounds are monitored with serial ultrasounds for the remainder of the pregnancy. Up to 62% of children found to have intestinal malrotation have other congenital abnormalities. Most strongly associated congenital abnormalities include abdominal wall defects such as gastroschisis and omphalocele, congenital diaphragmatic hernia and congenital heart disease, all of which may be identified on antenatal ultrasounds. Intestinal malrotation may also be seen with other congenital disorders of the GI tract, including intestinal, oesophageal and biliary atresia, Meckel diverticulum and anorectal malformations. Intestinal malrotation may also be seen as part of the VACTERL association of congenital anomalies. VACTERL association refers to a constellation of non-syndromic congenital abnormalities which frequently occur in conjunction with each other. It incorporates Vertebral anomalies, Anal atresia, Cardiac Anomalies, Tracheo-oEophageal fistula, Renal anomalies and Limb anomalies. Additionally, other congenital abnormalities not covered in the above list have also been seen with VACTERL association, including ear anomalies, laryngomalacia, laryngeal or tracheal stenosis, ambiguous genitalia, omphalocele, single umbilical artery and duodenal atresia.

Examination

- The infant appears **lethargic, irritable and unwell** [1].
- They are **saturating at 96%** [2] on air, their **respiratory rate is 55 breaths per minute** [3] and there is **no increased work of breathing** [4] evident.
- Their **heart rate is 190bpm** [5] and their **blood pressure is 125/85mmHg** [6].
- Their **temperature is 37°C** [7].
- The infant's **fontanelles are soft and not sunken and their capillary refill time is 3 seconds** [8].
- The **heart sounds are dual and there are no murmurs and the chest is clear** [9] to auscultation.
- Upon general inspection of the abdomen, there is no evidence of an **abdominal wall defect** [10].
- The abdomen is **mildly distended** [11].
- The abdomen is **tender to palpation with guarding** [12] present.
- A **dark red stool** [13] is in the infant's nappy.
- The **anus is patent and in a normal position** [14].
- The patient does not have any **facial or form features associated with genetic or congenital anomalies** [15].

1 The infant may present distressed, inconsolable and irritable due to severe abdominal pain associated with volvulus. As their condition worsens, they may become flat and lethargic and have an altered conscious state.

2 In an infant under 3 months of age, oxygen saturation should be ≥94%.

3 Normal respiratory rate for an infant under 3 months of age is 25–60 breaths per minute. Tachypnoea may develop as a response to a metabolic acidosis.

4 Increased work of breathing may not be evident in the absence of a primary respiratory pathology; however, in infants and children breaths may become short and shallow to try to reduce movement of the abdomen in an attempt to prevent aggravating their abdominal pain.

5 Normal heart rate for an infant under 3 months of age is 110–170bpm. Tachycardia is a response to extreme abdominal pain due to intestinal malrotation with volvulus. The tachycardia may be further precipitated by developing intestinal ischaemia.

6 Normal systolic BP range for an infant under 3 months of age is 60–105mmHg. Initially, infants and children may present hypertensive as a response to extreme abdominal pain due to intestinal malrotation with volvulus, in addition to tachycardia. Later, hypotension may develop as part of a septic response to ischaemic and infarcted bowel.

7 Fever is not a typical presenting feature of intestinal malrotation or of intestinal malrotation with volvulus. Fever may be a late-stage symptom in the event of volvulus as part of a septic response to ischaemic and infarcted bowel.

8 Fluid balance assessment should be performed as part of the initial examination. Other signs to identify are evidence of oliguria or anuria, poor skin turgor, dry mucous membranes and altered conscious level, all suggestive of severe dehydration. Patients with intestinal malrotation with volvulus can quickly become shocked.

9 Cardiac examination may identify added sounds or murmurs suggestive of a congenital heart defect. In most cases, significant cardiac defects are identified before the neonate is discharged from hospital. Heterotaxy syndrome, otherwise known as situs ambiguus, is a rare syndrome affecting one in 10 000 people globally that affects the positioning of internal organs. The structure of organs can also be affected, most commonly the heart, lungs, spleen, liver and biliary tree and bowel, with malrotation in the latter. Of all congenital heart defects worldwide, 3% are due to heterotaxy syndrome. The likelihood of an infant with heterotaxy syndrome having intestinal malrotation is so high that many paediatric specialists frequently screen these infants with upper GI contrast studies while they remain asymptomatic.

10 Most abdominal wall defects will be picked up on antenatal ultrasounds from 10 weeks' gestation. Omphaloceles, where internal abdominal organs protrude through an opening where the umbilical cord joins the abdomen enveloped in a membranous sac of peritoneum, affects 2.5 per 10 000 births. Gastroschisis, where bowel may protrude through the abdominal wall without a membranous covering, affects 2–6 per 10 000 births. Omphalocele is more frequently associated with intestinal malrotation than gastroschisis. Prune belly syndrome, a rare congenital disorder that affects 1 per 40 000 births, is another abdominal wall defect that is sometimes associated with intestinal malrotation. Prune belly syndrome consists of three key features: urinary tract abnormalities, undescended testes

and complete or partial absence of anterior abdominal wall muscles, giving the abdomen a wrinkled, 'prune-like' appearance.

11 Abdominal exam may initially be relatively normal due to the acuteness of the presentation of intestinal malrotation with volvulus. An infant or child presenting with vomiting and acute abdominal pain with a non-distended abdomen should raise suspicion for intestinal malrotation with volvulus. Abdominal distension may progress as the volved bowel becomes more ischaemic. Abdominal distension is a more prominent feature of other causes of bowel obstruction in the infant, including intestinal atresia and Hirschsprung disease.

12 The abdomen will be tender and may have features of peritonitis in the setting of intestinal malrotation with volvulus. Peritonitis is a concerning finding as it indicates likely bowel necrosis with perforation. Other abdominal pathologies can also present with a tender abdomen and peritonitis, including acute appendicitis.

13 Patients with intestinal malrotation with volvulus may develop haematochezia which signals bowel ischaemia and potential necrosis. In older infants, intussusception may present similarly to intestinal malrotation with volvulus, with acute abdominal pain, vomiting and blood in stool. Classically, these episodes of pain come in waves rather than being constant, as is seen with volvulus. Intussusception can be identified on abdominal ultrasound with the classical target sign finding.

14 Anal atresia may be seen as part of VACTERL associations in which intestinal malrotation can also occur. Assessment of anus position and patency is a standard part of pre-discharge baby exams. In the setting of an infant presenting acutely unwell from the community who has been stooling well at home, an assessment of the anus at this time is unlikely to provide any diagnostic benefit or aid in guiding management.

15 In an acute, time-sensitive presentation assessing for physical indications of chromosomal anomalies or congenital malformations can be delayed until the neonate is stabilised. Physical features that may be observed clinically in VACTERL association include cleft palate and limb anomalies such as radial aplasia or hypoplasia, polydactyly, syndactyly and hypoplastic thumb, clubfoot and tibial hypoplasia, and anal atresia. For an infant presenting from the community, it is likely they would have already had relevant investigations if VACTERL association or other congenital defects were suspected prior to discharge. The operating surgeon and anaesthetist should be informed if the patient has any known congenital abnormalities, as it may affect surgical approach and anaesthesia. Any patient with known congenital anomalies that have associations with intestinal malrotation who develops vomiting should raise suspicion for the presence of malrotation if not previously diagnosed.

Investigations

- An **FBE** [1] is normal.
- A VBG demonstrates a **metabolic acidosis** [2] .
- **Coagulation studies** [3] are normal.
- The infant's **blood type** [4] is A+.
- An **abdominal plain film** [5] demonstrates no free air in the abdomen.
- An **upper GI contrast study** [6] shows beaking of the bowel and a malrotated bowel configuration.
- An **abdominal ultrasound** [7] and **CT scan** [8] are not performed.
- **Genetic screening** [9] is completed.

[1] Haemoglobin and platelet counts should be available as part of the preoperative blood panel.

[2] A metabolic acidosis may be evident on venous gas due to lactic acidosis from impaired bowel perfusion, lowering the serum pH. A VBG gives an overall idea of the patient's physiological and electrolyte status, to help guide and monitor resuscitation measures.

[3] Coagulation studies should be also obtained as part of a pre-operative work-up.

[4] Blood type and available compatible blood that is readily available should be organised preoperatively, particularly if the infant or child is proceeding to invasive emergency surgery, as risk of blood loss and consequential need for blood transfusion is high.

[5] Abdominal plain films are not diagnostic of intestinal malrotation. They may be performed in settings of suspected malrotation with volvulus to identify the presence of a pneumoperitoneum. In some cases, volvulus may appear with a 'double-bubble' sign similar to that seen in duodenal atresia due to duodenal obstruction. The finding of a pneumoperitoneum on plain film warrants urgent surgical intervention.

[6] If a pneumoperitoneum is excluded on plain film, an upper GI contrast study is the next imaging modality of choice when investigating for causes of bowel obstruction in the neonate. The study can confirm the presence of intestinal malrotation with volvulus which may appear with a 'corkscrew sign', named for the appearance of coiled duodenum and jejunum, or with a 'beak sign', which describes the way tapering of the bowel lumen in complete obstruction appears like a bird's beak. A dilated stomach and proximal duodenum are also often demonstrated. Upper GI contrast study is also well-equipped to identify intestinal malrotation without volvulus demonstrating the malrotated bowel configuration. 75% of cases of symptomatic intestinal malrotation are able to be identified on upper GI contrast study. Two in every thousand upper GI contrast studies performed for other clinical indications have an incidental finding of non-rotation. Individuals with non-rotation are low risk for midgut volvulus, as the mesentery has a wider base than what is seen in malrotation.

[7] Abdominal ultrasounds are not routinely used as part of the work-up for intestinal malrotation with volvulus, except in some specialised paediatric centres. An ultrasound may be ordered if symptoms are thought to be due to intussusception. If volvulus is present, a 'whirlpool' sign due to twisting of the superior mesenteric artery and vein may be seen. A dilated duodenum or dilated, fluid-filled loops of small bowel may also be visualised. Some centres may use abdominal ultrasound for screening for intestinal malrotation. Intestinal malrotation may be suspected if the duodenum is abnormally located and reversal of the superior mesenteric artery and superior mesenteric vein relationship is viewed. In up to 70% of cases, the superior mesenteric artery will be on the right and the superior mesenteric vein will be on the left. In normal anatomy, the superior mesenteric vein always sits to the right of the superior mesenteric artery.

[8] CT is an imaging modality not frequently used in infants and children due to risks associated with radiation exposure, and is considered only when benefits of the scan outweigh the risks. Similar findings to those seen on abdominal ultrasound may be identified, and it can sometimes give a clearer visualisation of the malrotated bowel configuration or demonstrate free air in the setting of a pneumoperitoneum. MRI is an alternative modality to CT that can be used to identify intestinal malrotation without radiation concerns. MRI is often not readily available and scanning takes several minutes at a minimum, so it is not a useful imaging modality in an emergency situation. Infants and young children may also require sedation in order to remain still long enough to perform the MRI scan. For these reasons, MRI is still not widely used. CT scans are utilised more in adolescents and adults.

[9] Outside of the acute presentation and particularly if other congenital anomalies are evident or suspected, formal karyotype testing and microarray should be performed to identify any potential underlying genetic disorders as a cause for congenital abnormalities. VACTERL association is not associated with an underlying genetic defect and its occurrence is thought to be sporadic. Further imaging, such as an echocardiogram, renal tract ultrasound, chest radiograph and skeletal plain films may be considered if intestinal malrotation is thought to be present as part of a VACTERL association.

Management

Immediate

Refer to the paediatric surgical team [1]. Gain **IV access** [2]. Administer **analgesia** [3]. Commence **resuscitation** [4] measures. Start **antibiotics** [5]. Keep **fasted** [6]. **Insert an NGT** [7]. **Monitor vital signs and fluid status** [8].

Short-term

Consider if imaging is required [9]. Proceed to an **emergency laparotomy** [10] for surgical exploration.

Transfer the patient to the **ICU** [11]. Remain **nil by mouth** [12]. Regularly review the patient's **surgical wounds** [13]. Once well, **discharge** [14] the patient home.

Long-term

The patient should be followed up in the **paediatric surgical outpatient clinic** [15].

---

[1] The paediatric surgical team should be contacted urgently due to the time-sensitive nature in which intervention is required in the setting of volvulus. The patient will require ongoing management in a centre that has a neonatal or paediatric ICU for ongoing support. In regional and rural settings, the patient should be stabilised and urgent transfer arranged. Detorsion of the volvulus is the only definitive management for the patient.

[2] Rapid establishment of IV access is required in order not to delay provision of adequate analgesia and antibiotics and so fluid resuscitation measures can be urgently commenced. Baseline bloods are able to be obtained with the insertion of the peripheral access. Establishing a secondary access or insertion of an arterial line should be considered if intensive haemodynamic support is required.

[3] Due to the severe pain associated with volvulus due to malrotation, the infant or child should be provided with adequate analgesia to provide some relief from the pain. While IV access is being established, alternative routes for pain relief should be considered, including intranasal administration.

[4] The patient will require aggressive fluid resuscitation measures with 0.9% sodium chloride boluses if presenting with haemodynamic instability. Boluses are normally given in 10–20ml per kg increments, but more aggressive resuscitation may be required based on the patient's clinical picture. Ionotropic support should be considered if there is ongoing circulatory compromise in the setting of shock. Venous or arterial blood gas results can help guide the patient's response to initial management measures and to observe for any further deterioration in their condition.

[5] Broad-spectrum antibiotics should be given intravenously due to the risk of sepsis from bowel ischaemia leading to necrosis and perforation and subsequent spillage of bowel contents into the peritoneum.

[6] The patient should be made nil by mouth as they will require emergency surgery.

[7] An NGT should be inserted and left on free drainage to provide gastric decompression.

[8] The patient should be commenced on continuous monitoring while awaiting surgery in order to observe response to initial management interventions, including changes in heart rate and BP as a response to initial fluid resuscitation measures. Ongoing assessment of fluid status is required while rapid fluid resuscitation is given and to monitor maintenance of intravascular volume.

[9] In a neonate or child presenting acutely unwell with haemodynamic instability, paired with a clinical history and examination findings highly suggestive of intestinal malrotation with volvulus and peritonitis, evaluation with imaging is not required as it would only delay definitive management. These patients should receive rapid resuscitation and proceed immediately to surgery for exploration. Patients presenting with suspected intestinal malrotation with volvulus but who are otherwise systemically stable with no haemodynamic instability should have an abdominal plain film. If pneumoperitoneum is identified on plain film, the patient should also proceed immediately to surgery for exploration. If a pneumoperitoneum is not identified and the patient remains stable, either an upper GI contrast study or ultrasound should be performed, depending on local protocols and availability. This may confirm the presence of intestinal malrotation with or without volvulus, or may point towards an alternative pathology to explain the patient's symptoms.

[10] During surgical exploration, the volvulus is untwisted and areas of infarction, necrosis and perforation are resected. Stoma formation may be required. If the viability of some segments of bowel is unclear, the remaining bowel is repositioned in a position of non-rotation and the abdomen is closed, allowing up to 36 hours of observation to see if

the bowel recovers or becomes necrotic, before returning to theatre for resection of any necrotic segments. Once non-viable segments have been removed, the rest of the procedure for correction of malrotation is performed. Known as the Ladd procedure, this intervention involves an appendicectomy, passing a tube through the duodenum to identify any other anomalies causing obstruction, dividing any Ladd bands and dividing any adhesions between the duodenum and caecum at the base of the mesentery, in order to widen the base of the mesentery and to create adhesions that can help to hold the bowel in the position it was placed in. Outside of acute presentations where volvulus and bowel ischaemia are not present but intestinal malrotation is confirmed, the Ladd procedure may be performed laparoscopically as an elective procedure. The objective of the Ladd procedure is to put the bowel in a position of non-rotation and reduce the risk of volvulus occurring. There is an overall risk of recurrent volvulus following Ladd procedure, as anatomically it is impossible to ever reposition the bowel into a normal anatomical position due to its embryological origins, although this risk is small. For all intestinal malrotation surgery, there is an overall mortality rate of 9%. Mortality is much higher in those patients with associated congenital anomalies, those that are preterm and those that presented with volvulus and associated bowel necrosis.

11 Postoperatively, the patient should be monitored in an intensive care setting. There is the potential for ongoing haemodynamic instability and requirement for ongoing circulatory support as well as high fluid shifts and losses. The additional risk of sepsis from spillage of abdominal contents means that care requirements are usually higher than can be provided in a ward setting.

12 The patient should remain nil by mouth to provide ongoing bowel rest in the acute postoperative period. As signs of bowel function, including passing flatus and audible bowel sounds, become apparent, the patient can slowly reintroduce clear fluids and continue gradual diet upgrades as tolerated.

13 The patient should be observed for any postoperative complications including anastomotic leak or iatrogenic bowel injury. As with any surgical wound, they should have regular review of the surgical site to ensure good wound healing and no evidence of dehiscence or secondary skin infection.

14 Once the patient has recovered from their surgery and are tolerating food and fluid intake, have passed stool, postoperative pain is controlled and they no longer require any IV supports, they are able to be discharged home. Parents should be educated on care in the postoperative period and instructed on concerning features that would warrant re-presentation to the ED, including features of recurrent volvulus. Patients with a stoma may require ongoing stoma care and education and should be linked in with community stoma nursing.

15 Patients should have review in paediatric surgical outpatient clinic after they have been discharged from hospital. Aside from reviewing surgical scars, the child should be assessed to ensure they are growing and gaining weight appropriately, tolerating food and achieving age-appropriate developmental milestones. 89% of patients who were symptomatic of intestinal malrotation will have full resolution of symptoms following a Ladd procedure. The patients should be observed for any postoperative complications, including short gut syndrome and adhesional small bowel obstruction. Patients with short gut syndrome, where <25% of bowel length is retained post resection leading to significant malabsorption, will require coordinated MDT management to ensure they are growing and gaining weight appropriately, as these patients usually require long-term parenteral nutrition.

CASE 56: Intussusception

History

- A **2-year-old** [1] **boy** [2] with no significant **past medical history** [3] is brought into the ED by his parents with a **12-hour history of colicky abdominal pain** [4].
- The episodes last **1–2 minutes** [5] and the parents have noticed he becomes **very distressed and draws his legs up** [6] while they are happening.
- These episodes are occurring at 15–20 minute intervals and he seems **back to his usual self** [7] between episodes.

- He has **vomited yellow** [8], food-like material at home several times and passed a few **loose, brown stools** [9].
- His parents have noticed that he also seems to be becoming more **lethargic** [10] as the day goes on.
- He has not been **unwell recently** [11].
- He hasn't had a **fever** [12] and has not had any **sick contacts** [13].
- He last had the **rotavirus vaccine** [14] at 6 months of age.

[1] Intussusception refers to the telescoping of part of the intestine into a more distal segment. 90% of cases are ileocolic, where the terminal ileum invaginates into the proximal caecum through the ileocaecal valve. The condition typically presents between 6 months and 3 years of age and is the most common cause of intestinal obstruction in this age group. Approximately 10% of cases will occur in children over 5 years of age, and 1% of cases in infants under 3 months. When intussusception is occurring outside of the usual age range it is more likely to be associated with a pathological lead point, a lesion or variant of the intestine protruding into the lumen that becomes trapped by peristalsis, thereby causing intussusception.

[2] There is a slight male predominance with a male to female ratio of 3 to 2.

[3] Most episodes of intussusception occur in otherwise healthy and well children. Risk factors for intussusception include recent, resolved intussusception, recent bowel surgery or a pathological lead point, such as Meckel's diverticulum or lymphoma. In patients with cystic fibrosis, thick stool may act as the lead point.

[4] The history of pain is usually reasonably short as the distress of the child during episodes is quite significant, warranting parents to seek expert opinion quickly. The colicky nature of the pain is associated with the peristaltic movements of the bowel.

[5] The pain recurs in episodes lasting approximately 1–2 minutes as the bowel undergoes peristalsis, worsening the intussusception and causing venous congestion and oedema, which subsequently worsens the intussusception further.

[6] Children will become inconsolable during episodes and classically draw their legs up to their chest to help ease

pain. Pain may often seem out of proportion to history or examination.

[7] Often between these distressing episodes children will behave normally as the pain fully resolves. This can sometimes make diagnosis of intussusception challenging.

[8] Vomiting is a prominent feature in intussusception and usually begins with the first episode of pain. Bile-stained vomiting is a late sign and indicates bowel obstruction.

[9] Diarrhoea is also common initially and in combination with the other symptoms may lead more towards a diagnosis of gastroenteritis. The classic 'redcurrant jelly stools', or passing of frank blood per rectum, suggests late-stage disease and may be associated with a prolonged history of symptoms. Bleeding suggests underlying mucosal oedema, ulceration and ischaemia.

[10] Lethargy may sometimes be the only presenting complaint, particularly in younger age groups. Lethargy may be progressive, constant or episodic. Therefore in young patients presenting with what appears to be sepsis, intussusception is an important differential to be excluded.

[11] 75% of cases of intussusception are considered idiopathic as there is no clear trigger or lead point. Recent viral infections may cause hypertrophy of the Peyer's patches in the terminal ileum, which may act as a lead point for ileocolic intussusception.

[12] A fever is more commonly associated with other intra-abdominal pathologies such as appendicitis or gastroenteritis. Fever may be seen in late-stage intussusception if a section of bowel has become necrotic, leading to perforation and sepsis.

13 Sick contacts with similar symptoms may suggest gastroenteritis rather than intussusception.

14 Recent rotavirus vaccination is a risk factor for intussusception.

Examination

- The child appears **tired and pale** [1] but is **settled currently** [2] on his mother's lap.
- **Observations are within normal limits** [3] for age and the patient is **afebrile** [4].
- Abdominal exam reveals a **non-distended abdomen** [5] **without tenderness or guarding** [6].
- A **sausage-shaped mass** [7] is palpable on the right side of the abdomen crossing the midline to the epigastrium.
- Inspection of the nappy reveals a **loose, brown stool but no frank bleeding** [8].

1 Pallor may be seen in >50% of cases, and is worst during painful episodes.

2 It is important to examine the patient between episodes, as this allows for a more accurate examination and is also less distressing for the child.

3 Assessing the haemodynamic status of the child is important as part of a full work-up. In 5–10% of cases, infants will present in hypovolaemic shock secondary to intestinal ischaemia or perforation.

4 A fever is more commonly associated with other intra-abdominal pathologies, such as appendicitis or gastroenteritis. Fever may be seen in late-stage intussusception if a section of bowel has become necrotic, leading to perforation and sepsis.

5 Abdominal distension suggests bowel obstruction.

6 Tenderness or guarding may suggest perforation and subsequent peritonitis.

7 The abdominal mass may be subtle, which is why it is important to look for it while the child is settled. It is sometimes easier to palpate with the child lying on their side.

8 It is important to check the nappy to assess for any frank blood in stools, of which would indicate a later-stage intussusception. Rectal examinations are not indicated in the paediatric population.

Investigations

- **Blood tests** [1] are performed.
- An FBE reveals a normal haemoglobin, mildly **elevated WCC** [2] and normal platelets.
- A **UEC** [3] is normal.
- **Venous blood gas** [4] is normal.
- A **group and hold** [5] finds a blood group of A+.
- An **abdominal ultrasound** [6] is performed, which demonstrates a **single hypoechoic ring with a hyperechoic centre** [7] in the right lower quadrant.
- **Doppler** [8] flow is normal.
- A **pathological lead point** [9] is not identified.
- An **abdominal plain film** [10] does not show any intra-peritoneal **free air** [11] and does not show large **distended bowel loops** [12].

1 Blood tests are not routinely performed for suspected intussusception, but are indicated if the child appears unwell, febrile or haemodynamically unstable.

2 White cell count may be elevated due to recurrent vomiting, or as a marker of infection from necrotic or perforated bowel.

3 UECs may identify any electrolyte abnormalities that should ideally be corrected prior to surgery.

4 A VBG may show a metabolic acidosis or raised lactate if the bowel has become obstructed and necrotic.

5 If taking bloods, a group and hold should be taken in case the patient needs to be taken to theatre for operative management.

6 Ultrasound is the gold standard investigation to diagnose intussusception. It has a sensitivity and specificity of >98% and a negative predictive value of 100% when performed by an experienced sonographer. Ultrasound offers the benefit of no radiation exposure for the child and can also be used to exclude other alternative causes for symptoms concurrently, such as appendicitis.

7 The classical appearance of intussusception on ultrasound is the so-called target sign, which demonstrates that a portion of bowel has been drawn into the lumen of an adjacent part of bowel. In ileocolic intussusception, the target sign is usually in the right lower quadrant.

8 Mesenteric blood flow can be assessed on ultrasound. Lack of perfusion indicates the development of ischaemia, bowel wall necrosis and irreducibility.

9 Ultrasound can also be used to identify a possible pathological lead point as a precipitant for the intussusception.

10 An abdominal plain film should be part of intussusception work-up only if obstruction or perforation is suspected clinically.

11 If free air is present, indicating perforation, this would change the management approach to the intussusception and would lead to operative management in the first instance to correct the intussusception, rather than trialling non-operative measures.

12 Distended bowel loops and absence of colonic gas may be present on plain film as evidence of intestinal obstruction. Other findings on plain film in patients with intussusception may include an obscured liver margin, lack of air in the caecum and a crescent sign – a soft tissue density projecting into the gas of the large bowel, indicating the intussusception.

Management

Immediate

Analgesia [1] and **resuscitation** [2] should precede investigation. Establish **IV access** [3] early. Some hospital protocols may recommend administering **IV antibiotics** [4] at this time. Monitor **vital signs** [5]. Keep the child **nil by mouth** [6]. If there is evidence of bowel obstruction or perforation, a **nasogastric tube** [7] should be inserted and the patient should be started on **IV fluids** [8] and **IV antibiotics** [9]. Alert the **paediatric surgical team** [10] and **radiology** [11] department about need for urgent abdominal ultrasound and enema.

Short-term

Patients with ileocolic intussusception, normal vital signs and no evidence of bowel perforation can be managed with non-operative **enema reduction** [12]. In patients where non-operative reduction is wholly unsuccessful or who are unstable or have evidence of bowel perforation, **surgical reduction** [13] should be attempted in the first instance.

Long-term

Monitor the patient post reduction of the intussusception for signs of **recurrence** [14]. **Antibiotics** [15] may be continued in some cases. Patients are encouraged to drink clear fluids initially, then diet is upgraded as tolerated. Perform regular **abdominal examinations** [16]. For patients who required operative management, regular **wound inspections** [17] should be performed. Patients are suitable for discharge once they are haemodynamically stable, have tolerated a **regular diet** [18] and their **bowels are opening** [19]. Patients' parents are advised to return to the ED if symptoms re-occur and to see their **GP** [20] 1–2 days post discharge. Patients who required surgical management should be followed up in **outpatient clinic** [21].

1 Usually intranasal fentanyl or IV morphine is required to help settle the patient's extreme pain and distress.

2 Treat patients with hypovolaemic shock with 10–20ml/kg boluses of 0.9% sodium chloride.

3 Rapid IV access is important in order not to delay ongoing management. IV access should be established before diagnostic imaging.

4 It is important to consult local hospital protocols in regard to antibiotic use in intussusception. Some guidelines suggest that a dose of broad-spectrum antibiotics covering intra-abdominal pathogens must be given prior to enema reduction, due to risk of bacteraemia and potential perforation. In other hospitals, pre-procedural antibiotics are not routinely used.

5 Patients can decompensate quickly, particularly while undergoing imaging. Children must always be accompanied by medical or nursing escorts capable of providing urgent resuscitation when they are away from the ED.

6 Patients must remain nil by mouth in the event they require operative management. This is to reduce the risk of aspiration during anaesthesia induction.

7 NGTs must be inserted if there is evidence of bowel obstruction or perforation on abdominal plain film, to help decompress the bowel. It is also important to place an NGT if the patient needs to be transferred to a larger centre to pre-empt the possibility of deterioration.

8 Commencing regular fluids should be done for unwell patients due to their risk of deterioration and nil by mouth status. Fluids should be 0.9% sodium chloride + 5% glucose.

9 Broad-spectrum antibiotic treatment should be commenced in patients demonstrating evidence of shock, perforation, peritonitis or bowel wall necrosis.

10 The paediatric surgical team needs to be alerted as soon as intussusception is suspected in order to help arrange for air enema and the possible requirement of theatre space. In rural areas, a patient may need urgent air transfer as the risk of requiring laparotomy demands that appropriately trained paediatric surgeons are immediately available.

11 Alerting the radiology department early also helps them to schedule the patient in for abdominal ultrasound and enema reduction as soon as possible.

12 Enema reduction has a high success rate in children with ileocolic intussusception. Most radiologists perform enema reduction without sedation or general anaesthesia. Reduction is usually done under fluoroscopic guidance using hydrostatic (saline or contrast) or pneumatic (air) pressure. In some institutions, abdominal ultrasound may be skipped and enema reduction is used as a both a diagnostic and therapeutic procedure. The risk of perforation with non-operative reduction is 1%, but is an acute surgical emergency if it occurs. Risk factors for perforation include age <6 months, >3 days of symptoms and evidence of small bowel obstruction. If perforation occurs, needle decompression of the abdomen may be necessary, as a large pneumoperitoneum may compromise a patient's respiratory status. Non-operative reduction is successful in up to 85% of cases. If the non-operative reduction is successful in reducing part of the intussusception and the patient remains stable, a delayed repeat enema may be performed in 30 minutes to 3 hours later. This may help to avoid surgical management for some patients in whom successful reduction is achieved on subsequent enema attempts. Small bowel–small bowel intussusception will usually spontaneously reduce and does not require reduction.

13 Indications for urgent surgical intervention include unstable patients, peritonitis, perforation or unsuccessful non-operative reduction. Prophylactic antibiotics must be given prior to skin incision. Most surgical reductions can be performed via laparoscopy but an open approach may need to be utilised. The intussusception is reduced manually and the bowel can be inspected. In some cases, it may be necessary to perform a bowel resection and anastomosis in the instance that manual reduction is not successful or if a pathological lead point is identified. The risk of recurrence is 1% after manual reduction and negligible after surgical resection.

14 Intussusception re-occurs in 10% of children after successful non-operative reduction, with approximately half of these within the first 72 hours. Each recurrence should be handled as if it were the first episode, including prompt abdominal ultrasound if the child is still an inpatient.

15 Antibiotics should be continued if there is suggestion of sepsis or findings of perforation and peritonitis intra-operatively. A low grade fever may be noted in the first few hours after enema reduction due to transient bowel ischaemia causing a systemic inflammatory response.

16 Abdominal examinations should be performed to ensure resolution of any features of peritonitis and also to identify any signs of postoperative ileus, which may be suggested by abdominal distension and hypoactive bowel sounds. In these cases, diet should be upgraded more slowly.

17 Wound inspections should be performed to ensure there is no dehiscence or evidence of development of wound infection.

18 It is important to ensure children are tolerating their regular diet prior to discharge to prevent the risk of dehydration in the community if oral intake is not well established.

19 It is important to ensure bowels are opening normally prior to discharge to ensure postoperative ileus has resolved.

20 Follow-up with a GP soon after discharge is recommended for further evaluation, wound inspection and to ensure there are no symptoms present that might suggest recurrence.

21 Follow-up in paediatric surgical outpatient clinic is advised to ensure adequate wound healing and that the patient has been able to return to their premorbid level of function.

CASE 57: Necrotising enterocolitis

History

- A **12-day-old** [1], **very preterm neonate** [2] is reviewed in the **neonatal ICU** [3] as they have developed **increasing abdominal distension** [4], **new bilious vomiting** [5] and **loose stools** [6] over the past 24 hours.
- They were born at **31 weeks' gestation** [7] with a corrected age of 32+5 weeks via a normal vaginal delivery following a spontaneous onset of labour.
- The mother received **antenatal corticosteroids** [8].
- Their **birthweight was 1450g** [9].
- They have been **receiving feeds** [10] exclusively via NGT of **expressed breast milk** [11].

- They had been **making good progress** [12] in terms of weight gain and feeding up until one day ago.
- They have seemed more **lethargic** [13] over the past day.
- Following birth, they received empirical **antibiotics** [14] for 2 days.
- This is the mother's first pregnancy, there were no concerning features on her **routine antenatal screening** [15] and no concerns on her antenatal ultrasounds.
- There is no significant **family history** [16].

[1] The development of necrotising enterocolitis (NEC) in a neonate leads to ischaemic necrosis of intestinal mucosa, and is an emergency requiring prompt identification and treatment. It can affect the entire bowel but most commonly affects the colon and distal ileum. The timing of the onset of symptoms varies depending on the gestational age of the neonate. For neonates born at <26 weeks' gestation, the median time of onset of symptoms is >3 weeks, and for neonates born at a gestation >31 weeks the median time of onset of symptoms is before 2 weeks.

[2] Neonates can be divided into categories based on the gestational age at which they were born. Term neonates are those born between 37 and 41 weeks of gestation. Preterm neonates are those born before 37 weeks of gestation. This can be broken down further into late preterm for those neonates born between 32 and 36+6 weeks' gestation, very preterm for those neonates born between 28 and 31+6 weeks' gestation, and extremely preterm for those neonates born earlier than 28 weeks' gestation.

[3] Neonates who are delivered prematurely are always cared for in a neonatal intensive care unit or special care nursery. Any neonates born earlier than 32 weeks' gestation will generally be monitored in a neonatal intensive care unit, while those delivered at 32 weeks' gestation and above may require monitoring in a special care nursery. However, this is often hospital-dependent and local hospital protocols should be observed when identifying the best-equipped place to care for a preterm neonate. Preterm neonates are at risk of temperature instability due to their relatively large surface area, limited stores of brown fat and glycogen, and an underdeveloped neurological response to cold, and

consequently should be wrapped well and nursed in an incubator. Preterm infants are also at risk of hypoglycaemia and require blood glucose monitoring and stabilisation of blood sugars with regular feeds, buccal glucose gel, IV dextrose or IM glucagon, depending on the infant's particular circumstances and risk factors. Depending on how preterm the neonate is and other maternal and neonatal factors, they may also require respiratory support, enteral feeding support, vitamin and mineral supplementation, phototherapy, IV antibiotics and neonatal eye examination, among others.

[4] Symptoms of necrotising enterocolitis can be non-specific. Abdominal distension is a key abdominal finding to look out for when suspecting NEC.

[5] Bilious vomiting is another sign to identify when considering NEC. Differentiating the presence of bilious vomiting from birth or developing later in life is important. As NEC presents sometimes weeks after the neonate is born, new bilious vomiting would lend itself more to a diagnosis of NEC. Bilious vomiting present from birth may suggest an alternative cause, such as an intestinal atresia, Hirschsprung disease or intestinal malrotation.

[6] New diarrhoea can be another indicator of an abdominal pathology. The presence of haematochezia is a concerning finding and requires prompt investigation and intervention.

[7] The incidence of NEC decreases with increasing gestational age. The incidence of NEC in neonates born earlier than 32 weeks' gestation is 2–7%. Of total cases of NEC, 10–15% are seen in term infants, but these infants usually have other risk factors that predispose them to developing NEC, such as congenital heart disease, other GI pathology,

sepsis, low birthweight, respiratory disease, endocrine disorders, polycythaemia or exclusive formula feeding.

8 Women thought to be at risk of preterm labour and early delivery should be given a course of antenatal steroids. Local hospital or governmental protocols should be followed in regard to the administration of antenatal corticosteroids, but in general for a woman thought to be at risk of preterm delivery, two doses of antenatal corticosteroids given 24 hours apart should be administered. Antenatal corticosteroids offer many benefits for the preterm neonate, including reducing the risk of respiratory distress syndrome, intraventricular haemorrhage, retinopathy of prematurity and NEC. Overall they have benefits in reducing preterm neonatal morbidity and mortality.

9 The incidence of NEC decreases with increasing birthweight. Of total cases of NEC, >90% occur in neonates with a birthweight <1500g (termed very low birthweight), and also born at <32 weeks' gestation.

10 NEC occurs in only 10% of neonates who have never received enteral feeding.

11 Breast milk is preferred to cow's milk-based formulas as it is believed it reduces the risk of NEC by stimulating the neonate's developing immunity and promoting GI motility. There is a dose-dependent relationship, with higher levels of intake of breast milk conferring a higher level of protection against developing NEC.

12 Most preterm neonates who develop NEC have generally been stabilised on feeds and are tolerating feeds and growing well prior to developing symptoms. Feed intolerance is an early sign of developing NEC.

13 Lethargy is a non-specific, systemic symptom which may be identified in neonates with NEC. Other non-specific systemic symptoms include new or increased apnoea or need for respiratory support, and temperature instability.

14 Preterm neonates may receive empirical antibiotics post delivery; due to their early gestational age they are at risk for early-onset sepsis. Other maternal factors play a role in determining the risk of sepsis in the neonate, such as if they are known to have Group B streptococcus, had a fever in labour, received antibiotics during labour or had prolonged rupture of membranes. Retrospective studies suggest that prolonged IV antibiotic administration for >5 days within the first 14 days of life, particularly in the setting of cultures without growth, may contribute to intestinal microbial imbalance and in turn increase risk of developing NEC.

15 Taking a full maternal history is important whenever called to review a neonate. Particular findings on maternal and birth history may raise or reduce suspicion for various differentials.

16 NEC is not known to have any familial link but taking a family history is a part of robust history taking and should be included as part of the work-up.

Examination

- The neonate is lying in an **incubator** [1] and appears **flat and unwell** [2].
- They are of a **small size** [3].
- They are having brief periods of **halted respirations** [4].
- They are demonstrating evidence of **temperature instability** [5].
- Their **BP and heart rate** [6] are within the normal range.
- There is **bilious drainage** [7] from their NGT.
- The neonate has a **delayed capillary refill time and sunken fontanelles** [8].
- Their **heart sounds are dual and there are no murmurs** [9].
- **Chest is clear** [10] to auscultation with no added sounds and good air entry throughout.

- Upon general inspection of the abdomen, there is **no evidence of previous abdominal surgeries** [11].
- The **umbilicus** [12] is clean and dry.
- There is a patch of **erythema** [13] on the anterior abdominal wall.
- The **abdomen is distended** [14].
- The abdomen is soft to palpation, but the neonate becomes **distressed** [15] by the exam.
- There are **no palpable masses** [16].
- **Bowel sounds are absent** [17].
- The patient's **nappy contains a loose stool with no visible blood** [18].
- The **anus is patent and in a normal position** [19].

1 Due to their premature age and temperature instability, the neonate must be nursed in an incubator to maintain an optimal body temperature.

2 General inspection of the neonate can be a good overall indicator of how they are progressing. Neonates with NEC may appear lethargic or irritable. They may handle poorly, particularly if they have a peritonitic abdomen.

3 The incidence of NEC is greater in preterm and low birthweight neonates. This may be due to an immature immune system and GI tract, which increases their susceptibility to infections. Immature gut motility leads to increased transit time for feeds, which increases the chance of intraluminal bacterial overgrowth. An underdeveloped mucosal barrier may allow bacteria to penetrate into the intestinal wall.

4 Apnoea or increasing respiratory requirements requiring respiratory support are non-specific features that can be seen with NEC.

5 Temperature instability is another non-specific sign that may be seen in NEC. Due to their relatively high surface area, low birthweight neonates are at increased risk of rapid heat loss.

6 Hypotension and bradycardia may be present in advanced presentations of NEC.

7 If there is new feed intolerance associated with abdominal distension, the NGT should be placed on free drainage with regular aspirations. Bilious drainage or aspirates raise suspicion for NEC.

8 Neonates are particularly susceptible to rapid volume depletion as a consequence of vomiting, particularly when combined with diarrhoea, so a careful fluid balance assessment should be performed. Other signs to identify are evidence of oliguria or anuria, poor skin turgor, dry mucous membranes and altered conscious level.

9 A full assessment of the neonate should be performed, particularly when the presentation is undifferentiated. Cardiac examination may identify added sounds or murmurs suggestive of a congenital heart defect, which is a risk factor for the development of NEC, particularly in term neonates.

10 Lung field auscultation may indicate signs of pneumonia, which may have developed due to aspiration following repeated vomiting. Lung field auscultation may also identify an alternative cause for the changing respiratory requirements of the neonate and should be included as part of a full assessment of an unwell neonate.

11 Particularly in term neonates, previous abdominal surgery, such as for correction of gastroschisis or intestinal atresia, is a risk factor for subsequent development of NEC. There is a theory that a period of insufficient intestinal perfusion and subsequent reperfusion may contribute to bowel wall injury. This may also be the case for neonates with other comorbidities affecting circulation, such as congenital heart disease or polycythaemia.

12 Omphalitis, or infection of the umbilical cord stump, is a serious infection in the newborn, with a mortality rate of 10%. It generally presents in neonates <14 days old with purulent discharge from the umbilical stump with surrounding cellulitis. The infection can spread from the umbilical vessels to the systemic circulation, causing sepsis.

13 Anterior abdominal wall erythema or cellulitis is a feature of NEC. Crepitus and induration of the anterior abdominal wall may also be present.

14 Abdominal distension is a prominent feature of NEC.

15 Tenderness during palpation of the anterior abdominal wall is another feature of NEC. It can be difficult to determine pain in neonates so cues must be taken from the patient's behaviour. The neonate may cry and become distressed during palpation. They may also be sensitive to handling, such as during nappy or position changes, as handling aggravates their pain. In very rare cases, neonates can develop appendicitis which presents almost identically to NEC. Often a diagnosis of neonatal appendicitis will only be made macroscopically during laparotomy.

16 Occasionally fixed bowel loops can be palpated through the anterior abdominal wall. Ascites may also be identified on abdominal palpation.

17 Ileus is an early feature of NEC. In early presentations of NEC where features are non-specific, the presence of ileus does not help to distinguish NEC from other causes of ileus, such as sepsis.

18 Diarrhoea is a feature of NEC. A late feature is that of haematochezia or blood in stools.

19 The anus should be inspected for evidence of an anal fissure, an alternative source of rectal bleeding. Anal fissures are generally benign.

Investigations

- An FBE reveals a **mildly elevated WCC and low platelets** [1].
- **UEC** [2] demonstrates low sodium.
- A VBG shows a **metabolic acidosis and a high lactate** [3].
- **BGLs are elevated** [4].
- Coagulation studies demonstrate **normal clotting profiles** [5].
- **A blood culture is pending** [6].
- A **peritoneal fluid culture** [7] and **stool culture** [8] are not obtained.

- An **abdominal plain film** [9] is ordered, which reveals **dilated bowel loops** [10] and **bubbles of gas in the wall of the small bowel** [11].
- There is **no free air** [12].

- Based on the history, examination and investigation findings, the **Modified Bell's staging criteria** [13] are used to assess the severity of NEC.

[1] Thrombocytopenia is a common finding on blood work for neonates suspected of having NEC. A typical trend shows decreasing platelet counts as the disease progresses, increasing the risk of potential catastrophic bleeding for the neonate. Once management has been instigated, a rising platelet count is a marker of improvement. WCC is often non-specific. A WCC differential can be more useful, with a high leucocyte count associated with intestinal perforation due to NEC. Neutropenia in low birthweight neonates contributes to their increased risk for developing NEC.

[2] Electrolyte abnormalities are often non-specific. A persistent hyponatraemia may be observed in neonates with NEC.

[3] A metabolic acidosis with high lactate can be markers of both NEC and of sepsis. An ABG may also be performed, particularly if the neonate also has increased respiratory support requirements. Performing serial blood gases can be good indicators of disease progression and subsequent improvements.

[4] Increasing BGLs are another marker of possible developing NEC.

[5] Coagulation studies should be performed if thrombocytopenia is noted on the FBE or if the infant has evidence of bleeding, such as haematochezia or bruising. In severe NEC, the neonate may develop disseminated intravascular coagulation (DIC). Prolonged APTT and PT, decreasing fibrinogen levels, increased D-dimer and the presence of thrombocytopenia are all suggestive of DIC.

[6] A blood culture should be obtained as part of a panel of investigations for NEC. Sepsis may develop due to NEC, or the neonate's symptoms may be attributable to sepsis from an alternative cause. It can take >24 hours for blood culture results to demonstrate any bacterial growth, so there should be no delay in commencing antibiotic therapy after the culture has been obtained. Antibiotic therapy can be rationalised based on culture results and sensitivities as they become available. 20% of cases of NEC are associated with a positive blood culture result. If clinical suspicion for NEC over any other cause of sepsis is not absolute, then a full septic work-up including CSF culture and urine microscopy and culture should also be performed.

[7] In settings of peritonism or high volume ascites, abdominal paracentesis may be performed to obtain a peritoneal fluid sample for microscopy and culture. If GI organisms are identified in the peritoneal fluid culture then this suggests bowel wall perforation as a cause of peritonitis.

The results of the culture and sensitivities can also be used to guide antibiotic therapy.

[8] Stool cultures are generally not a useful investigation in suspected NEC as the results are non-specific. Frank blood suggests an acute intestinal pathology such as NEC or intestinal malrotation with volvulus. The presence of occult blood in stools is non-specific, as it is possible for occult blood to be present in the stools of healthy, low birthweight, preterm neonates. Other causes of blood in stools include infectious neonatal enterocolitis caused by pathogens such as *Clostridioides difficile*, salmonella, shigella or campylobacter, anal fissures, cow's milk protein allergy and swallowed maternal blood.

[9] Abdominal plain films are the imaging modality of choice for identifying and staging NEC as well as monitoring progression of the disease. They should be interpreted in conjunction with clinical features, and to a lesser extent, laboratory markers, which can often be non-specific but can give an indication of disease severity. The findings on abdominal plain film tend to be clearer and present more typically the higher the gestational age of the neonate. Plain films should be taken supine and additional views, including a lateral or lateral decubitus view, may also be obtained. These extra views can be useful when assessing for evidence of pneumoperitoneum or sentinel loops. Lateral decubitus view is used to look for free air over the liver. Serial abdominal plain films will be obtained 2–3 times a day for monitoring of disease progression and the frequency can be reduced as the neonate demonstrates clinical improvement.

[10] Dilated bowel loops may be seen in early presentations of NEC. Dilated bowel loops may also be present with a septic ileus, so dilated bowel loops on plain film alone are not enough to confirm the presence of NEC. The bowel loops may have an asymmetrical distribution in the abdomen. Sentinel bowel loops, where a dilated loop of bowel remains in a fixed position and is visible on multiple views, are suggestive of necrotic or perforated bowel due to NEC. Bowel wall oedema and thickening may also be noted.

[11] Bubbles of gas in the wall of the small bowel is known as pneumatosis intestinalis and it is present in most cases of confirmed NEC. In a preterm neonate, the presence of pneumatosis intestinalis is NEC until proven otherwise. Other conditions can also cause a similar finding on plain radiograph, including ischaemic bowel, cow's milk protein allergy and typhlitis (inflammation of the caecum), but NEC must be excluded before pursuing alternative diagnoses. Cow's milk protein allergy is rarely seen in preterm neonates

and especially before 6 weeks of life; however, it can present similarly with abdominal distension and diarrhoea, which if severe can result in frank blood in stools as well as the presence of pneumatosis intestinalis on plain film. Changing to a non-cow's milk-based feed will reverse symptoms.

12 In advanced NEC causing a bowel wall perforation, pneumoperitoneum may be evident on plain film. In supine views, a large pneumoperitoneum may appear as a 'football sign' with air outlining the falciform ligament. Rigler sign, otherwise called the double-wall sign, where gas is visible both within the bowel lumen and within the peritoneal cavity, may also be seen. Portal venous gas may also be recognised on plain film. Another cause of pneumoperitoneum is spontaneous intestinal perforation of the newborn. Similar to NEC, it typically affects low birthweight neonates but generally affects neonates in their first week of life and is independent of feeding, which distinguishes it from NEC. A blue discolouration of the anterior abdominal wall is a classic sign of spontaneous intestinal perforation of the newborn. Pneumatosis intestinalis will not be present on imaging.

13 Suspected or stage 1 NEC incorporates non-specific symptoms and signs, such as temperature instability, bradycardia, lethargy, apnoea, abdominal distension, vomiting, and either normal plain film or evidence of dilated loops on plain film. It is divided into stage 1A or stage 1B by the absence or presence, respectively, of gross blood in stools. Definite or stage 2 NEC has the same non-specific features as in stage 1 but includes absent bowel sounds, anterior abdominal wall tenderness and the presence of pneumatosis intestinalis; these features are categorised as stage 2A. Stage 2B has the same features as stage 2A and also includes metabolic acidosis and thrombocytopenia on laboratory evaluation as well as anterior abdominal wall cellulitis and the presence of a right lower quadrant mass and portal venous gas on plain film. Advanced or stage 3 NEC will also have hypotension, DIC and neutropenia, signs of generalised peritonitis and ascites. The absence or presence of a pneumoperitoneum divides stage 3 into A and B, respectively. Approximately 30% of cases of NEC do not progress past stage 1 and symptoms gradually improve and resolve. In these cases, it cannot be said definitely whether the neonate did or did not have NEC. Up to 40% of cases of NEC will progress to stage 3.

Management

Immediate

Manage patient in the **neonatal intensive care unit** [1]. **Stop feeding** [2]. Insert an **NGT** [3]. Ensure patient has **IV access** [4]. Continuously **monitor vital signs** [5]. Perform **baseline investigations** [6]. Commence **empirical antibiotics** [7]. **Monitor fluid status** [8]. **Correct any laboratory abnormalities** [9]. **Refer to the paediatric surgical team** [10].

Short-term

Commence **total parenteral nutrition** [11]. Perform **serial abdominal examinations** [12], **laboratory markers** [13] and **abdominal plain films** [14]. Proceed to **peritoneal drainage** [15] or **laparotomy** [16] if required. **Monitor** [17] the neonate and their surgical wounds in the postoperative period.

Long-term

Once discharged from hospital, the infant should have **regular follow-up** [18] in outpatient clinic and in the community.

1 If NEC is suspected, medical management should be commenced immediately due to the highly fulminant nature of the disease and the high risk of rapid deterioration. Where a neonatal ICU or local paediatric surgical team are not readily available, transfer to a tertiary centre should be arranged before the possibility that the neonate becomes too unstable to transfer.

2 Feeding should be discontinued immediately in order to provide bowel rest. The neonate will remain nil per oral for an extended period of time, often up to 2 weeks. As the neonate

begins to show clinical improvement, feeds can gradually be reintroduced.

3 If not already present, an NGT should be inserted for gastric decompression. It should be left on free drainage with regular aspirates.

4 In general, most preterm neonates already being cared for in the neonatal intensive care unit will have established peripheral IV access. If not, urgent insertion of a peripheral venous cannula is essential so as not to delay ongoing management. Establishing a secondary access should be considered.

5 Monitoring of vital signs is essential as they may be the first indication of deterioration of the patient's condition. The neonate may require cardiovascular and respiratory support, including inotropes or mechanical ventilation.

6 An initial abdominal plain film and baseline bloodwork, including a blood culture, should be obtained. This helps to stage the suspected NEC and provides a marker to guide response to treatment and improvement or deterioration in patient condition.

7 Local hospital protocol should be followed in regard to antibiotic treatment choice for NEC. Generally, a combination of broad-spectrum antibiotics is initiated and the antibiotic regimen is narrowed once previously obtained cultures and sensitivities are available. Antibiotics may be continued for up to 2 weeks, although this course may be longer, especially in the setting of intra-abdominal abscess formation. In stage 1 NEC, if the disease does not progress further and the neonate shows clinical improvement, antibiotics may be ceased and feeds reintroduced earlier when compared to later stages.

8 The neonate should receive adequate fluid resuscitation and replacement, especially in the setting of repeated vomiting, being nil by mouth and third space losses. Bowel wall inflammation promotes capillary leakage and the loss of fluid from the circulating intravascular volume.

9 Any electrolyte, acid–base or haematological abnormalities seen on laboratory results should be corrected if possible.

10 Evaluation and management of suspected or definite NEC should be a multidisciplinary approach between both the neonatal and paediatric surgical teams.

11 Due to the extended time the neonate will need to be nil by mouth, they should be commenced on parenteral nutrition until feeds can be reintroduced. This should be done in conjunction with the neonatal team and the neonatal dietitian. A longer-term point of vascular access such as a central venous catheter may need to be inserted.

12 Regular examination of a neonate with suspected NEC should be performed due to the potential for rapid deterioration and disease progression over a short space of time.

13 Repeating laboratory markers gives an indication as to whether the neonate's condition is deteriorating or whether they are showing improvement with medical management. Repeat lactate levels should be obtained once to twice daily.

14 Serial abdominal plain films are used in conjunction with physical examination and laboratory studies to monitor response to treatment. They should be done 2–3 times a day in the initial phase of the illness and repeated if there has been a change in clinical condition. As the neonate begins to demonstrate improvement, the frequency of abdominal imaging can be reduced. Once the bowel gas pattern returns to normal and there is no more pneumatosis intestinalis, serial abdominal plain films can be stopped.

15 Pneumoperitoneum is an absolute indication for surgical intervention. In critically unwell neonates who are not well enough for a general anaesthetic or invasive abdominal surgery, primary peritoneal drainage can be performed within the neonatal intensive care unit. This procedure can help reduce abdominal tension and distension by evacuating free air and meconium-stained ascites. IV analgesia and local anaesthetic are used to manage pain associated with the procedure. Under sterile technique, the peritoneal cavity is entered via the anterior abdominal wall at McBurney's point, cultures are taken and the peritoneal cavity is irrigated with warmed normal saline. A drain is then left *in situ*. If the neonate's clinical condition improves and there is no ongoing drain output, the drain can be removed. If bowel function appears to have returned to normal, the neonate can have a trial of feeding.

16 Laparotomy is performed for neonates who develop a bowel perforation, but is also considered for neonates who are not improving on maximal medical therapy. Between a quarter and half of neonates with NEC will require surgical intervention. During the procedure, the involved section of bowel is excised. Where only a short segment is affected, primary anastomosis may be done during the initial surgery. For longer affected bowel segments, often the proximal end of bowel is brought out as an enterostomy while the distal segment is formed into a mucous fistula. If the neonate recovers well and is able to undergo a second surgery, the re-anastomosis of the two ends will be done 4–6 weeks after the initial procedure. To ensure there are no intestinal strictures in the remaining bowel prior to re-anastomosis, a contrast enema should be organised prior. In severe cases with multiple affected segments of bowel, only segments with clear necrosis or perforation should be resected to try to prevent short gut syndrome. A repeat laparotomy should be done in 2–3 days to re-explore the bowel and resect any further necrotic segments.

17 As with any surgical procedure, the neonate's abdominal wounds should have regular review to ensure they are healing well and not showing evidence of secondary infection or dehiscence. If present, stomal output should be recorded and these losses accounted for in fluid balance calculations. Continue with serial examinations, laboratory evaluations and abdominal plain films. In a small number of cases, necrotising enterocolitis can recur so a decline in clinical condition should warrant re-investigation for necrotising enterocolitis or other causes. The neonate should continue with IV antibiotics and nil by mouth until both the neonatal and paediatric surgical teams feel the NEC has resolved and the neonate can gradually have feeds reintroduced. Even once the neonate has recovered from their acute NEC, they may still require an extended stay in the neonatal intensive care unit or paediatric ward for ongoing monitoring and management of other comorbidities associated with prematurity, or any complications from their NEC, such as short gut syndrome. Mortality from NEC increases in neonates born at an earlier gestation or low birthweight or those that undergo surgical intervention.

18 The infant should have regular review in both the paediatric surgical outpatient clinic and in the paediatric medical clinic for follow-up of their recovery from NEC, as well as any comorbidities associated with prematurity. Approximately 50% of infants affected by necrotising enterocolitis will have no long-term effects from the disease. The others may experience short- or long-term GI complications, as well as issues with age-appropriate growth and development. Up to a quarter of neonates who have

had NEC may develop areas of intestinal stricture formation, resulting in luminal stenosis, with most occurring within the first 3 months. These infants may present with features of bowel obstruction or failure to thrive. Stricture formation is not related to severity of the NEC and may need to be resected surgically. Infants with short gut syndrome, where <25% of bowel length is retained post resection leading to significant malabsorption, will require coordinated MDT management to ensure they are growing and gaining weight appropriately, as these infants are usually on long-term total parenteral nutrition. The infant's GP and maternal and child health nurse also play an important role in coordinating care and monitoring growth and development in the community.

CASE 58: Neonatal bowel atresias

History

- A **36-hour-old** [1] **neonate** [2] is transferred from a rural hospital to a tertiary centre with **repeated non-bilious vomiting** [3] .
- They were **born at term** [4] via a normal vaginal delivery.
- They have not **passed meconium** [5] .
- They have not had any **fevers** [6] .
- There is **no significant family history** [7] .

- The patient's mother did not take any **medications or illicit drugs** [8] or **smoke** [9] during her pregnancy.
- The patient's mother reports her **antenatal testing** [10] was normal but she did have **polyhydramnios** [11] on her antenatal ultrasounds.
- The mother states she also underwent **maternal screening tests** [12] for congenital abnormalities.

[1] An intestinal atresia is a congenital defect along the GI tract resulting in complete or partial obstruction of the lumen of the bowel. It can occur anywhere from oesophagus to rectum. Vomiting due to small bowel intestinal atresia will begin 24–48 hours after birth.

[2] The term 'neonate' encompasses any newborn in their first 28 days of life.

[3] In duodenal atresia the vomiting may or may not be bilious, depending on whether or not the defect is proximal or distal to the hepatopancreatic ampulla. For jejunal, ileal and colonic atresia, the vomiting is always bilious. Intestinal atresias range in incidence from approximately 1.3–3.5 per 10 000 live births. Of these, the most common is duodenal atresia, making up 60% of all atresias. This is followed by jejunal and ileal atresias, representing 20% of all atresias, while colonic atresia contributes <10% of all atresias.

[4] The majority of neonates with intestinal atresias are born at term or near term. Term refers to a gestation of 37–41 weeks. A gestation <37 weeks is referred to as preterm and a gestation >41 weeks is referred to as post-term.

[5] While it is more common for a neonate to not pass meconium after birth, it is still possible for infants with intestinal atresia to pass meconium despite their bowel obstruction. This is more commonly seen in more proximal obstructions, such as duodenal atresia, but can also occur with ileal or jejunal atresia if meconium is present in the bowel distal to the obstruction. Neonates with colonic atresia are unlikely to pass meconium.

[6] Fevers may indicate sepsis as a possible alternative cause of the patient's symptoms. Sepsis could also develop from an aspiration pneumonia caused by the repeated vomiting.

[7] Familial genetic factors do not play a large role in the development of intestinal atresias in the foetus. However,

there have been some cases of familial atresia syndromes, as well as newborns being more likely to have atresias in families with known thrombophilia. A family history of cystic fibrosis may also point towards the same diagnosis in the neonate. During foetal development, thick inspissated meconium may cause a segmental volvulus affecting the mesenteric vascular supply of the developing bowel, causing failure of that portion of the bowel to develop. Most jejunal and ileal atresias are acquired from impaired vascular supply.

[8] The use of vasoconstrictive medications such as pseudoephedrine found in over-the-counter decongestants or methylenedioxymethamphetamine (MDMA) triples the risk of intestinal atresia in the newborn. It is thought this could be due to interruption of mesenteric vessel blood flow during development. Significant vomiting is also a feature of neonatal abstinence syndrome in neonates whose mothers used opioids during the pregnancy.

[9] Similar to vasoconstrictive medications, smoking in the first trimester of pregnancy also triples the risk of formation of intestinal atresias in the foetus, thought to be by a similar mechanism of interrupting blood flow.

[10] Antenatal testing and screening are a routine part of antenatal care for an expectant mother to ensure a safe pregnancy and delivery for mother and baby, and to try to pre-empt and correct any issues early should they arise. Antenatal testing involves regular reviews with GPs, midwives and obstetrician gynaecologists. During these reviews, general physical check-ups including assessment of height, weight and BP for the mother, as well as fundal height measurements for an estimation of the development of the foetus, are performed. The mother will also be referred for antenatal ultrasound scans for monitoring of foetal morphology and growth as well as observation of amniotic fluid volume and blood flow in the foetus and placenta. Urine samples are taken to look for evidence of infection or

pre-eclampsia. Glucose tolerance testing is performed to identify early evidence of gestational diabetes mellitus. Blood tests are carried out, including for mother's blood group and antibodies, haemoglobin levels, vitamin D levels, and to identify the presence of or immunity to various infections that could be passed on to the foetus or neonate by vertical transmission. This includes rubella, varicella, CMV, parvovirus, herpes simplex virus, toxoplasmosis, hepatitis B and C, syphilis and HIV. The above collection of conditions may lead to infant morbidity and mortality through a variety of means including various neonatal infections leading to sepsis, congenital abnormalities, rashes, intrauterine growth restriction and developmental delays. A swab of the vagina late in pregnancy assesses for the presence of Group B streptococcus. Group B streptococcus can be a cause of early-onset sepsis in the newborn, and a positive finding of Group B streptococcus on swab or urine microscopy and culture means a woman should receive antibiotic coverage during labour to prevent infecting her newborn during delivery. For an unwell, vomiting neonate, sepsis as a cause of their symptoms must always be excluded.

11 Antenatal ultrasounds have a low sensitivity for detecting GI atresias and fewer than half of neonates with an atresia will be picked up on routine screening. During the third trimester, there may be a high suspicion for the neonate having duodenal atresia if a dilated, fluid-filled stomach and proximal duodenum are visualised on ultrasound. They appear like large 'bubbles', hence the term 'double bubble' sign. In up to 50% of cases of duodenal atresia polyhydramnios is present on antenatal ultrasounds, usually developing well into the second trimester. Jejunal and ileal atresias also may have findings of polyhydramnios

on antenatal ultrasounds, as well as findings of ascites and dilated bowel loops.

12 Maternal serum screening tests are blood tests available to women during their pregnancy to help identify the likelihood of their unborn baby having Down syndrome (trisomy 21), Edwards syndrome (trisomy 18) or a neural tube defect. Small bowel intestinal atresias can be associated with chromosomal abnormalities or other congenital anomalies. Fewer than 5% of neonates with Down syndrome will have duodenal atresia, but they represent 30% of total cases. Duodenal atresia may also be seen as part of the VACTERL association of congenital anomalies. VACTERL association refers to a constellation of non-syndromic congenital abnormalities which frequently occur in conjunction with each other. It incorporates Vertebral anomalies, Anal atresia, Cardiac Anomalies, Tracheo-oEophageal fistula, Renal anomalies and Limb anomalies. Additionally, other congenital abnormalities not covered in the above list have also been seen with VACTERL association, including ear anomalies, laryngomalacia, laryngeal or tracheal stenosis, ambiguous genitalia, omphalocele, single umbilical artery and intestinal malrotation. As VACTERL is an association and there is no identified genetic cause, it cannot be tested for with any currently available maternal screening tests. Some features of VACTERL may be identified antenatally on ultrasounds when looking at foetal morphology. With this in mind, isolated duodenal atresia is present in up to half of all cases without any other anatomical or karyotypical abnormalities. In contrast, only 5% of cases of jejunal and ileal atresia are associated with chromosomal abnormalities. Jejunal atresia may be seen with cardiac or other GI malformations. Ileal atresia and colonic atresia are less commonly associated with other major anatomical malformations.

Examination

- The neonate appears **flat and unwell** [1].
- The **heart rate is 190bpm** [2].
- The **respiratory rate is 60 breaths per minute with mild work of breathing** [3] evident. **Oxygen saturations on air are 95%** [4].
- The **temperature is 37°C** [5].
- The neonate has **sunken fontanelles and a sluggish capillary refill time** [6].
- Their **skin is mildly tinged yellow** [7].
- Their **heart sounds are dual and there are no murmurs** [8].
- **Chest is clear** [9] to auscultation with no added

sounds and good air entry throughout.
- Upon general inspection of the abdomen, there is **no evidence of an abdominal wall defect** [10].
- The **abdomen is mildly distended** [11].
- The abdomen is soft to palpation with **no guarding or rigidity and the neonate tolerates the examination** [12] of the abdomen well.
- The patient's **nappy is dry** [13].
- The **anus is patent and in a normal position** [14].
- The patient does not have any **facial or form features associated with genetic or congenital anomalies** [15].

1 Due to repeated vomiting the neonate is unable to sufficiently absorb any fluids such as breast milk or formula that they have been taking orally, and thus the neonate may present in hypovolaemic shock. Repeated vomiting

may also be a sign of sepsis, which is a critical differential to consider in an unwell neonate. Bilious, but occasionally non-bilious vomiting is also part of the presentation of intestinal malrotation with volvulus.

2 Normal heart rate for a term neonate is 110–170bpm. A tachycardia may be present as a response to hypovolaemia, sepsis, pain or distress.

3 Normal respiratory rate for a term neonate is 30–60 breaths per minute. Respiratory compromise may be evident due to abdominal distension causing diaphragmatic elevation that is preventing adequate chest expansion. Respiratory changes may also be present in the setting of an aspiration pneumonia caused by the repeated bouts of vomiting. Increased respiratory rate may also be seen with dehydration and a subsequent metabolic acidosis.

4 In term neonates, oxygen saturations should be ≥95%. If saturations are <95% further investigation is warranted, for example looking for signs of sepsis, an airway or respiratory pathology or a cardiac pathology.

5 A fever is not usually seen in an isolated presentation of a small bowel intestinal atresia. However, a fever may be present in other diagnoses such as sepsis or aspiration pneumonia.

6 Neonates are particularly susceptible to rapid volume depletion as a consequence of vomiting, so a careful fluid balance assessment should be performed. Other signs to identify are evidence of oliguria or anuria, poor skin turgor, dry mucous membranes and altered conscious level.

7 Jaundice may be present in presentations of intestinal atresia, as intestinal obstruction increases the distribution of bilirubin in the enterohepatic circulation. Jaundice may also be intensified in the setting of associated volume depletion.

8 A full assessment of the neonate should be performed, particularly when the presentation is undifferentiated. Cardiac examination may identify added sounds or murmurs suggestive of a congenital heart defect which may be associated with a small bowel atresia. Atrioventricular septal defects are the most common cardiac defect seen in patients with Down syndrome, and may be found along with an intestinal atresia in these patients.

9 Lung field auscultation may indicate signs of pneumonia, which may have developed due to aspiration following repeated vomiting.

10 A finding of an abdominal wall defect on abdominal inspection may indicate the presence of other GI abnormalities. Most abdominal wall defects will be picked up on antenatal ultrasounds from 10 weeks' gestation. There are two main types of abdominal wall defects – omphalocele and gastroschisis. Omphalocele, also known as exomphalos, is where internal abdominal organs – most frequently the stomach, liver and bowel – protrude through an opening where the umbilical cord joins the abdomen. This results in the organs being enveloped in a membranous sac of peritoneum. Omphalocele is seen in only 2.5 per 10 000 births and is largely associated with genetic and chromosomal abnormalities and congenital cardiac defects.

The abdominal wall defect in gastroschisis is not associated with the umbilical cord and small and large bowel may protrude through the abdominal wall without a membranous covering, exposing them to the surrounding amniotic fluid. Gastroschisis is seen in 2–6 per 10 000 births. It is rarely associated with genetic and chromosomal abnormalities and less commonly with other congenital defects. 10% of cases of gastroschisis are associated with a small bowel atresia. During development, the extracorporeal intestine may volve or be compressed at the opening in the anterior abdominal wall. Due to the impaired blood supply, the affected bowel will undergo necrosis and subsequently be reabsorbed, causing an atresia.

11 Abdominal distension is a frequent finding in presentations of intestinal atresia. The more distal the atresia, often the greater the level of abdominal distension. Visible or palpable loops of bowel may also be present. In cases of colonic atresia, symptoms and examination findings may present later than in more proximal atresias.

12 The abdomen should be assessed for evidence of peritonism, which may be present in the setting of a bowel perforation or intra-abdominal cause of sepsis. Assessing for the presence of abdominal tenderness in a neonate and infants can be challenging, so paying close attention to their behaviour during palpation, palpating when they are settled and performing serial examinations may be required for an accurate assessment.

13 The neonate's nappy should be inspected to assess for any passed meconium, and as part of a fluid assessment to ensure urine is still being produced. Haematochezia may be visible in an infant's nappy in cases of intestinal malrotation with volvulus, indicating bowel ischaemia and necrosis.

14 Anal atresia can be associated with more proximal GI atresias as well as part of VACTERL associations. Therefore, assessment of anus position and patency should be performed.

15 A full top-to-toe assessment of the child should be completed, looking for physical indications of chromosomal anomalies or congenital malformations. In an acute presentation this assessment can be delayed until the neonate is stabilised. External features that may be present in neonates with Down syndrome include small low-set ears, brachycephaly, epicanthal folds, a low nasal bridge with a short nose and small nostrils, a small down-turned mouth, single palmar creases and a wide space between the first and second toes. Other structural malformations to identify, which may or may not be evident on physical examination, include cardiac, other GI, renal and skeletal abnormalities. Physical features that may be observed clinically in VACTERL association include anal atresia, cleft palate and limb anomalies such as radial aplasia or hypoplasia, polydactyly, syndactyly and hypoplastic thumb, club foot and tibial hypoplasia.

Investigations

- **Urinalysis** [1] is unremarkable.
- A **full blood examination** [2] is normal.
- A VBG demonstrates a **metabolic acidosis** [3] and **urea, electrolytes and creatinine** [4] show electrolyte disturbances.
- There is no growth seen on **blood microscopy and culture** [5].
- **Coagulation studies** [6] are normal.
- The neonate's **blood type** [7] is O+.
- Liver function testing shows a raised **bilirubin** [8] level.

- An **abdominal plain film** [9] is performed, which reveals dilatation of the stomach and proximal duodenum and an absence of distal gas.
- There is no **free air** [10].
- An **upper GI contrast study** [11] is performed which correlates the findings of the abdominal plain film.
- A **contrast enema** [12] is not required.
- A **CXR, renal ultrasound and echocardiogram** [13] are all normal.
- **Genetic screening** [14] is performed.

[1] A urinalysis is a quick and simple test that can be done to screen for signs of a urinary tract infection. A formal microscopy and culture should also be sent, as part of a septic work-up for an unwell neonate presenting with vomiting.

[2] An FBC may reveal an elevated WCC in the setting of infection and sepsis. Haemoglobin and platelet counts should also be on hand prior to proceeding to operative management.

[3] A metabolic acidosis may develop in the setting of severe dehydration due to ongoing losses from vomiting.

[4] Deranged electrolytes may develop due to ongoing losses from vomiting, as well as due to altered volume status.

[5] If sepsis is suspected, a blood culture should be obtained as part of a septic work-up. Results of a blood culture will take >24 hours to return, so if sepsis is suspected antibiotics should be commenced immediately following collection of blood samples. Antibiotics should be rationalised after results of the culture and sensitivities are known.

[6] Coagulation studies should be performed as part of a preoperative work-up to evaluate potential coagulopathies.

[7] Blood type and available compatible blood on hand should be organised preoperatively, particularly if the neonate is proceeding to invasive abdominal surgery, as risk of blood loss and consequential need for blood transfusion are high.

[8] Bilirubin levels will be elevated in intestinal atresia as bilirubin is unable to be faecally excreted and therefore remains in enterohepatic circulation. A bilirubin panel will show increased levels of unconjugated bilirubin. Raised bilirubin levels may also be seen in sepsis or in biliary atresia, another GI malformation that may be present with intestinal atresia, among many other pathologies causing raised bilirubin.

[9] Abdominal X-rays should be ordered in all suspected cases of neonatal bowel obstruction. The findings on plain film can be diagnostic in some cases. A classical finding on plain film is the 'double bubble' sign. Combined with an absence of distal bowel gas, this appearance is strongly suggestive of duodenal atresia. The double bubble sign may also be seen with other pathologies causing high grade duodenal obstruction. Intestinal malrotation may also present with a similar-appearing double bubble sign. Rare causes of neonatal bowel obstruction, including duplication cysts and duodenal webs, can in some cases also present with similar abdominal radiograph findings. Dilated small bowel loops with air–fluid levels is suggestive of a more distal bowel obstruction, such as a jejunal or ileal atresia.

[10] A finding of free air, or pneumoperitoneum, on plain abdominal radiograph indicates intestinal perforation, a surgical emergency requiring urgent treatment and management.

[11] An upper GI contrast study is the next investigation to proceed with if plain film confirms suspicions of obstruction, providing there is no evidence of pneumoperitoneum. A duodenal atresia would demonstrate similar findings on contrast study to those seen on radiography, with a dilated stomach and proximal duodenum and pooling of contrast in those areas and lack of contrast movement into the more distal small bowel. An upper GI contrast study is important to differentiate between a small bowel atresia and an intestinal malrotation with volvulus. Signs of malrotation on contrast study include a displaced duodenojejunal junction and coiling of the bowel. Malrotation occurs during embryonic development due to interruption of the normal rotation of the embryonic gut. This leads to the eventual midgut being supported on a narrow vascular pedicle instead of the wide-based mesentery that is normally seen, increasing the risk of volvulus. The development of volvulus is a surgical emergency as it leads to small bowel ischaemia, necrosis and intestinal perforation causing peritonitis. Presentation is often within the first year of life, but it can be diagnosed at any age. More than half of cases are associated with other congenital anomalies.

12 If a diagnosis has not been reached from both the plain film and upper GI contrast study, a contrast enema study is the next modality used to identify the cause of the bowel obstruction. Often, a microcolon may be present in cases of small bowel atresia or meconium ileus, due to lack of use of this section of the GI tract. A distal small bowel atresia is confirmed by the inability for contrast to move into the dilated loops of more proximal small bowel. Meconium ileus, an obstruction of the distal ileum due to thick, impacted meconium, may be confirmed by intraluminal filling defects on the contrast enema. The contrast enema may also be a therapeutic study, with meconium being passed post the enema in approximately 60% of studies. Meconium ileus is commonly seen in neonates with cystic fibrosis. Colonic atresia may be identified on contrast enema with limited to no filling with contrast of more proximal sections of colon with a distal microcolon. A contrast enema is also included as part of the work-up for Hirschsprung disease. Colonic atresia and Hirschsprung disease may occur together.

13 If a finding of a small bowel atresia is confirmed, particularly if it is a duodenal atresia, the neonate should be evaluated for any evidence of other congenital anomalies.

This includes anomalies associated with Down syndrome, particularly if a concurrent diagnosis of Down syndrome is suspected or confirmed, most importantly being any evidence of cardiac anomalies. An echocardiogram should be performed to identify any possible cardiac malformations. It is essential that this is done prior to proceeding to operative management for a small bowel atresia. Further imaging is required to identify any other anomalies that may not be immediately apparent or that have not revealed themselves so far.

14 To confirm a clinical suspicion of Down syndrome, FISH (fluorescence *in situ* hybridisation) and formal karyotype testing should be ordered. For neonates with a small bowel atresia and particularly if they also had meconium plugs, cystic fibrosis mutation testing should be performed. A microarray to look further into the neonate's genetic make-up will also be performed in certain cases to identify any underlying genetic disorders leading to congenital abnormalities. VACTERL association is not associated with an underlying genetic defect and its occurrence is thought to be sporadic.

Management

Immediate

Gain **IV access** [1]. **Stop feeding** [2]. **Insert an NGT** [3]. **Correct fluid and electrolyte balance** [4]. Monitor **vital signs** [5] and **urine output** [6]. Commence broad-spectrum **antibiotics** [7]. **Refer** [8] to the paediatric general surgical team.

Short-term

Once the neonate is **stable** [9], proceed to **operative management** [10] of the atresia. Postoperatively, the neonate should be **monitored closely** [11] in

the neonatal ICU. Commence **feeding** [12] 3–5 days postoperatively.

Long-term

Once the neonate has been established on full feeds, is making good weight gains, and has been fully investigated for any other congenital malformations, they are suitable for **discharge home** [13]. They should continue to be **reviewed** [14] in the community by their GP and maternal and child health nurse and should be reviewed in the **paediatric surgical outpatient clinic** [15].

1 It is important to establish IV access early. It will be an essential route for fluids and medications since the neonate is not able to have anything orally.

2 The neonate must be made nil by mouth until definitive management of the atresia has been undertaken. This will also reduce the risk of further vomiting, in turn reducing the chance of the neonate developing an aspiration pneumonia.

3 A nasogastric or orogastric tube should be inserted to decompress the stomach. It should be left on free drainage with regular aspirates.

4 It is important to ensure optimisation of fluid and electrolyte status before proceeding to operative

management. It is likely that the neonate will be hypovolaemic from repeated vomiting and failure to absorb anything enterally and in turn will have altered electrolytes and acid–base status.

5 Continuous monitoring of vital signs helps guide response to treatment, ensures the patient remains stable while preparing for surgery and can identify any new issues that may arise and need to be addressed. These may include a new fever or change in oxygen saturations, which could indicate the development of an aspiration pneumonia from the repeated vomiting.

6 Monitoring of urine output is important as part of ongoing fluid status assessments, particularly when replacing losses and trying to ensure the patient remains euvolaemic.

7 Antibiotics may be commenced, particularly if surgery is imminent, to reduce the risk of postoperative infection. They are continued for several days postoperatively as well.

8 Neonates presenting with a small bowel obstruction should be managed in a tertiary centre in a neonatal intensive care unit under joint care of the neonatologists and the paediatric surgical team.

9 If an acute surgical emergency, such as a malrotation with volvulus, has been excluded on imaging, then surgery for correction of the atresia can be scheduled once the neonate has been optimised for surgical intervention. This includes adequate fluid and metabolic status and investigation for any other present congenital abnormalities. There are risks associated with waiting longer for surgical correction, however, including further vomiting leading to aspiration and potential sepsis; and complications of extended use of total parenteral nutrition, such as oral aversion, hyperlipidaemia, bone demineralisation and rebound hypoglycaemia.

10 A transverse right upper quadrant incision is made to access the duodenum in cases of duodenal atresia. Duodenal atresia is corrected by forming a duodeno-duodenostomy, either by a side-to-side or end-to-side anastomosis. Jejunal and ileal atresias are approached via a para- or transumbilical incision and are repaired primarily, usually with an end-to-end anastomosis. During the correction of atresias, the remaining bowel must be checked for the presence of other, previously unidentified, atresias. Primary repair is preferred when resecting multiple atresias, and care is taken to preserve adequate length of bowel to prevent short-gut syndrome – ideally >75cm, but some children may tolerate much less. While repairing colonic atresia, biopsies of the bowel wall should be taken intraoperatively to evaluate for evidence of Hirschsprung disease. Usually, the proximal end of the colon is externalised as a colostomy and anastomosis of the colon is delayed for several months. Babies tolerate colostomies well and this delayed anastomosis allows time for the dilated proximal colon to be decompressed and recover its tone, as well as allow time for biopsy results to demonstrate whether Hirschsprung disease is present.

11 Postoperatively, neonates should remain nil by mouth and continue with IV hydration and parenteral nutrition. The nasogastric or orogastric tube should also remain *in situ* for ongoing decompression. This allows for ongoing bowel rest in the initial days postoperatively. The neonate should be observed for any potential postoperative complications, e.g. peritonitis from an anastomotic leak or iatrogenic bowel injury.

12 Feeding can be reintroduced 3–5 days postoperatively and slowly increased until full oral feeds are established. Parenteral nutrition should be gradually weaned down as feeding is re-established.

13 Most neonates do well after repair of an intestinal atresia. Morbidity and mortality in these infants are more commonly attributable to concurrent issues, such as prematurity or other congenital anomalies, or the presence of multiple atresias or short-gut syndrome. If the neonate has required formation of a colostomy, they should be linked in with stomal therapy or hospital in the home to provide information and guidance for the care of colostomies in the community.

14 Neonates with small bowel atresias should have good follow-up in the community to ensure ongoing good feeding and weight gain is being maintained.

15 Regular review in the paediatric outpatient clinic is important, again to ensure good feeding and weight gain is being maintained. Surgical wounds should be reviewed to ensure adequate healing has occurred and there is no evidence of dehiscence or associated infection. The neonate should also be reviewed for the potential for late postoperative complications, such as anastomotic dysfunction or delayed emptying, or stricture or adhesion formation causing further full or partial obstructions. Reoperation should be considered if obstruction is confirmed on imaging, but return to theatre must be at least 3 weeks following the initial operation date.

CASE 59: Ovarian torsion

History

- A **15-year-old female** [1] with **no significant past medical history** [2] presents with a **4-hour history** [3] of **acute left-sided abdominal pain** [4].
- She has been having **waves of nausea associated with the pain and has vomited** [5] a few times.
- She had been **sitting** [6] in school when the pain came on. She has not had any **fevers** [7] at home.
- She has not had changes with **urination** [8].
- Her last **menstrual period finished a week ago and she is not sexually active** [9]. She has not had any abnormal **vaginal bleeding** [10].
- She has **no regular medications and no allergies** [11].

[1] Ovarian torsion is an acute surgical emergency. It can affect women of any age from the neonatal period to postmenopausal but is most likely to affect women of reproductive age. Most paediatric general surgeons will manage ovarian torsion up until the age of 16, after which the adult obstetrics and gynaecology team will guide management. The ovary is suspended by the infundibulopelvic ligament (also known as the suspensory ligament of the ovary) which is a fold of the broad ligament. It is through the infundibulopelvic ligament that the ovarian vessels travel to reach the ovary. Due to this mobile nature, the ovary may sit laterally or posteriorly to the uterus depending on the position of the patient. It is on these ligamentous supports that the ovary can twist, obstructing its own blood supply. Often the Fallopian tube will twist with the ovary if this occurs.

[2] Ovarian torsion is much more likely to occur due to the presence of an ovarian mass or cyst. The asymmetric size and weight of an affected ovary predisposes it to twist on its ligamentous supports. Masses or cysts >6cm in size are most likely to precipitate torsion. Approximately 40% of cases of ovarian torsion are due to ovarian neoplasms, the most common of which are benign, such as teratomas and adenomas. Up to 2% of ovarian torsions in adults are due to malignant neoplasms, but this percentage is much lower in children. Another 40% of cases of ovarian torsion are due to the presence of ovarian cysts. In the paediatric population, however, half the presentations of ovarian torsion are in females with normal ovaries, particularly if they are pre-menarchal. It is important to obtain a full past history from the patient to identify if there are any acute or chronic health problems that must be considered should the patient require surgery or to help refine the list of differentials for the presentation, such as if the patient has previously had any abdominal surgery as an infant or child, as this may make certain diagnoses such as bowel obstruction from adhesions or appendicitis more or less likely.

[3] The time from symptom development to presentation is often short due to the severity of the symptoms.

[4] Pain associated with ovarian torsion is acute, of a sudden onset, and may be constant or intermittent. The pain may be generalised abdominal pain or localised to the side of the affected ovary. The patient may report that the pain radiates to the groin, flank or back.

[5] Nausea and vomiting are frequently seen with a presentation of ovarian torsion. However, these symptoms are non-specific and can also be present with many different pathologies. Diarrhoea is another non-specific symptom that may be present. Gastroenteritis can also present with abdominal pain, nausea, vomiting and diarrhoea, although usually the abdominal pain will begin after the other symptoms, unlike in ovarian torsion, and is usually much less acute. As the presentation of torsion can be very non-specific, it should always be considered when a female presents with abdominal pain. Ovarian torsion presents similarly from children to older adults although pre-menarchal children are more likely to present later after the onset of symptoms with diffuse pain and fever. Ovarian torsion can be challenging to identify in neonates whose only symptoms may be abdominal distension, irritability, vomiting and feed intolerance.

[6] Some cases of ovarian torsion may be precipitated by sudden movements such as with strenuous exercise or brief, sudden increase in intra-abdominal pressure, such as when coughing, hiccuping or straining on the toilet.

[7] Fever may be seen in cases of ovarian torsion but is uncommon. A fever associated with a presentation of ovarian torsion could indicate that the ovary is undergoing necrosis. The presence of a fever may also suggest an infective cause for the symptoms, such as appendicitis or a UTI.

[8] Pyelonephritis can also present similarly to ovarian torsion with unilateral back, flank or abdominal pain. Fevers

are more likely to be a significant feature on history. Renal colic may also present with a similar picture of acute onset, unilateral back or flank pain with nausea and vomiting. Pain in renal colic is more likely to be intermittent and moving loin to groin, but will not always present with this classical history.

9 An ectopic pregnancy can present similarly to ovarian torsion so must be considered as part of the work-up for abdominal pain in females. Pregnancy itself is also a risk factor for ovarian torsion, with up to 20% of ovarian torsion cases occurring in pregnant women. Enlargement of the uterus as the foetus grows may displace the nearby ovary causing it to tort, particularly if it is already enlarged, such as due to a mass or a cyst. Most cases occur prior to 20 weeks'

gestation. In the adolescent population it is important to obtain a gynaecological, menstrual and sexual history from the patient as part of the work-up for abdominal pain. Pelvic inflammatory disease can also present with non-specific diffuse abdominal pain and should be considered in females who are sexually active.

10 Abnormal vaginal bleeding is not commonly seen in ovarian torsion; however, it can be seen with an ectopic pregnancy, a differential that is important to exclude.

11 It is important to elicit a complete medication history to minimise any drug interactions or to avoid causing adverse reactions during management.

Examination

- The patient appears very **uncomfortable** [1] but **not unwell** [2].
- She is **mildly tachycardic** [3] and **hypertensive** [3].
- The respiratory rate and oxygen saturations are within normal limits for age. Her **temperature is 36.5°C** [4].
- The patient has **moist mucous membranes, peripheral and central capillary refill of <2 seconds and good skin turgor** [5].
- **Heart sounds are dual with no added sounds and the chest is clear** [6].
- Abdominal inspection is unremarkable, with **no previous surgical scars** [7] visible.
- There is **diffuse tenderness to palpation** [8] across the lower abdomen.
- There is **no guarding or rigidity** [9].
- An **exquisitely tender mass** [10] is palpable deep in the left iliac fossa.

1 Ovarian torsion is incredibly painful so patients will appear in pain. Younger patients may be restless or inconsolable.

2 Due to the acute onset and presentation of ovarian torsion, patients may still appear relatively well when they attend the ED.

3 Mild tachycardia and/or hypertension may be present as a response to the acute pain the patient is experiencing. In rare cases, haemorrhage may be seen with ovarian torsion, in which case evidence of hypovolaemia with tachycardia and hypotension may be present.

4 Often patients are afebrile but a low grade fever may be seen in some patients with ovarian torsion. The presence of a fever can indicate that the ovary is undergoing necrosis. A fever may also suggest an infective cause for the symptoms, such as appendicitis or a UTI. Children are more likely to present with fever in cases of ovarian torsion.

5 A fluid balance assessment is important as part of the examination, particularly if the patient has been experiencing losses, such as through vomiting and diarrhoea.

6 A general physical assessment of the patient, including cardiovascular and respiratory assessment, should be performed, particularly as part of a pre-theatre assessment.

7 The presence of previous surgical scars may make a diagnosis of a bowel obstruction secondary to adhesions higher on the list of differentials.

8 In 66% of presentations of ovarian torsion, the patient will experience abdominal or pelvic tenderness during palpation. This may be localised to the side of the torsion or the pain may be diffuse.

9 Signs of peritonism may be present in a few patients and raise concern for the presence of ovarian necrosis.

10 A palpable, tender adnexal mass raises the suspicion for ovarian torsion. The adnexa may be palpable due to swelling from venous congestion or due to the presence of an associated mass or cyst. However, this finding is not present in all examinations where the patient has ovarian torsion. An adnexal mass may also suggest other pathologies such as an ectopic pregnancy or a tubo-ovarian abscess.

Investigations

- **Urinalysis** [1] is unremarkable.
- A **urinary and serum pregnancy test** [2] is negative.
- An **FBE is normal**. Urea, creatinine and electrolytes are normal [3].
- **Serum tumour markers** [4] are taken and pending.

- An **abdominal ultrasound reveals an enlarged left ovary with probe tenderness and decreased Doppler flow** [5] within the ovary.
- There is a small amount of **free fluid** [6] in the pelvis.
- A **normal appendix** [7] is visualised.

[1] Urinalysis should be performed to look for evidence of white cells and nitrites and red blood cells, which may be present in UTI, or for isolated red blood cells which may be present in nephrolithiasis, causing renal colic.

[2] Pregnancy testing is important as torsion is more common in pregnant women and an ectopic pregnancy needs to be excluded as a differential. hCG (human chorionic gonadotrophin) is also elevated with some ovarian tumours.

[3] In most cases of ovarian torsion, laboratory studies will be normal. In rare cases, a drop in haemoglobin may be seen as a result of haemorrhage associated with the torsion or from a large, ruptured ovarian cyst. A white cell rise may be present with ovarian necrosis but is also non-specific and may be seen in many other alternative pathologies such as appendicitis, gastroenteritis, a UTI or a tubo-ovarian abscess. Thrombocytosis may also be seen in ovarian malignancies in children and adolescents.

[4] If a mass is found on examination or further investigation, tumour markers should be ordered in consultation with the paediatric surgical or obstetrics and gynaecological team to investigate for ovarian tumours. In the paediatric population malignancy is unlikely, so senior advice should be sought before exploring further. Generally, tumour markers may only be ordered if a mass is confirmed on ultrasound and appears suspicious for malignancy. Examples of tumour markers include CA-125, a sensitive but not specific marker for epithelial ovarian cancer; AFP, an antigen produced by teratomas and mixed germ cell tumours; LDH, which is elevated with dysgerminomas; CEA, which is produced by germ or epithelial cell tumours; and inhibin and MIS (Müllerian-inhibiting substance), which are elevated in children with granulosa-theca cell tumours.

[5] Ultrasound is the imaging modality of choice for patients with ovarian torsion. An abdominal and transvaginal approach is preferred, but in children only an abdominal ultrasound should be performed. A full bladder is needed for best visualisation, which can sometimes be difficult for children, particularly when they are already in pain and distressed. Findings on ultrasound can vary depending on duration of symptoms and degree of torsion, but can include an enlarged ovary relative to the other side due to lymphatic and vascular congestion causing oedema; visualisation of an ovarian mass; abnormal ovarian location; absent or reduced Doppler flow (although the presence of Doppler flow does not rule out torsion); heterogeneous appearance of ovarian stroma due to oedema and haemorrhage; multiple small peripheral follicles as they have been displaced by oedema (this finding is also seen in polycystic ovarian syndrome but is not associated with acute pain or oedema); and a 'whirlpool sign' caused by side-by-side arrangement of vessels with opposing directions of blood flow, representing twisting of the vascular pedicle. CT is not typically used to diagnose ovarian torsion, but may be performed when another cause of acute abdominal pain, such as appendicitis, is thought to be more likely. Its findings are similar to those seen on ultrasound, with an enlarged, abnormally placed ovary, and with contrast enhancement the whirlpool sign may also be visible. However, CTs are rarely used in the paediatric population unless essential, due to the associated radiation exposure. MRIs are another modality that can be used to diagnose ovarian torsion, especially if the findings on ultrasound are equivocal, although due to time, cost and centre availability it may not be frequently used. In the neonatal population, ovarian cysts are often diagnosed on antenatal ultrasounds and will then be followed up with serial ultrasounds in the prenatal and neonatal period and beyond to track progress/resolution. Most cysts are expected to resolve by 6 months of age. If cysts do not resolve, continue increasing in size or become symptomatic they may be excised surgically, or if the cyst is simple and >4mm in size the fluid from the cyst can be aspirated. Parents and carers should be informed of the signs of ovarian torsion in a neonate and instructed to present to the ED immediately if their child is displaying concerning symptoms for torsion.

[6] Both ovarian torsion and a ruptured ovarian cyst can have findings of free fluid in the pelvis on ultrasound.

[7] Appendicitis can present similarly to ovarian torsion with abdominal pain, nausea and fever. Differentiation between the two should be made on history, examination and investigations. In this case a normal appendix has been visualised on ultrasound, which lowers clinical suspicion for appendicitis being the cause of the pain, particularly with the other imaging findings present being suggestive of ovarian torsion.

Management

Immediate

Gain **IV access** [1]. Provide **analgesia and anti-emetics** [2]. Keep patient **nil by mouth** [3]. Monitor **vital signs** [4]. Commence **IV fluids** [5]. Refer to **paediatric surgical team** [6].

Short-term

Patients should proceed **as an emergency** [7] to the **operating theatre** [8] for exploration of suspected ovarian torsion. Postoperatively they should be monitored [9] and have **examination of the abdomen** [10] and **surgical sites** [11]. They should be started back on a **full diet** [12].

Long-term

Patients are suitable for discharge if their **observations remain stable, they are pain-free and tolerating a full diet** [13]. They should be **educated** [14] on signs of ovarian torsion. They should be followed up in **paediatric surgical outpatient clinic** [15].

[1] IV access should be established quickly so as not to delay getting the patient to theatre, and it also provides an access for IV medication and fluid administration.

[2] Effective analgesia should be provided to the patient to help ease the pain from a torted ovary. Anti-emetics can help settle nausea and vomiting.

[3] Patients should be kept nil by mouth due to the urgent requirement for surgery to reduce the risk of aspiration while under anaesthetic.

[4] Vital signs should be observed to ensure the patient remains haemodynamically stable.

[5] While the patient is fasting, provide fluids in the form of 0.9% sodium chloride with 5% glucose at full maintenance hydration. Consider fluid boluses of 0.9% sodium chloride if the patient appears hypovolaemic.

[6] Refer to the paediatric surgical team for all patients ≤16 years presenting with suspected ovarian torsion for urgent surgical intervention. If a paediatric service is not available, consider transfer to a tertiary centre or alternatively referral to the obstetrics and gynaecology team.

[7] Surgical intervention should be performed swiftly in order to preserve ovarian function and reduce the chance of other adverse effects associated with ovarian necrosis, such as haemorrhage, peritonitis and subsequent formation of adhesions.

[8] A diagnosis of ovarian torsion can only be made once visualised intraoperatively. A laparoscopic approach is usually used. The ovary should be detorted and viability assessed. In most cases the ovary is viable even with a blue–black appearance, and should be left in situ, particularly in young patients and those who are premenopausal, to preserve fertility. A necrotic ovary or Fallopian tube may appear gelatinous or have loss of its usual structure. If an ovary is clearly necrosed, an oophorectomy should be performed. For patients with a large ovarian cyst identified, cystectomy can be done at the same time as the detorsion procedure. For patients in whom malignancy is suspected, unless malignancy is confirmed at the time of procedure via frozen section, the mass should be excised and the ovary reconstructed. However, if malignancy is confirmed, a salpingo-oophorectomy should be performed on the affected side. It is better in a paediatric population, if malignancy is suspected but not definitively diagnosed, to manage only the torsion and excision of the lesion and then confirm malignancy with specimens and serum tumour markers. It is preferable to have the patient undergo a second procedure for salpingo-oophorectomy rather than remove them without absolute confirmation of the diagnosis.

[9] Observations should be monitored postoperatively to ensure haemodynamic stability. Tachycardia or hypotension may indicate postoperative bleeding, while the concurrent presence of a fever could indicate sepsis from a retained necrotic ovary, something that warrants urgent re-exploration.

[10] The abdomen should be examined for any evidence of guarding or rigidity, indicating peritonitis which may also be present with a retained necrotic ovary.

[11] Surgical wounds should be observed to ensure good wound healing, and that there are no signs of dehiscence or wound infection.

[12] Patients can be restarted on a normal diet as tolerated postoperatively and encourage children to resume feeding as normal as soon as able.

[13] Once the patient appears well and is back to their usual baseline functioning, they are suitable for discharge from hospital.

[14] Patients, parents and carers should be advised of the symptoms of ovarian torsion and instructed to re-present if the symptoms re-occur. Ovarian torsion may re-occur but the incidence and risk factors for recurrence are not known.

[15] Patients should be followed up in the outpatient clinic to ensure they have been able to resume their usual activities, to review their surgical wounds to ensure good healing and to review any outstanding pathology from their admission.

CASE 60: Pyloric stenosis

History

- A **6-week-old** [1] **male** [2] infant with **no significant past medical history** [3] is sent in to the ED with his parents by his maternal and child health nurse, due to a 2-week history of recurrent vomiting and **irritability** [4].
- His parents describe a progressive history of **forceful milky vomiting not long after feeding** [5].
- There is no **blood** [6] noticed in the vomits.
- They have tried **multiple different formulas** [7] over the past couple of weeks but there has not been any improvement in symptoms.
- The maternal and child health nurse has documented that **weight gain** [8] has stagnated over the past few weeks.

- The infant has **not opened his bowels** [9] for two days and his **wet nappies** [10] have been lighter and less frequent.
- His mother had an unremarkable pregnancy and the infant was born at **term** [11] via a normal vaginal delivery.
- She is a **non-smoker** [12].
- The infant has had no **sick contacts** [13].
- This is the couple's **first child** [14].
- The infant's **mother had pyloric stenosis** [15] as a baby.

[1] Most infants with hypertrophic pyloric stenosis present within 3–6 weeks of age and very rarely after 12 weeks of age. Hypertrophic pyloric stenosis, also known as infantile hypertrophic pyloric stenosis or simply pyloric stenosis, occurs at a rate of 2–3.5 per 1000 live births on average, but is often region-dependent, with pyloric stenosis more common in western populations as opposed to those in Africa and Asia.

[2] Pyloric stenosis is more common in males, with a male to female ratio of 4:1.

[3] Infants with a history of previous abdominal surgery who develop vomiting may have their symptoms initially attributed to adhesions causing bowel obstruction.

[4] Infants with pyloric stenosis are often irritable, crying and difficult to console as they are hungry due to ineffective feeding. They will often want to feed again soon after vomiting.

[5] Vomiting is the most common symptom seen in pyloric stenosis. It is projectile in nature, non-bilious as only food products are being regurgitated, and occurs following feeds. Sometimes this may be mistakenly assumed to be gastroenteritis, though other features of gastroenteritis such as loose stools and fever are not present. UTI can also present in a similar way, with repeated vomiting and irritable infants, and it is an important differential diagnosis to exclude as part of the work-up. The presence of bilious vomiting is indicative of a more distal intestinal obstruction, such as malrotation with volvulus or Hirschsprung disease.

[6] In approximately 10% of cases, parents may notice blood stains in the vomit.

[7] Early pyloric stenosis can be easily confused with intolerance to certain formulas or gastro-oesophageal reflux, and may be misdiagnosed before later stage symptoms present. Vomiting in gastro-oesophageal reflux tends not to be projectile and occurs 10 or more minutes after finishing feeding. Pyloric stenosis is also seen more often in bottle-fed infants as opposed to exclusively breastfed infants.

[8] There is often inadequate weight gain in these infants due to insufficient ingestion and retention of food, and consequently poor nutritional absorption.

[9] Constipation may develop in late stages of pyloric stenosis, secondary to dehydration due to poor oral intake, as most food is being vomited rather than digested.

[10] Decreased wet nappies is another sign of dehydration secondary to poor oral intake.

[11] Preterm delivery is a risk factor for pyloric stenosis, though diagnosis is usually at a later chronological age than term infants, and it can be more difficult to reach the diagnosis due to atypical symptoms or investigation findings. Term infants are more likely to present with classical features of pyloric stenosis with non-bilious, postprandial projectile vomiting.

[12] The risk of an infant developing pyloric stenosis is increased by 1.5–2 times in children whose mothers smoked during their pregnancy.

13 Contact with other patients with GI symptoms such as diarrhoea and vomiting may make a diagnosis of gastroenteritis more likely.

14 Pyloric stenosis is most likely to affect the first-born in a family, as opposed to later children, at a rate of 2:1.

15 There is a strong familial risk involved in developing pyloric stenosis and it is seen more often when the mother had pyloric stenosis.

Examination

- The infant appears **flat** [1] and lethargic.
- His **heart rate** [2] is 190bpm.
- **Blood pressure** [3] is 75/50mmHg.
- **Respiratory rate** [4] is 40 breaths per minute. Oxygen saturation is 97% on air.
- The **temperature** [5] is 37°C.
- The infant has **sunken fontanelles and dry mucous membranes** [6].
- There are **no changes to the skin or sclera** [7].

- **Heart sounds are dual** [8] with no added sounds.
- **Chest is clear** [9] to auscultation.
- **Inspection of the abdomen** [10] is normal with **no surgical scars visible** [11].
- Careful palpation of the abdomen reveals a **small, firm mass in the right upper quadrant, lateral to the rectus abdominis** [12].
- **Bowel sounds** [13] are present.
- The **nappy is dry** [14].

1 A change in conscious state is a sign of shock from severe volume depletion.

2 Tachycardia is seen in severe dehydration associated with prolonged course of symptoms and delayed presentation.

3 The infant may be in hypovolaemic shock due to severe volume depletion. In some cases, infants with a delayed presentation of pyloric stenosis need to be stabilised in the ICU before they are suitable for surgery.

4 Respiratory rate may be increased in dehydration states.

5 Fever is not usually an examination finding in pyloric stenosis and if present, may suggest an alternative diagnosis.

6 A fluid balance assessment is an important part of the work-up for pyloric stenosis to assess hydration status, as infants can become severely dehydrated from repeated vomiting and inability to absorb feeds. Other features of the fluid balance assessment include assessing skin turgor, urine output and capillary refill time.

7 The presence of eczema raises suspicion for a food allergy as the cause of the patient's symptoms. Additionally, jaundice or icterus may be seen in infants with pyloric stenosis due to hyperbilirubinaemia. The presence of jaundice would also warrant an investigation into the possibility of underlying liver disease. Mottled skin is a sign of severe dehydration.

8 A full physical work-up is necessary as part of assessing suitability for surgery. A flow murmur may be appreciated during tachycardia which resolves after adequate volume repletion.

9 Repeated vomiting increases an infant's risk of aspiration during these episodes. Assessment of the lungs should be completed to rule out a concurrent pneumonia.

10 Visible peristalsis may be observed as waves travelling from left to right across the abdomen as the stomach attempts to force contents across the hypertrophied pylorus and narrowed pyloric outlet. It can be seen just prior to vomiting in some infants. Abdominal distension may indicate obstruction rather than pyloric stenosis.

11 Previous abdominal surgery may cause adhesions and bowel obstruction, which can also present with repeated vomiting.

12 A small, firm mass in the right upper quadrant lateral to the rectus abdominis described as an 'olive-shaped mass' is pathognomonic for pyloric stenosis and its presence confirms a clinical diagnosis without need for imaging. It is most easily palpable when the infant is settled and immediately post vomiting so that its presence is not obscured by tensed abdominal muscles. In earlier presentations of pyloric stenosis, the olive-shaped mass may be difficult to palpate.

13 High-pitched bowel sounds are suggestive of bowel obstruction, and if concurrently associated with bilious rather than non-bilious vomiting, should be investigated with a plain film to identify an obstruction.

14 A dry nappy may also be a sign of volume depletion as urine output is reduced. Stool should be inspected for evidence of bleeding. Occult blood may be present in otherwise healthy-appearing infants with a cow's milk protein allergy, while frank blood PR may suggest intussusception, particularly if the symptoms are of a shorter duration.

Investigations

- **Urinalysis** [1] is normal.
- An **FBE** [2] is normal.
- A VBG shows a **raised pH and bicarbonate levels and low serum chloride and potassium** [3].
- Formal UECs confirm low serum chloride and potassium and **mildly elevated creatinine and urea** [4].

- There is a finding of **unconjugated hyperbilirubinaemia** [5] on liver function testing.
- An **abdominal ultrasound** [6] confirms the diagnosis of pyloric stenosis.

[1] A urine dipstick is a quick way to test for signs of a UTI that may be causing vomiting and irritability. A full urine microscopy and culture should be sent, as infants presenting in severe dehydration present similarly to those in sepsis, so investigating for all possible causes while the diagnosis is not confirmed is important.

[2] FBE is usually normal in pyloric stenosis. There may be a mild WCC rise as a response to repeated vomiting. A large inflammatory marker rise may indicate symptoms are more likely due to an infection rather than pyloric stenosis. Patients with early presentation and diagnosis will often still have normal pathology results, as changes due to repeated vomiting and dehydration are seen in delayed presentations.

[3] A hypochloraemic hypokalaemic metabolic alkalosis is a typical finding in late presentations of pyloric stenosis. It has a positive predictive value of 88% in diagnosing pyloric stenosis when the infant's main presenting symptom is vomiting. The degree of abnormality on the blood samples is proportional to the duration of symptoms prior to presentation.

[4] Raised urea and creatinine are also a marker of dehydration status and give an assessment of effects of dehydration on renal function.

[5] 14% of cases of pyloric stenosis are associated with unconjugated hyperbilirubinaemia – the combination of which is termed icteropyloric syndrome. In many cases it is an early manifestation of Gilbert syndrome. Hyperbilirubinaemia resolves quickly after surgical correction of the pyloric stenosis.

[6] If a diagnosis of pyloric stenosis cannot be made clinically then abdominal ultrasound is the gold standard to confirm the suspected diagnosis. The sensitivity and specificity for diagnosing pyloric stenosis on ultrasound is >95%. If the ultrasound is negative or equivocal for pyloric stenosis but based on history and examination pyloric stenosis still seems the most likely diagnosis, ultrasonography is repeated in a few days to see if classical imaging findings of pyloric stenosis develop with more time.

Management

Immediate

Gain **IV access** [1] and begin **fluid resuscitation** [2]. **Stop feeding** [3]. Consider **NGT insertion** [4]. Monitor **vital signs** [5] and **urine output** [6] and escalate to intensive care team if required. **Repeat blood gases every 6 hours** [7]. Refer to **paediatric surgical team** [8] or **transfer** [9] to nearest paediatric surgical service if in a rural area.

Short-term

Once the patient has been stabilised with hydration status, acid–base status and electrolyte disturbances all corrected, they can proceed to definitive management

in the form of a **pyloromyotomy** [10]. Postoperatively patients should receive **apnoea monitoring** [11] for at least 24 hours. **Feeding** [12] can be resumed within a few hours after surgery. Examine the **abdomen** [13] and review surgical **wounds** [14].

Long-term

Patients are suitable for discharge once they are pain-free and **tolerating full oral feeds** [15]. They should be monitored in the community by their maternal and child health nurse or GP to ensure adequate **weight gain** [16] is made. They should be followed up in **surgical outpatient clinic** [17].

1 Ensure quick establishment of IV access to begin fluid replacement and electrolyte correction as quickly as possible.

2 Initial fluid resuscitation should be with 10–20ml/kg bolus of 0.9% sodium chloride. Not all children will require fluid resuscitation if they have presented early, appear clinically euvolaemic, have good urine output and normal vital signs. Replace any ongoing deficits and commence maintenance fluids using 0.9% sodium chloride with 5% glucose.

3 Feeding must be stopped as preparation preoperatively and to ensure emesis episodes subside.

4 If copious vomiting persists despite stopping feeds, an NG should be inserted to decompress the stomach.

5 Monitor vital signs to ensure tachycardia resolves, hypotension improves and respiratory rate is stable as fluid and electrolyte correction is provided.

6 Once urine output reaches 1–2ml/kg/hour, 20mmol of potassium can be added to maintenance fluids.

7 Blood gases should be repeated regularly so that fluids can be adjusted accordingly. Fluid and electrolyte deficits should be fully corrected within 48 hours from presentation. Serum bicarbonate levels should be fully corrected prior to surgery as ongoing metabolic alkalosis puts the patient at risk for hypoventilation and apnoea postoperatively.

8 A paediatric general surgical team should review and admit the patient for definitive management of their pyloric stenosis.

9 All patients with pyloric stenosis should be managed in a tertiary centre with paediatric surgical and paediatric intensive care capabilities. Once management has been initiated a patient should be transferred to a tertiary centre urgently.

10 To correct the pyloric narrowing due to the hypertrophic pylorus and therefore allow stomach contents to pass into the duodenum, a longitudinal incision is made in the pylorus and then blunt dissected down to the level of the submucosa. When an open approach is used this is referred to as a Ramstedt procedure, although a laparoscopic approach is typically favoured when possible.

11 Apnoea monitoring should be a routine part of postoperative monitoring, as infants are at higher risk for apnoea due to their young age, effects of anaesthetic and if the patient's alkalosis was not fully corrected preoperatively.

12 Infants may still demonstrate some regurgitation postoperatively, but the projectile-type vomiting should now have resolved. The rate of incomplete pyloromyotomy is 1%.

13 Routine abdominal examination should be a part of postoperative reviews. Ensure there is no evidence of abdominal distension, rigidity or abdominal tenderness out of proportion with surgical wounds, as this may be concerning for an intraoperative perforation and consequent peritonitis. However, the rate of mucosal perforations intraoperatively is <1%, and easily identified and corrected at the time.

14 Surgical wounds should be reviewed to ensure adequate wound healing, no signs of dehiscence or developing infection.

15 Feeds should be back at expected amount for age before discharge, to ensure the infant will receive adequate nutrition and hydration in the community.

16 Infants with delayed presentation may have had weight loss due to inadequate feeding at initial presentation. It is important to ensure the infant is having steady weight gain after correction of the pyloric stenosis, and length and weight should be plotted on child growth charts.

17 Patients should be reviewed in surgical outpatient clinic for review of wound healing and to ensure the child is gaining weight and reaching expected milestones. If infants are still having issues with vomiting or inadequate weight gain despite correction of the pyloric stenosis, a referral to a paediatrician or inpatient admission for further investigation is warranted in order to identify other causes to explain their persisting symptoms. Gastro-oesophageal reflux is common but no more so than in infants who have not had pyloric stenosis, and should only be investigated if the reflux is severe or causing other symptoms.

CASE 61: Breast lump and lymphoedema

History

- A **70-year-old** [1] **female** [2] has been referred to the outpatient plastic and reconstructive surgery clinic of a tertiary hospital with a **right-sided breast lump** [3] .
- She has not yet had any investigations and tells you that she found the lump **about 6 months ago whilst showering** [4] .
- She is up to date with her **mammography** [5] and has always had **'dense breasts'** [6] .
- Throughout her teens and early 20s, she had **breast mice** [7] but nothing more serious.
- Her **sister and mother both died of breast cancer** [8] , her sister aged 49 and her mother aged 74.
- She has a **BMI of 30** [9] , **T2DM** [10] and **hypercholesterolaemia** [11] .

- She is a retired **nurse** [12] , and spends her spare time making small handicrafts for the local market.
- She has been married for 50 years and her husband has recently pointed out that she has **lost a lot of weight** [13] and on prompting, she says perhaps her **appetite has been low** [14] for the last year.
- She has not had **drenching night sweats or fevers** [15] .
- When she first found the lump, it was about the size of a pea, but **grew rapidly** [16] over the last 6 months to now be the size of a golf ball.
- The patient has also noticed her **nipple has turned in** [17] .
- She denies **any pain or tenderness** [18] in the lump and has not experienced any **nipple discharge** [19] .

1 Breast cancer occurs most commonly in women over 50 years old and in men over 60 years old. Risk increases with age.

2 Both males and females can develop breast cancer.

3 A breast lump is a localised bulge or swelling in the breast that feels different from the surrounding breast tissue or compared with the other breast.

4 Knowing the time period that the breast lesion developed can be helpful in diagnosis and determining how aggressive a cancer is; the faster it has been growing, the more likely it is to be metastatic.

5 Mammography is a radiographic technique where the breasts are sandwiched between X-ray plates and imaged to view the ducts, the breast tissue and the nipple. Regular screening mammography is recommended for women after age 45.

6 Dense breast tissue comprises milk glands, supportive tissue and milk ducts as seen on a mammogram. Non-dense breast tissue is fat. Having 'dense breasts' means that there is less fat than breast tissue and breast cancer may not be able to be seen easily on a mammogram; it is more common in women with a lower BMI, taking hormone therapy for menopause or who are of a younger age. Levels of breast density are described using a reporting system called Breast Imaging Reporting and Data System (BI-RADS):

- A: almost entirely fatty; 1 in 10 women have this result
- B: scattered areas of fibroglandular density, most of the tissue is non-dense (fat); 4 in 10 women have this result
- C: heterogeneously dense (majority of breast tissue is dense tissue); 4 in 10 women have this result
- D: extremely dense (nearly all the breast tissue is dense); 1 in 10 women have this result.

7 'Breast mice' are breast fibroadenomas. Simple fibroadenomas are the most common and do not increase the risk of breast cancer; however, the complex subtype does. The latter has calcification, enlarged lobules (glands) and cysts. There can be one or several and can occur in one or both breasts. Both types are often tender and enlarge during the period of menstruation and are most common in women aged 20–30 years.

8 The majority of inherited cases of breast cancer are associated with two genes, *BRCA1* and *BRCA2* (which stands for BReast CAncer gene 1 and 2). These normally repair cell damage. Female carriers of a germline mutation in BRCA1 have a lifetime risk of breast cancer >80% and ovarian cancer risk of 60%. Female carriers with a germline mutation in *BRCA2* have a similar lifetime risk of breast cancer to this but a higher ovarian cancer risk in their lifetime.

9 Obesity increases incidence and mortality from multiple cancer types, including breast and endometrial. The current thought is that through a multitude of various endocrine factors, adipose tissue contributes to a high inflammatory response and resultant tumorigenesis.

10 People with T2DM have much higher rates of all types of cancer compared to non-diabetics.

11 Hypercholesterolaemia is not a risk factor for breast cancer, but an overall reflection of general health.

12 Some studies suggest people who work night shifts long-term, such as nurses, have a higher risk of breast, GI and lung cancer than people who do not.

13 Loss of weight can be a sign of cancer or chronic inflammatory disease.

14 Loss of appetite can be a symptom of cancer but can also be a reflection of stress, anxiety, depression or other chronic disease (e.g. lung disease, heart failure, chronic kidney failure).

15 Drenching night sweats and fevers are symptoms of cancer (typical of Hodgkin's disease but can be any neoplastic process) or infectious disease (e.g. TB or HIV).

16 Rapid growth of a mass in any region is a concern for a neoplastic process.

17 Inverted nipples can be a symptom of breast cancer but also can be due to increased age, mammary duct ectasia (a non-cancerous occurrence during perimenopause), or Paget's disease of the nipple.

18 Breast cancers are not typically tender.

19 Nipple discharge (clear or bloody) is the most common presentation for intraductal papilloma. It is a wart-like tumour that develops within the breast ducts which are close to the nipple.

Examination

- The patient has a right breast mass about **3cm in diameter at 3 o'clock** [1].
- It is **firm** [2] to the touch and **adherent to the overlying skin** [3].
- It feels **irregular** [4], but is **non-tender** [5], and there is **no erythema or change in temperature** [6] when compared with the surrounding skin.

- There is no evidence of **tethering** [7] or **peau d'orange** [8] but the **nipple is partially inverted** [9].
- There are no dilated veins or ulceration of the breast and the **nipple looks otherwise normal** [10]. It is not possible to express anything from the nipple.
- The left breast does not have any masses. On a lymphatic examination, there is **one enlarged lymph node** [11] at **axillary node level I** [12].

1 When describing a breast lesion or skin change, it is reported using a clock face where the nipple is in the centre.

2 Texture of a breast mass can aid diagnosis. For example, breast mice are round, smooth, and move underneath the examiner's hand easily, which is why they are colloquially called mice. Concerning for malignancy are masses that are firm, irregular in shape or fixed to the skin.

3 This is a concerning feature for malignancy as the mass underneath has tethered to the skin overlying it.

4 Irregular breast masses are suspicious of cancer.

5 Non-tender breast lumps can be lipomas, a milk cyst (galactocele), a malignant breast cancer (e.g. lobular or ductal carcinoma) or lymphoma. Tender breast masses can be an abscess, mastitis, fibroadenoma (more common in those aged 20–30 years), or phylloides tumour (these can also be non-tender, but grow rapidly as a firm, round mass that is rarely malignant but treated with wide local excision).

6 This is looking for inflammatory lesions (such as a breast abscess or cellulitis) and inflammatory breast cancer. The latter is more common in younger women and those of African heritage, becoming clinically apparent when the

cancer cells block the lymph vessels in the skin of the breast and cause it to become erythematous and swollen. It is highly aggressive and is often metastatic when diagnosed.

7 Tethering is highly suggestive of breast cancer.

8 Peau d'orange is an orange peel appearance of the skin caused by lymphatic blockage.

9 As mentioned above, nipple inversion can be due to age, mammary duct ectasia (a non-cancerous occurrence during perimenopause), Paget's disease of the nipple and breast cancer.

10 Clinical findings in Paget disease of the nipple include:
- crusting, scaling or flaking of the nipple
- erythema of the nipple and areola
- burning or itching in the nipple and breast
- bleeding or discharge from the nipple
- nipple inversion or flattening
- a lump felt underneath or around the nipple.

11 Enlarged lymph nodes are >1cm and can be smooth, rubbery or hard in consistency.

12 Lymphatic drainage of the breast is to internal mammary nodes and via axillary lymph nodes. The latter is surgically divided into:
- level I – inferior and lateral to pectoralis minor muscle
- level II – posterior to the pectoralis minor muscle and inferior to the axillary vein
- level III – infraclavicular, medial to the pectoralis minor and against the chest wall; involvement of these lymph nodes carries a poor prognosis.

Investigations

- Breast lesion work-up is often called the **'triple assessment'** [1].
- **FBE and UECs** [2] are unremarkable and a **group and hold** [3] is ordered in preparation for surgery.
- **Coagulation studies** [4] are considered for ordering.
- **Mammography** [5] is ordered for this patient and the results show a **spiculated, irregular mass** [6] at 3 o'clock in the right breast **just next to the nipple** [7].
- It has **microcalcifications and areas of hyperdensity** [8].

- The left breast does not have any suspicious features. The mammography findings that are suspicious for breast cancer are conveyed to the patient at the next outpatient visit.
- **Core biopsy** [9] of the lesion is organised under ultrasound guidance and the results return as **invasive ductal carcinoma** [10].
- After the core biopsy has been taken to aid diagnosis, a **PET scan or CT chest** [11] will be further organised.

1 The 'triple assessment' consists of the clinical examination, imaging of the breast and a biopsy of the lesion.

2 In this patient, an FBE could be taken in order to have a baseline haemoglobin level in the event she needs blood transfusion after surgery. UECs are useful in this patient for a baseline, as many medications and anaesthetics are dosed based on renal excretion.

3 A blood group and hold tests for blood type and a few units are put aside in preparation for surgery. It is performed preoperatively in major surgeries; for example, a mastectomy or reconstruction.

4 Coagulation studies should be ordered if the patient has a history of liver disease, chronic alcoholism (with undiagnosed liver disease), has a clotting disorder or is on anticoagulation. Peri-operatively, these tests are used to guide whether the patient will require medications or blood products to reverse their anticoagulation in order to minimise blood loss during and after surgery.

5 Mammography is used in fatty breasts, but ultrasound and MRI are more sensitive for detecting breast cancer in non-fatty breasts.

6 These features suggest cancer. Spiculated lesions mean that the lesion's edges have spikes, like the sun, but can be found in benign processes such as a post-surgical scar, a Desmond tumour, an abscess or fat necrosis, but can be suspicious of malignancy (where the lesion is invading surrounding tissue).

7 Lesions next to the nipple can be papillomas or ductal carcinomas.

8 Microcalcifications, asymmetry and architectural distortion are suspicious features for malignancy but can also be seen in fat necrosis (from trauma to the breast) and scarring. Benign causes of hyperdense breasts are after breast irradiation, in pregnancy, and in breasts with minimal fat. Malignant and infective causes of hyperdense breasts include diffuse involvement with lymphoma, inflammatory carcinoma and mastitis (the latter two secondary to lymphatic or venous drainage obstruction in that breast).

9 A core biopsy is performed under ultrasound guidance and is the least invasive way to diagnose a breast lesion and therefore whether the patient requires surgery.

10 Invasive ductal carcinoma is the most common type of invasive breast cancer and metastasises via the lymphatics. Invasive carcinomas of the breast are reviewed on histopathology using the Nottingham Criteria that assess gland formation, nuclear atypical and mitosis counts in order to give the lesion a 'grade' – higher grades correspond to a lesion that is more invasive, more aggressive and has a higher risk of metastasis.

11 A PET scan uses a radioactive tracer administered through the vein which is taken up by tissues that have a high metabolic rate (e.g. cancerous lesions, the thyroid) and excreted through the kidneys. In breast cancer, it has been recently shown that PET and PET/CT imaging have low sensitivity and specificity in staging axillary lymph nodes or metastases and also have high false-positive results.

Management

Immediate

The patient should be offered **psychological support** [1] . Breast cancer resection, whilst important, is not an emergency so the patient should be **consented for surgery** [2] and placed on the **waiting list** [3] .

Short-term

Treatment is by surgical excision +/– **sentinel node biopsy** [4] or **axillary node dissection** [5] . A **suction drain** [6] may be left in place after a mastectomy with axillary dissection to reduce the dead space and allow a path for **fluid to drain** [7] . Postoperatively, the patient may be fitted with a **compression garment** [8] to wear around their chest for 1–2 weeks to reduce formation of **seroma or haematoma** [9] . She should be presented at a multidisciplinary meeting where the **full course of treatment** [10] can be determined. Adjuvant treatment options include **chemotherapy** [11], **radiation therapy** [12] and **targeted hormone treatment** [13] . Reconstructive options after mastectomy include a **TRAM** [14] or **DIEP flap** [15] or **tissue expanders and breast implants** [16] .

Long-term

If the patient develops lymphoedema post axillary lymph node dissection then **compression garments** [17] can be worn and venepuncture or vascular access **should be avoided** [18] in this region. They should be followed up **every 3–6 months** [19] initially to monitor response to treatment and recurrence. Often, follow-up imaging is in the form of mammography. If *BRCA1* or *BRCA2* gene positive, first-degree relatives should be offered **genetic screening and counselling** [20] .

[1] Psychological support should be long-term, as the diagnosis and treatment of breast cancer can understandably cause grief, stress, depression and anxiety. Additional long-term effects of the diagnosis and treatment of any cancer can be pain, fatigue, loss of appetite, weight loss, hair loss and other medication side-effects.

[2] Surgical excision of breast cancer can be in the form of a wide local excision, lumpectomy or segmentectomy (i.e. breast-conserving surgery) or total mastectomy, depending on the type of breast cancer, the tumour stage, patient preference and breast size, and geographic region (i.e. surgeons that are available in that city or country, and if reconstructive options are offered in that region).

[3] Time on the wait list for surgery depends on the geographical location of the hospital, but generally cancer surgery is urgent, warranting <30 days of waiting before the surgery date.

[4] Sentinel node biopsy is performed when there is one lymph node that is involved by metastasis – the 'sentinel node'. Lymphatic mapping with technetium-99 or blue dye can be injected into the region that the breast cancer is occupying and the lymph drainage to this lymph node can be detected with a hand-held gamma probe during the operation. Risks involved in sentinel lymph node biopsy (SLNB) are reactions to the dye (e.g. anaphylaxis), lymphoedema and false-negative results.

[5] Axillary lymph node clearance has higher morbidity than an SLNB as more lymph nodes are being removed. It is performed when there is evidence of metastasis on imaging or if the lesion is high risk for metastasis, such as invasive ductal carcinoma. During the procedure, the patient should be under general anaesthesia but not paralysed, so that the large motor nerves can be tested during the dissection.

[6] Examples of surgical drains include:
- Jackson–Pratt – a perforated round or flat tube connected to negative pressure collection bottle
- Blake – round silicone radio-opaque drain with four channels along the sides connected to a negative pressure bottle
- Penrose – a flat, thin malleable tube that is put in a wound to hold it open; it cannot be attached to a drain bottle.

[7] Fluid from any wound after an operation can be serous (yellow watery proteinaceous fluid), bloody, or haemoserous (blood-tinged serous fluid). Placing a drain in a wound that is on suction allows dead space to collapse down and promote internal wound healing, whilst also allowing any slow bleeding or build-up of serous fluid to drain.

[8] Compression garments can be tailor-made or by using a Tubigrip sock in a size as large as the patient's chest and cut to size.

[9] A seroma is a collection of a clear (serous) fluid collection under a skin flap and frequently occurs after mastectomy and axillary dissections. A haematoma is a collection of blood.

[10] Whilst resection is the primary treatment for invasive ductal carcinoma, after histology has returned, an MDT

should discuss whether adjuvant chemo- or radiotherapy is required and what reconstructive options can be employed for this patient.

11 Chemotherapy for breast cancer includes doxorubicin, carboplatin and cyclophosphamide, among others, and can be used in combinations.

12 Radiation therapy can be delivered via external beam radiation or partial breast irradiation, being aimed at the chest and the lymph nodes in the chest, shoulder and axilla. This aims to eradicate residual disease that is not macroscopically seen during surgical resection of the tumour or where margins are considered close after resection. Some risks associated with radiotherapy include a rash, pain and change in colour or texture of the skin.

13 Targeted hormone therapy depends on what receptors the cancer expresses and are used only in postmenopausal women. These are:
- Herceptin (trastuzumab, a monoclonal antibody against HER2 receptors) for breast cancers that express HER2 (human epidermal growth factor-2).
- Anastrozole (Arimidex) and letrozole (Femara) for breast cancers that express oestrogen receptors (called ER-positive) or progesterone receptors (called PR-positive). Around 80% of breast cancers are ER-positive.
- Tamoxifen (a selective oestrogen receptor modulator) used in ER-positive breast cancers (largely replaced by anastrozole and letrozole).
- Palbociclib (Ibrance) – therapy in combination with letrozole for HER2-negative, hormone-receptor positive (ER- or PR-positive) breast cancer.

14 A TRAM (transverse rectus abdominis myocutaneous) flap is the surgical method of removing skin, fat and part of the rectus abdominis muscle from the abdomen to the chest with the superior epigastric artery.

15 A DIEP (deep inferior epigastric perforator) flap is the surgical method of removing skin and fat in the infraumbilical part of the abdomen to reconstruct a chest wall defect from a mastectomy. The benefits of a DIEP flap are that the rectus abdominis muscle is preserved, therefore reducing abdominal hernias in future.

16 In some patients who have small breasts or who have a mastectomy, tissue expanders are inserted under the skin and pectoralis major to slowly stretch the skin overlying it in preparation for a prosthetic breast implant.

17 Compression garments for upper limb lymphoedema are Tubigrip stockings which fit to the arm and aim at milking the lymph up the arm.

18 In patients without lymphoedema of the upper limb, there is minimal evidence to suggest venepuncture precipitates lymphoedema. Current suggestions state that if a venepuncture cannot be achieved on the contralateral arm, then venepuncture in the ipsilateral arm (the side of the axillary lymph node dissection) should be attempted rather than in sites with higher infection rates, such as the foot. The concern in arms that have had an axillary lymph node clearance is that it is at higher risk of infection and venous thrombosis due to slow or absent lymphatic clearance.

19 Frequency of follow-up depends on the tumour grade and staging and the treatment the patient undergoes.

20 Genetic counselling involves a healthcare practitioner trained in cancer genetics guiding patients and their families through genetic testing and helping them understand their risk and options for prevention in various hereditary conditions.

CASE 62: Burns in a child and non-accidental injury

History

- A **3-year-old** [1] girl is brought in to the ED by her parents **3 days after** [2] sustaining **burns to both of her hands and legs to mid-shin** [3].
- The parents state that the child went into the bathroom and **turned the hot tap on by herself** [4], and they **came in when they heard her yell** [5].
- They state they **ran her hands and feet under tepid water afterwards for 20 minutes** [6] and gave her paracetamol and thought it would be fine.
- However, after the following few days, **she complained of more pain, and blisters developed** [7].

- On further history, the parents state she was **born at term** [8], had **Apgar scores of 9 and 9 at birth** [9], and has **no known medical issues or allergies** [10].
- She is **up to date with her immunisations** [11] and has no known allergies.
- They have **left their other two children at home** [12] with the maternal grandmother today.
- This is a **peripheral hospital** [13] 3 hours away from the nearest burns centre.

[1] Thermal burns in a child are the most common type of burn for this age group.

[2] Always be wary of delayed presentations to the ED or local doctor. Most parents (with medical background or not) will present almost immediately after an accident has occurred to their child.

[3] Burns in a glove and stocking distribution is a major warning sign that this child has had a non-accidental injury (NAI). These occur when the patient's hands or feet are held in hot water for a prolonged period of time, causing a line of demarcation. This is contrary to normal thermal burns where there is no clear line of demarcation (a splash is seen) where the patient has pulled their affected body part away from the hot water.

[4] Consider if the child's age and level of development fits with the carer or witness account of the injury. For example, a 3-year-old can walk, and may be able to turn taps on, but likely will not be tall enough to be able to reach a pan of hot water.

[5] Whilst brief moments of lack of supervision may be normal, be suspicious when a prolonged period of no supervision of a young child is given by their carers.

[6] Initial first aid for a thermal burn is running cool tap water over the affected region(s) for 20 minutes. If it has not been applied, it is still effective for up to 3 hours post burn injury.

[7] Blistering of the skin is typical of a superficial dermal burn.

[8] Being born premature means developmental calculations need to be adjusted for the weeks or months the child was born preterm.

[9] To know what state of development the child is, questions to ask are whether they were born at term, their Apgar (Appearance, Pulse, Grimace, Activity, Respiration) scores and any medical issues. Apgar scores do not predict further health issues but are a useful aid in the case of developmental delay.

[10] Medical comorbidites are important to know in any patient. Of note in children who have had a burn, immunodeficiencies, skin conditions requiring steroid creams or genetic disorders can all affect their body's response to the injury.

[11] Immunisations are an important factor in development and retention of major infections; noteworthy in burns is vaccination against tetanus toxoid.

[12] It is important to ask if there are other children and who is taking care of them. This is not only for the safety of the other children, but to assess if the parents need help with taking care of their children whilst they are currently with the one they brought to hospital. They may require discussion with social work for some additional support at home, should their child require admission.

[13] When performing initial assessment and management, it is important to remember the capabilities and services of the geographical location. If it is not equipped to deal with burns, in any age group, let alone a paediatric burn, then be sure to refer early to the nearest large burns unit. The British Burn Association has a list of criteria of when to refer burns patients to tertiary burns centres.

Examination

- The child isn't able to be **comforted by the parents** [1] and looks **underweight** [2] and **pale** [3].
- She weighs **12kg** [4] and has a height of **85cm** [5].
- She is tachycardic at **150bpm** [6], has an **unrecordable BP** [7] and a temperature of **38.7°C** [8].
- Both of her hands and feet are erythematous with a **glove and stocking distribution** [9], a **brisk capillary refill** [10], and some areas have formed **fluid-filled blisters** [11].
- These are particularly **painful** [12].
- On parts of her palms, there are **blotchy, creamy-looking, non-blanching regions** [13].

- These seem **not to be causing the child any pain** [14].
- The burns are estimated as **8% total body surface area (TBSA)** [15].
- The rest of her body is unaffected by burns but there are some **old bruises on both her arms and chest** [16] where the parents state she fell a few weeks prior.
- She has a **nappy rash** [17] with a **thick, white, malodorous build-up in the groin** [18].

[1] If the parents aren't reacting to the child when she is distressed, this is a warning that the child may be being neglected or abused at home. Equally, children who are not comforted by their carer or do not seek their carer for comfort is suspicious for neglect. A less sinister reason for not being comforted is that the child is in considerable pain and therefore cannot be distracted from this.

[2] Children who 'look thin' are usually in a normal weight range – beware here though and plot any paediatric patient on a height and weight chart for their age.

[3] Children can easily have iron-deficiency anaemia when fed cow's milk or formula instead of a varied diet.

[4] A weight of 12kg in a 3-year-old girl is within the 25th centile for her age, on the UK-WHO growth chart for girls. The parents should be asked what centile she was or her weight and height when she was born, to compare.

[5] A height of 85cm is below the 3rd centile for a 3-year-old on the UK-WHO growth chart for girls. This indicates malnutrition and needs to be dealt with promptly.

[6] Tachycardia can be due to pain, crying, dehydration or the fever. Treat the pain, assess dehydration status and comfort the child.

[7] Unrecordable or false blood pressures are common in children due to screaming, moving, or trying to remove the BP cuff.

[8] Febrile episodes are common in the early post-burn phase due to the inflammatory response of the body to the injury. Additional findings such as increased pain, cellulitis or malodour would be used to determine if the burn wound is infected.

[9] See Note 3 in *History* regarding glove and stocking burns.

[10] Superficial epidermal and superficial dermal burns have brisk capillary refill. Skin that is erythematous without blistering is called a superficial (epidermal) burn and will spontaneously resolve without scarring, as in the case of a sun burn.

[11] Blanching erythematous burns that develop blisters within minutes of the injury are superficial dermal burns. They only involve the epidermis and upper part of the dermal papillae and are very painful, as the area affected now has exposed nerve endings. As the epidermal layer is lost, both the barrier against infection and the ability to contain fluid are lost, resulting in moderate oedema (causing the blistering).

[12] Superficial dermal burns are exquisitely tender.

[13] Partial thickness burns (mid to deep dermal) involve destruction of the entire epidermal layer and variable thickness of the dermis. These look mottled with a slightly delayed capillary refill from normal. A superficial partial thickness burn will regenerate the epidermal layer but will take longer to heal than a superficial burn. A deep partial burn will affect the sweat glands and hair follicles and will leave a scar if untreated. These burns take 7–10 days to declare themselves as superficial or deep partial thickness.

[14] Non-blanching, white, leathery, charred black or cherry red burns that are insensate or lack much sensation are deep dermal burns. This is because the layer of nerves and capillaries has been removed. As such, they do not blanch under pressure (have no capillary refill) and will not heal by themselves as they do not have an epidermal layer to regenerate from. They are associated with underlying tissue oedema and fluid loss and require grafting.

[15] Percentage of TBSA is calculated on partial thickness burns and greater, not superficial dermal burns. For children, each hand is roughly 1% of TBSA. It is related to the 'Rule of 9s' but is modified for paediatric use. As per British Burn Association criteria, any child with TBSA >5% burns is

recommended to be referred to a tertiary burns centre, and any with TBSA >10% requires IV fluid resuscitation.

16 Bruising on a child's limbs is usually not a sign of NAI. However, bruises of varying ages and on parts of the body easily hidden (chest, back, abdomen) are more suspicious of non-accidental injury.

17 A child of 3 years old should be toilet trained. If they are in nappies, suspect a developmental delay, parental neglect or chronic disease.

18 Nappy rash and *Candida albicans* infection point towards poor toileting practice, irritants being used on the skin, friction between the nappy and the skin, infrequent changing of nappies and/or neglect.

Investigations

- FBE [1] reports a **mildly elevated WCC** [2].
- UEC results are normal [3].
- CRP is elevated [4].

- Urine MC&S grows **candida with some squamous cells** [5].
- X-rays of the chest, upper and lower limbs show **old fractures in the humeri and ribs** [6] but clear lungs.

1 In a story where there is no suspicion of child abuse, no investigations are required for a burn. However, in this case, the patient has a delayed presentation for burns, multiple previous bruises in regions suspicious for abuse, and possible infection (tachycardia and fever).

2 Mildly elevated WCC is expected in a burn due to the inflammatory response and therefore is unreliable in this context unless a clear infective source is found.

3 If the child is not dehydrated, septic or vomiting then UEC is likely to be normal.

4 CRP would be elevated whether the child had a superimposed infection or not, as an injury has occurred and the body mounts an inflammatory reaction in response.

5 Squamous cells are most often a contaminant, and in this case, candida infection may well be from the nappy rash, not a UTI.

6 X-rays would not commonly be performed unless inhalational burns or thoracic injury has occurred during the burn injury. In this case, it would be performed as maltreatment is suspected and therefore X-rays of the bruised arms and chest were taken.

Management

Immediate

Start with **first aid** [1] [2] – in any situation. Determine if this child **requires nasogastric or IV fluid resuscitation** [3]. Use the **Modified Parkland Formula** [4] to guide fluid administration. Maintain an **accurate fluid balance chart** [5]. Monitor vital signs, **clinical response to management** [6] and **urine output** [7]. Give **adequate analgesia** [8] – this includes paracetamol regularly and **may require opioid analgesia or nitrous oxide** [9] for examination and burns treatment. However, it is worth utilising **non-pharmacological techniques for analgesia** [10]. Remember to **keep the child warm** [11]. **Do not deroof the blisters** [12] but cover the affected region **in a sterile dressing** [13]. Seek advice from the **paediatric plastic surgery or burns team** [14]. Find out if the child's **tetanus status is up to date** [15], and if the parents are unsure, give a tetanus booster. If there

are **circumferential burns** [16] she will **need prompt escharotomy** [17].

Short-term

The plastic surgery team will admit the patient and prepare for **debridement and skin grafting of the full thickness burns** [18]. The blisters **(superficial dermal burns) are usually left alone** [19] but the partial thickness burns will require 7–10 days **to declare themselves** [20]. **Topical antibiotics** [21] may be used for partial or full thickness burns but unless septic or superinfection of the burn is suspected, **IV antibiotics are not routine** [22]. **Burns dressings** [23] will be applied postoperatively. This child may require a **nutritionist** [24] to be involved for a high protein diet. Burns involving joints will require **early physiotherapist involvement** [25] to improve mobilisation and prevent contracture formation.

Long-term

Link the family in with **social work** [26] and have a low threshold for **notifying the relevant child health protection agency** [27]. The child will need burns dressings management in the community, whether this be in a burns outpatient clinic or via the GP. After the burn has healed, there are many dressing options to **reduce scar formation and appearance** [28]. Parents should be **vigilant in UV protection** [29] of their child's burn wounds and skin grafts. As the child grows, any of the regions affected by burns **may form contractures or be cosmetically unappealing** [30] and may need re-referral by their GP to a plastic surgery unit for treatment.

1 First aid is guided by ABCDE. Assess if the airway is patent or if there are signs of inhalational injury (soot around the mouth or face, facial burns, respiratory distress, hoarse voice) and apply humidified oxygen at 100% FiO_2 via a non-rebreather mask. Have one person focus on the airway and breathing and perform simple manoeuvres such as jaw thrust. Decide early if this patient requires intubation or add airway adjuncts such as a guedel or laryngeal mask airway.

2 Remember that in a child there are anatomical differences in the oropharynx compared with adults. Their head is proportionally larger relative to body size and has a prominent occiput so when lying supine on a flat surface, their neck is flexed and therefore predisposes them to airway obstruction. A folded towel or shoulder roll is often required to achieve a neutral neck position to open up the airway. They are also more difficult to ventilate and intubate because of their airway anatomy. Start with a guedel to prevent the posterior displacement of the tongue if the patient cannot maintain an open airway. If the child requires intubation, the gold standard is direct laryngoscopy. Traditionally, uncuffed endotracheal tubes were used in neonates to young children to prevent pressure trauma to the subglottis. However, it is becoming more common to use cuffed endotracheal tubes to achieve better ventilation and this is associated with a lower incidence of laryngospasm than uncuffed tubes.

3 A child with >10% TBSA burns should have an NGT or IV line inserted for fluid resuscitation and indwelling urinary catheter for close urine output measurement.

4 Where required, use the modified Parkland Formula to calculate resuscitation fluid. This is 3–4ml IV fluid x (weight in kg) x (%TBSA) = IV fluid in 24 hours. Maintenance fluid for paediatric patients is calculated by the 4/2/1 rule: 4ml/kg/hour for the first 10kg of weight plus 2ml/kg/hour for the next 10kg of weight, then 1ml/kg/hour for the remaining kgs of weight. Half the volume is administered in the first 8 hours from the time of injury and the second half over the next 16 hours. The IV fluid may change depending on the local protocol. Never give normal saline alone to children as they have a higher metabolic rate than adults and will quickly become hypoglycaemic when fasting.

5 Fluid balance charts are a nursing chart to record fluid administration and output.

6 Children may have completely normal vital signs seconds before deterioration. It is far more important to observe the child's behaviours, what they look like at the end of the bed, urine output, and oral intake, to guide clinical management.

7 Urine output is one of the most accurate measures of dehydration and to determine fluid resuscitation requirements. Aim for 1–2ml/kg/hour of urine output for paediatric patients <30kg, and 0.5–1.0ml/kg/hour for weight >30kg.

8 For children with >10% TBSA, the British Burn Association recommends IV morphine 0.1mg/kg every 5 minutes with an upper limit of 0.3mg/kg and reassess pain score, adjusting accordingly. Consider the use of a morphine infusion if ongoing pain relief is required. For children with <10% TBSA, simple analgesia such as paracetamol and ibuprofen may be adequate.

9 Nitrous oxide, administered by mask or inhalational mouthpiece, has a quick onset and can be sedating. Its main adverse side-effect in children is vomiting and requires the administrator to be familiar with its use.

10 Non-pharmacological analgesic methods include deep breathing, hypnosis, music therapy and distraction (e.g. encouraging the child to play with their favourite toy, watch a film, use a virtual reality headset, or talking with the child about their favourite hobby).

11 Hypothermia is quick to develop in burns victims, especially children who have a large surface area to body mass ratio. Hypothermia has been shown to increase risk of sepsis, wound infection and mortality in burns patients.

12 Debridement or deroofing of blisters is not usually required as they will burst on their own, and deroofing will likely cause the child more distress and pain, and increases the risk of infection.

13 Sterile dressings are used first before the child can be assessed by plastic or general surgeons who specialise in burns treatment, as the dressings will be repeatedly removed and reapplied. A simple example is a non-stick layer such as Jelonet, covered by sterile gauze and loosely wrapped by a crepe bandage. If this was a burn that happened on the day of presentation, cling film wrap is often used to cover the burn sites as it reduces hypothermia and is non-stick.

14 Referral criteria to a tertiary burns criteria as per the British Burn Association is of note in this case – this includes burns >5% TBSA in children, burns of special areas (face, hands, feet, genitalia, perineum, major joints and circumferential limb or chest burns) and non-accidental burns.

15 Tetanus immunisation should be within the last 10 years, and should be given if the patient cannot recall their last vaccination. In burns injuries, tetanus immunisation is recommended in any age with burns deeper than superficial thickness.

16 Circumferential burns have a high risk of developing compartment syndrome. Assess the limb for the 6 Ps: Pain, Paraesthesia, Paralysis, Pallor, Pulseless and Perishingly cold. The first sign is usually pain, but have a low threshold for suspicion and elevate the affected region to reduce risk.

17 Escharotomy involves an incision through the skin and dermis down to subcutaneous fat, in order to release the constricting eschar. This is to prevent or treat compartment syndrome as it releases tension across the affected region and thus allows reperfusion and space for muscle and tissue to swell.

18 Full thickness burns cannot regenerate epidermis and require skin grafting to close the wound.

19 This type of burn may not require surgical intervention. Management is with an occlusive, waterproof, non-stick dressing for comfort for the child and parents. Timing of dressing changes can be every 2nd day to every week, depending on the body region affected, the amount of exudate, presence of infection and burn team preference.

20 Laser Doppler, whilst expensive, is used in some tertiary centres to diagnose partial thickness burns in a short period of time as it monitors microvascular blood flow within the dermis. In Jackson's Burn Model, the zone of stasis of a partial thickness burn can convert to full thickness a few days after the injury; prevention of this is dependent on adequate fluid resuscitation to improve blood flow to the wound.

21 Choice of topical antibiotics should be discussed with the burns team. These include bacitracin, polymyxin B or neomycin, but a simple antimicrobial agent is also topical silver sulfadiazine.

22 Septic shock can rapidly develop in this setting where there is decreased barrier function, increased inflammatory mediators and bacterial translocation across the GI system; this is higher in larger TBSA and with increased severity of burn type.

23 There are many types of dressings used for burns. Some include silicone-based dressings, foam dressings, alginate dressings, hydrogel-containing dressings and hydrocolloid dressings. They are used in different situations based on many wound characteristics. Integra biodegradable temporising matrix (BTM) is a form of biological wound dressing that can be placed into the wound after the burn is excised and before skin grafting is performed. BTM is left in the wound bed and covered with a simple dressing for 3–9 weeks. It promotes collagen deposition, fibroblast invasion and neovascular ingrowth to the wound bed called a neo-dermis, allowing for better graft healing.

24 Burn injury increases the body's catabolism, resulting in loss of muscle and BMD. A specialised high protein diet is therefore required for wound healing and rebuilding muscle bulk.

25 Early mobilisation for any scar region, particularly those crossing joints, is critical for reducing contractures and gaining premorbid function.

26 A social worker can link the family in to support if they are struggling with parenting or anger management, aid them with searching and applying for financial assistance or help them find accommodation whilst the child is being treated in the hospital.

27 Anyone can make a report to a child protection agency if they have a belief that a child is likely to suffer, or has suffered, significant harm in the form of abuse or neglect and their parents are unable to protect them from this harm. Doctors, nurses, police officers and other professional groups are legally mandated to report this suspicion as soon as practicable.

28 Long-term compression garments can be used to reduce scar thickness and prevent contractures. Massage, moisturising with moisture-rich creams and silicone-impregnated dressings or gels are also used to reduce scar thickness, promote collagen fibre reorientation and prevent keloid scarring. In fact, silicone sheeting or gel is the gold standard treatment for hypertrophic or keloid scars.

29 Ultraviolet (UV) light protective techniques should be employed in the first 1–2 years after any burn injury or skin grafting as this skin is hypersensitive to UV damage and resultant pigmentation and skin cancer formation. UV protection involves wearing factor 50+ sunscreen, protective clothing, a hat and sunglasses, and encouraging the patient to stay in the shade even on cloudy days.

30 Scar revision can be grouped into resurfacing, excision and lengthening or reorientation. Resurfacing involves microneedling, laser therapy and microdermabrasion. Excision of scar tissue may be able to be closed primarily, or with another graft or flap. Reorientation involves incising the scar and moving it with geometrical flaps to reorient the fibres, such as in the case of contracture release.

CASE 63: Carpal tunnel syndrome

History

- A **60-year-old female** [1] **right-hand dominant** [2] **car mechanic** [3] presents to the GP clinic with right hand numbness and weakness.
- Her main complaint is numbness, particularly at night, in her **thumb, index and middle fingers** [4], and she often has **shooting pains and tingling** [5] from her right hand that radiates up her arm.
- She states sometimes she will be holding a tool at work and **drop it** [6] which is increasingly frustrating.

- This issue has progressed over the last few years and does not affect **the left hand** [7]. This issue has altered her ability to hold even the car steering wheel when driving, as it exacerbates her pain and numbness.
- Nothing seems to help relieve the issue apart from **resting the hand for a few minutes when symptoms occur** [8].

[1] Middle-aged females have the highest incidence of carpal tunnel syndrome. However, it is important through history and examination, in addition to clinical testing, that carpal tunnel syndrome be distinguished from median nerve damage or compression at a higher level in the arm.

[2] It is important in any upper limb complaint to establish handedness. The patient's livelihood and general use of their hand will be affected by the management plan.

[3] Manual workers, desk workers and people who have repetitive strain injuries are at high risk of developing carpal tunnel syndrome.

[4] Sensory innervation to the thumb, index, middle and radial side of the ring finger is provided by the median nerve. Sensory innervation to the region over the thenar eminence itself is supplied by the palmar branch of the median nerve or occasionally by the lateral cutaneous nerve of the forearm – both of these enter the palm superficial to the flexor retinaculum and therefore are not compressed in carpal tunnel syndrome.

[5] Shooting and tingling pains are neuropathic pain from compression of the median nerve. However, shooting up the arm may be due to compression higher up the path of the median nerve, rather than at the carpal tunnel.

[6] The power of the thenar eminence muscles (opponens pollicis, abductor pollicis and flexor pollicis brevis) and lateral two lumbricals can be reduced in severe median nerve compression. The thenar eminence is supplied by the muscular (recurrent) branch of the median nerve, whilst the lateral two lumbricals are innervated by the median nerve. The flexor digitorum superficialis and profundus tendons run through the carpal tunnel but are innervated before the flexor retinaculum. The former is innervated by the median nerve, whilst the latter is innervated by the anterior interosseous branch of the median nerve and by the ulnar nerve.

[7] Carpal tunnel syndrome can be uni- or bilateral.

[8] Night-time bracing can help reduce symptoms but not much else can relieve compression of the carpal tunnel except surgical release.

Examination

- There is **thenar eminence wasting on the right hand** [1] compared with the left.
- Sensation is decreased in the **right thumb, index and middle finger** [2] compared with the rest of the hand.

- Pincer grip strength on her right hand is 3/5 [3].
- **Tinel's and Phalen's signs** [4] are positive on the right and negative on the left.
- She can **flex the interphalangeal joint of the thumb with 5/5 power** [5].

1 The thenar eminence is innervated by the motor (recurrent) branch of the median nerve.

2 See Note 4 in *History* for sensation of the hand.

3 Pincer grip strength is dictated by the thenar muscles of the hand. These are affected in carpal tunnel syndrome.

4 Tinel's sign is performed by tapping over the flexor retinaculum. A positive result is reproducing the patient's

pain, whether this be shooting, stabbing or pins and needles. Phalen's sign is performed by having the patient putting their palms together as in prayer, with their wrists at 90° to their forearms. A positive result is reproduction of the patient's pain.

5 Power in the IPJ of the thumb (performed by the flexor pollicis longus) is lost with more proximal lesions of the median nerve.

Investigations

- Baseline blood tests are unremarkable.
- Bilateral **nerve conduction studies** [1] show results consistent with moderate to severe compression

of the right radial nerve at the level of the flexor retinaculum.

1 Carpal tunnel syndrome is a clinical diagnosis. However, nerve conduction studies (electromyography) are helpful to determine if nerve conduction is inhibited at the level of the carpal tunnel or higher in the arm. Further imaging is only

indicated if there is suspected brachial plexus or cervical spine (C-spine) neuropathy. This would include an MRI of the C-spine.

Management

Immediate

Consider **conservative treatment** [1]. Refer to the **hand therapy unit** [2] for night-time splinting. Seek advice from the hand surgery team.

Short-term

If deemed appropriate, perform a nerve decompression by **open carpal tunnel release** [3]. Prescribe **vitamin C (500–1000mg daily) for 90 days** [4] for these patients in addition to postoperative simple analgesia.

Long-term

If the wound is **closed with non-dissolvable sutures** [5], these will need to be removed at 7–10 days post procedure. Once the wound has fully healed, the patient can **massage the scar** [6] and **gradually increase use of the affected hand** [7]. Patients will be unable to drive for at least 2 weeks whilst their hands are swollen and painful. Some patients will require referral to a hand therapist in the first 2 weeks postoperatively to start gradual ROM exercises and strength training.

1 Untreated carpal tunnel syndrome can spontaneously resolve in up to one-third of patients, particularly after pregnancy (which has a known association with carpal tunnel syndrome). If the patient has multiple medical comorbidities, does not wish to have surgery, or has a long waiting time for a surgeon to perform decompression, then night-time splinting is an option. Thermoplastic splints with the wrist in neutral or 20° extension has no difference in benefit for the patient apart from the latter being more comfortable to wear. Its use may limit the patient in their ADLs but is recommended to be worn initially at night then progressing to continuously for a month, to see if this improves their symptoms.

2 Hand therapy units may be part of a plastic surgery unit or by themselves in the public sector. They can also give the patient minor aids for the house such as kettle tippers,

long-handled shoehorns or jar openers, in order to prevent exacerbation of the symptoms.

3 This involves referral to a private or public service of general, plastic or orthopaedic surgery. The relevant nerve conduction studies should be sent with the referral. The procedure takes around 15 minutes and involves a small linear incision over the flexor retinaculum, careful dissection through the palmar fascia and the flexor retinaculum. Identification and preservation of the median nerve and its recurrent branch are highly important in this procedure to ensure no damage is incurred and full function can be restored to the patient's hand.

4 There has been recent evidence that administering oral vitamin C reduces the risk of chronic regional pain syndrome in carpal tunnel release and some other procedures, such as ankle and foot surgeries.

5 Debate exists around whether non-dissolvable (e.g. proline, nylon) versus dissolvable (e.g. monocryl, Vicryl Rapide) sutures are best to close hand wounds. The choice often reflects the particular hospital or Consultant surgeon's preference.

6 Massage of any scar with any cream, such as one containing vitamin E, can reduce the thickness of scar formation, as it is thought to help reorganise the collagen.

7 Strength of the affected hand from prolonged median nerve compression can take up to a year to recover to pre-compression levels. It is important that patients do not lift heavy objects more than 2kg or 'overdo' ROM exercises with their hands in the first 2–6 weeks, as there is evidence this can delay wound healing and recovery in the long term.

CASE 64: Cleft lip and palate

History

- A **36-year-old** [1] **Thai** [2] female has just delivered her first newborn at full term, which is a **girl** [3].
- She has noted an issue in breastfeeding in the first few hours of life. On review of her obstetric history, she never had a **morphology ultrasound** [4] and states she **smoked throughout her pregnancy** [5] as she was worried about a large child with a **vaginal birth** [6].
- The mother did not take any specific perinatal vitamins apart from **folic acid** [7] and **is not on any medications** [8].
- She did not **drink alcohol before or during her pregnancy** [9]. She also discloses that **her sister had a 'hole in her lip'** [10] and had to have it surgically treated as a child.
- When asked about feeding difficulties, she states her baby doesn't seem to be able to suckle properly and she has noticed when it cries that there is a 'black hole' in her mouth. Sometimes when feeding, the **milk comes out of the child's nose** [11].
- The mother also states that she noticed her infant moving to one side when she is speaking with her and is wondering if she **cannot hear out of her right ear** [12].

[1] Rates of orofacial clefts are highest in American Indians followed by Alaska Natives, then intermediate prevalence in whites, Hispanics, Asians and Pacific Islanders.

[2] Maternal age >35 years is associated with a higher risk of oral clefts in the foetus.

[3] Females are more likely to have cleft palate without cleft lip. The opposite is true for males.

[4] Cleft lip and palate are orofacial defects involving one or both sides of the lip and/or palate. It is the result of the hard and soft palate not joining in the midline during the first 6–9 weeks of pregnancy. However, the foetal face cannot be clearly visualised via ultrasound transabdominally until 13–14 weeks' gestation.

[5] Incidence of cleft lip and palate is higher when the mother smokes during pregnancy.

[6] Smoking in pregnancy has been shown to stunt foetal growth.

[7] Some association between taking folate and reduced risk of cleft lip and palate has been shown but evidence is weak. However, maternal perinatal multivitamin use has been shown to be protective against cleft lip and palate in some genotypes.

[8] Prevalence of cleft lip and palate is also higher in mothers who have diabetes, are obese, or take certain medications such as anti-epileptics during their pregnancy (e.g. phenytoin, sodium valproate and topiramate).

[9] Alcohol consumption by the mother during pregnancy (>6 units per week) has been associated with a higher incidence of cleft lip and palate.

[10] Often the cause of cleft lip or palate is not known but it has a genetic component. Parents without clefts whose child has cleft lip or palate have a 4% recurrence rate in future pregnancies, and the risk increases with further affected children.

[11] This is because in cleft palate the oropharynx and the nasal cavity are communicating.

[12] Children with cleft lip and palate often have long-standing conductive hearing loss due to Eustachian tube malfunction. They can also have sensorineural or mixed hearing losses, especially if the cleft lip and palate is part of a clinical syndrome.

Examination

- The newborn has normal weight, length and head circumference for her gestation and sex. Whilst attempting to suckle, the newborn is able to latch well to the nipple, but she **coughs and splutters often** [1].
- She **tires easily** [2] [3] and cries after feeding, **pulling her legs up to her chest** [4].
- There is a **right unilateral cleft** [5] in her lip which **extends down the hard and soft palate** [6] on the right-hand side.
- The child does not otherwise **look syndromic** [7].

[1] Coughing and spluttering whilst feeding occurs when a baby is trying to drink too much too quickly.

[2] Cleft lip and palate can result in fatigue during feeding due to excessive energy expenditure whilst trying to increase negative pressure within the mouth to draw milk in. Children with cleft lip alone usually are able to feed well, as their suction is not affected. With a cleft palate, air leaks from the mouth into the nose during feeding and therefore cannot create enough suction during feeding to draw milk easily from the breast or bottle.

[3] Swallowing difficulties during feeding can manifest as inability to establish suck–swallow–breathe sequence, coughing, choking or gagging, an increased respiratory rate or oxygen desaturation.

[4] Infant colic can be increased in cleft lip and palate due to inhalation of air whilst trying to feed.

[5] There are various classifications for orofacial clefts. The most recent is the Tessier classification from 1976 which is universally used – where the clefts are related to the orbit anatomically and are numbered as they progress periorbitally. However, the simplest way to describe orofacial clefts is:
- unilateral or bilateral
- complete, incomplete or microform
- clefting of the lip or palate, or both
- atypical craniofacial clefts.

[6] The newborn screening examination includes looking in the mouth but also using the little finger to palpate the palate, as defects may not be able to be clearly seen.

[7] Over 90% of isolated cleft palate cases are non-syndromic; however, cleft lip with or without cleft palate is associated with over 300 syndromes. The most common are oculoauriculovertebral spectrum, oro-facial-digital syndrome, Treacher Collins syndrome and Pierre Robin sequence, among others.

Investigations

- **Hearing tests** [1] are organised at 4 weeks as a baseline and find a **conductive deficit** [2] on the right.
- The newborn also undergoes a **transthoracic echocardiogram** [3], which is normal.
- She also has a **FISH** [4] for various facial syndromes, which come back normal.
- Other testing **is not performed** [5].

[1] Hearing tests are performed at 4 weeks and 12 weeks of age in newborns with cleft lip and palate, as they are more likely to develop otitis media with effusion and consequently conductive deafness if untreated. Other complications of otitis media with effusion include cholesteatoma formation, ossicular fixation and retraction pockets.

[2] Auditory brainstem response testing can be performed if an audiogram is inconclusive, to assess for hearing loss.

[3] Congenital cardiac malformations are commonly associated with cleft lip and palate, such as tetralogy of Fallot, transposition of the great vessels and tricuspid valve atresia, among many others.

[4] Genetic testing involving fluorescence *in situ* hybridisation (FISH) should be performed in patients with suspected genetic disorders such as velocardiofacial syndrome, which is associated with a cleft palate.

[5] If hemifacial microsomia is present with a cleft lip and palate, spinal X-rays can assess hemivertebrae and other spinal abnormalities associated with this.

Management

Immediate

Special **broad-based teats or bottles** [1] are used for this child in consultation with a **lactation consultant** [2] . The mother also decides to breastfeed so she is encouraged **to express** [3] . The child's care team consists of an **ear, nose and throat surgeon** [4] , **plastic surgeon** [5] , **paediatrician** [6] , **speech pathologist** [7] , **dental specialist** [8] , **oral and maxillofacial surgeon** [9] and **audiologist** [10] .

Short-term

At 4 months old, the child is started on solids just like other children her age. She is linked in with a **general paediatrician and nutritionist** [11] familiar with cleft lip and palate defects, in order to avoid malnutrition. Her mother is followed up in the plastic surgery clinic and recommended to make the **solids more liquid consistency** [12] in order to be swallowed. The first surgical intervention to **repair cleft lip** [13] [14] is performed at 6 months of age. In the interim, **dentofacial alignment** [15] using orthopaedic appliances is carried out. At the time of the cleft palate repair **grommets are inserted bilaterally** [16] . Post-

surgical management of the child includes **hand and arm immobilisation** [17] , avoiding dummies and bottle feeding to reduce **pressure on the wound** [18] and application of **silicone gel** [19] for scar management. Postoperative wound care involves using a wet cotton bud or swab to wipe parallel to the scar if **crusting** [20] occurs, use of **topical antibiotic gel** [21] and to return to the plastic surgery department for removal of non-dissolvable sutures **around day 7** [22] . The child's food is kept to a **more liquid consistency** [23] for the first 3 weeks after surgery and her carers are reminded to be vigilant with **hygiene** [24] of their hands and the utensils used to feed the child, to reduce postoperative infection rate.

Long-term

When the child is 5 years old, **revision of the lip and nose** [25] is offered to improve aesthetics. At age 9 years, associated nasal and bony parts of the alveolus require **bone grafting** [26] [27] for union. At 15 years she discusses a **rhinoplasty** [28] with the paediatric plastic surgeon to improve cosmetic issues. She is linked in with her local GP and counsellor due to bullying and resultant impacts on **mental health** [29] .

---

[1] There are many types of artificial teats and malleable bottles for cleft lip and/or palate that assist the mother in squeezing milk into the child's mouth and allow a large flow rate at a time. Another option is feeding plates that can bridge the gap between the oral and nasal cavity to reduce regurgitation and give a ridge for the child to push against the breast.

[2] Lactation consultants are specialised midwives that aid mothers in breastfeeding techniques. Various methods of feeding are suggested for a baby with cleft lip and/or palate, including sitting them up, positioning the nipple of the breast or bottle away from the side of the cleft if possible, squeezing the bottle to deliver milk into the mouth and having several breaks during feeding for burping.

[3] Expressing milk is encouraged because poor feeding by the newborn may cause low milk supply from the mother and because children with cleft lip and/or palate cannot generate enough suction to propel the milk into the mouth.

[4] Commonly, children with cleft lip and palate have recurrent otitis media from Eustachian tube dysfunction and therefore should be linked in with an ENT surgeon.

[5] Plastic and reconstructive surgeons are the primary surgeons that repair the child's cleft lip and palate and can revise the scar down the track if cosmetically it requires it.

[6] General or specialised paediatricians may be involved with this patient's care, as they have a multitude of associated congenital abnormalities such as cardiac or limb defects or chromosomal abnormalities.

[7] Speech can be affected as patients can have difficulty pronouncing consonants and hard sounds such as 'ch' and 'sh' as well as having a nasal-sounding voice. Cleft lip and palate can result in delays in the onset of babbling and other prelinguistic sounds, which have been linked to delays in speech and language development.

[8] Many children with cleft lip and palate may have missing teeth in the midline. It is therefore important that they see a dentist when their first teeth come through. They may be recommended braces or other dental options to improve their appearance and eating.

[9] Maxillofacial surgeons can also be involved in cleft lip and palate repair.

10 These children should have a hearing test at 4 weeks and 3 months of age with an audiologist.

11 A general paediatrician or paediatric nutritionist can follow the child through their growth and support them as needed with special high protein, high vitamin diets. Protein deficiency can result in stunted growth, oedema, increased infection rate, and changes in skin colour and hair colour and texture. As children with cleft lip and palate are most often bottle-fed (due to difficulty in generating suction on the breast), around one-third develop iron deficiency and consequent anaemia.

12 This prevents regurgitation of food content through the cleft palate and into the nose.

13 Surgical treatment of cleft lip and palate is a soft tissue procedure involving a flap of muscle and mucosa to cover the defect. Surgical repair of a cleft lip and/or palate is recommended in the first 12 months of life. This is because it will improve breathing, speech and language development as well as feeding and therefore growth. It usually involves either an overnight stay or a few days in hospital, depending on the complexity of the procedure. The operation usually involves dissolvable sutures in and around the mouth and the lip may be swollen and red. Healing takes 3–4 weeks and it is important the parents are counselled that there will always be a scar, but it may fade over time.

14 Complications after cleft lip and/or palate repair are wound dehiscence, bleeding, wound infection, fistula formation and irregular healing of scars, including thickening, overgrowth or shortening that may require revision.

15 Dentofacial alignment is also known as naso-alveolar moulding (NAM) and is used to facilitate a tension-free labial repair.

16 Grommets allow fluid in the middle ear to drain externally and are surgically placed to prevent and treat chronic middle ear infections. They are left in the ear canal to slowly push their way out as the eardrum heals; a process that takes 6–9 months.

17 Depending on the centre, hand and arm immobilisation may or may not be recommended. These can be in the form of mittens or swaddling, or elbow immobilisation. The aim is to prevent contamination and disruption of the wound by the child.

18 To avoid wound breakdown and infection, dummies, bottles and hard teething instruments are not recommended in the first few weeks post cleft lip repair. In isolated cleft lip surgery, resuming breast- or bottle-feeding immediately postoperatively is a contentious issue.

19 Silicon-based gel products have been shown to reduce visible appearance of scars and flatten them. It can also be used to reduce pruritus. They can also be used in burns management after epithelialisation or healing of a graft and to reduce the appearance and thickness of keloid or hypertrophic scarring.

20 Crusting is the dried haemoserous exudate from the wound that occurs with healing.

21 The most common topical antibiotic gel is chloramphenicol for prevention of infection. It is usually applied to the wound three times a day for the first 1–2 weeks post-surgery.

22 Mild sedation may be required to remove sutures. Healing time varies on the body, from around 5–7 days on the face, 7 days on the neck, 10 days on the scalp, 10–14 days on the trunk and upper extremities and 14–21 days on the lower limbs. It takes less time to heal those regions that have better blood supply and those that have less friction or use (hands are in contact with the environment and clothing, and are used much more than the face).

23 Mastication of hard foods increases friction and mobility of the wound edges. Such foods may also irritate the wound, resulting in pain and wound dehiscence. Feeding by bottle is also not generally recommended as it grazes against the palatal repair.

24 Simple routines by the carer for the child such as hand washing after going to the toilet, before feeding the child, or before and after cleaning the child, can reduce the risk of wound infection postoperatively. Additional instructions given to the carer(s) may include avoiding use of tissues on the wound, ensuring the child's clothes are clean, and washing utensils before every use.

25 Some surgical interventions include flattening the nasal tip or ala, reducing vermillion border mismatch and resecting widened scars. These are often at the request of the parents.

26 Bone grafts from the hip are usually used and placed in the alveolus (gum) to allow adult teeth to grow through. These are after the molars have erupted at age 6 and cleft tooth buds are also near eruption. Bone grafting of the alveolar cleft aims to close oronasal fistula and complete the alveolar ridge.

27 Orthognathic surgery is performed after most of the mid-face and mandibular growth has occurred and aims to achieve optimal occlusion of the jaw.

28 Rhinoplasty is often the last surgical procedure for cleft lip and palate. Nasal and alar issues due to the cleft lip can be a widened nostril on the cleft side, septal deviation or alar malpositioning, amongst other issues.

29 Children who have cleft lip and/or palate and their families should be supported with psychological counselling and long-term follow-up to assist them with this.

CASE 65: Electrical burns in an adult

History

- A **28-year-old** [1] **right hand dominant** [2] **male** [3] **electrician** [4] is brought in by ambulance to the ED after sustaining an **electrical shock whilst at work** [5].
- He is **unconscious** [6] so the history is taken from his colleagues.
- He was working on **electrical wiring in a roof** [7] when there was a **spark from the equipment** [8] he was working with **at around 1.30pm today** [9].
- It was **not raining** [10] today and the patient had not been working for long.
- One co-worker immediately **called the ambulance** [11] whilst the other **safely removed** [12] the patient from the roof.
- The ambulance officers state that when they arrived at the scene, the patient was on the ground next to his co-worker who was **feeling for a pulse** [13].
- **No CPR was required** [14], but his GCS has been 9 since they arrived at the ED, around 45 minutes ago.
- The patient's co-workers state that he is usually well but **smokes around 20 cigarettes a day** [15] and has consistently done so during the time he has been working with them, which is around 6 years.
- They don't know if he is taking **any medication** [16], has any known **medical history** [17], but they believe he does not take **illicit drugs** [18].
- He **last ate at 10am** [19].

1 The average age of patients sustaining electrical burn injuries is between 27 and 40 years.

2 There is no clear documentation of handedness and risk for electrical injuries. In any trauma through the hands, however, it is important to establish the dominant hand of the patient for functional implications.

3 In adults, 90% of electrical injuries occur in men. In children, boys are twice as likely than girls to sustain an electrical injury.

4 The majority of electrical burns occur at work in adults and at-home accidents in children usually younger than six years. Electrical burns in older children and adolescents are usually whilst climbing trees or utility poles and coming into contact with power lines. In two-thirds of electrical injuries, the patient is an electrician or construction worker.

5 In electrical injuries, it is important to know what type of current (direct current (DC) or alternating current (AC)) the patient was in contact with, whether it was high or low voltage, and what stimulus created the electricity (e.g. lightning, a fuse box or power lines). Low voltage is considered <600 volts or current <240 amps; most of low voltage is AC which causes ventricular fibrillation and muscle tetany. Resultant rhabdomyolysis is common but acute mortality is low and may result in superficial burns. High voltage is >1000 volts but a current of <1000 amps, and can be DC or AC. An example is power lines. Burns are common and penetrate deeply, with consequent

rhabdomyolysis and moderate mortality rate. DC current injuries have a short duration of exposure as it results in a single muscle contraction and throws the victim from the source. Secondary trauma is the main cause of morbidity in DC current injuries.

6 This patient may have sustained secondary head injury after falling from a height or striking his head against the beams of the roof during or after tetanic muscle contractions.

7 Electrical wiring is usually AC current and low voltage.

8 There are four types of electrical injury that need to be ascertained on history.
- Contact with an electrical current – when the body becomes part of the circuit, there are classically entry and exit wounds which can cause cardiac damage and rhabdomyolysis as it passes through the flesh.
- Flash or arc burns – occur when the current jumps to the skin but does not enter the body, causing a flash of light.
- Flame injuries – from clothing catching fire from an electrical source.
- Lightning injuries – caused by high voltage DC current (greater than 30×10^6 volts), rarely causing burns but has a high mortality rate secondary to immediate cardiac or respiratory arrest.

9 Time of the injury, time that any first aid was performed and time that emergency services arrived is crucial in any trauma scenario, as it paints a picture of what care the patient received prior to reaching the final treatment destination (i.e. the ED).

10 Dry skin has a high resistance, but this lessens by a factor of 40 when wet. Low resistance means more current can penetrate through the skin and cause more damage.

11 Ambulance arrival and transit time helps to understand how long the patient was without first aid and what has been done en route.

12 It is worth asking how the patient was retrieved, how long it took to retrieve them post injury and if anyone else was injured.

13 Feeling for a pulse and looking for signs of breathing are one of the first steps of basic first aid before commencing CPR.

14 This is important in the history as high voltage electrical injuries can cause arrhythmias and asystole.

15 Smoking delays wound healing, increases wound infection rates and risk of pulmonary emboli, cardiac events

and stroke. A medication list is important to understand both what the patient's medical history is and resultant effects this has on the patient – for example, knowing a patient has high BP and is on a beta blocker means that their heart rate will not increase with hypovolaemia or sepsis.

16 Always take a medical history including allergies. This helps to guide treatment goals and assess for risk of complications or prognosis.

17 When taking a history of any injury, it is important to know the time of the injury, the mechanism, other associated injuries, medications, comorbidities and last meal, to plan for surgery.

18 Illicit drugs that are sympathomimetic, such as cocaine, increase cardiac arrhythmias and asystole.

19 Knowing when the patient last ate and drank is asked to ascertain if they are at risk of aspiration if they cannot maintain their airway or require intubation or anaesthesia. Fasting times to reduce risk of aspiration during anaesthesia are 6 hours for food and 2 hours for clear fluids.

Examination

- In the ambulance, the patient had a run of **ventricular fibrillation** [1] that spontaneously resolved within a few seconds, and has been **tachycardic** [2] since.
- He is **mildly hypotensive** [3], **tachypnoeic** [4] and his oxygen saturations are within normal limits but they have applied a **Hudson mask at 15L/min** [5] en route.
- The ambulance officers have **inserted a large-bore cannula** [6] into the cubital fossa of his right arm and **started IV Hartmann's solution** [7], of which 500ml has been administered so far.
- He has a small **contusion to the occiput** [8] but no obvious bleeding or overlying fracture.
- His pupils are **equal and reactive** [9] and he has no other obvious **signs of injury on his head or neck** [10].
- On **cardiorespiratory examination** [11] his **trachea is midline** [12] and **air entry is equal bilaterally** [13].
- The patient has small **partial thickness burns on both palms** [14].
- Continuing the primary survey, his abdomen is soft and has no obvious injuries, **Cullen or Grey Turner's signs** [15].
- By looking and feeling over his limbs, there are **no occult fractures or exsanguination** [16].
- On a **log roll** [17] there is no acute pathology, but due to the patient's altered GCS, the **spine cannot be cleared** [18].

1 Ventricular fibrillation occurs from an AC current and is the most common fatal arrhythmia from electrical injuries. It occurs when the current pathway travels from one hand to another, essentially crossing through the heart.

2 Tachycardia in an adult is from 120bpm. This patient could have sinus tachycardia, premature ventricular contractions or ventricular fibrillation (which has a ventricular rate of >300bpm).

3 This patient is hypotensive, which may be due to tissue oedema secondary to the electrical injury.

4 Normal respiratory rate is 12–20 breaths/min. This tachypnoea could be due to pneumothorax or pain from concomitant injuries.

5 Application of a Hudson mask (also known as a non-rebreather) is part of first aid in order to give the patient as much oxygen as possible; 15L/min is maximum delivery of supplemental oxygen.

6 A large-bore cannula is considered an 18 gauge or higher. These are used in trauma situations in order to administer fluid as quickly as possible via a peripheral line.

7 Hartmann's solution (also known as CSL – compound sodium lactate, or lactated Ringer solution) is a crystalloid fluid that is isotonic. In trauma or resuscitation situations, using this fluid or 0.9% sodium chloride (also known as 'normal saline' or 0.9% NaCl) is current practice.

8 This may have occurred from the force of the electrical stimulus throwing the patient into an overhead beam in the roof.

9 Shining a pen torch into the patient's eyes quickly assesses pupillary size and reaction to light. This is part of a quick neurological examination in a trauma survey.

10 A primary trauma survey includes examining for signs of base of skull fractures, characterised by haemotympanum, Battle sign (bruising behind the ear indicative of a base of skull fracture) and around the periorbital region for raccoon eyes (bruising around the orbit indicative of a base of skull fracture or subgaleal haematoma). Examination of the face may also reveal conjunctival haemorrhages, blow-out fractures, hyphaemas and pupillary size and shape.

11 This is a quick combined cardiac and respiratory examination encompassing JVP, heart rate and pulse character at the radial or carotid pulse (one at a time), respiratory rate, oxygen saturation, BP, listening to the lungs anterolaterally and listening to the heart sounds.

12 Tracheal deviation is a late sign of tension pneumothorax.

13 Decreased air entry to one lung or segment of a lung could be due to obstruction in a main bronchus from vomitus (aspiration) or foreign body (a tooth or food), or from pneumothorax. The latter also clinically results in hyper-resonance to percussion and decreased breath sounds.

14 These are entry and exit wounds from the electrical current. As they have crossed the cardiac axis, he is at high risk of arrhythmias and cardiac death. Partial thickness burns are mid to deep dermal and involve destruction of the epidermal layer with variable thickness of the dermis. They have a delayed capillary refill (>3 seconds) and are mottled in colour.

15 Cullen sign is periumbilical bruising and Grey Turner sign is flank bruising, both caused by retroperitoneal haemorrhage. Both signs can take 24–48 hours to develop and can also be seen in severe acute necrotising pancreatitis with retroperitoneal or intra-abdominal bleeding, as well as several other intra-abdominal pathologies.

16 Fractures and consequent bleeding can occur in high voltage electrical injuries due to the electrical stimulus, from secondary trauma (e.g. being thrown against a wall) or from tetanic muscle contractions.

17 A log roll is the moving of a patient in one movement onto their side and back again without flexing the spine. One person is stationed at the head and controls the cervical spine and dictates the timing of the roll. The process is used to move a patient or to feel down their spinal column, one vertebra at a time, in order to ascertain if there is pain, a step (from a retro- or anterolisthesis) or obvious fracture.

18 Clearing the spine means the patient may be allowed to resume sitting up, weight bearing or walking, as the examiner is clinically or radiographically reassured there is no acute injury. For the cervical spine, the NEXUS criteria or the Canadian C-spine rule can be used. The NEXUS criteria are used to determine whether or not imaging is required to assess cervical spinal injury. Low risk criteria (i.e. not requiring imaging) include no posterior midline cervical-spine tenderness, no intoxication, a normal alertness, no focal neurological deficit and no painful distracting injuries. The Canadian C-spine rule has more criteria than this to determine whether or not the patient needs C-spine immobilisation and imaging.

Investigations

- A VBG reveals a **mild respiratory alkalosis, normal haemoglobin count, and mildly elevated lactate** [1].
- FBE shows a **normal haemoglobin count and a mild leucocytosis** [2].
- **UECs are unremarkable** [3].
- **CK is moderately elevated** [4].
- An ECG shows a **sinus tachycardia** [5].
- A **mobile chest X-ray** [6] reveals no obvious rib fractures or haemopneumothorax.
- A **CT of the brain and C-spine** [7] shows no intracranial or C-spine injury.

1 A VBG can be tested in a few minutes within the ED or ICU. It gives a haemoglobin level, sodium, potassium, chloride, bicarbonate and lactate, among other information. In this case, the patient may have respiratory alkalosis secondary to tachypnoea.

2 A full blood examination is used to obtain a haemoglobin level, a WCC and a platelet count. In this case, this would be performed to have a baseline in the event the patient undergoes further procedures. A mildly raised WCC is not unexpected in the setting of trauma.

3 A UEC would be performed in this case to ascertain baseline renal function and response to fluid administration. This patient's renal function should be normal; however, due to rhabdomyolysis it may decline rapidly.

4 A CK is elevated in rhabdomyolysis and cardiac damage. In this case, it may be serially measured to observe response to fluid administration.

5 Electrical burns can result in cardiac arrhythmias and asystole. As this patient is tachycardic, an ECG should be performed to ascertain whether it is sinus tachycardia or an arrhythmia.

6 A mobile, inspiratory CXR is performed in this case to investigate for haemopneumothorax and rib fractures. Ideally, this should be performed in the erect position, but this may not be possible in the setting of spinal precautions.

7 A CT of the brain and cervical spine in this context is looking for cerebral contusions, intra- and extracranial haematomas and vertebral fractures from trauma.

Management

NB.: Initial management, investigations and examination are usually carried out concurrently in a trauma situation by various team members.

Immediate

This patient should be classified as a **trauma call** [1] and be managed with **full spinal precautions** [2]. Place **defibrillation pads** [3] on his chest and constantly reassess his **GCS** [4]. Of vital importance is to **maintain a patent airway** [5]. Obtain vascular access with 2 large-bore cannulas to start **IV fluid rehydration** [6] and place a **urinary catheter** [7]. Monitor **vital signs** [8], **clinical response to management** [9] and urine output. Give **adequate analgesia** [10] and **keep the patient normothermic** [11]. Place the patient on **continuous cardiac monitoring** [12]. Seek advice from the **plastic surgery, trauma or burns team** [13] applicable to the current hospital. This patient may require **prompt fasciotomy** [14].

Short-term

The partial thickness burns may take 7–10 days to **declare themselves** [15]. In the interim, this patient should be managed in the **ICU** [16] with **multiple teams consulting** [17]. He may require **temporary haemofiltration** [18], **escharotomy** [19] or **debridement** [20] of the burn wounds. After the burn has healed, there are many dressing options to **reduce scar formation and appearance** [21]. In extreme cases, the patient may require **limb amputation** [22].

Long-term

Long-term complications of electrical burns include **neurological issues** [23] and **psychological illness** [24]. It is therefore important that the patient seek **psychological aid** [25] and have continuous follow-up with **their GP** [26]. The patient should be **vigilant in UV protection** [27] of the regions that were burned and any skin grafts in the first year.

1 A trauma call, trauma alert or bat call are codes used in the ED to alert relevant team members to attend to that patient urgently. For example, a trauma call might be called for a high-speed motor vehicle accident to alert the general surgery registrar, the anaesthetic registrar and the intensive care registrar to assemble in the ED and assist with assessment and management of a patient, in addition to the Emergency physicians and nursing staff.

2 It is unknown whether this patient has sustained head or neck trauma during or after the electrical shock, so a cervical spine immobilisation collar (also known as a C-spine collar) should be fitted. Full spinal precautions mean the patient has to be lying down at all times, is not allowed to walk around or bear weight until his spine has been cleared either through NEXUS criteria or Canadian C-spine rules, or via imaging (CT, MRI).

3 Defibrillation pads should be applied as this patient is at risk of cardiac arrhythmias and asystole.

4 The GCS is reported as a maximum score of 15 through combined eye response (E, maximum score of 4), verbal response (V, maximum score of 5) and motor response (M, maximum score of 6). Serial assessment is vital, as a GCS of ≤8 suggests an inability for the patient to maintain their own airway, and the need for intubation.

5 Have one person focus on the airway and breathing and perform simple manoeuvres such as jaw thrust and chin lift. They should also check the airway for vomit, blood, dislodged teeth and foreign bodies and can administer suction if required to remove these. As this patient has a low GCS, he may require a guedel airway or a laryngeal mask airway to maintain patency and for adequate oxygen delivery.

6 IV fluids in a trauma situation depends on geographic location but general guidelines include sodium chloride 0.9% or CSL (also known as Hartmann's solution) as they are isotonic.

7 In adults, urine output should be 0.5–1.0ml/kg/hour. In this case, electrical burns cause rhabdomyolysis and the patient's urine may be tinted red from myoglobinuria and so IV fluid administration and urine output aims should be higher to prevent acute kidney injury (AKI).

8 Vital signs are BP, HR, respiratory rate, temperature and oxygen saturation.

9 Clinical response can be an alteration in GCS, urine output, pain worsening or lessening, as well as vital signs.

10 Adequate analgesia may include 'simple analgesia' such as paracetamol or ibuprofen, in addition to opioid analgesia such as morphine.

11 Hypothermia is quick to develop in patients with altered GCS, especially trauma patients whose clothes are removed for adequate assessment.

12 Cardiac monitoring should be standard for all electrical burns that have crossed through the cardiac axis. In this case, the patient has an entry wound from the electrical current on his left hand and an exit wound on his right hand, so he is at high risk of cardiac damage, arrhythmias and death.

13 It is important to understand the capabilities of the hospital and referral criteria to major trauma centres or those with experience in treating electrical burns victims.

14 Fasciotomy is the process of incising the skin down to the fascia (past the subcutaneous fat) in particular lines. It is performed in high voltage electrical injury due to high risk of compartment syndrome in the affected body parts. In this case, fasciotomy may be indicated in both arms and the trunk.

15 These burns take 7–10 days to declare themselves as superficial or deep partial thickness. A superficial partial thickness burn will regenerate the epidermal layer but will take longer to heal than a superficial burn. A deep partial burn will affect the sweat glands and hair follicles and will leave a scar if untreated.

16 This patient should be managed in the ICU or high dependency unit (HDU) in a major tertiary centre which treats electrical burns.

17 Multidisciplinary management may include cardiology for the risk of arrhythmias, ICU or general medicine for rhabdomyolysis and nephrology for AKI secondary to rhabdomyolysis.

18 Haemofiltration may be required due to rhabdomyolysis causing AKI, acute tubular necrosis and prerenal azotemia.

19 Escharotomy is performed where there are circumferential burns that are causing a constriction around the affected region. It is a surgical procedure of making an incision through the skin and dermis down to subcutaneous fat in order to prevent or treat compartment syndrome.

20 Debridement of burns is performed in partial to full thickness burns. Skin grafting is required for full thickness burns but deep dermal burns may be managed with dressings and healing by secondary intention if they are in a small region.

21 Burns dressings are chosen based on the wound's characteristics, such as ooziness, size and depth. This is discussed in further detail in *Case 62*.

22 Limb amputation may be required if there is deep muscle necrosis or sequestration of bone and cartilage from more severe electrical burns.

23 Early intervention with psychological counselling could reduce the rates of depression, anxiety or post-traumatic stress.

24 Neurological issues associated with electrical injury include memory difficulties, peripheral neuropathy, chronic pain, poor concentration, loss of balance or gait ataxia, seizures, dizziness, tremor and tinnitus.

25 Many electrical burns victims struggle with returning to work, possibly because of the traumatic event occurring there or behavioural changes such as anger, frustration or irritability. In the literature, as many as 78% of people who have sustained an electrical injury later developed a psychiatric illness such as post-traumatic stress and depression.

26 Although many of the long-term sequelae of electrical injuries are difficult to treat, the GP can refer the patient to neurologists or chronic pain specialists, or prescribe chronic pain medication. They can also help the patient apply for disability support or industrial injuries compensation.

27 UV light protective techniques should be employed in the first 1–2 years after any burn injury or skin grafting, as this skin is hypersensitive to UV damage and resultant pigmentation and skin cancer formation. UV protection involves wearing factor 50+ sunscreen, protective clothing, a hat and sunglasses, and encouraging the patient to stay in the shade even on cloudy days.

CASE 66: Hand contractures and trigger finger

History

- A **60-year-old** [1] **right hand dominant** [2] **female** [3] **medical receptionist** [4] is referred to the plastic surgery outpatient clinic for management of bilateral hand complaints.
- She states her right little finger has been **getting 'stuck' in flexion episodically** [5] for some years now and she finds it difficult to grasp items.
- She has to **manually release** [6] her finger when it locks, and that process is sometimes painful when it releases.
- Her right hand has a similar issue – **the little and ring finger are stuck in flexion** [7] – she can't pull them out of this position.

- She feels a **thickened cord** [8] in her palm over the tendons of these fingers, but it isn't painful.
- She recalls **her father** [9] has the same thing but never had it treated.
- He lives in his **home country of Ireland** [10].
- She denies **tingling or numbness** [11] in either arm.
- She doesn't smoke but **she drinks a bottle of wine a night** [12] and has done so for 30 years or more.
- She doesn't have any **chronic diseases** [13].
- She has the same sort of thickened feeling in the **arches of her feet** [14], but they don't affect her walking.

[1] Dupuytren's contracture is more prevalent after 50 years of age. Trigger fingers are more prevalent in ages 40–60 years but can occur in children.

[2] Dupuytren's can affect both hands in 80% of affected people but affects the right hand twice as often as the left. Trigger fingers can affect either hand equally, and can affect multiple digits in the one hand. It is also important to establish handedness in any patient with a hand injury or issue, as its function directly affects their livelihood and quality of life.

[3] Men are more likely to develop and have more severe Dupuytren's contractures than women. This has been postulated to be due to expression of androgen receptors in Dupuytren's fascia.

[4] There is an association between manual work and vibration exposure and the development of Dupuytren's contractures.

[5] Trigger fingers are digits that lock or catch during active flexion and extension activities due to thickening of the flexor tendon in the distal palm which interrupts normal smooth gliding through the first annular pulley (A1). The flexor pulleys are ligaments that hold the flexor tendons against the bones of the hand and are numbered A1 to A5 proximal to distal. The A1 pulley overlies the head of the metacarpal bone for each digit. The patient may have fixed flexion deformities in late presentations, particularly at the proximal interphalangeal digit.

[6] Trigger fingers require manual manipulation by the patient or examiners to achieve extension. The patient may feel pain over the distal palm, tenderness over the A1 pulley of the affected finger, or a palpable snapping sensation over the A1 pulley.

[7] The digits affected by Dupuytren's, in order of most to least frequently, are: ring, little, middle, then index finger.

[8] Dupuytren's contracture is a disease of unknown cause but results in abnormal proliferation and differentiation of fibroblastic cells in the fascia with excess production of type III collagen.

[9] Dupuytren's contracture is thought to have a genetic predisposition, but also a number of other risk factors including being male, having an ancestry from northern Europe, heavy alcohol intake, diabetes or being on anti-epileptic medications, age >50, thyroid disease and hypercholesterolaemia. The exact cause of trigger fingers is not known but risk is increased in patients with RA, gout or diabetes.

[10] People of northern European heritage have a higher incidence of Dupuytren's disease.

[11] Around a quarter of affected people have a sensation of tenderness, burning or itching in the affected hand. It is important to differentiate this from a median, ulnar or radial nerve palsy by a neurological examination of the affected upper limb.

12 Heavy alcohol intake increases the risk of Dupuytren's contractures.

13 Some systemic diseases that have higher rates of trigger fingers include RA, gout, psoriatic arthritis, amyloidosis, hypothyroidism and sarcoidosis.

14 Other areas affected by the same process as Dupuytren's are Garrod pads (nodules that develop on the knuckles), Ledderhose disease (thickening of the plantar fascia of the foot) and Peyronie's disease (dartos fascia of the penis thickens, leading to a painful curvature).

Examination

- The patient is a **thin** [1] **Caucasian** [2] female with **light blonde hair and blue eyes** [3].
- Her **right ring and little fingers** [4] have a **fixed flexion deformity at the level of the metocarpophalangeal joints (MCPJ)** [5].
- Along the palmar surface, they have a **thickened feeling** [6] where the flexor tendons run and **nodules** [7] palpable over the MCPJs.
- These nodules have **pitting in the skin** [8] near them.
- Her left little finger locks on flexion but **can be manipulated into full extension** [9] with a slight twinge felt by the patient.

- The patient is unable to perform a **Hueston tabletop test** [10] with her right ring and little finger but the left little finger lies flat.
- She has a strong **pincer grip** [11] with both hands and **no sensory deficit** [12] in the radial, ulnar or median nerve distributions on either hand.
- She does not have **Froment sign** [13] in either hand and can perform all **directions of movement with both thumbs** [14] with no weakness. She is diagnosed with Dupuytren's contracture of the right hand affecting her ring and little fingers, and a left little trigger finger.

1 There is no association between obesity and Dupuytren's or trigger fingers.

2 Dupuytren's contractures affect 4–6% of Caucasians worldwide.

3 These features suggest northern European descent, which have the highest prevalence of Dupuytren's disease.

4 This is in keeping with the most common digits affected by Dupuytren's disease.

5 Palmar fascial thickening in Dupuytren's most commonly forms contractures at the metacarpophalangeal and proximal interphalangeal joints.

6 The thickened feeling in Dupuytren's disease is due to excess collagen III in the palmar fascia. The normal longitudinal components of the superficial palmar aponeurosis are called bands. If diseased, they are referred to as cords.

7 Diagnostic features of Dupuytren's disease include the nodule, the cord and the flexion contracture of the digit. A nodule is a small, rounded lesion fixed to the overlying skin that develops from the superficial fibres of the palms–digital fascia and precede the formation of cords and contractures.

8 Pitting of the skin is due to small vertical fibres (called Grapow fibres) that connect the dermis to the palmar fascia, that are distorted in Dupuytren's disease.

9 Trigger fingers require manual manipulation to achieve full extension as they become stuck in flexion due to the thickened flexor tendon being unable to glide as normal

through the various pulleys. There may also be a palpable nodule distal to the MCPJ along the line of the flexor digitorum superficialis.

10 The Hueston tabletop test involves having the patient lay their palms down flat on a tabletop. If the fingers cannot be laid flat, the test is considered positive for a Dupuytren's contracture.

11 Pincer grip is weak or lost in a low ulnar nerve palsy (at or near the wrist) due to loss of innervation to the deep head of the flexor pollicis brevis, adductor pollicis and the first dorsal interosseous. However, there can be communication between the anterior interosseous branch of the median nerve and the ulnar nerve called the 'Martin–Gruber communication' that will result in retaining some intrinsic muscle motor function in the affected hand. An ulnar nerve palsy can be investigated with nerve conduction studies or an MRI of the arm to find the level of the lesion.

12 Froment sign is when the patient is asked to adduct the thumb and the patient will instead flex the IPJ to compensate for loss of motor to the adductor pollicis.

13 Sensation to the first dorsal webspace is innervated by the superficial branch of the radial nerve. The sensation to the thenar eminence is primarily by the palmar cutaneous branch of the median nerve, and radially by the superficial branch of the radial nerve. The cutaneous branch of the ulnar nerve supplies the palmar side of the little finger and ulnar half of the ring finger and their nailbeds, so the little finger is the region to test for ulnar nerve sensation.

14 Thumb extension is performed by the extensor pollicis longus muscle, which is a test of the posterior interosseous branch of the radial nerve. Opposition, abduction and flexion of the thumb is performed by the median nerve (via the innervation of opponens pollicis, abductor pollicis brevis and flexor pollicis brevis and longus, respectively).

Investigations

- No investigations are needed for Dupuytren's disease or trigger fingers as they are clinical diagnoses.
- Differentials for flexion contractures of the fingers include **abnormal sesamoid bones, loose bodies within the MCPJs, osteoarthritis spurs over the metacarpal head and collateral ligament avulsion fractures** [1].
- This appearance is not in keeping with **ulnar claw** [2].

1 Hand X-ray may be used to look for these issues radiographically.

2 Ulnar claw hand results from compression at the cubital tunnel or in Guyon's canal (in the hand). The resulting defect is that the ring and little finger are hyperextended at the MCPJs and flexed at the proximal and distal IPJs, due to loss of the ulnar nerve innervation to the lumbricals. The difference between this and Dupuytren's disease is that the latter has flexion at the MCPJs.

Management

Immediate

Medications to release the Dupuytren's contractures are not an option. First-line treatment for trigger fingers is non-operative, in the form of **corticosteroid injections** [1]. If the patient does not wish to have either of these performed, a custom-made **thermoplastic splint** [2] can be used to avoid the use of the finger in question.

Short-term

Counsel the patient on non-operative and operative management options. Non-operative options for Dupuytren's contractures include **corticosteroid injections** [3] or **needle aponeurotomy** [4]. Surgical treatment for Dupuytren's includes **fasciotomy** [5] or subtotal **palmar fasciectomy** [6]. Expected postoperative results are pain, swelling and stiffness, which will improve with time. If two corticosteroid injections (**separated by at least 6 weeks** [7]) do not resolve the trigger finger, then offer **surgical release** [8]. Risks and complications of both surgical procedures include pain, scarring, injury to surrounding neurovascular structures (although care is taken to identify and preserve these), **wound infection** [9], **alterations in sensation** [10] and loss of the affected finger(s).

These surgeries are day cases, so postoperative analgesia should be simple, but some patients may require a script for **opioid analgesia** [11]. Postoperative instructions include keeping any **bulky top dressing** [12] clean and dry for at least the first 3–5 days and keeping the **small dressing underneath** [13] intact until suture removal. The patient may be instructed to keep their **affected hand elevated** [14] where possible. They can also start **slow finger exercises** [15] immediately postoperatively but avoid heavy lifting for the first 2–4 weeks to avoid wound breakdown. Suture removal, if non-absorbable, is performed around **10–14 days** [16] postoperatively. **Topical antibiotics** [17] are not usually required unless the patient is at high risk of infections, such as heavy smokers or the immunosuppressed. In Dupuytren's disease, the affected fingers can be **splinted** [18] postoperatively for up to 6 weeks or have **hand therapy** [19].

Long-term

There is no cure for Dupuytren's disease, and it may recur after surgical treatment.

1 Similar to corticosteroid injections for Dupuytren's contractures, a small volume of this is injected into the thickened part of the flexor tendon sheath.

2 A thermoplastic splint in this case can be made, with the affected finger at 10–15° of flexion; this allows the proximal and distal IPJs to remain free but prevents the finger from further flexion and therefore from locking in place.

3 A small volume of corticosteroid is injected into a painful nodule and is thought to slow the progression of the contractures, but this has variable success.

4 Needle aponeurotomy is the process of passing a hypodermic needle in a few regions through the cord to weaken and break apart the thickened tissue.

5 This involves making a volar incision over the thickened cords to divide them. It can be done under local anaesthetic with sedation or general anaesthetic, depending on the patient preference. Closing the wound is with a Z-plasty, and splinting in extension for several weeks postoperatively may be recommended. Recurrence rates are about 20% of patients who have had surgical release. Choice of suture depends on surgeon preference.

6 Subtotal palmar fasciectomy is a more intensive, time-consuming procedure that aims to only resect diseased parts of the fascia, leaving non-diseased portions behind. It requires a larger exposure of the fascia, with more incisions, commonly in a zigzag pattern for better cosmetic outcome. It generally involves more wound care, physical therapy and longer healing time.

7 Corticosteroid injections may take up to 6 weeks to have an effect.

8 Surgical release of a trigger finger involves a volar incision over the A1 pulley. It is then divided under direct vision, either with a tenotomy scissor or a scalpel. Resection of any associated nodules is not recommended as it can weaken the flexor tendon. The wound is usually closed directly with non-absorbable or absorbable sutures (depending on surgeon preference).

9 Postoperative infection and wound breakdown is higher in diabetics, smokers and immunosuppressed patients, whereas bleeding risk is higher in patients on anticoagulation or who have abnormal coagulation (e.g. due to liver disease).

10 After stretching the finger back to neutral, the neurovascular bundle may also be stretched, leading to altered sensation.

11 Simple analgesia includes regular paracetamol and ibuprofen. Opioid analgesia can come in many tablet forms, e.g. tramadol, tapentadol or oxycodone.

12 For hand surgeries, the patient's top dressing may be a soft Velband then crepe, or gauze and crepe.

13 For the inner dressing, waterproof, absorbable padded dressing such as an Opsite or padded Tegaderm can be used.

14 Elevation of the hand aids venous return and reduces wound oedema.

15 For trigger fingers, tendon gliding exercises are recommended several times a day in the first month. For Dupuytren's contractures, hand exercises aim at increasing extension range.

16 Healing time varies on the body, from around 5–7 days on the face, 7 days on the neck, 10 days on the scalp, 10–14 days on the trunk and upper extremities and 14–21 days on the lower limbs. Some regions require less time to heal because of better blood supply and/or less friction or use (i.e. the face is used much less than hands, which are in contact with the environment and clothing).

17 Topical antibiotics such as chloramphenicol (a bacteriostatic antibiotic) are sometimes used on skin wounds for prophylaxis, despite being recommended for ophthalmic and otic treatment only.

18 Static night-time splinting in maximal extension of the digits operated on aims to reduce scar tissue contraction postoperatively whilst avoiding tension on the wound.

19 Hand therapists work to reduce oedema and pain, and give the patient flexion and extension exercises to gain as much function in the operated digit as possible. Scar management techniques include massage and use of vitamin E cream in order to lessen scar thickness and scar contracture and improve appearance.

CASE 67: Hand injuries and digit amputation

History

- A **53-year-old** [1] **right hand dominant** [2] **male** [3] **carpenter** [4] is brought in by his friend to the ED with a bloody rag around his right hand.
- He has sustained **a dog bite** [5] after trying to separate his German shepherd from another dog at the park **one hour ago** [6].
- The bite cut off the **tip of his right index finger** [7], which he is **holding in a plastic bag that is sitting within another bag filled with ice cubes** [8].
- He has **a few other puncture sites on his right thenar eminence** [9].
- The patient states he **smokes fifteen cigarettes a day** [10] and has done so for the past 40 years.

- He **isn't on any anticoagulation** [11] and **isn't taking any medications** [12].
- He states he hardly sees a doctor unless it is life-threatening.
- He **last ate at midday** [13], but he was recently given some water with analgesia in the ED.
- He can't recall the last time he had **a tetanus booster** [14].
- In his spare time, he **plays cricket** [15]; he asks you if he will be able to get back to work tomorrow.

[1] The age distribution of hand injuries peaks in children aged 3–6 years (door-related crush injuries and dog bites), adolescence (closed fractures and deep hand lacerations), and adults aged 45–64 years.

[2] When taking a history of a hand injury, it is important functionally to know the handedness of the patient.

[3] Digit amputations are 4 times more likely in males than in females.

[4] In adults, digit amputation is most commonly secondary to power tools during woodworking and at home in the kitchen or performing DIY projects. In children, digit amputation is often from being caught in a door as it is closing or in a dog bite injury.

[5] Animal and human bites result in infection (including flexor tenosynovitis and septic arthritis), disfigurement and disability. Dog bites to the hand are the most common site in adults, with the incident usually occurring at home or whilst separating two dogs fighting. In children, bites are most often on the face.

[6] Once a finger has been amputated, ischaemic tolerance time is 24 hours if cold, and half that if warm. For more proximal amputations (i.e. at the level of the MCPJ vs. the DIPJ) these times are halved. This is due to more muscle tissue being involved which is less tolerant of ischaemia.

[7] Fingertip and partial digit amputations are more common than complete digit and multiple digit amputations.

[8] To avoid tissue damage from direct contact with ice, the amputated part should be covered in a normal saline-soaked gauze, sealed in a plastic bag and submerged in icy water.

[9] Penetrating injury to the fingers can cause flexor tenosynovitis – an infection caused by *Staphylococcus aureus* most commonly, followed by MRSA and *Pseudomonas* spp. (in immunocompromised patients). This infection affects the flexor tendon sheath of the digit and there are four cardinal signs of it:
- finger held in flexion
- pain with passive extension of the digit
- tenderness along the flexor tendon sheath
- fusiform swelling.

[10] Smoking is associated with surgical site infection, pulmonary complications such as pneumonia and pulmonary embolism, as well as slower wound healing due to a reduced inflammatory response and vasoconstriction mediated by nicotine.

[11] Patients who are on anticoagulant medications may need reversal in the setting of trauma to reduce blood loss. It is important to discuss this with a haematology team, as blood products may be required to reverse certain medications and dose is dependent on the current circulating level of the anticoagulant medication.

[12] When taking a history of any injury, it is important to know the time of the injury, the mechanism, other associated injuries, medications, comorbidities and last meal, to plan for surgery.

13 Optimal fasting times to reduce risk of aspiration during anaesthesia are 6 hours for food and 2 hours for clear fluids.

14 Tetanus can be transmitted from animal or human bites and is a serious and potentially life-threatening illness.

15 In addition to a patient's occupation, it is important in any injury to know how the patient spends their leisure time, as it contributes to their overall quality of life.

Examination

- The patient is observed to be **lying down on the bed** [1] in a patient cubicle.
- He has his amputated index finger beside him, **not touched yet by any medical staff** [2].
- The tip of the index finger **is amputated from the DIPJ (a Zone 1 injury)** [3] and the **thenar eminence and index finger are not oedematous** [4] but bruised.
- The middle finger of the right hand has **a subungual haematoma** [5] but is otherwise intact and there are **puncture marks in the right thenar eminence** [6] that correspond to some on the 1st dorsal web space.

- He has **normal sensation on his thenar eminence, 1st dorsal webspace and palmar surface of the little finger** [7].
- He cannot make a **pincer grip** [8] with his thumb and index finger due to the injury but **can move the thumb in all planes except for flexion** [9].
- He has **full ROM of all other fingers** [10] at their respective joints.
- The amputated index fingertip is **cool but not frozen** [11].

1 It is important to have the patient lying down on a bed rather than in a chair to prevent injury from a vasovagal reaction whilst examining them or inserting cannulas. It is also important to place their injured limb on a sterile surface (the Huck towel) and examine with sterile gloves after the examiner's hands are washed thoroughly to reduce risk of infection.

2 It is imperative that the patient hold their own amputated digit with them, to prevent it being lost or kept in a refrigerator – so long as it is properly packaged in a plastic bag inside a separate bag with ice in it. Ideally, the amputated tip would be wrapped in sterile saline-soaked gauze.

3 Sebastian and Chung classification of finger amputations is a subdivision of the flexor zones of the hand, explained below.
- Zone 1 distal amputations
  - Zone 1A – distal to the lunula (the white crescent at the proximal nail bed) and through the sterile matrix (the most distal part of the nail, above which sits the nail plate)
  - Zone 1B – between the lunula and nail bed
- Zone 1 proximal amputations
  - Zone 1C – between the flexor digitorum profundus (FDP) insertion and neck of the middle phalanx
  - Zone 1D – between the neck of the middle phalanx and insertion of the flexor digitorum superficialis (FDS).

4 It is important to know the fascial planes of the hand where potential spread of infection can occur. Of relevance to this case, the index flexor tendon sheath is in communication with the thenar space.

5 A subungual haematoma is a collection of blood underneath a nail often caused by a crush injury. The pressure of this causes severe pain. If elevation and application of ice does not relieve the pain or pressure, then nail trephination can be performed.

6 The puncture wounds to the thenar eminence is a zone TIII injury which may have affected the flexor pollicis longus tendon or brevis muscle, causing the patient to be unable to flex his thumb. Zones of the flexor tendons of the hand serve as a guide to what structures may be injured. Zone I is most distal – from the fingertip to the insertion of FDS, containing only FDP tendon and associated neurovascular bundles. This zone ends about halfway between the DIPJ and PIPJ. Zone II is from the insertion of FDP to the A1 pulley and therefore contains both the tendons of FDS and FDP. Zone III is the region between the A1 pulley and the distal end of the carpal tunnel and contains the origins of the lumbricals from the FDP tendons, and the superficial and deep palmar arches (the arterial supply to the hand and digits). Zone IV is within the carpal tunnel (which contains the tendons of all four tendons of FDS and FDP and the median nerve and includes the hypothenar eminence) and Zone V is between the entrance of the carpal tunnel and the musculotendinous junction (seen as the volar wrist crease). For the thumb, the zones are T1–TIII (T standing for Thumb), where Zone T1 is from the tip of the finger to the IPJ proximally, Zone TII is from the IPJ to the A1 pulley and Zone TIII is the thenar eminence.

7 Sensation to the first dorsal webspace is innervated by the superficial branch of the radial nerve. The sensation to the thenar eminence is primarily by the palmar cutaneous branch of the median nerve, and radially by the superficial branch of the radial nerve. The cutaneous branch of the ulnar nerve supplies the palmar side of the little finger and ulnar half of the ring finger and their nail beds, so the little finger is the region to test for ulnar nerve sensation.

8 Pincer grip is mediated by the ulnar nerve through the adductor pollicis and the first dorsal interosseous. In this case it is unlikely to be affected unless there were wounds over the wrist, elbow (where the ulnar nerve runs through the cubital tunnel) or hypothenar eminence (where the ulnar nerve travels through Guyon's canal).

9 Testing the different actions of the thumb assesses different muscles – in this case, the flexor pollicis longus tendon or flexor pollicis brevis muscle is likely to be injured.

10 Flexion at the DIPJ is performed by the FDP tendons, whereas flexion at the PIPJ is performed by the FDS tendon. Flexion at the MCPJs is mediated by the interossei and the lumbricals, in addition to the flexor tendons.

11 Frozen tissue cannot be rewarmed as it has died and will no longer be able to be reattached.

Investigations

- Baseline **FBE and UECs** [1] are ordered.
- A **group and hold** [2] is also performed, along with **coagulation studies** [3] which are unremarkable.
- X-rays of the affected hand show an amputation at the level of the distal phalanx of the index finger,

with **associated crush injury to the remaining middle phalanx** [4].

1 An FBE (also called FBC) is to ascertain baseline haemoglobin and assess for acute blood loss. A UEC is to test the patient's renal function and any electrolyte abnormality; in this patient taking no medications, and previously fit and well, it should be normal. A normal creatinine for a healthy adult male is 110μmol/L and 90μmol/L for females. A normal urea in a healthy adult (male and female) ranges from 3.0–8.5mmol/L depending on dietary protein intake.

2 Group and hold is a blood test used to ascertain the patient's blood group in the event they need blood products transfused. In a digit amputation, blood loss may be substantial.

3 Coagulation studies are performed in patients who have a clinical suspicion of a coagulation disorder, such as chronic

alcoholics, patients on anticoagulant agents (e.g. warfarin, rivaroxaban), those with liver disease (e.g. hepatitis B, hepatitis C, liver tumours) or those cannot accurately state what medication they are on (e.g. in the case of an altered GCS or an elderly patient with dementia).

4 Simple X-rays ordered for any limb are AP and lateral views. These X-rays of the affected region are to evaluate associated bony injury and bone quality, and therefore to aid surgical planning. Dog bites usually cause crush injuries of the tissue and bones due to their blunt teeth, whereas cat bites inject bacteria into deep tissue spaces due to their long, sharp teeth.

Management

Immediate

The **Plastics and Reconstructive Surgery** [1] registrar on call should be alerted and relayed the history and examination. Keep the patient **nil by mouth** [2]. **Obtain haemostasis** [3] in the amputated stump with external compression. Insert **a large-bore cannula** [4] into the cubital fossa and after taking the blood tests above, **start IV fluids** [5] for resuscitation and maintenance. Start regular **IV antibiotics** [6], give **tetanus injection** [7] and if the dog's immunisation status is not known, and depending on territory, then a **rabies immunisation** [8] may also be administered. **Perform a**

ring block [9] of the affected finger and **prescribe oral analgesia** [10]. If the subungual haematoma in his middle finger becomes painful, then **nail trephination** [11] should be performed. The patient is recommended to **cease smoking** [12]. The Plastic and Reconstructive Surgery team will consent him **for surgery** [13]. The digit may require **K-wiring** [14] but due to the nature of the injury, it is more likely he will have the **digit terminalised** [15]. The patient should be made aware that the digit and his remaining index finger will be inspected in the operating theatre and **may not be amenable to replantation** [16].

Short-term

After surgery, the patient would be continued on IV antibiotics for **at least 24 hours** [17]. If the amputated digit was replanted, it would be on **vascular obs** [18] in order to closely monitor its blood supply and healing. **Range of motion exercises** [19] for the injured digits would depend on whether any tendons were repaired. Short-term complications of a replanted digit include infection, haematoma, poor wound healing, **arterial or venous congestion** [20] requiring return to surgery, and loss of viability of the amputated part. The wounds on this patient's thenar eminence **may need multiple washouts** [21] before definitive closure or **healing by secondary intention** [22]. The digit itself, if not replanted, **may be closed with a flap** [23] of skin or surrounding tissue and may also need multiple washouts before definitive closure and recovery can fully begin. The patient should be **on preventive anticoagulation** [24]. The recovery of this patient requires **skilled nursing staff** [25] who are familiar with amputated and replanted digits or flaps, as well as **hand and occupational therapists** [26] to facilitate early recovery and engagement of the patient. Remember to always offer **counsel with a psychology team** [27] in any injury or amputation; grieving for the amputated part, anger or shock at the event and subsequent surgery, anxiety or post-traumatic stress can all occur in this setting.

Long-term

Follow-up after wound healing involves **intensive hand therapy** [28]. Long-term complications of a replantation are stiffness, bony malunion, abnormal nail growth, altered sensation, neuroma formation and cold intolerance. If the digit was terminalised, the patient can develop neuropathic pain (associated with neuroma formation) or phantom sensations. Long-term complications of a tendon repair are contractures and stiffness (issues with smooth tendon gliding due to scar tissue).

1 Depending on the hospital, hand injuries will be admitted under the Orthopaedics or Plastic Surgery team.

2 This patient needs surgery and therefore must be kept fasted until a definitive timing for surgery can be ascertained by the appropriate surgical team.

3 Haemostasis of the amputated part should not be obtained by clamping vessels, as it will cause additional damage.

4 Inserting a large-bore cannula (18 gauge or larger) is necessary to administer IV fluids rapidly, should they be needed for haemodynamic stability.

5 If the patient is haemodynamically unstable or hypotensive secondary to blood loss, give isotonic crystalloid fluid intravenously and rapidly, such as sodium chloride 0.9%, CSL (otherwise known as Hartmann's), or what is appropriate to the hospital protocol.

6 Intravenous antibiotic combinations should cover for *Staphylococcus*, *Streptococcus*, anaerobes and *Pasteurella* spp. Choice is dependent on the geographic location of the hospital and the availability of the antibiotic, such as:
- ampicillin + sulbactam
- ticarcillin + clavulanate
- piperacillin + tazobactam
- carbapenems (meropenem, imipenem, ertapenem).

7 Dog bites can lead to tetanus in addition to the many bacteria inoculated from the dog's oral cavity. As tetanus is a life-threatening, easily preventable illness, it is vital to ascertain the patient's tetanus status and give a booster if the last dose was more than 10 years ago or if the patient is unsure of their last dose.

8 Rabies is a virus that is transmitted by the saliva of various animals, historically via domestic dogs. This virus attacks the CNS and causes paralysis, encephalitis, coma and death.

9 A ring block is the name of the procedure where local anaesthetic is used to block nerves of the digit and there are several techniques to do this.

10 Oral analgesia should begin with simple analgesia such as paracetamol and NSAIDs, followed by opioids or opioid-like analgesics if required. If pain still cannot be controlled with oral options, the Acute Pain Service or equivalent should be consulted to consider IV alternatives.

11 Nail trephination is performed in the case of a subungual haematoma. It involves using a sterile large-bore needle (or in remote areas, a sterilised sewing needle or paperclip can be used) to burrow into the nail at 90° to the nail plate, over where the haematoma lies.

12 Some contraindications to reimplantation include smoking status (as this increases wound complications including dehiscence, infection and tissue necrosis, and prolongs wound healing time), severe crushing injury, heavy contamination (with animal or human bites, or debris such as car shrapnel from a motor vehicle accident), prolonged warm ischaemic time (i.e. the amputated part was not preserved properly), the patient being medically unfit for the procedure, multiple level injuries in the same digit, previous surgery to the affected finger, frozen amputated part or prolonged normothermic ischaemia time. In the operating theatre, signs of severe damage to the neurovascular bundle and prediction of unsuccessful replantation include the 'ribbon sign' where the artery to the amputated digit is twisted. This is a sign of significant avulsion injury to the vessel.

13 Surgery would involve a washout of the dog bites +/– exploration of the wounds +/– repair of any injured tendons +/– replant of the amputated tip +/– K-wiring +/– terminalisation of the index finger. Replantation of an amputated part of the body is time-sensitive and therefore the operating theatre and relevant surgical teams should be organised urgently. Clean fingertip amputations (e.g. from a power tool) are usually replanted. Dirty wounds (i.e. from multitrauma or animal bites) may not be replanted depending on the viability of the amputated part. In contrast to adults, fingertip amputations in children generally do very well, even with concurrent bony injury, due to their rapid healing. Often, they are not surgically treated, but closely monitored by the surgical team in an outpatient setting with regular dressing changes.

14 Fixation of the bony structures of the amputated part to its previous alignment and articulations involves Kirschner wiring (known more commonly as K-wiring). These are malleable thin rods of metal with sharp ends that are inserted via power drill and can be easily removed. Their advantage in replant injury is that they can be easily removed if infection occurs, whereas fixation with plates or screws can easily become a nidus of infection and subsequent formation of osteomyelitis. Fixation of the replanted digit may require shortening osteotomies to cleanly align the two parts.

15 In some cases, the patient might choose to have the digit terminalised rather than replanted for various reasons – not wanting to go through the risks of the surgery or anaesthetic, unwillingness to engage with hand therapy postoperatively, or to return to work sooner (e.g. a self-employed handyman). The patient should be counselled on both treatment options.

16 The final decision to replant an amputated part of the hand, digit or limb in major trauma should be made in the operating theatre. This is because the stump and amputated parts can be inspected and explored in this environment under the microscope.

17 IV antibiotics are recommended prophylactically for animal and human bites. These are most beneficial if initiated within 12–24 hours after injury and are commonly continued for 3–5 days post injury. Dog bites commonly isolate anaerobic bacteria (specifically *Fusobacterium*, *Prevotella*, *Bacteroides* and *Peptostreptococcus* spp.), Gram-positive bacteria (*Streptococcus* and *Staphylococcus* spp.) and Gram-negative bacteria (*Pasteurella canis* being the most common). An important bacterium from dog bites that causes sepsis, gangrene, meningitis and endocarditis, particularly in children with immunodeficiency, is *Capnocytophaga*

canimorsus. Cat bites commonly isolate *Pasteurella multocida* (aerobic Gram-negative), *Streptococcus* and *Staphylococcus* (aerobic Gram-positive) and anaerobic organisms (*Fusobacterium*, *Porphyromonas*, *Bacteroides*, *Prevotella* and *Propionibacterium*). Human bites commonly isolate aerobic Gram-negative *Eikenella corrodens* and Gram-positive bacteria (*Staphylococcus*, *Streptococcus* and *Corynebacterium* spp.).

18 Vascular observations include capillary refill, colour and temperature of the affected part – in this case, the digit. In some circumstances, it includes the presence of a Doppler arterial signal – measured with a bedside Doppler ultrasound probe – such as in the case of breast reconstruction.

19 ROM exercises are important immediately postoperatively for the unaffected fingers. In the replanted digit, ROM may not be recommended for the first few weeks in order to allow the wound edges, bone and neurovasculature to heal. After such time, exercise programmes for mobilising the digit at the various joints are important to regain function and are taught to patients by hand therapists.

20 Arterial insufficiency and venous congestion present differently – the first typically presents as a pale, cool, pulseless digit, whereas the latter presents as a purple or blue digit with brisk capillary refill but which is swollen. Both can be due to anastomosis failure or thrombosis. Complications of a wound washout are similar but as the vessels are not involved, they do not have the risk of arterial or venous congestion.

21 Any dirty wound, including those caused by human or animal bites, is immediately infected with various bacteria, and may need multiple washouts and debridement procedures to allow the infection to drain in order to heal. The likelihood of a cat bite becoming infected, for example, is double that of a dog bite.

22 Healing by secondary intention means to leave the wound open and allow it to heal on its own.

23 Flaps used for tissue arrangement over the amputated stump are volar or bilateral V–Y advancement flaps, homodigital island flaps and fillet flaps. 'Dog ears' should be left to eliminate tension and prevent compromising the blood supply to the flap. These will either disappear over time or be revised once the flap has healed.

24 Anticoagulation is not solely for the prevention of DVT or PE, but to prevent clotting within the anastomosed vessels of the newly replanted digit.

25 Skilled nursing staff are vital as they are the front line to realise the complications and alert the surgeon and obviously are the primary carers of the patient after surgery. Of note to this case, wound dressing changes are usually not performed in the first 48–72 hours of the replant, in order to prevent damage to the anastomotic repair.

26 If flexor tendons were injured and repaired, extension past neutral is not recommended, to allow the flexor tendons to heal. A dorsal blocking plaster or thermoplastic splint can aid to comply with this restriction, which is made by a hand therapist.

27 Any trauma situation, let alone amputation of a digit, may leave the patient with fear, anger, guilt, depression or post-traumatic stress. Offering psychological counselling early is important to support return to work and daily activities that improve quality of life.

28 This may include heat and massage and desensitisation of the affected region as well as ROM exercises to regain prior function. Full recovery to premorbid function is dependent on the patient – they should be made aware of this, but also that their sensation in this replanted digit may not return to its premorbid state.

CASE 68: Pressure ulcers

History

- An **80-year-old** [1] **obese** [2] female has **been an inpatient in hospital for many weeks** [3] after a fall.
- The plastic and reconstructive surgery team is consulted to see her because of a **sacral pressure ulcer** [4] that has not been improving with **conventional padded dressings** [5].
- She was a pack-a-day **smoker** [6] for 60 years, having quit when she was placed in a nursing home with **dementia** [7].
- Her BMI is 47 and she has known **peripheral vascular disease** [8] with **a stent in her right femoral artery** [9].

- The patient also has **T2DM on insulin** [10] with **peripheral neuropathy and moderate renal impairment** [11] and **emphysema** [12].
- She is **allergic to penicillin** [13], which gives her a rash.
- She is **doubly incontinent** [14], wearing nappies, is **mostly bed-bound** [15] due to her obesity and general deconditioning, and requires hoist transfer to the chair.
- Her nursing notes state her **Braden Scale score** [16] was 13.

[1] Pressure ulcers are most common in those aged 60–80 years.

[2] Obesity is one of the risk factors for pressure ulcers due to immobility and occluding blood flow when seated or lying down.

[3] Deconditioning (sarcopenia) occurs when patients are unwell, bed-bound, or have limited mobility for a period of time – in the elderly, this can be just 2 days!

[4] Pressure ulcers/sores develop from a combination of localised ischaemia and reperfusion injury to the tissue involved and impaired lymphatic drainage. They occur over bony prominences that are more likely to compress tissues when the patient is in extended contact with hard surfaces, such as the sacrum, elbows, ischium, scapula or the heels.

[5] There are particular padded foam dressings with adhesive edges that are designed to protect such pressure points as the sacrum and heels (e.g. Mepilex Border Sacrum and ALLEVYN Heel).

[6] Patient risk factors for the development of pressure ulcers include increasing age (ageing skin has decreased elasticity, cutaneous blood flow and subcutaneous fat), diabetes, smoking, malnutrition, immunosuppression, congestive cardiac failure, vascular disease, contractures, limited mobility and poor skin hygiene. Environmental risk factors include lying on hard surfaces, being in a nursing home, poorly fitting limb prostheses and physical restraints.

[7] Patients with dementia are particularly at risk for pressure ulcers because they are unable to ask the carer to move them, they don't remember how long they have been in a particular

position for or when they last walked around, and they can have incontinence due to anatomical or memory-related issues.

[8] Peripheral vascular disease is associated with ischaemic ulcers on the legs and heels, but this also reflects the patient's overall atherosclerosis and therefore their skin is generally at higher risk of ischaemia.

[9] Placing a metal stent or opening a narrowed vessel by percutaneous transluminal angioplasty (PTA) is the treatment for a blocked or narrowed vessel secondary to atherosclerosis. This aims to prevent downstream ischaemia of the affected limb.

[10] Diabetic peripheral neuropathy also contributes to pressure ulcer development, as they cannot feel when an injurious source comes into contact with their feet or hands, and this insensate region may progress up the legs.

[11] Diabetes causes micro- and macrovascular complications. Microvascular complications include retinopathy, nephropathy, autonomic neuropathy and peripheral neuropathy. Macrovascular complications include cardiovascular disease, cerebrovascular disease and peripheral vascular disease (mediated by atherosclerosis and autonomic neuropathy).

[12] In addition to severe obesity, this patient's multiple medical comorbidities are significant and may mean she is at too high a risk of peri-operative and anaesthetic complications to justify surgical intervention.

[13] Penicillin allergies are common, but not all are life-threatening. It is worth clarifying and considering penicillin

desensitisation in future and ask if the patient has had cephalosporins before and if they tolerated them well.

14 Incontinence increases the risk of pressure ulcers as it leads to moist skin.

15 Being bed- or wheelchair-bound or having poor mobility all increase the risk of pressure ulcers due to prolonged ischaemia and reperfusion injury to the tissues (e.g. the sacrum and the heels).

16 The Braden Scale is a way to measure pressure ulcer risk based on sensory perception of the patient, moisture of their skin, activity level, mobility, nutrition level and if they have issues with friction and shearing such as in bedsheets or clothing. Each section has a score from 1–4, where 1 is the worst outcome. A score of 15–18 is a mild risk of pressure ulcers, 13–14 is moderate risk, 10–12 is high risk, and ≤9 is very high risk.

Examination

- The patient is **afebrile and has been haemodynamically stable** [1] for several days.
- She has a 5 x 4cm pressure ulcer on her sacral region with a **depth** [2] of about 3cm.
- The skin around it is **voluminous and mobile** [3].
- When **probing the wound** [4], bone is felt underneath the layer of slough and debris.

- The overlying skin is necrotic, ulcerated in some regions, **sloughy** [5] in others and has **no capillary refill** [6] in the centre.
- It is **malodorous and highly exudative** [7] but there is no pus extruding.
- This is diagnosed as a **stage IV to unstageable** [8] sacral pressure ulcer.

1 It is important to note whether the patient is haemodynamically stable. Findings otherwise may indicate shock, and a fever may also indicate whether infection is more likely in the wound.

2 Measurement of an ulcer should be length (from head to toe at its longest point), width (from edge to edge at the widest point, perpendicular to length) and depth (perpendicular to the patient's skin to the base at the deepest point).

3 Mobility of skin is an observation of elasticity – if the wound requires surgical debridement and closure, it is an observation of whether the wound could be primarily closed or would require grafting or a flap.

4 Probing into a wound is performed with a linear metal, dull-ended object that is used to assess depth and whether bone can be felt through the wound bed. Feeling bone under a probe suggests a high risk of osteomyelitis.

5 Slough is dead tissue, macrophages and other inflammatory immune cells on top of a wound.

6 Assessing capillary refill is important to ascertain blood flow to the ulcerated region. No capillary blood flow means

the wound is deeper and has poor or absent vascular supply to the wound bed. This has a poor prognosis for wound healing and survival.

7 A malodorous wound may be from the surrounding incontinence or secondary to the necrotic tissue. A wound with high exudate does not necessarily imply infection.

8 The staging system for pressure ulcers has been made by the National Pressure Ulcer Advisory Panel (NPUAP), from stage I to unstageable.
- Stage I – intact skin with non-blanchable redness of a localised area, usually over a bony prominence.
- Stage II – partial thickness loss of the dermis presenting as a shallow, open ulcer with a pink–red wound bed, without slough. Can also appear as an intact or open or ruptured serum-filled blister.
- Stage III – full-thickness tissue loss. Subcutaneous fat may be visible but not bone, tendon or muscle. Slough may or may not be present.
- Stage IV – full-thickness tissue loss with exposed bone, tendon or muscle. May have slough or eschar on some wound beds, often with undermining and tunnelling.
- Unstageable – full-thickness tissue loss with the base of the ulcer covered by slough or eschar.

Investigations

- No blood tests are usually required in pressure ulcer care; however, consider **FBE** [1], **UEC** [2], **CMP** [3], **ESR** [4], and **albumin** [5] level.
- As she is a diabetic, the most **recent HbA1c** [6] would be helpful to monitor her diabetic control

as this will markedly affect wound healing and susceptibility to infection, sepsis and opportunistic pathogens such as *Pseudomonas*.
- An **MRI** [7] scan of the sacrum is ordered and is equivocal for osteomyelitis.

1 The WCC may be elevated due to the chronic inflammatory response to the pressure ulcer or due to an infection within the ulcer bed. It could also be normal or low in elderly patients even in the setting of infection, as they often do not mount an appropriate response.

2 In this setting, chronic renal impairment may be evident from her diabetes. Some studies also suggest hyponatraemia as a risk factor for pressure ulcer development.

3 CMP stands for calcium, magnesium and phosphate. These electrolytes are important in wound healing.

4 The erythrocyte sedimentation rate is used to ascertain chronic inflammation.

5 Albumin, a protein within the blood, is a marker of nutritional status over a month and should be at least 35g/L to aid wound healing.

6 An HbA1c is a blood test for glucose saturation of haemoglobin (glycated haemoglobin) roughly over the last 120 days (the lifespan of the red blood cell) and is used as a marker of diabetic control. Optimal HbA1c (known as the 'target' HbA1c) is <7.0% and higher levels increase the risk of micro- and macrovascular complications of diabetes. This is measured every 3 months if targets are not met or if there is a change in therapy, and every 6 months if the HbA1c target is being met.

7 An MRI scan can observe sinus tracts or tunnelling of the wound to the underlying bone, any abscesses or drainable fluid collections. It can also identify granulation tissue and osteomyelitis, but sometimes cannot differentiate osteomyelitis from bone remodelling.

Management

Immediate

The nursing staff are advised to perform **positional changes** [1] every 2 hours and avoid the patient lying flat (supine) as much as possible, to allow the region to heal. Non-operative management is used initially, with **enzymatic debridement** [2] dressings changed twice a day. Toileting measures including **more frequent pad changing** [3] and **sitting out of bed and mobilising** [4] should also be employed to reduce infection as well as a **pressure-reducing hospital mattress** [5]. An Endocrinology consult is requested for **controlling her diabetes** [6] and supporting **weight loss** [7]. The patient and **her next of kin** [8] are advised that it is largely up to her diabetic control, her mobility and her vascular supply to that region that will help her to heal, but it will take months if not years.

Short-term

To confirm the diagnosis of osteomyelitis, a bone biopsy of the affected region is taken to **examine histopathologically** [9]. As the MRI is equivocal, **IV**

antibiotics [10] are not recommended unless the patient is febrile. **Surgical debridement** [11] is performed when conservative management fails but **reconstructive options** [12] are not performed due to the high risk of failure.

Long-term

A multidisciplinary approach to this patient is utilised, including a nutritionist or dietitian to aid both diabetic control and combat malnutrition. **Nursing staff** [13] educated on pressure ulcer prevention liaise with the nursing home and patient's family on how to prevent further ulcerations. **Foam wedges and pressure-reducing cushions** [14] and pillows are used for prevention of pressure ulcers in other areas. The patient's family or next of kin are informed of the pressure ulcer and the **plan of treatment and prevention** [15].

1 Hallmarks of prevention and treatment for pressure ulcerations are keeping the wound clean and well perfused. This may involve position changes (every 2 hours) in a bed-bound patient to rotate the sides that are compressed on the bedside. In surgery predicted to last >4 hours, patients should have gel pads in areas at risk of pressure ulceration.

2 Various forms of debridement techniques exist. Enzymatic debridement uses chemical agents to break down necrotic tissue or eschar. Issues with this include high cost, secondary dressings may be required to absorb exudate, the patient may experience a burning sensation or increased wound pain, and care must be taken with application so that healthy tissue is not in contact with the enzymatic dressing. If this patient had a less exudative wound or a stage II–III ulcer, autolytic debridement can be used. This does not damage healthy skin and takes a long time (days to weeks) to take effect. The process involves using transparent films, hydrogels or hydrocolloids to keep wound fluids in direct contact with the wound to promote debridement. However, the wound can become infected as anaerobic bacteria can grow under the occlusive dressing.

3 A Cochrane review showed there was insufficient evidence to suggest a relationship between nutrition and pressure ulcer prevention; however, a dietitian consultation and the use of skin moisturisers may be considered.

4 Positional change also includes sitting out of bed and mobilising.

5 Pressure-reducing hospital mattresses can be air or gel mattresses that reduce pressure over the body and can be dynamic, that alternate pressure.

6 Diabetic control is crucial to wound healing due to micro- and macrovascular complications caused by hyperglycaemia that prevent ulcers from healing as quickly as in patients without diabetes.

7 Weight loss may be difficult in this patient as she is not only diabetic but morbidly obese, has dementia and is in a nursing home – encouraging exercise and a nutritional low-calorie diet will likely be difficult.

8 Discussion with the patient and their family is vital to any management plan as the family can support and encourage the patient along the treatment regimen. It is important in patients who have intellectual disability or memory issues to relay the plan to their carers and next of kin, as well as documenting it.

9 Osteomyelitis is infection of the bone. Due to the chronic wound breakdown, poor vascular supply to the region and slough, an MRI of the region may misdiagnose osteomyelitis.

10 This is a contentious issue – whether Stage IV sacral pressure ulcers should be treated with IV antibiotics because of the high risk of osteomyelitis. The decision should be made in discussion with the plastic surgeon or general medicine physician who is overseeing the care of the patient. Organisms cultured in osteomyelitis are most commonly *Staphylococcus aureus*, coagulase-negative staphylococci, aerobic Gram-negative bacteria, and anaerobes.

11 Surgical debridement may be required if enzymatic or autolytic debridement is not adequate to remove the slough. In most cases of deep pressure ulcers, as in this case, conservative management is often the choice as these wounds take months if not years to heal, and surgical debridement carries anaesthetic risks, pain and bleeding.

12 Reconstructive options are reserved for younger patients with more mobility, better nutrition and a higher chance of success. This can be a flap from the buttock to close the wound, either as a skin flap or with a myocutaneous gluteus maximus flap.

13 Skilled nursing staff are vital in preventing and treating pressure ulcers. They should be performing wound assessments and Braden scores at least once a week.

14 Measures to manage and prevent pressure areas include repositioning every few hours even if in a chair, using pillows or a soft wedge to offload the weight on the heels when in bed, and using pillows between legs when lying on the side. Emollients (moisture creams) for the skin, washing the patient with non-drying products and ensuring adequate hydration or nutrition also help prevent pressure ulcers.

15 Although the treatment and prevention plan are important to discuss with next of kin and carers, nearly 70% of patients with a pressure ulcer die within 6 months.

CASE 69: The purple spot

History

- A **3-month-old** [1] **Caucasian** [2] **girl** [3] is brought to the plastic surgery outpatients by her mother, having been referred by their GP for a **rapidly enlarging blueish mass on her face** [4]. The mother is visibly distressed, worried about what her child has and asks you if it is cancer and if she will be 'scarred for the rest of her life' if you remove it.
- Apart from the mother being **40 years old** [5], the pregnancy was uncomplicated, but the child was born at **34 weeks** [6] from early rupture of membranes by vaginal delivery but she is **meeting developmental milestones** [7] in adequate time.
- This lesion was **not present at birth** [8].

- On prompting, the mother tells you she started snoring at night in the last few months and sometimes **'stops breathing for a few seconds'** [9] before snoring again.
- She hasn't shown any **difficulty in feeding or swallowing** [10] and has had **no change in activity** [11] since the lesion has grown.
- The mother has two other children, aged 4 and 10 years, who are at home with her husband and **do not have any skin lesions like this** [12].

[1] Infantile deep haemangiomas (historically called 'cavernous') become apparent at 2–3 months old with a subcutaneous swelling that has a blue hue to it. These involve the deep dermis and subcutaneous tissue. Superficial lesions become apparent weeks after birth, presenting as an elevated, bright red papule or plaque (these used to be called 'strawberry' or 'capillary' lesions). These only involve the superficial dermis. There can be mixed or combined lesions composed of both superficial and deep components.

[2] Caucasians have a higher incidence of haemangiomas than other populations.

[3] Females are more likely to have haemangiomas than males.

[4] Infantile haemangiomas are the most common vascular mass in infants and children and become clinically apparent within the first few days to months of life. They are benign vascular neoplasms formed from endothelial cells and have a characteristic life cycle of rapid proliferation, then regression, but size and duration of existence are variable.

[5] Minor risk factors to development of haemangiomas include:
- a child of multiple gestation pregnancy
- advanced maternal age at pregnancy
- infants born via *in vitro* fertilisation (IVF)
- first-born infants
- complications in pregnancy, e.g. pre-eclampsia, breech presentation or placenta praevia.

[6] Infantile haemangiomas are more common in premature infants.

[7] Developmental milestones are a way to ascertain if the child has any concomitant organ anomalies that are affecting motor or speech development or growth.

[8] Infantile haemangiomas are not present at birth. However, in 50% of cases, premonitory marks are visible at birth. These include a pale macule, fine telangiectasia or a subtle ecchymotic patch. Haemangiomas that are present at birth are called congenital haemangiomas and are fully grown at this time. They are subtyped into rapidly involuting or non-involuting congenital haemangiomas (RICH and NICH, respectively).

[9] Snoring and cessation of breathing is concerning for obstruction and sleep apnoea.

[10] Difficulty feeding and swallowing can be a symptom of complicated facial or airway haemangiomas.

[11] Change in activity may be due to airway compromise or a systemic cause. Hepatic haemangiomas, for example, can cause high-output cardiac failure, whereas malignant lesions may cause anaemia, fatigue and failure to thrive.

[12] Most cases of haemangiomas are sporadic – there are no definitive familial inheritance patterns.

Examination

- The child looks happy and well. She is playing on her mother's lap with a toy and there is **no evidence of stridor or tachypnoea** [1].
- There is **one well-defined blue-hued swelling of skin** [2] [3] over her right cheek that **encroaches on her nasal bridge and right naris** [4]. It measures about 2cm in width, 2cm in length and around 3cm in height from her surrounding cheek.
- It does **not approach her eyes** [5].
- It is **firm** [6] and **non-tender** [7].
- There is **no crusting or bruising** [7] around the lesion and the skin overlying it **looks otherwise healthy** [8].

- The child weighs **6kg and has a height of 60cm** [9].
- Her **red reflex is normal** [10], she **does not have any other haemangiomatous lesions** [11] or **skin tags, naevi, lipomas or hair tufts** [12].
- On a **cardiovascular examination** [13], she does not have any murmurs nor is she tachycardic, and she has a regular strong radial pulse with no **radio-femoral delay** [14].
- Her **abdomen is soft and non-tender** [15], she has a **perforate anus** [16] and no clinical signs of **hip dysplasia** [17].

[1] Stridor, tachypnoea or hoarseness present evidence of airway obstruction.

[2] Blue-hued swellings with a normal thickness of skin overlying are deep haemangiomas. The differential here is a tufted angioma, which are erythematous or purple patches, plaques or nodules, that grow more slowly than haemangiomas and are often found over the neck or upper throat. They can be differentiated from haemangiomas in that they often have excess hair growth (called hypertrichosis) and form across all paediatric ages. Tufted angiomas without Kasabach–Merritt syndrome that are small can be left alone. Those that are larger may be treated by oral aspirin, laser therapy (the same type used for port wine stains), immunosuppressive agents or surgical excision. Another differential is a venous malformation, but these are compressible and soft, and may increase in volume with increased venous pressure (e.g. in exercise or Valsalva). In venous malformations, sclerotherapy, endovenous laser therapy or venous embolisation with or without resection is the mainstay of treatment.

[3] Localised haemangiomas are well-defined and contained in one region, appearing to grow from a single focus. These account for around 80% of infantile haemangiomas and are most commonly located on the head and neck, followed by the trunk. Segmental haemangiomas are elevated and plaque-like, and seem to form over a specific cutaneous region; they are most commonly found on the face. These are often more difficult to treat and are more likely to ulcerate with inevitable scarring. They are separated into 4 discrete zones:
- zone 1 = frontotemporal
- zone 2 = maxillary
- zone 3 = mandibular
- zone 4 = frontonasal.

[4] This location may result in airway obstruction and may conceal an internal nasal haemangioma. This lesion location is also at high risk of cosmetic disfigurement.

[5] Lesions that encroach around the periorbital region require urgent referral to an ophthalmologist as they can incur serious visual complications (e.g. amblyopia, ptosis, displacement of the globe).

[6] Indurated, warm lesions can be kaposiform haemangioendotheliomas. Compressible, bluish discoloured lesions can be a venous malformation. Firm lesions that are fixed to surrounding structures with or without systemic signs of illness (weight loss, failure to thrive, petechiae or anaemia) are suspicious of malignant tumours such as rhabdomyosarcomas, but these rarely look like haemangiomas at presentation.

[7] Urgent consultation with a paediatric dermatologist, plastic surgeon or specialty surgeon (ENT or ophthalmologist) are for haemangiomas that are painful, may cause functional impairment or disfigurement (i.e. those around the periocular or periauricular region, on the nasal tip or genitalia), are ulcerated or have systemic involvement (e.g. hepatic haemangiomas or cardiac anomalies).

[8] This is looking for ulceration, which is the most common complication of haemangiomas. It most commonly occurs when the lesion is rapidly proliferating and is located in pressure- or trauma-prone locations. An early white discolouration of the surface can herald ulceration.

[9] The aforementioned height and weight measurements are both within the 50–75th percentile for a 3-year-old female.

[10] A normal 'red reflex' means the child does not have a cataract or retinoblastoma. Checking for ophthalmic anomalies from a clinical syndrome or from encroachment of the haemangioma is critical. One such clinical syndrome is called PHACES and is most common in infant females with

large segmental haemangiomas in the head and neck region. It stands for:

- **P**osterior fossa brain malformations (present in 90% of children with this condition, most commonly cerebellar hypoplasia)
- **H**aemangiomas on the face
- **A**rterial anomalies (8% of children with PHACES will have a stroke in infancy)
- **C**ardiac anomalies (e.g. coarctation of the aorta)
- **E**ye abnormalities (e.g. optic nerve hypoplasia, cataracts)
- **S**ternal malformations.

Eye examination in an infant includes measuring the pupil, testing pupillary response with a pen torch, and their ability to focus on and follow a toy or object (which tests visual acuity).

11 Children with multifocal lesions can have clinical syndromes. For instance, those with low lumbar segmental lesions should be screened for LUMBAR syndrome (**L**ower body haemangioma or other cutaneous defects, **U**rogenital anomalies or ulceration, **M**yelopathy, **B**ony deformities, **A**norectal malformations/arterial anomalies and **R**enal anomalies). These children can have occult spinal and urogenital lesions.

12 Hair tufts, lipomas, skin tags and naevi can be found in children with LUMBAR syndrome.

13 A cardiovascular examination is important in any child with haemangioma as they can have cardiac anomalies (such as coarctation of the aorta) and hepatic haemangiomas that result in high-output cardiac failure.

14 Radio-femoral delay is suggestive of coarctation of the aorta.

15 This is to feel for hepatomegaly and abdominal compartment syndrome caused by hepatic haemangiomas. Other abnormalities within the abdomen that are associated with LUMBAR syndrome cannot be felt (single kidney, pelvic kidney, hydronephrosis or a hypoplastic kidney) and will instead need visualisation via ultrasound.

16 Imperforate anus or rectal fistulae are associated with LUMBAR syndrome.

17 Hip dysplasia, foot deformities and scoliosis are bony deformities found in LUMBAR syndrome. Screening for developmental dysplasia of the hip involves the Ortolani test and Barlow manoeuvre. The first test is performed to promote dislocation, whilst the second aims to reduce a posteriorly dislocated hip.

Investigations

- This is an infantile haemangioma and investigations are rarely required. This child's lesion extends over the airway and thus warrants an **ultrasound** [1].
- In this case, perform a **screening X-ray of the airway** [2] [3] whilst in the outpatient department as they are high risk for airway obstruction.
- She does not have 5 or more haemangiomas so does not require a **liver ultrasound** [4].
- She should be discussed with an ENT surgeon to arrange a **screening bronchoscopy** [5] to investigate for **airway haemangioma** [6].
- **Biopsy** [7] of the lesion is rarely indicated.

[1] Ultrasound is preferred for initial diagnosis than MRI as it is a quicker test and does not require sedation (which MRI may require as the nature of the test places the patient in a very loud, round tubular structure and takes around an hour or more to complete).

[2] Indications for imaging include:
- suspicion of organ involvement or associated anomalies (e.g. in patients with 5 or more cutaneous haemangiomas or who have a beard-like distribution)
- to define the extent or depth of the lesion (e.g. in periocular haemangiomas)
- to assess treatment efficacy (usually in deep lesions)
- to exclude alternative diagnoses for the lesion
- to plan for surgical excision.

[3] More specifically, this is known as a high-kilovolt plain neck X-ray, used to diagnose subglottic haemangiomas.

[4] Up to 15% of infants with 5 or more cutaneous haemangiomas also have hepatic haemangioma(s). If there are diffuse or multifocal hepatic haemangiomas, there is a risk of consumptive hypothyroidism and therefore thyroid function should be tested.

[5] Screening bronchoscopy is the preferred modality to directly visualise the airway.

[6] Airway haemangiomas are more common in haemangiomas that have beard-like distribution.

[7] Biopsy of a haemangioma will cause bleeding that may be difficult to control and will not aid diagnosis for this lesion. It is only performed in lesions where diagnosis is unclear; in those that are firm, have an unusual appearance or are found to have radiological features of concern.

Management

Immediate

Ensure the lesion is not causing **airway obstruction** [1] and **assess vision** [2]. Refer this patient urgently to an **ENT surgeon** [3]. Consider further referral to an **ophthalmologist** [4] if the lesion extends to the periorbital region. This lesion **may enlarge further** [5] but will eventually slow down over mid to late infancy and will **spontaneously shrink** [6] in size from age 1–4 years. Some children may not have full regression until age 10, but after this there will not be any further changes to the skin, and it will not recur.

Short-term

Continue regular follow-up with **serial photographs** [7] and **intensive observation** [8]. Non-surgical treatment includes **systemic propranolol** [9], **systemic corticosteroids** [10], **phototherapy** [11], **topical beta blockers** [12], **topical corticosteroid** [13] or intralesional **injections of corticosteroid** [14]. Specific **wound care** [15] is indicated if this lesion ulcerates. **Surgical treatment** [16] is not indicated here. She does not have a life-threatening haemangioma so does not require **interferon-alpha or vincristine** [17].

Long-term

After involution, minor residual skin changes can be altered with **surgery or laser treatment** [18] if requested by the parents or child.

---

[1] Airway obstruction can present as biphasic stridor, a barking cough, hoarseness or wheeze or can be observed as nasal flaring, increased recruitment of accessory respiratory muscles (intercostals, sternocleidomastoid), or tripoding (leaning forward on their hands to breathe). This may occur in the absence of a skin finding (i.e. the haemangioma is located within the nasal, subglottic or laryngeal space) and should be treated with corticosteroids immediately.

[2] Eye movements in an infant can be examined by moving a toy and observing their tracking of that toy in space. Pupillary reactions and presence of cataracts can be examined with a pen torch.

[3] Referral to an ENT surgeon is indicated in patients with multiple haemangiomas in the cervical region or lower face or with airway obstructive symptoms (e.g. progressive biphasic stridor, sleep apnoea). They might perform a microlaryngoscopy within the outpatient department or under anaesthesia to investigate for subglottic haemangioma(s).

[4] The type of surgeon referred to is dependent on the geographic region and hospital protocol.

[5] Between 3 and 6 months of age, around 80% of the final size of the haemangioma is commonly reached, and it completes its growth by 9–12 months.

[6] Active observation for haemangiomas is the only treatment required for most lesions and involves weekly or monthly check-ups in the outpatient setting during the proliferative phase, and annually when the lesion stabilises or is in involution. Treatment is warranted only if the lesion ulcerates, it impairs function or vital structures, or if the lesion has the potential of disfigurement.

[7] Serial photographs are used to provide an unbiased visual aid and observe clinical progression over time.

[8] Intensive observation is best for small, focal, non-facial lesions without ulceration and allows the haemangioma to naturally involute. This often results in the best cosmetic outcome.

[9] Oral propranolol is first-line medical therapy for haemangiomas and is continued until age 8–12 months. Indications for use are large or medically complex lesions, those at risk of functional impairment or disfigurement from the lesion, and lesions refractory to other initial therapies. Contraindications to propranolol use are:
- sinus bradycardia
- congenital cardiac conditions or arrhythmias
- maternal history of connective tissue disease
- hypotension
- heart block
- heart failure or cardiogenic shock
- asthma or other airways disease
- hypersensitivity or allergy to beta blockers
- intracranial vascular anomalies
- PHACE syndrome (relative contraindication as can have cardiac or vascular anomalies).

[10] Systemic corticosteroids are an alternative therapy to systemic propranolol but have more adverse effects, including hypothalamic–pituitary–adrenal axis suppression, growth deceleration, gastric irritation, behavioural change, immunosuppression and cushingoid features. This therapy is generally administered for a period of 4–12 weeks at full dose

then tapered over weeks to months and completed by age 9–12 months.

11 Phototherapy or laser treatment is administered via selective pulsation of light between 585–595nm to the vascular mass whilst sparing the surrounding tissue. It only penetrates 1.2mm of depth and requires multiple treatments over 2–6-week intervals. It may require general anaesthetic to administer to large lesions or those in sensitive anatomic areas (such as the perineal region). It is only used in combination with other therapies to treat a haemangioma, or by itself to treat refractory ulceration or residual telangiectasia after the haemangioma has involuted.

12 Topical beta blockers come in the form of timolol 0.25% and 0.5% and propranolol 1%.

13 Topical corticosteroid (mometasone furoate) can be used for small, thin, superficial haemangiomas (<5cm) at a high dose.

14 Intralesional injections of corticosteroid (triamcinolone acetonide) are used in small, thick, well-circumscribed lesions but may require multiple injections at 4–6-week intervals to have an effect. Complications include fat or dermal atrophy, local hypopigmentation, and if used in the upper eyelid, can result in retinal embolus.

15 Ulcerated infantile haemangiomas can be managed with barrier dressings in order to reduce trauma, bleeding, infection and prevent drying. These include hydrocolloid or silver-impregnated dressings or petroleum gauze. Topical barrier creams, ointments with zinc or topical antibiotics may be used in ulcerated regions as well.

16 Surgical treatment includes reconstruction of damaged tissue, excision of fibrofatty tissue after haemangioma involution, and resection of scarring or excess skin. It is rarely indicated and reserved for the involution phase, when blood loss, iatrogenic injury and anaesthetic risks are lessened.

17 Interferon-alpha is an angiogenesis inhibitor. Vincristine is a chemotherapy agent and is used at low doses for treatment of haemangiomas.

18 Surgical resection is most often used in facial venous malformations in order to restore normal facial contours, after the previous less invasive treatments have reduced the bulk of the mass.

CASE 70: The skin lesion

History

- An **83-year-old** [1] **male** [2] presents to the GP practice with a lesion on his scalp that has been annoying him.
- He states it crusts up, and it **bleeds readily when scratched** [3].
- He has been treated in the past for similar regions diagnosed as psoriasis, but it **never improved** [4] with typical psoriatic treatment.
- When prompted about other skin lesions, he states he has had many removed in his life which have come back as **some sort of skin cancer** [5].

- He was a **farmer** [6] in **Australia** [7], **did not apply sunscreen** [8] as it "wasn't known in those days" and swam in the sea for leisure, but now he plays golf.
- He has never had **radiation therapy** [9].
- His past medical history includes cardiac disease on aspirin with an **acute MI 7 years ago** [10], managed with coronary artery bypass grafting, **emphysema** [11] (**he was a smoker** [12] of about 60 pack years but quit 10 years ago when he had grandchildren).
- He does not have any immunosuppressive disease nor is he taking any **immunosuppressive agents** [13].

[1] Most skin cancers arise in the age group of ≥50 years.

[2] Squamous cell carcinomas (SCC) affect men more commonly than women at a ratio of 2:1.

[3] SCC are hyperkeratotic with crusting and ulceration. They are the second most common type of skin cancer and appear on sun-exposed regions such as the face, ears and backs of the hands. Actinic (also known as solar) keratoses are the precursors to cutaneous SCC – scaly, crusty lesions that form in areas most exposed to the sun (face, scalp, lips and backs of the hands). The most common type of skin cancer is basal cell carcinoma (BCC). They are shiny, pearlescent and nodule-like with a rolled edge (otherwise known as having an umbilicated centre) and telangiectatic. It does not have a precursor and only occurs on the skin. Melanoma is the most dangerous skin cancer as it metastasises early. They present most commonly on sun-exposed skin but also can develop under such regions as the nail bed (acral or subungual melanomas) and the sole of the foot. The precursors to melanomas are 'atypical moles' (dysplastic naevi).

[4] Superficial BCC and SCC *in situ* (Bowen's disease) can be misdiagnosed as a patch of psoriasis or eczema. When the patch doesn't improve with conservative treatment, reinspection with magnification and a biopsy can help with diagnosis.

[5] One of the risk factors for having a skin cancer is a personal history of precancerous or cancerous skin lesions.

[6] UV radiation damages DNA. If the damage cannot be repaired, and multiple alterations occur, then the cell undergoes malignant transformation. One of the genes that are damaged by UV radiation is the p53 tumour suppressor

gene, which is mutated in an estimated 45–60% of cutaneous SCCs. When taking a history of a skin lesion it is important to ask about other episodes of UV exposure such as tanning beds, outdoor exercise or gardening. This is to estimate the cumulative sun exposure of the patient.

Cumulative sun exposure increases the risk of all skin cancers, but in particular, intense intermittent sun exposure (for example sunburn repeatedly in childhood) is the most important risk factor for BCC and melanoma formation.

[7] UV rays are strongest in areas closer to the equator.

[8] Sunscreen with sun protection factor (SPF) of 30 will protect against 97% of UVB radiation. The ingredients block and scatter the UV rays before they enter the skin. Only recently has it been found that SPF with oxybenzone is readily absorbed in the skin but also pollutes the water that is swum in or showered in after application, which is harmful to animals and vegetation in the sea, including coral.

[9] Ionising radiation (such as is used in cancer treatment, acne or other skin diseases) increases the risk of both SCC and BCC.

[10] In any patient, taking a past medical history is important to rationalise treatment goals and assess for risk of other complications in the diagnostic or treatment plan. For example, this patient will bleed more after any invasive procedure as he is anticoagulated, a recent cardiac event or symptoms of angina may delay surgical intervention in order to reduce the risk of perioperative cardiac events, and obstructive lung disease may mean general anaesthesia will carry a high risk of pneumonia or death.

[11] It is important to clarify if the patient is currently a smoker as it significantly delays wound healing and increases

risk of wound infection, wound breakdown, pulmonary embolism, stroke, and cardiac events, let alone pulmonary complications after hospitalisation or general anaesthesia.

12 Other risk factors for SCC include smoking tobacco, HPV, having a burn injury in the past, chronically inflamed skin (when SCC develops within a chronic wound it is called a Marjolin's ulcer) and genetic disorders such as xeroderma pigmentosum, albinism or epidermolysis bullosa. Risk factors for BCC are similar except for HPV. The latter is also higher in people with arsenic and coal tar exposure. All types of skin cancers have a higher incidence in people with fair or red hair, blue or green eyes and light skin colour.

13 Immunosuppression increases the risk of SCC by up to 250 times and BCC by up to 6 times that of the immunocompetent. Melanoma risk in immunosuppressed patients is around 2 times higher than the immunocompetent.

Examination

- He is a well-looking man with a **bald scalp** [1] and a few **crusting lesions** [2] over the vertex.
- The one he is concerned with is a **discrete** [3] **nodular** [4] lesion with a shallow base and an ulcerated edge over the vertex of his scalp.
- It has no **telangiectasia or pigmentation** [5].
- It is symmetrical, has clearly defined borders and a **diameter of approximately 2cm** [6].
- His skin type is a **Fitzpatrick type II** [7].
- Both of the **dorsa of his hands** [8] have rough, scaly-looking lesions with no **ulceration or bleeding** [9].
- He has a few **palpable lymph nodes at the occiput** [10] but no others around the **parotid, submandibular or mastoid region** [11].

1 The sites on the body most exposed to sun are the face, ears, back, shoulders, arms and backs of hands. These regions have a higher incidence of all types of skin cancers – see Note 6 in *History* regarding UV exposure and skin cancer development.

2 Crusting lesions could be SCCs, keratocanthomas or solar keratoses. Rarely, this could also be primary cutaneous B-cell lymphoma. Nodular prurigo can also be a raised, scaly lesion but occurs in areas of recurrent trauma and treatment is with topical steroids.

3 Types of configurations of skin lesions or rashes can be described as:
- discrete (individual lesions, clearly separated from each other, e.g. melanoma, solar keratoses)
- confluent (lesions that appear to merge together, e.g. systemic mastocytosis or mast cell activation syndrome)
- discoid (coin-shaped, e.g. lupus or eczema)
- target (resembling a bull's-eye, e.g. in erythema multiforme), or
- annular (ring-like lesions, e.g. in psoriasis, tinea corporis or lichen planus).

4 Descriptions of lesions depending on size and content are:
- macule – flat area of altered colouration <1.5cm in diameter
- patch – flat area of altered colouration >1.5cm in diameter
- papule – solid raised lesion <0.5cm in diameter
- nodule – solid raised lesion >0.5cm in diameter
- plaque – palpable flat lesion >1cm in diameter that is raised or thickened
- vesicle – a clear fluid-filled, raised lesion <0.5cm in diameter
- bulla – a clear fluid-filled, raised lesion >0.5cm in diameter
- pustule – a pus-containing raised lesion <0.5cm in diameter
- abscess – an accumulation of pus >0.5cm in diameter
- boil or furuncle – staphylococcal infection within a hair follicle
- carbuncle – multiple boils/furuncles, or
- wheal – oedematous papule or plaque caused by dermal oedema.

5 See Note 3 in *History* regarding the typical features of various skin cancers.

6 When examining a pigmented lesion (melanocytic), the ABCDE method is used to evaluate and detect malignant melanoma. It can also help as a guide to describing other non-pigmented lesions.
- **A**symmetry or irregularity
- is the **B**order uneven?
- **C**olour (does it have one block of colour or many shades?)
- **D**iameter (>6mm in a mole may be malignant)
- **E**volving (changes) over time.

For example, a melanoma is asymmetrical, has an uneven border, multiple shades of brown/grey/white/blue/black or red, a diameter usually of >6mm and evolves (e.g. grew in size over 6 months).

7 The Fitzpatrick scale classifies human skin pigmentation from types I–VI to help assess risk of skin cancers. Type I always burns, never tans (palest skin, often with freckles; UV sensitive – therefore has the highest risk of skin cancers). Type II usually burns and tans sometimes. Type III tans uniformly, only sometimes mildly burning. Type IV burns minimally and always tans well. Type V tans very easily and rarely burns (dark brown) and type VI never burns (darkest brown; UV resistant – therefore has the lowest risk of skin cancers).

8 See Note 1 in *Examination* regarding areas of skin cancer predominance.

9 Remember that the precursors for SCCs are solar keratoses.

10 The posterior scalp drains to the posterior auricular (mastoid) and occipital lymph nodes.

11 The region of the face anterior to the ears drains to the parotid, submandibular and deep cervical lymph nodes.

Investigations

- After taking a **punch biopsy of the lesion** [1] with a 3mm **surgical punch** [2] , the histopathology returns as poorly differentiated **squamous cell carcinoma** [3] .

- It could not comment on whether there was perineural or lymphatic spread due to the **size of the sample** [4] .

1 The most important diagnostic test is a biopsy. It can be performed in a few ways:
- punch biopsy (often performed as it is a quick procedure under local anaesthetic and does not require closing with a stitch until 4mm wide)
- local excision (taking the tissue and 1–2mm of healthy tissue around it)
- wide local excision (taking a cuff of normal tissue with the specimen).

2 When taking a punch biopsy, a width of 3mm is usually adequate to make a pathological diagnosis. However, a few pointers for taking a biopsy:
- If there is dry or flaky skin around the lesion, gently remove this and take the biopsy from the underlying skin.
- If there is an ulcerated region, avoid taking a biopsy here as it may be largely necrotic tissue and therefore is

not specific. It may also bleed heavily, and this may not be amenable to suturing.

3 The differentiation of SCC correlates well with its clinical behaviour. Well-differentiated lesions invade locally, whilst poorly differentiated SCCs are more commonly infiltrative and metastatic. If this were a melanoma, one of the most important histological findings is the tumour thickness, which is called the Breslow thickness, as it helps in prognostication. If a melanoma thickness is <1mm from the skin surface, then it is classed as a stage 1A and has a 97% 5-year survival rate. If a melanoma is >2mm then it has invaded into the dermis and is a stage 3 or above. This drastically lowers 5-year survival rate to 60–75%.

4 Spread of any skin cancer into nearby or distant locations drastically reduces survival. For SCC, regional lymphatic spread reduces overall survival by half.

Management

Immediate

The histological findings are discussed with the patient and **surgical excision** [1] [2] is recommended. If the patient consents, refer to a **plastic or general surgeon** [3] . For the actinic keratoses, **cryotherapy** [4] , topical application of **5-fluorouracil** [5] or **photodynamic therapy** [6] is the mainstay of treatment.

Short-term

Prior to excision, this patient requires a few **peri-operative investigations** [7] . The first are blood tests

including **FBE, UEC and coagulation studies** [8] . He should be referred to a respiratory physician and cardiologist to optimise his comorbidities **prior to surgical intervention** [9] . Given the high risk features in his initial punch biopsy, **a CT or MRI scan** [10] of his head and neck should be ordered for peri-operative planning. The histological report of the lesion and any nearby lymph node(s) (sentinel node) will guide **further investigations and management** [11] [12] [13] . Should the lesion have lymphatic invasion, a **sentinel lymph node biopsy** [14] or **lymph node clearance** [15] will be offered.

Long-term

In most cases, simple excision with or without adjunct **chemo- or radiotherapy**[16] will be sufficient for treatment. Patients in cases of invasive SCC have a **poor prognosis**[17] and **high morbidity**[18] from lymph node clearance, but may be offered **immunotherapy**[19] or **reconstruction**[20] of a defect left after surgical resection. Patients with a previous skin cancer should have a **yearly skin check**[21]. The patient should avoid sun exposure by utilising **preventive measures**[22].

1 Standard (elliptical) excision of an SCC with a cuff of at least 4mm of normal skin is usually adequate for the non-invasive type. Usually these can be closed primarily (i.e. no need for a graft or flap). Moh's micrographic surgery can be employed for regions of cosmetic importance as it is a tissue-sparing procedure. It is when a surgical excision is undertaken and sent to the pathologist to determine if the lesion has been excised with adequate margins. This procedure has the lowest overall rate of recurrence compared with other surgical excision techniques.

2 Choice of sedation or general anaesthetic is dependent on the patient's comorbidities and size of procedure. In this case, this patient has multiple comorbidities with a significant pack year history and cardiac complications and will likely be more appropriate for sedation with local anaesthetic to surgically remove the lesion.

3 Complications of a biopsy are like any other surgical intervention: bleeding, scarring, damage to surrounding structures (in this case, nerve or vessel injury), wound breakdown, infection and anaesthetic reactions.

4 Cryotherapy is the local or general use of low temperatures for medical therapy, used to treat a variety of skin lesions including plantar warts, superficial BCCs and Bowen disease.

5 5-fluorouracil blocks DNA synthesis and therefore cell proliferation, and is used to treat small, superficial BCCs in low risk areas such as the trunk of the body, arms, legs, cheeks, forehead, temples and scalp, and solar keratoses.

6 Photodynamic therapy can be used to treat actinic keratoses, superficial BCCs and some types of low risk nodular BCC.

7 These tests ultimately are to aid the operating anaesthetist to assess whether this patient would be able to survive surgery with minimal complications, such as pneumonia, PE, acute pulmonary oedema, etc. This is known as being 'fit for surgery'.

8 This patient may have anaemia of chronic disease, chronic renal failure from atherosclerosis, hypertension or medications. The former is important in oxygen delivery and wound healing, but also in major surgery if he requires transfusion pre- or postoperatively, while the renal function is crucial knowledge to adequately dose certain medications such as propofol or morphine.

9 Peri-operative 'optimisation' in patients with a history of cardiac events involves an ECG, review by a Cardiologist (to manage any angina, possibly for an angiogram to see if the stent is still patent), and a TTE or TOE to assess heart function. Given this patient has chronic lung disease, referral and review by a Respiratory physician with recent respiratory function tests is important.

10 CT and MRI can be used separately or in combination with PET in order to assess local structures for invasive disease. For example, in patients who do not have palpable lymph nodes with cutaneous SCC, certain factors increase the need for further imaging for evaluation of metastases, such as if the lesion is larger than 2cm, located near major nerves in the head and neck, or invading deep structures (bone, cartilage, etc.), among others.

11 Results from histopathology usually take around 1–2 weeks. If concerned about a melanoma, the result can be escalated as 'urgent' with the local pathology department, but a diagnosis may still take 24–72 hours.

12 Biomarkers are tumour markers found on special staining of the lesion during the histopathological examination, in high risk SCC. If there is elevated expression of various tumour markers, this has been shown to correlate with increased risk of nodal metastases or death.

13 TNM is the universal staging system used for various cancers, created by the AJCC. It stands for Tumour burden (how the tumour has invaded local tissues), Nodal involvement (ranging from local to peripheral) and Metastatic disease, and higher numbers indicate worse prognosis.

14 The sentinel lymph node is the one that is most commonly be involved by metastasis. To find this lymph node, lymphatic mapping is performed using either blue dye or technetium-99 (Tc-99) injected into the region that the skin cancer is in. If using blue dye, the sentinel node will become blue, but if using Tc-99 it will emit gamma radiation which can be detected with a hand-held gamma probe intra-operatively. This is most often used in melanoma but can be used for high risk SCC, Merkel cell carcinomas and pigmented epithelioid melanocytoma. Adverse reactions to SLNB are reactions to the dye (e.g. anaphylaxis), lymphoedema and false-negative results.

15 A lymph node clearance has higher morbidity than an SLNB but is performed when there are high risk features on histopathology for metastasis or evidence of local lymphatic metastases on imaging such as PET, CT or MRI.

16 Chemotherapy can be topical or systemic. Topical chemotherapy includes imiquimod used for small BCCs that are outside of the head and neck region, 5-fluorouracil for superficial BCC and solar keratoses, among others. Radiotherapy is often given in high risk BCC, SCC, melanoma and Merkel cell cancer. Adverse reactions to this include skin infections, urticaria, pruritus and skin colour changes.

17 Survival rate in poorly differentiated SCC is around 25% at 5 years (post diagnosis). Patients in this category are therefore usually offered SLNB or locoregional lymph node clearance.

18 Morbidity from lymph node clearance includes seroma, venous thromboembolism, wound infection, wound necrosis and lymphoedema.

19 Immunotherapy or biologic therapy aims to increase the immune system's defence against the cancer. Some are approved for use and others may require recruitment into a trial. These are usually reserved for locally advanced or metastatic skin cancers such as metastatic melanoma or SCC.

20 Reconstruction can be as small as a localised skin flap to a large craniofacial surgery. In this case, for example, if the patient has invasion into the underlying occipital bone, it will require either resection through part of the bone or to the meninges. This can be performed by the appropriately trained Plastic and Reconstructive Surgeon and Neurosurgeon. Reconstructive options for this will involve a bone graft and flap.

21 For patients who have had a high risk skin cancer (melanoma, or a squamous or basal cell carcinoma with invasion or poor differentiation) follow-up is every 3 months until a consultant surgeon deems it safe to lengthen review intervals. A skin check is usually performed by a Dermatologist.

22 Preventive measures include broad-spectrum sunscreen (with both UVA and UVB protection, applied 30 minutes before going outside and every 2 hours minimum), wearing a brimmed hat and covering the scalp, wearing sunglasses, wearing clothing that covers the shoulders and arms, and seeking shade.

CASE 71: Fournier's gangrene

History

- A 56-year-old **male** [1] presents with a **4-day history** [2] of worsening **scrotal cellulitis and pain** [3].
- His past medical history is significant for **T2DM** [4], obstructive sleep apnoea, chronic obstructive airway disease and **obesity** [5] with a BMI of 40.

- The patient reports **worsening of redness and pain over the scrotum despite oral antibiotics** [6] prescribed by his GP.
- He denies abdominal pain, change in bowel habits and urinary symptoms. He is a **non-smoker** [7].

[1] Fournier's gangrene is much more common in males compared to females, with a ratio of 7:1.

[2] Cellulitis and pain over the scrotal or perineal region are the typical presentation. Buttock, thigh, penile and lower abdominal regions are also commonly involved. However, the disease can essentially affect any region as it progresses.

[3] It is common to see a relatively delayed presentation because patients often initially present to their GP or local ED and are diagnosed with simple cellulitis. There is difficulty differentiating early Fournier's gangrene from cellulitis.

[4] Fournier's gangrene patients are often immunosuppressed due to diabetes, malignancy, alcohol abuse, malnutrition, HIV, advanced age or immunosuppressive medications. However, healthy patients can also be affected.

[5] Fournier's gangrene commonly affects obese patients, as they often have other comorbidities that predispose them to the disease. Poor personal hygiene is another contributing factor.

[6] This part of the history is important. Worsening cellulitis despite antibiotic treatment should raise red flags that this may be much more serious than just simple cellulitis and requires urgent attention.

[7] Smoking is also a risk factor for Fournier's gangrene. It not only causes various malignancies, but has been shown to be an immunosuppressive agent.

Examination

- The patient appears **unwell and a foul odour is detected on observation** [1].
- His vital signs demonstrate a **mild tachycardia, hypotension, tachypnoea, a small oxygen requirement to maintain saturations and a moderate fever at 38.6°C** [2].
- There is extensive **cellulitis of the scrotum and perineum, as well as the inner thigh** [3].
- The affected tissue is **indurated and crepitus** [4] can be felt.

- There are small **black and necrotic areas** [5] detected.
- The patient's **testicles are non-tender** [6] and the penile skin is not involved.
- No **abdominal tenderness** [7] is elicited and **no inguinal lymphadenopathy** [8] is palpable.
- Systematic examination of the **cardiorespiratory system** [9] is unremarkable.

[1] Patients with Fournier's gangrene can look very unwell and this is a late sign. Sometimes one can detect a distinct foul smell emanating from necrotic tissue. All these point to a serious underlying pathology.

[2] This set of vital signs point to the fact that the patient is in septic shock – hypotension and tachycardia. These changes are driven by a hyper-inflammatory response to endotoxins or exotoxins. There is mass release of inflammatory mediators such as cytokines which leads to dilatation of vasculature as well as increased vascular permeability, leading to decreased intravascular volume and tissue hypoperfusion. Tachypnoea suggests that the patient may also be acidotic, likely due to build-up of lactic acid from prolonged tissue hypoperfusion.

This patient needs urgent resuscitation, as sepsis can be life-threatening.

3 This is the common distribution of cellulitis seen in Fournier's gangrene. The disease can progress quickly and involve many other regions.

4 Fournier's gangrene is a clinical diagnosis. Severe induration and crepitus are classic findings and are essentially diagnostic of the disease. It is a result of infection with gas-forming organisms.

5 Areas of necrosis signal advanced disease, and urgent surgical debridement is required because infection can progress rapidly.

6 Infection spreads along dartos, Colle's and Scarpa's fasciae and generally does not involve deep fascial planes and muscle. Therefore, the testicles themselves are usually spared.

7 It is important to examine the anterior abdomen to look for spread of infection as well as ruling out other concurrent pathology.

8 Inguinal lymphadenopathy may not be present but positive findings will not change management.

9 Complete cardiorespiratory examination is essential to assess cardiovascular reserve for general anaesthesia.

Investigations

- FBE shows a **significantly raised WCC** [1].
- **UEC** [2] results are normal.
- **CRP is high at 340mg/L** [3]. LFT results are normal.
- Venous blood gas shows a **lactate of 4.2mmol/L and pH of 7.21** [4].
- **Urine dipstick** [5] is unremarkable.
- **CT scan of the pelvis** [6] reveals **extensive induration of the tissue of scrotum and perineum; gas is detected in the subcutaneous tissue** [7].

1 Raised WCC is expected in the setting of severe sepsis. This certainly is the case with Fournier's gangrene.

2 Renal function can usually be maintained in early stages. However, as sepsis progresses and organ hypoperfusion begins, acute tubular necrosis can occur and significantly affect renal function.

3 CRP is a general reflection of infection and inflammation. Higher levels tend to indicate severe infection.

4 The VBG findings are consistent with severe sepsis causing acidosis as well as tissue hypoperfusion, which drive up the lactate.

5 Urine dipstick can be useful to detect underlying UTI as a source of infection that progressed to Fournier's gangrene.

6 Fournier's gangrene is a clinical diagnosis, but CT scan can assist to confirm the diagnosis. Imaging can be useful to assist in equivocal patients without overt signs of sepsis.

7 These are classic findings on CT scan of the areas of Fournier's gangrene. Gas-forming organisms cause gas to form in subcutaneous tissue and these findings are diagnostic.

Management

Immediate

Monitor vital signs and resuscitate [1] the patient. Obtain IV access, administer **fluids and broad-spectrum IV antibiotics** [2]. Insert an **indwelling catheter** [3] for monitoring of urine output. Keep the patient **fasted** [4]. Seek review from the **ICU, Urology and General Surgery** [5] teams.

Short-term

Perform **emergency surgical debridement** [6] of Fournier's gangrene. Send **specimens for culture** [7].

Arrange for **re-look debridement** [8] in 24–72 hours and ensure **meticulous wound care** [9]. Monitor the patient in **ICU** [10], including optimising fluid and glycaemic control. Consider **hyperbaric oxygen therapy** [11]. Involvement of the **plastic surgery team for reconstruction** [12] of debrided areas is recommended.

Long-term

Continue **plastic surgery** [13] follow-up for wound assessment. Involve **Endocrinology** [14] follow-up for diabetic control.

1 Resuscitate the patient according to EMST (Early Management of Severe Trauma) and stabilise the patient's airway, breathing and circulation. This is a medical emergency that carries a mortality rate of 17–30%.

2 Ensure IV access is obtained early so fluid resuscitation can be initiated in the setting of septic shock. Broad-spectrum antibiotics in this setting should include meropenem, vancomycin and clindamycin.

3 An indwelling urinary catheter (IDC) should be inserted to closely monitor fluid levels. This is particularly important in sepsis. Decreasing urine output in septic patient indicates progression of tissue hypoperfusion and decreasing kidney function. This is often a poor prognostic sign in a septic patient.

4 Ensure the patient is fasted to facilitate general anaesthesia and reduce aspiration risks.

5 Management of Fournier's gangrene requires input from multiple teams. Surgical debridement is often led by the Urology and General surgery teams, especially if there is suspicion that debridement may involve the rectum. If extensive debridement is required of tissue on the limbs or abdominal wall, Plastic Surgery may also need to be involved. ICU needs to be involved to resuscitate the patient as well as for postoperative monitoring.

6 Urgent and aggressive surgical debridement of devitalised tissue is key. Debridement needs to be continued until bleeding/healthy tissue is reached, to ensure complete removal of necrotic/infected tissue.

7 Tissue is sent for culture to find the offending organisms. Most cases are caused by polymicrobial infection. *Escherichia coli* is usually the most commonly cultured organism.

Other commonly cultured organisms include *Enterococcus*, *Staphylococcus*, *Streptococcus*, *Bacteroides fragilis* and *Pseudomonas*. Aerobes and anaerobes may be present.

8 The patient needs to be brought back to theatre in 24–72 hours to reassess the tissue and perform additional debridement if initial debridement is incomplete or if there is progression of infection.

9 Wound care is an important part of management. It can be challenging, often due to the extensive debridement areas. Temporary colostomy and suprapubic catheter should be considered to avoid contamination of the wound as well as facilitate complete seal of the dressings.

10 The patient will likely stay in the ICU for a period of time due to the complex nature of the disease.

11 Hyperbaric oxygen therapy for Fournier's gangrene is controversial. Theoretically, it enhances healing of damaged tissue by improving angiogenesis and formation of granulation tissue, it can reduce bleeding by enhancing vasoconstriction, as well as enhancing efficacy of antibiotic therapy and immune function.

12 Following satisfactory debridement of devitalised tissue and stabilisation of the patient, the Plastic Surgery team is often asked to be involved to consider reconstructing the debrided areas with skin grafting and tissue flaps.

13 Ongoing Plastic Surgery follow-up is required post discharge to ensure the tissue reconstruction is healing satisfactorily.

14 Endocrinology follow-up should also be arranged to ensure stable diabetic control and reduce the risk of diabetes-related complications.

CASE 72: Haematuria

History

- A 73-year-old female presents with a 2-day history of **frank haematuria** [1] and **difficulty voiding** [2].
- She has a past medical history significant for T2DM, **previous TIA** [3] on **clopidogrel** [4], and hypertension.
- She had a hysterectomy 10 years ago but reports **no other previous surgery or radiation therapy** [5].
- She is an **ex-smoker** [6].
- The patient also reports **dysuria** [7] and **suprapubic discomfort** [8].
- She denies **infective symptoms** [9], **flank pain** [10], **constitutional symptoms** [11] or recent **overseas travel** [12].

1 Haematuria can be classified by site of origin: nephrologic (intrinsic renal diseases), urologic (upper and lower urinary tract) and pseudohaematuria (menstruation, medication-related, etc.). Urological malignancy is more common in patients with gross haematuria (23%) than in patients with microscopic haematuria (5%).

2 Symptoms of difficulty voiding may suggest clot retention in the setting of macroscopic haematuria. Ask the patient about passage of clots when assessing haematuria.

3 Full past medical history should be obtained, including previous history of urological malignancies and procedures performed on the urinary tract.

4 Medication history is important especially for anticoagulants and antiplatelets, both of which can complicate haematuria. Some medications can cause haematuria such as nitrofurantoin, ibuprofen, phenytoin and levodopa.

5 Previous surgeries may indicate previous pathology the patient has had and the possibility of recurrence or complications. Radiation therapy can cause radiation cystitis that can cause severe haematuria which can be difficult to manage.

6 Smoking is the greatest risk factor for bladder cancer. Other risk factors include chronic cystitis, chemical exposure of aromatic amines (occupational exposure from textile, dye, rubber or paint industries), radiation and chemotherapy (cyclophosphamide).

7 Irritative lower urinary tract symptoms can suggest underlying UTI.

8 Suprapubic discomfort in the setting of frank haematuria likely indicates the patient is in clot retention.

9 Infective symptoms include irritative lower urinary tract symptoms such as dysuria, frequency and urgency of urination. Also enquire about symptoms such as fever, chills and rigors.

10 Flank pain with haematuria can suggest urolithiasis, and upper tract bleeding causing clot colic.

11 Constitutional symptoms of fevers, weight loss and night sweats can be a sign that there is underlying advanced malignancy.

12 Enquire about overseas travel for differential diagnoses such as TB and schistosomiasis as causes for haematuria.

Examination

- The patient appears **uncomfortable** [1].
- Her vital signs are unremarkable apart from a **mild tachycardia** [2].
- The **conjunctivae are pale** [3] and her **mucous membranes are dry** [4].
- Examination of the **cardiorespiratory system** [5] is unremarkable.
- The patient's **abdomen appears mildly distended** [6] and **tender to palpate over the suprapubic region** [7].
- There is **dullness on percussion** [8] just inferior to the umbilicus.
- There is **no flank tenderness** [9] on palpation.
- **Post-void bladder scan** [10] demonstrates residual urine of 700ml.

1 Patients can be in severe discomfort when in urinary retention.

2 Elevated HR can be due to pain of urinary retention. Her other observations suggest that the patient is stable and not septic.

3 Pale conjunctivae can be due to blood loss in the urine causing anaemia.

4 Dry mucous membranes suggest that the patient is dehydrated. This can be secondary to decreased oral intake during time of illness.

5 A systematic examination should include the cardiorespiratory system to ensure no significant abnormalities exist to put patients at risk during general anaesthesia.

6 Abdominal distension can be secondary to urinary retention, or possibly concurrent bowel pathology.

7 When the patient is in retention, the abdomen – especially the suprapubic region – is often tender on palpation.

8 A full bladder is dull on percussion. If the patient's bladder is palpable up to the umbilicus this means she is in retention with a large volume.

9 Flank tenderness can suggest urolithiasis or upper tract clot colic in setting of haematuria.

10 Bladder scan immediately after voiding is an excellent simple bedside test to detect urinary retention.

Investigations

- FBE reports a **haemoglobin level of 79g/L [1]** and a **mildly elevated WCC [2]** .
- UEC shows **creatinine level of 110µmol/L, eGFR 65ml/min/1.73m² [3]** , and normal electrolyte levels.
- Urine dipstick demonstrates **haematuria, trace leucocytes and no nitrites [4]** .
- **Urine cytology [5]** is suspicious for malignant cells.
- **CT IVP [6]** reveals a **3cm mass on left lateral wall of the bladder [7]** .
- **No upper tract dilatation or filling defects [8]** are detected.

1 The low haemoglobin level suggests significant haematuria which is exacerbated by antiplatelet agent. Haemoglobin level needs to be carefully maintained, especially in patients with cardiac history where low haemoglobin can put significant stress on limited cardiac function.

2 Mildly elevated WCC does not always mean there is an infection. Systemic inflammatory reaction can also cause this picture.

3 There is mild renal impairment. This needs to be compared to the patient's previous readings and could be a chronic change. Transient renal impairment could be due to prerenal issues such as dehydration, intrinsic renal issues such as acute tubular necrosis or postrenal obstruction.

4 Detection of leucocytes and nitrites can indicate UTI. UTI can cause haemorrhagic cystitis.

5 Urine cytology has high sensitivity in detecting high grade transitional cell carcinoma or carcinoma *in situ*. Low grade tumours do not cause positive urine cytology results.

6 CT intravenous pyelogram (IVP) is the gold standard imaging modality for investigation of haematuria. The delayed phase which allows the contrast to opacify the collecting system and the lower urinary tract can outline filling defects that may suggest malignancy.

7 This finding is highly suspicious of a large transition cell carcinoma of the bladder as the cause of the patient's symptoms.

8 No filling defect in the upper urinary tract is reassuring that the patient does not have any obvious pathology in that area.

Management

Immediate

Insert a **3-way urinary catheter** [1] and begin **bladder irrigation** [2]. **Withhold clopidogrel** [3]. Obtain IV access, administer **fluid** [4] and **transfuse packed RBCs** [5]. Seek advice from the **urology team** [6].

Short-term

Perform emergency or urgent elective **transurethral resection of bladder tumour** [7]. Following the procedure, a 3-way catheter is inserted to commence **bladder irrigation** [8] to ensure bleeding settles. The patient's **vital signs and haemoglobin levels** [9] need to be monitored. Depending on the pathology, **staging CT chest and whole-body bone scan** [10] should be performed. The patient can be discharged home after **trial of void** [11].

Long-term

The patient's case should be discussed at an **MDT meeting** [12]. Follow the patient up in an outpatient clinic to **inform patient of the histopathology, MDT recommendation and ongoing management** [13] of her bladder cancer.

---

1 A 3-way IDC should be inserted in setting of clot retention. These catheters have an inflow channel as well as an outflow channel, along with the balloon channel. Through the larger-bore channel and the fluid inflow, they allow for evacuation of clots and debris whilst providing continuous irrigation of the bladder.

2 When the 3-way IDC is initially inserted, manual washout should be performed first to evacuate all blood clots from bladder. Bladder irrigation helps to stop bleeding for several reasons. Firstly, urine contains urokinase (an enzyme that converts plasminogen to plasmin, which ultimately leads to clot lysis). Urokinase can cause persistent urinary bleeding because it impairs clot stability. Irrigation constantly washes out urokinase to promote clot stability. It also allows collapse of bladder after large clots have been evacuated to allow haemostasis from pressure.

3 Any coagulopathy should be corrected and antiplatelets withheld to assist in treating haematuria. This should be done in conjunction with advice from the Neurology team, weighing the risk of further TIA or stroke against the risk of bleeding.

4 The patient is likely dehydrated, and fluids are important to minimise the negative effects of dehydration and improve renal function.

5 The patient is anaemic from haematuria and should be transfused packed red cells. In patients with cardiac history, this is especially important due to limited cardiac reserve.

6 The Urology team should be managing this patient as they will be operating on her bladder tumour.

7 Transurethral resection of the bladder tumour is performed under general anaesthesia. A resectoscope is used to remove the tumour to obtain tissue diagnosis as well as assess depth of invasion.

8 A 3-way IDC is again placed postoperatively to ensure bleeding stops.

9 Vital signs are monitored to ensure the patient recovers well from anaesthesia and to look for immediate signs of complication such as sepsis. Postoperative haemoglobin is also monitored and transfused as required.

10 Sites of bladder cancer metastasis include pelvic lymph nodes, liver, lung and bone. CT chest, abdomen and pelvis as well as bone scan are standard staging scans.

11 After the catheter is removed, patients are asked to void into a bottle. The void volume, as well as their bladder residuals, is measured. Factors taken into consideration during a trial of void include void volume, residuals (whether it increases, decreases or remains stable) and the patient's comfort level with the residual urine volume.

12 Management of bladder cancer requires a multidisciplinary approach. Imaging and pathology results should be discussed at the MDT meeting which consists of surgeons, radiation and medical oncologists, radiologists and pathologists. Further management of bladder cancer depends on grading of cancer, depth of invasion and presence of metastatic disease.

13 The patient should be seen in the outpatient clinic to be informed of the histopathology result and the recommendation from the MDT meeting. Further follow-up surveillance, treatments or procedures can be explained to the patient at this time.

CASE 73: Prostate cancer

History

- A **68-year-old** [1] male is referred to the Urology clinic with a recent **prostate-specific antigen (PSA) reading of 6.3** [2].
- **Previous PSA is 4.8** [3] six months ago.
- He does not report any **lower urinary tract symptoms** [4].
- The patient denies **constitutional symptoms** [5] such as loss of weight and night sweats.
- He does not have any **bony tenderness** [6].
- His **past medical history** [7] is significant for hypertension and hypercholesterolaemia.
- He has no **surgical history** [8].
- He does not **smoke** [9].
- The patient's **father and uncle have both previously been diagnosed with prostate cancer** [10].

[1] Prostate cancer is the most commonly diagnosed cancer in males in the UK. Patients usually present after the age of 65 but it may also occur in younger men.

[2] There are no universally accepted total PSA threshold value above which is considered abnormal. Normal PSA values vary with age and ethnicity. The upper limit of normal PSA value in a 68-year-old Caucasian male is 4.5. PSA on its own is not capable of diagnosing prostate cancer – it only estimates the risk.

[3] A single abnormal PSA should not prompt prostate biopsy. A number of other causes can elevate the PSA, such as genitourinary infection, ejaculation, prostate examination, catheterisation, urethral instrumentation and cycling. It is important to verify the trend of abnormal PSA with serial tests.

[4] The patient's baseline lower urinary tract symptoms need to be established. This may alter management in the setting of prostate cancer. Radiotherapy as first-line treatment for prostate cancer can worsen obstructive lower urinary tract symptoms and may require transurethral resection of the prostate prior to commencing treatment.

[5] Constitutional symptoms can manifest in the setting of metastatic cancer.

[6] Bone is the second most common metastatic location in patients with prostate cancer, first being the pelvic lymph nodes. Bony tenderness, especially in the back, is not an uncommon initial presenting symptom for patients with advanced prostate cancer.

[7] Past medical history is not only important for completeness of the patient's clinic picture, but it will also dictate the type of treatment the patient will receive for their malignancy. Radical surgery is mainly indicated in patients with good functional reserve.

[8] Previous surgeries can complicate surgical management of prostate cancer. Patients who have had previous inguinal hernia repaired with mesh may be difficult radical prostatectomy candidates because the mesh can often obliterate the extra-peritoneal plane that needs to be reached during prostatectomy.

[9] Smoking not only puts patients at higher risk for general anaesthesia, but also slows or impairs wound healing after surgery. Patients should be encouraged to quit or at least reduce smoking prior to treatment.

[10] Family history of prostate cancer is the most important risk factor. The risk of prostate cancer increases the closer the relative, if they were diagnosed at a younger age, and the number of relatives with diagnosis. The risk of prostate cancer increases over 2-fold when a first-degree relative has prostate cancer.

Examination

- The patient appears well on **general examination** [1].
- There are no signs of **cachexia** [2].
- **Heart sounds** [3] are dual with no murmurs.
- **Auscultation of the chest** [4] reveals normal breath sounds and equal air entry.

- The abdomen is **soft and no tenderness** [5] is elicited.
- No **surgical scars** [6] are detected.
- Examination of the **genitalia** [7] is unremarkable.

- **Digital rectal examination** [8] reveals a **moderately enlarged gland** [9] that is non-**tender** [10], and a **nodule** [11] is detected at the left base.
- There is no **pitting oedema** [12] in the lower limbs.

[1] General inspection is an essential start to every physical examination. It can reveal vital clues indicating that the patient is acutely unwell.

[2] Cachexia is often associated with patients with metastatic malignancy. Poor nutritional state is also associated with poorer outcomes post major surgery. If a cachectic patient is being worked up for surgery, it would be important to seek advice from a dietitian.

[3] Cardiac examination is required as part of a general work-up of the patient's comorbidities as well as pre-anaesthetic assessment. Further investigations such as ECG and echocardiogram should be obtained along with advice from the cardiology team.

[4] Similarly, the patient's respiratory reserve needs to be determined, especially prior to major surgery. Patients who are obese or have a smoking history should have preoperative CXRs, as well as spirometry testing and sleep studies as indicated.

[5] Examination of the abdomen should be carried out to ensure no concurrent pathology exists. Patients with advanced prostate cancer can sometimes present with flank pain secondary to obstructed kidneys.

[6] Surgical scars give an indication of previous surgical history. Of particular relevance to prostate surgery is previous mesh repair of inguinal hernia, which can sometimes significantly complicate radical prostatectomy.

[7] Genitalia should be examined to rule out issues such as phimosis or meatal pathology which could impact on future procedures.

[8] DRE is an essential part of work-up for prostate and bowel pathology. Patients need to be properly counselled prior to examination, informing them of the indication, likelihood of discomfort, and small risk of bleeding, especially in patients with haemorrhoids or anal fissures. There are two common ways to position patients: lateral position with legs tucked or standing and bent over at the hips. Liberal use of lubricants is encouraged to decrease the patient's discomfort. After warning the patient of commencement of exam, the examiner's index finger is inserted into the patient's rectum. Patients can be encouraged to focus on taking breaths to assist in relaxing them. The prostate bulge is felt at the anterior wall of rectum. DRE is also useful in clinical scenarios where bowel obstruction or bleeding is suspected. At completion of the examination, residual lubricant should be wiped away for the patient as a courtesy. Efficacy of DRE can be limited in obese or non-compliant patients, as well as examiners with short index fingers.

[9] Size of the prostate is the first characteristic to be assessed. After examining both lobes of the prostate, a rough estimation of size can be established. A young man's prostate is about the size of a walnut. Prostate size is not a reliable indicator of a patient's lower urinary tract symptoms – small prostates may sometimes cause significant symptoms.

[10] Tenderness on prostate examination can suggest underlying prostatitis, which can cause elevated PSA levels. It is important to distinguish the pain from digital insertion through the anus and pain on palpation of the prostate. Other associated features of prostatitis can be bogginess and fluctuance, which may indicate prostatic abscess. Suspect abscess formation if there are ongoing symptoms with fevers despite appropriate antibiotic treatment.

[11] Prostate cancer is suspected if nodules, irregularities or firmness are detected on DRE. An abnormal DRE with an elevated PSA should trigger consideration for prostate biopsy.

[12] Examination of the lower limbs should be performed to complete the cardiovascular examination. Pitting oedema suggests underlying cardiac failure which needs to be further investigated and managed before major surgery.

Investigations

- **FBE and UEC** [1] are within normal limits.
- **LFT** [2] results are also normal.
- **Urine dipstick and culture** [3] does not suggest UTI.
- A **multiparametric MRI** [4] scan of the prostate shows the prostate size to be **52cc** [5], and a 1.4cm lesion in the **peripheral zone** [6] at left base is detected.

- The appearance is consistent with **PI-RADS 4** [7].
- A **transrectal ultrasound-guided prostate biopsy** [8] revealed **Gleason 4+4=8** [9] prostate cancer.
- Subsequent **CT scan of abdomen and pelvis, as well as whole body bone scan** [10] were negative for metastatic disease.

1 Baseline FBE and UEC detects WCC abnormalities which can indicate infective/inflammatory process. Renal impairment in patients suspected with prostate cancer needs to be further investigated with CT scan to rule out postrenal obstruction.

2 Patients with prostate cancer and bony metastasis may have a deranged ALP level.

3 Urine culture should be performed to rule out infective processes, such as UTI or prostatitis, as causes of elevated PSA.

4 Multiparametric MRI (mpMRI) combines anatomical and functional MR sequences in a single examination and has become an established tool in prostate cancer work-up. MRI has high sensitivity (>90%) when it comes to detecting clinically significant prostate cancer, which is defined as Gleason score ≥7. It also has very high negative predictive value, meaning that if MRI is negative for prostate cancer, there is a high chance that there is no significant underlying cancer.

5 MRI can accurately assess the prostate size. PSA density can then be calculated by dividing serum PSA level by prostate volume. PSA density has been used as another predictive tool in the diagnosis of prostate cancer, and the cut-off used most commonly is 0.15 or 0.20ng/ml.

6 The prostate is divided into 4 zones: transition zone, central zone, anterior fibromuscular stroma and peripheral zone. The most common location of prostate cancer is the peripheral zone, comprising around 70% of prostate cancers.

7 The overall PI-RADS score is a weighted calculation on a 5-point scale. It is based on the probability that a combination of the MRI parameters correlates with the presence of a clinically significant cancer at a particular location of the prostate. PI-RADS 4 score indicates that there is an 80–85% probability of the lesion being clinically significant prostate cancer.

8 Prostate biopsy can be obtained transrectally under sedation or local anaesthetic using ultrasound guidance. Biopsy can also be performed transperineally with transrectal ultrasound. The latter technique requires general anaesthesia but has reduced rates of sepsis.

9 The Gleason grading system is based on architectural pattern of the prostate gland. The two most abundant patterns of tumour are graded from 1–5, and two grades are added to give the Gleason score. Therefore, the Gleason score is reported as the most abundant grade plus the second most abundant grade. The higher the score, the worse the prognosis.

10 CT and bone scan are the traditional methods of staging for prostate cancer. Staging is usually reserved for prostate cancer with a Gleason score of ≥7. A PSMA PET scan is a more contemporary method of detecting metastatic disease and is highly sensitive, but is only available at certain centres.

Management

Immediate

Counsel the patient [1] on the results of investigations to date. Offer support [2] and give the patient further information [3] to aid the patient's understanding of his disease.

Short-term

Present the patient's case at the MDT meeting [4] and discuss radical prostatectomy [5] or radiotherapy [6] as curative options. Arrange treatment after obtaining informed consent [7] from the patient.

Long-term

Monitor PSA [8] for cancer recurrence. Evaluate and manage side-effects of treatment [9].

1 Appropriate patient counselling is very important, especially for cancer diagnosis. Breaking bad news is a complex communication task that involves verbal components as well as responding to emotional reactions, empowering the patient in decision-making, involving loved ones and giving hope.

2 The patient is likely to be in shock due to the bad news and should be offered support not only during the consultation but also longer-term by offering to link the patient up with an organisation such as Prostate Cancer UK. Such bodies have connections to a comprehensive network of services for cancer patients.

3 Patients are often bombarded with information during the consultation and likely to remember only a small portion of the conversation. Excellent literature exists in booklet form, in a simple and easy to read format to allow patients to understand their disease at their own pace. This is vital to ensure the patient is well informed before making treatment decisions.

4 Multidisciplinary involvement for prostate cancer is the standard of practice. The MDT should include surgeons, radiation and medical oncologists, radiologists and pathologists. During the case discussion, all aspects of the patient's disease are discussed ranging from diagnosis, staging, treatment and adjuvant therapy, taking into consideration the patient's conditioning, preferences and social situation.

5 Radical prostatectomy is the mainstay curative surgical treatment of localised prostate cancer. It can be performed via open approach, robotically and less commonly, via laparoscopic approach.

6 Radiotherapy is another treatment option for localised prostate cancer with a similar success rate to surgery. This is a good option for patients who decline surgery or those who are not suitable for surgery due to their comorbidities.

7 Informed consent begins with the patient having a good understanding of their disease. This is followed by comprehensive discussions of treatment options, including short- and long-term side-effects. This allows patients to evaluate their options and make an informed decision based on their individual situation.

8 After treatment, patients are followed up with interval PSA monitoring. Detectable or rising PSA post treatment can indicate residual disease or disease recurrence.

9 Long-term side-effects of surgery include urinary incontinence and erectile dysfunction. Radiation side-effects are related to effects of radiation to surrounding organs such as rectum (proctitis), bladder (radiation cystitis) and genitalia (sexual dysfunction, strictures, etc.).

CASE 74: Pyelonephritis

History

- A 42-year-old **female** [1] presents to the ED with a 12-hour history of **right flank pain, dysuria and urinary frequency** [2].
- Her past medical history is significant for **T2DM** [3] and dyslipidaemia.

- She also reports **chills and rigors** [4], and **nausea but no vomiting** [5].
- She **denies haematuria** [6] or **smoking history** [7].
- She has **not had any change in bowel habits** [8].

[1] Most cases of pyelonephritis occur in women, and around 75% of patients have a previous history of cystitis or recurrent UTIs.

[2] These are typical presenting symptoms of pyelonephritis. Most presentations range from mild cystitis with flank discomfort to sepsis.

[3] Patients with diabetes are immunosuppressed and more susceptible to UTIs.

[4] Chills and rigors indicate the patient is febrile. Pyelonephritis can make the patient septic and very unwell.

[5] Patients can often have nausea, likely secondary to the pain and infection.

[6] Patients can have haemorrhagic cystitis from severe UTI.

[7] It is important to ask about smoking history to establish risk for urothelial carcinoma.

[8] Bowel pathology should always be ruled out in patients with acute abdomen.

Examination

- The patient appears **unwell** [1].
- Her vital signs are within normal limits **apart from a mild tachycardia, tachypnoea and a fever to 39.2°C** [2].
- Examination of the **heart and respiratory system is unremarkable** [3].

- The abdomen is **soft and moderately tender at the right flank** [4].
- There is no sign of **peritonism** [5].
- Her **bowel sounds are present** [6].
- **Post-void bladder scan** [7] demonstrates residual volume of 80ml.

[1] Patients with pyelonephritis can be septic and look very unwell.

[2] This set of vital signs (febrile, tachycardic and tachypnoeic) may indicate the patient is septic. It is important to note that the patient is relatively young and has a decent cardiorespiratory reserve and thus, her BP is currently stable. However, if not appropriately treated, patients can decompensate into septic shock.

[3] Systematic examination of the cardiorespiratory system is important. Severe lower lobe pneumonia may sometimes present with upper abdominal pain if atypical, and needs to be ruled out.

[4] Patients with pyelonephritis can often have tenderness on the side of the infection. This is a consequence of ascending UTI and subsequent oedema of the kidney.

[5] Pyelonephritis does not produce symptoms of peritonitis. Kidneys, ureters and bladder are extraperitoneal organs and do not irritate peritoneum.

[6] The presence of bowel sounds helps to rule out bowel obstruction as a cause for this patient's abdominal pain.

[7] It is important to perform a post-void bladder scan to assess a patient's ability to empty their bladder. Urinary retention can be a cause of UTI, which can lead to pyelonephritis.

Investigations

- FBE reports high **WCC count of 19.3 x 10^9/L** [1].
- UEC results show **mildly deranged renal function** [2] with eGFR of 80ml/min/1.73m^2. Electrolytes are normal.
- A **urine dipstick is positive for microscopic haematuria, leucocytes and nitrites** [3].

- **CT KUB shows mild hydronephrosis with perinephric stranding** [4].
- **No obstructing lesion or stones are detected** [5].

[1] Infection and inflammation can cause an elevated WCC. In this patient, pyelonephritis is a severe ascending infection of the upper urinary tract and can cause this.

[2] Mildly deranged renal function can occur with upper tract infection. However, significantly deranged renal function can signal postrenal obstruction.

[3] Urine contains nitrate from protein metabolism. Some bacteria have reductase enzymes that reduce urinary nitrate to nitrite. A positive nitrite test indicates that certain bacteria are present in urine. Bacteria that typically generate a positive nitrite test include *Escherichia coli*, *Klebsiella*, *Enterobacter*, *Serratia*, *Proteus* and *Staphylococcus*. Microscopic haematuria

and leucocytes are expected findings in a patient with pyelonephritis.

[4] A non-contrast CT of the kidneys, ureter and bladder (KUB) is indicated in a patient presenting with flank pain and sepsis. This is to rule out an infected ureteric stone. Mild hydronephrosis and perinephric stranding are common findings in pyelonephritis. Perinephric stranding refers to the appearance of oedema within the perinephric fat on imaging. It is non-specific but can indicate renal inflammation.

[5] Pyelonephritis is the diagnosis of exclusion after an infected obstructed ureteric stone has been ruled out.

Management

Immediate

Monitor **vital signs** [1]. Obtain IV access and **administer broad-spectrum antibiotics** [2] **and fluids** [3]. Insert **2-way indwelling catheter** [4] and monitor urine output.

Short-term

Continue **antibiotic therapy** [5]. The patient can have **diet as tolerated** [6]. Monitor **vital signs, symptoms,**

inflammatory markers and renal function [7]. Chase **urine and blood cultures and taper antibiotic regime** [8] accordingly. Patient can be safely discharged if **fevers settle and bloods have normalised** [9].

Long-term

Follow the patient up in outpatient clinic for further investigations such as **renal tract ultrasound scan and cystoscopy** [10].

[1] Close monitoring of vital signs is important in the initial period. The patient can become septic and develop shock. ICU may need to be involved, depending on how the patient responds to resuscitation.

[2] Broad-spectrum antibiotics such as gentamicin or ceftriaxone (to cover Gram-negative organisms) and ampicillin (to cover *Enterococcus*) are good initial antibiotics.

[3] IV fluid is important in the resuscitation of septic patients. Its primary goal is to ensure adequate intravascular volume to maintain tissue perfusion.

[4] An IDC should be inserted to ensure maximal drainage of infected urine. It also allows for close fluid monitoring in a septic patient.

[5] Antibiotic therapy is the mainstay management in patients with pyelonephritis.

[6] The patient can have solid diet if tolerated, unless there is any coexisting bowel pathology.

[7] A patient's recovery is judged clinically as well as biochemically. If any deterioration in either of these parameters is detected, a repeat CT scan should be performed to look for the development of abscess or postrenal obstruction.

8 Urine and blood culture results should be noted. Highest yield samples are taken prior to commencement of antibiotic therapy and when the patient is febrile. Positive cultures allow targeted antibiotic therapy and potentially decrease development of bacterial resistance.

9 When patients improve symptomatically and biochemically, they are ready for discharge.

10 Ascending upper tract infection is serious and should be investigated further with imaging such as renal tract ultrasound scan and cystoscopy elective to look for anatomical causes of the infection. Recurrent UTI should also be managed in an outpatient setting.

CASE 75: Renal cancer

History

- A **68-year-old** [1] female presents to the Urology clinic with an **incidentally found 5cm renal mass** [2] on renal tract ultrasound.
- She has a **past medical history** [3] significant for T2DM, HTN and hypercholesterolaemia.
- The patient has been referred by her GP for further investigation of **recurrent UTI** [4].

- She does not report **abdominal or flank pain** [5].
- The patient denies **loss of weight, fevers and night sweats** [6].
- She does not have any **lower urinary tract symptoms including haematuria** [7].
- She is a **non-smoker** [8].

[1] The most common age of presentation for renal cell carcinoma (RCC) is 60–70 years of age.

[2] Many tumours are found incidentally during evaluation of unrelated medical issues. Renal tumours are often asymptomatic.

[3] It is also important to ask about hereditary syndromes that are associated with renal tumours such as Birt–Hogg–Dubé syndrome, tuberous sclerosis or von Hippel–Lindau syndrome.

[4] This is a very common scenario – renal tract ultrasound being done routinely for investigation of UTI incidentally finding a renal mass.

[5] Most renal tumours are asymptomatic. The classic triad of flank mass, haematuria and pain signifies advanced disease.

[6] Constitutional symptoms of weight loss, fever and night sweats can indicated metastatic disease or paraneoplastic syndrome. Approximately 20–30% of patients with RCC experience paraneoplastic syndrome and this includes: weight loss, cachexia, fever, elevated ESR, anaemia, HTN, hypercalcaemia, Stauffer syndrome, elevated ALP and polycythaemia.

[7] It is uncommon to see haematuria related to RCC, unless in very advanced disease. Haematuria is more commonly associated with bladder cancer or upper tract urothelial cancer.

[8] Risk factors for RCC include tobacco smoking, obesity, HTN, horseshoe kidney, acquired renal cysts from chronic renal failure and genetic risk factors.

Examination

- The patient appears **well** [1].
- Vital signs are **unremarkable** [2].
- Examination of the **heart and lungs is unremarkable** [3].
- **The abdomen does not appear distended** [4] and there are **no surgical scars** [5].

- No **tenderness** [6] on abdomen is elicited and **no obvious mass is felt on balloting of the kidneys** [7].
- **No lymphadenopathy** [8] is detected.

[1] General inspection of the patient does not reveal any acute pathology, as often renal masses are incidentally found.

[2] The patient's vital signs are within normal range and do not demonstrate signs of paraneoplastic syndrome.

[3] Thorough systematic examination of the cardiorespiratory system should be performed to assess the patient as a surgical candidate. Any obvious abnormalities

should be further investigated to ensure the patient is safe to undergo general anaesthesia for nephrectomy.

[4] Renal masses generally do not cause distension of the abdomen. Kidneys are retroperitoneal structures and do not involve the bowel which is intraperitoneal.

[5] Surgical scars indicate previous surgeries, which can help indicate how difficult the surgery will be if nephrectomy is being considered. Extensive abdominal surgeries can result

in significant adhesions and make transperitoneal approach nephrectomy challenging. In these cases, retroperitoneal approach should be considered.

6 Renal masses are not generally tender unless in very advanced disease which has invaded surrounding structures.

7 Some large renal masses are palpable on balloting of the kidney in thin patients.

8 Lymphadenopathy is not detected in patients with renal masses until in advanced disease with significant paraneoplastic syndrome.

Investigations

- FBE reports normal **haemoglobin level** [1] and WCC.
- **UEC results are normal** [2].
- **LFT results** [3] are within normal ranges.
- **Urine dipstick** [4] does not demonstrate microscopic haematuria.
- **CT IVP shows an enhancing solid 5cm renal mass arising from upper pole of left kidney** [5]; no other filling defects are detected in the upper tracts or the bladder. No lymphadenopathy is detected.
- **Staging CT chest and whole-body bone scan** [6] does not demonstrate any metastasis.
- **MAG3 scan** [7] shows symmetrical renal function, with both kidneys contributing equally.

1 Anaemia can be part of the paraneoplastic syndrome in patients with RCC.

2 Renal function is an important consideration when evaluating patients with RCC. In patients with poor renal function, renal-sparing surgery may need to be considered to prevent patients from needing renal dialysis; whereas in older patients with large tumour and normal renal function, total nephrectomy is more appropriate.

3 Stauffer syndrome is a reversible hepatitis associated with RCC. It is associated with RCC that has not metastasised to the liver.

4 Haematuria is generally not associated with RCC. It is more commonly seen in cases of upper tract urothelial carcinoma or very advanced RCC.

5 CT IVP is a triple-phase contrast scan which accurately evaluates in terms of size, location, solid or cystic and enhancing components. This is a classic description of a renal mass that is suspicious for malignancy.

6 CT chest, abdomen and pelvis as well as a whole-body bone scan are traditional staging scans for renal cell carcinoma. Sites of metastases for RCC include lung, bone, regional lymph nodes, liver, adrenal gland, contralateral kidney and brain.

7 MAG3 is a nuclear medicine scan that investigates differential renal function and obstruction. It is not part of the standard work-up for RCC but is helpful in determining the health of the contralateral kidney if renal impairment is suspected. This is taken into consideration when deciding whether total nephrectomy would put the patient at risk of needing dialysis.

Management

Immediate

Counsel the patient [1] on the results of the investigations. Discuss the patient's case at the next **MDT** [2] meeting. Discuss **surgical management** [3] with the patient.

Short-term

If the decision is for surgical management – **consent the patient and refer them to the anaesthetics clinic** [4] for preoperative work-up. Perform an **elective laparoscopic radical nephrectomy** [5]. Following the procedure, **monitor the patient's vital signs** and drain tube outputs, as well as haemoglobin level and renal function [6]. Patients can generally be **commenced on diet** [7] postoperatively. Patients can be discharged if IDC and drain tubes are safely removed, they are tolerating diet and have returned to **premorbid level of functioning** [8].

Long-term

The patient should be followed up in the **outpatient clinic** [9] for histopathology result and wound check. Ongoing interval follow-up should be arranged for **cancer surveillance** [10].

1 Appropriate patient counselling is very important, especially for cancer diagnosis. Ensure the consultation takes place in a quiet area and allow the patient time to digest the information. Offer the patient written information for further reading at home.

2 Patients with renal cancer should have their case discussed at an MDT meeting to ensure the patient receives optimal management for the disease. The MDT should include surgeons, radiation and medical oncologists, radiologists and pathologists.

3 This patient is likely to benefit from total nephrectomy to cure them of the disease.

4 Appropriate informed consent involves ensuring the patient has an adequate understanding of their disease, management options and their risks. Laparoscopic nephrectomy is considered to be major cancer surgery and the patient should be adequately assessed at anaesthetics clinic for work-up so they can safely undergo general anaesthesia.

5 Laparoscopic nephrectomy is performed using three-port technique with the patient in lateral position, either through transperitoneal or retroperitoneal approaches.

6 Patients are monitored postoperatively for any immediate complications of surgery. These include signs of bleeding, infection, DVT and PE, cardiac events, etc. Drain output can indicate if there is any significant bleeding. Haemoglobin and renal function is also closely monitored postoperatively, especially in case of significant intra-operative bleeding and to ensure the function of the solitary kidney, respectively.

7 Usually, a light diet can be commenced postoperatively following nephrectomy as there is minimal bowel involvement during the surgery. This also ensures adequate nutrition is received in order to recover from surgery more quickly.

8 The patient should ideally be able to function at the level that they were able to prior to surgery. The allied health team (primarily physiotherapy, occupational therapy and social work) should be involved for further assessment on fitness for discharge home.

9 Patients should be seen 2–3 weeks postoperatively in the outpatient clinic to be informed of the final histopathology result, as well as assessing wound healing. This is also an opportunity to inform the patient of the long-term plan for surveillance.

10 Cancer surveillance usually involves monitoring for cancer recurrence with interval imaging, as well as monitoring the function of the solitary kidney. If there are concerns with health of the kidney, renal physicians should be involved early.

CASE 76: Renal colic

History

- A **49-year-old male** [1] with previous **history of renal stones** [2] presents with **left flank pain** [3] over the past **6 hours** [4].
- The patient reports **dysuria** [5] but **no macroscopic haematuria** [6].
- He does not report other **lower urinary tract symptoms** [7].
- He also notes **nausea** [8] without vomiting.
- He denies **fevers** [9] or any **change in bowel habits** [10]. He does not smoke.

1 Urolithiasis can occur in any age group. The age of peak incidence is between 20 and 50 years. The average lifetime risk is 3–8%, with males being more commonly affected.

2 Patients who have a history of renal stones are predisposed to future stone formation. First-time stone formers are at 50% risk of further stones in next 5 years, and 10% have higher recurrent disease.

3 Classic renal colic presents with 'loin-to-groin' pain on the affected side. However, other acute abdominal pathology can also present with similar symptoms, such as diverticulitis, pyelonephritis and aortic aneurysm. Interestingly, pain from renal colic can also be felt in the testicles in males.

4 Renal colic is usually acute and severe, as the ureter peristalses against the stone. Patients generally present to the ED within hours of onset due to its severity. Contrasting the peritonitic pain from bowel pathology where patients prefer to lie still, patients with renal colic usually cannot get comfortable and will often roll around in pain.

5 Dysuria can indicate urinary tract infection but is not a reliable indicator. General irritation of the lower urinary tract

from stones, infection, inflammation or malignancy can all cause dysuria.

6 It is not uncommon for patients to present with macroscopic haematuria in the setting of renal colic, especially those who are taking anticoagulants. Stones irritate the mucosa of ureter or kidney and can cause bleeding.

7 Complete the urological history by asking about general lower urinary tract symptoms.

8 Nausea can be secondary to pain, as well as a side-effect of strong opiate medications that might be given to a patient to control the pain.

9 Fevers in the setting of renal colic indicate an infected obstructed kidney, which is a medical emergency. Patients with urosepsis can deteriorate very quickly and the condition can be life-threatening if not managed appropriately.

10 Patients with flank pain can also have bowel pathology such as diverticulitis or appendicitis if pain is on the right side. Clinicians need to be mindful of these differentials when taking a history.

Examination

- The patient appears in **distress** [1].
- The patient is **mildly tachycardic** [2].
- **Blood pressure is normal** [3].
- He is **afebrile** [4].
- There are no signs of respiratory distress. Auscultation of the **heart and lungs is normal** [5].
- The abdomen does not appear **distended** [6], and no **pulsatile mass** [7] is identified.
- There are **no surgical scars** [8] on the abdomen.
- The patient is **tender over the left flank** [9] on palpation but there is **no rebound tenderness** [10].
- **Bowel sounds are present** [11] on auscultation.

1 Pain from renal colic is often severe, and patients usually find it difficult to stay still. Pain is sharp in nature and comes in waves. Patients can be seen clutching the affected side during episodes of pain.

2 Tachycardia can be associated with sepsis. This is part of the initial SIRS response before decompensation which leads to hypotension. Tachycardia can also be seen in the presence of severe pain.

3 In younger patients, BP can often be maintained in septic state due to their cardiovascular reserve. Hypotension is a late sign of a deteriorating patient.

4 Fever in patients with a ureteric stone is a sign that the kidney is infected obstructed and is a medical emergency. It's one of the absolute indications for intervention in a patient with ureteric stone.

5 It is important to assess the patient holistically to ensure they can safely undergo anaesthesia if required. Abnormal findings on cardiorespiratory system mandate further investigations.

6 Distension of the abdomen is more likely to be a sign of bowel pathology in patients with an acute abdomen. Isolated renal colic does not usually cause abdominal distension.

7 Abdominal aortic aneurysm (AAA) is an important differential in patients with abdominal pain, as the condition can be fatal if not picked up early. A large central pulsatile mass is a sign of AAA.

8 Previous surgical scars can identify important past history and give clues to current presentation. Open surgery for urolithiasis is not performed any more, but scars from percutaneous nephrolithotomy (PCNL) can be identified to suggest previous stone history.

9 Flank tenderness on palpation is not always elicited in patients with renal colic because the kidneys and ureters are deep retroperitoneal structures. In thin patients, the kidneys may be ballotable.

10 Renal colic does not produce the peritonitic signs that acute bowel pathology creates, because the kidneys and ureters are retroperitoneal structures and do not irritate the peritoneum.

11 Bowel obstruction needs to be ruled out in all patients with acute abdomen, and auscultation for bowel sounds is part of that work-up.

Investigations

- FBE demonstrates a mildly **raised WCC** [1].
- **Acute renal impairment** [2] is found on UEC.
- **CRP is elevated** [3] at 40mg/L. LFT results are normal.
- **Urine dipstick** [4] shows microscopic haematuria, but no leucocytes or nitrites are detected.
- A **non-contrast CT KUB** [5] demonstrates a **9mm proximal** [6] left ureteric stone, with associated left **hydronephrosis** [7] and **perinephric stranding** [8].
- There is also a **non-obstructive 6mm right intrarenal stone** [9].
- No **bowel pathology** [10] is found.
- Subsequent **X-ray KUB** [11] shows that the stones are **radio-opaque** [12].

1 Infection and inflammation are common causes of an elevated WCC. In this patient, renal colic with a likely obstructing ureteric stone can explain this finding.

2 Derangement of renal function is commonly seen in renal colic patients. Rising creatinine in patients with obstructing stones, stones in a patient's single kidney or bilateral ureteric stones are indications for prompt surgical intervention.

3 CRP is a generic marker of infection and inflammation and is commonly mildly raised in renal colic patients. Markedly raised CRP levels suggest sepsis.

4 Urine dipstick is an important component in an acute stone work-up. Microscopic haematuria is expected in renal colic but if negative, another differential diagnosis should be explored. Presence of leucocytes and nitrites indicates UTI and that is another indication for intervention in an acute stone episode.

5 Non-contrast CT kidneys, ureters and bladder (KUB) is the gold standard investigation for renal colic and should be the first obtained when urolithiasis is suspected. It detects all stones except for protease inhibitor stones, but these are rare. In pregnant females and children, renal tract ultrasound is recommended as the initial study.

6 Stones are likely to pass spontaneously when small in size and located in the distal portion of ureter. Stones ≤5 mm in width can usually be conservatively managed because of the high probability (68%) of spontaneous passage, which can take up to 4 weeks. At 9mm width, there is only a 3% chance that this stone can pass spontaneously, especially being at the proximal end of the ureter.

7 Hydronephrosis is dilatation of the renal pelvis and calyces due to increased pressure from distal obstruction. This is a common finding in renal colic cases, as all ureteric stones will produce upstream obstruction to some degree.

8 Perinephric stranding refers to the appearance of oedema within the perinephric fat on imaging. It is non-specific but can indicate renal inflammation or acute obstruction, and is commonly detected on CT in patients with stones.

9 Non-obstructing intrarenal stones are usually incidentally detected. They generally do not produce symptoms until they drop into the ureter or grow to a large size. These do not need to be treated in the acute setting.

10 CT KUB can also detect some bowel pathology, which is an important differential diagnosis in patients with acute abdomen.

11 X-ray KUB can be helpful in determining the stone composition, and useful in stone follow-up. This is not always obtained in the acute setting.

12 Calcium stones are the most common type of stones encountered and they are radio-opaque. Uric acid stones are radiolucent and can be dissolved with urinary alkalisation therapy.

Management

Immediate

Monitor **vital signs** [1] and provide **analgesia** [2]. Keep patient **fasted** [3]. Obtain IV access and administer **fluids** [4]. Seek advice from the **Urology team** [5].

Short-term

Perform **emergency cystoscopy and ureteric stent placement** [6]. Following the procedure, the patient should be kept in hospital for **monitoring** [7]. The patient can commence on a **full diet** [8]. Reviews should include the patient's vital signs and **level of pain** [9]. The patient can be discharged if stable and their **pain is manageable** [10] with oral analgesia.

Long-term

Patient will be booked for an **elective laser lithotripsy** [11] for removal of their stone. This is usually performed as a **day procedure** [12]. Further follow-up should be arranged in outpatient clinic for results of **stone analysis** and **further work-up** [13] of the patient's stone disease.

1 Ensure the patient remains haemodynamically stable prior to operative treatment. Patients with confirmed ureteric stones who spike a temperature require urgent surgical management.

2 Analgesia is an important part of stone management. Indometacin suppositories are effective for renal colic. Patients will also likely require opiates for break-through pain.

3 This patient has a stone that is unlikely to pass spontaneously and will require surgical intervention. Keep the patient fasted to ensure safety for anaesthesia and reduce aspiration risk.

4 Keeping a fasted patient hydrated is important. In patients with sepsis, fluids are required to ensure stability of BP.

5 Urolithiasis is managed by Urology and a prompt referral should be made.

6 Cystoscopy and stent insertion are performed under general anaesthesia with the patient in lithotomy position. Ureteric stent is a hollow plastic tube that has loops on either end to help it anchor to the renal pelvis as well as the bladder. Stents help to eliminate the obstruction by bypassing the stone and re-establish antegrade urine flow from the kidney. Contrast is used to outline the anatomy of the upper urinary tract and the stent is placed under intra-operative X-ray guidance.

7 Post stent insertion, the patient should be monitored for signs of sepsis in a phenomenon called 'septic shower', following the removal of the infected obstructing stone. This is more common in septic patients preoperatively.

8 In patients with no bowel pathology, a full diet can be commenced postoperatively.

9 After stent insertion, colicky pain from the stone should markedly improve. However, stents can cause irritation, especially when the patient voids.

10 The patient can be discharged when they are comfortable with simple oral analgesia.

11 Stone treatment is a stepwise process. Ureteric stents are placed in the first instance to allow the acute infection or inflammation to settle. Laser lithotripsy to fragment and remove the stone is performed electively. A small ureteroscope and holmium laser is used for this procedure.

12 Laser lithotripsy is an elective procedure performed under general anaesthesia. Patients can generally be discharged on the same day.

13 Stones removed during laser lithotripsy can be sent for analysis. This aids in the ongoing management of stone disease. Most stone disease is caused by dehydration, but uric acid stones can be managed with urine alkalisation. As a baseline, serum chemistries including sodium, potassium, chloride, bicarbonate, uric acid, calcium and creatinine should be obtained.

CASE 77: Renal trauma

History

- A 22-year-old male with no **past medical history** [1] presents with **right flank pain** [2] and **macroscopic haematuria** [3] over the past 4 hours.
- This is following a **football training accident** [4] where he was struck in the back on the right side during a tackle.

- He denies **head strike or loss of consciousness** [5] and does not report any **bony tenderness, nor neurological deficits** [6] in the limbs.
- He does not have any **pain in the chest or abdomen** [7].
- He denies other **lower urinary tract symptoms** [8].

[1] Past history is important to explore in the setting of trauma. Pre-existing renal lesions can increase the risk of renal injury from blunt trauma. Anticoagulants and antiplatelet agents can significantly complicate a bleeding patient in trauma.

[2] Flank pain/bruising is a common presentation in renal trauma.

[3] Haematuria is often present during renal trauma. However, haematuria can be absent even when significant renal injury exists.

[4] The kidney is the most common genitourinary organ injured by trauma and accounts for 5% of all trauma cases. Most traumatic renal injuries are caused by blunt trauma.

Penetrating renal trauma is often associated with other internal injuries.

[5] It is important to rule out other injuries, such as head trauma, when assessing this group of patients.

[6] Due to the mechanism of injury, fractures and spinal injury need to be assessed and ruled out.

[7] In severe injuries, patients can present with rib fractures and distended abdomen from an expanding haematoma.

[8] Complete the urological history by asking about other lower urinary tract symptoms, which can occasionally pick up issues such as urethral strictures in young patients, which can complicate catheter insertion.

Examination

- The patient appears **well** [1].
- His vital signs are **within normal limits** [2].
- **Primary survey** [3] of the patient does not reveal any immediate instability.
- Examination of the **head** [4] does not reveal any laceration or skull injuries; **cranial nerve** [5] examination is also normal.
- No soft tissue injury of the **neck** [6] is noted and **trachea** [7] is midline.
- Examination of the **chest** [8] reveals no tenderness of the ribs; auscultation of the lungs shows normal air entry and breath sounds.
- **Cardiac** [9] examination is also negative.

- The **abdomen is not distended** [10].
- The patient is **tender over the right flank with some overlying bruising** [11].
- No **rebound tenderness** [12] is elicited and bowel sounds are present.
- No bony tenderness can be elicited over the **pelvis** [13].
- **Spinal examination** [14] is negative for midline tenderness.
- Examination of the **limbs** [15] does not show any soft tissue or bony injuries, and no **neurological deficits** [16] are detected.
- **Post void bladder scan** [17] shows a residual of 15ml.

[1] General inspection of a trauma patient can often give clues to how severe the injury is. Young patients, however, can seem well despite severe underlying injuries, due to their cardiovascular reserve.

[2] Low BP is a late sign of severe trauma and can indicate significant bleeding. Tachycardia can be an early sign of hypovolaemia due to haemorrhage in trauma cases.

3 The primary survey is a rapid assessment of the trauma patient to identify any immediate life-threatening injuries. Any life-threatening abnormalities are identified and corrected during primary survey. The secondary survey, which is a head-to-toe assessment, is then carried out when the patient has been stabilised after primary survey.

4 The head is examined for any lacerations and bony injury to the skull.

5 Cranial nerve examinations can identify any intracranial injuries such as haematoma.

6 The neck is examined for bruising, soft tissue injuries, and penetrating injuries to great vessels, trachea or oesophagus.

7 Deviation of trachea can indicate tension pneumothorax, which is a medical emergency and requires prompt intervention.

8 Examination of the chest can reveal contusion, rib fractures, pneumothorax, haemothorax, etc.

9 Examination of the cardiovascular system is to rule out intrinsic cardiac abnormalities as well as for assessment of fluid status.

10 Renal trauma, especially when there are vascular injuries, can cause an expanding haematoma that leads to abdominal/flank distension, and is life-threatening. Urgent intervention is required.

11 Bruising and tenderness over the flank areas is an indication of possible renal injury.

12 Isolated renal injury in the absence of concurrent intraperitoneal injury does not usually produce peritonism.

13 Concurrent pelvic injury is important to rule out as a cause of haemorrhage. Pelvic bleeds can be devastating.

14 Spinal examination is essential in all trauma cases. Proper spinal precaution needs to remain in place before spinal injuries have been ruled out. Spinal examination should be performed with the assistance of a log-roll, and appropriate imaging with X-ray or CT needs to be carried out.

15 Fracture and soft tissue injuries of the limbs are also assessed on secondary survey. If indicated, X-rays should be performed.

16 Neurological examination is carried out as part of a spinal examination to identify any significant nerve damage.

17 Minimal post residual volume confirms that the patient is not in clot retention from haematuria. In patients with light haematuria, an IDC is not always indicated.

Investigations

- FBE shows a **haemoglobin level of 120g/L** [1] and a mildly **elevated WCC** [2], and UEC results are normal. CRP and LFT levels are within normal ranges.
- **INR level is 1.0** [3].
- **Urine dipstick** [4] shows haematuria.
- **CT IVP** [5] demonstrates a **2cm cortical laceration** [6] of the right kidney with a **small perinephric haematoma** [7], **without collecting system or vascular injury** [8].
- This is consistent with **grade III renal injury** [9].

1 Haemoglobin is an important indicator of severe haemorrhage secondary to renal trauma. The patient's blood should be taken for a blood group and hold, and cross-matched for transfusion if required.

2 Elevated WCC is associated with infection and inflammation. This can occur in the setting of renal trauma.

3 It is important to check patients' coagulation profile, especially those who are on anticoagulants. High INR level needs to be reversed with guidance from haematology, to reduce haemorrhage risks.

4 Urine dipstick can detect microscopic haematuria, which is a significant finding in context of renal trauma. However, haematuria is absent in up to 40% of renal and 25% of pedicle injuries.

5 CT IVP is a triple-phase CT scan that aims to illustrate the collecting systems, ureters and bladder with IV contrast. It has a non-contrast phase, nephrographic phase and delayed phase. The delayed phase allows the opacification of the collecting system to examine for contrast extravasation that indicates injury.

6 An isolated 2cm cortical laceration without collecting system or vascular involvement classifies this injury as grade III.

7 The perinephric haematoma is consistent with the cortical laceration. However, a haematoma medial to the kidney can suggest vascular injury.

8 Involvement of the collecting system or vascular injury upgrades the renal injury to grade IV. This increases the likelihood of requiring intervention and of long-term complications.

9 The American Association for the Surgery of Trauma grading of renal trauma is as follows:
- I – contusion or subcapsular haematoma
- II – <1cm deep cortical laceration without urinary extravasation
- III – >1cm deep cortical laceration without collecting system injury
- IV – laceration through to collecting system or renal artery/vein injury
- V – completely shattered kidney.

Management

Immediate

Obtain **IV access** [1]. Keep the patient limited to **bed rest** [2]. Monitor **vital signs** [3] and perform **serial Hb** [4] monitoring. Contact **ICU/HDU and Urology** [5] for review.

Short-term

Insert **IDC** [6] if patient has dark haematuria or clot retention. Confine patient to **strict bed rest** [7] until haematuria settles. Perform serial examination and Hb check. Consider **rescan** [8] of patient if they clinically deteriorate. **Discharge** [9] patient when haematuria settles, vitals and haemoglobin level remain stable.

Long-term

Follow the patient up in outpatient clinic in 6–12 weeks for **BP monitoring** [10] and **bloods** [11]. Consider **CT or renal tract ultrasound** [12] to exclude **complications** [13].

1 Obtaining IV access is necessary for administering fluids, taking bloods and for urgent transfusion if required.

2 Grade III injury can be conservatively managed by bed rest to allow the laceration to heal and prevent delayed bleeds.

3 Close monitoring of vital signs allows for early detection of deterioration of the trauma patient.

4 Serial haemoglobins every 6–12 hours is recommended for close monitoring of potential delayed bleeding, which occurs in 20% of grade III–V injuries.

5 Haemorrhagic complication from renal trauma can be life-threatening, so close monitoring in ICU/HDU is recommended. The Urology team should be involved in the care of the patient, as they will be responsible for the acute and long-term management of the patient.

6 An IDC is indicated in case of significant haematuria. However, if haematuria is light, patients can be encouraged to keep samples of urine for physicians to monitor urine colour.

7 Most renal trauma patients who are stable can be conservatively managed with bed rest to allow injuries to heal.

8 In the case of deterioration of vital signs, drop in haemoglobin or worsening haematuria, rescan with CT is indicated.

9 Patients can be discharged when vital signs and haemoglobin remain stable and haematuria resolves. Patients should be encouraged to not be involved in contact sport and perform light duties only at work for at least 4 weeks.

10 Late complications of renal lacerations such as hypertension occur in 5% of renal trauma patients. This is secondary to ischaemia causing renin release. There are two mechanisms. The first is related to compression of kidney by haematoma or fibrosis (Page kidney), and the second renal artery thrombosis or stenosis (Goldblatt kidney).

11 Renal function should be monitored for long-term renal dysfunction.

12 Follow-up scans should be considered to ensure resolution of injury and monitor for complications. Renal tract ultrasound is appropriate in younger patients and CT should be considered in older patients.

13 Late complications include HTN, fistula formation, persistent urinoma, infection and perinephric abscess formation.

CASE 78: Testicular cancer

History

- A **23-year-old male** [1] with no known past medical history is **referred to ED with a newly detected right testicular mass** [2] .
- This is in the setting of a **recent skateboarding accident** [3] where the patient was struck in the scrotum.
- He **denies any testicular pain** [4] .
- He does not report any symptoms of **fevers, loss of weight, night sweats or back pain** [5] .
- The patient does not **have history of cryptorchidism or family history of testicular cancer** [6] .

[1] Testicular cancer is the most common cancer in males aged 20–40 years. Testicular cancer comprises 1–1.5% of male neoplasms and 5% of urological malignancies.

[2] It is not uncommon for patients to see their GP with an incidentally detected mass in a testicle and be referred urgently to ED for management. Newly diagnosed testicular tumour should be managed with a sense of urgency.

[3] Trauma is not a cause of tumour but often prompts medical evaluation of the testicles and consequent incidental detection of tumours.

[4] Most tumours present with a painless mass or swelling in the testis. Testicular tumours can also present with hydrocele in 5–10% of the cases; and testicular pain is present in up to 27% of the cases, mainly due to infarction or haemorrhage.

[5] Presence of constitutional symptoms can signify advanced disease. Back pain or abdominal mass can occur with bulky retroperitoneal metastases.

[6] Risk factors for testicular cancer include cryptorchidism, personal history of testicular tumour, family history, HIV and Klinefelter syndrome.

Examination

- The patient appears **well** [1] .
- His vital signs are **unremarkable** [2] .
- Testicular examination reveals a **painless 1cm firm lump at the superior pole of the right testicle** [3] .
- Examination of the **contralateral testicle** [4] is normal.
- Examination of the **abdomen does not reveal any mass or tenderness** [5] .
- **Cardiac and respiratory examinations** [6] are unremarkable.
- No **lymphadenopathy** [7] is detected.

[1] Patients with testicular tumours are generally well unless significant metastatic disease is present.

[2] These vital signs indicate the patient is stable and not acutely unwell. This picture is not consistent with an infective cause of testicular mass.

[3] A painless solid lump of the testis is malignant until proven otherwise. Differential diagnoses of intra-testicular mass include lymphoma, leukaemia, metastasis (from prostate, lung, GI tract or melanoma), epidermoid cyst, haematoma and abscess.

[4] It is important to examine the contralateral testicle. Having a tumour of one testicle is a risk factor for developing a tumour in the contralateral testicle. Lymphoma can present as bilateral tumours in 35% of cases.

[5] In patients with advanced disease and bulky retroperitoneal disease, abdominal pain and mass may be detected.

[6] A systematic examination should include the cardiorespiratory system to ensure no significant abnormalities exist to put patients at risk during general anaesthesia.

[7] Lymph node examination should be included to assess for nodal spread from testicular malignancy. Firm, non-tender nodes that are tethered to surrounding structures are suggestive of malignancy. Tender and mobile nodes are suggestive of infection/inflammation.

Investigations

- **FBE reveals a normal haemoglobin and WCC** [1] . UEC results are normal.
- LFT results are normal. Tumour markers of **beta-hCG** [2] and **AFP** [3] levels are normal; **LDH** [4] level is mildly elevated.
- **Ultrasound** [5] demonstrates a 1.5cm homogenous solid vascular mass at the superior pole of right testicle.
- **CT of the chest, abdomen and pelvis** [6] is negative for metastatic disease.

[1] Normal WCC suggests that the mass is unlikely to be of infective origin.

[2] Tumour markers need to be checked prior to treatment. Elevation in hCG level is more commonly seen in non-seminomatous germ cell tumour (40–60%) than seminomas (10%). It is always elevated in choriocarcinoma. Other causes of elevated hCG include marijuana use and hypergonadotrophic hypogonadism. hCG has a half-life of 1–3 days.

[3] AFP is never elevated in pure seminomas and raised in 50–70% of non-seminomatous germ cell tumours. It is also elevated in pregnancy, infants <1 year old, liver disease and other malignancies. AFP has a half-life of 5–7 days.

[4] LDH is a non-specific tumour marker that increases in proportion to tumour volume. It has a half-life of 4 days.

[5] Testicular ultrasound is the gold standard investigation to confirm the presence of a mass, whether it is intratesticular or extratesticular, and its vascularity.

[6] CT staging is used to assess metastatic disease. Common sites of metastases include retroperitoneal lymph nodes, lung, liver, brain, bone, kidney, adrenal, GI tract and spleen.

Management

Immediate

Inform patient of the relevant **investigation findings** [1] . Seek advice from the **Urology team** [2] .

Short-term

Perform **emergency or urgent elective right inguinal orchidectomy** [3] . Following the procedure, the patient can be discharged as a day case or be monitored overnight. Review the patient's **vital signs and surgical site** [4] . The patient can be discharged if there is no **immediate complication from surgery** [5] .

Long-term

Follow the patient up in the outpatient clinic for a **wound check and to inform patient of the histopathology results** [6] . Discuss the case at the **MDT meeting** [7] and refer to a **medical oncologist** [8] for consideration of chemotherapy.

[1] It is important to update the patient on the results of the investigations, as the patient and his family are likely to be anxious about the diagnosis.

[2] Testicular tumour is managed by the Urology team and consult should be obtained for the patient.

[3] Orchidectomy for cancer is performed through an open inguinal approach. As the layers of the scrotum are contiguous with the layers of abdominal wall, there are risks of tumour seeding through the tissue planes if the surgery is performed through scrotal approach.

[4] Monitor the patient postoperatively to ensure he recovers well from the anaesthetic and there are no immediate complications from surgery.

[5] The main immediate complication of surgery is haematoma or haemorrhage. The incision site and scrotum should be examined for pain and swelling.

[6] Patients should be seen in the outpatient clinic to ensure healing of wound site and to examine for signs of infection or haematoma. The histopathology result should also be explained to the patient and his family during the consultation.

[7] Management of testicular cancer requires a multidisciplinary approach. Imaging and pathology results should be discussed at the MDT which consists of surgeons, radiation and medical oncologists, radiologists and pathologists.

[8] An appropriate referral needs to be made to medical oncology for consideration of chemotherapy to ensure cure of disease as well as to reduce likelihood of recurrence.

CASE 79: Testicular torsion

History

- A **15-year-old** [1] male with no known past medical history presents with **sudden** [2] onset **constant** [3] left testicular pain over the last **4 hours** [4].
- He also notes **nausea and vomiting** [5].

- He denies any **urinary symptoms** [6].
- He is not **sexually active** [7] and does not report any **history of trauma to the genital region** [8].
- He denies **similar episodes in the past** [9].

[1] Testicular torsion is most common in males between 12 and 18 years, but it can occur at any age.

[2] A sudden onset nature of pain is classic of torsion. Infective causes of acute testicular pain often produce a gradual worsening pattern of pain. A typical presentation, particularly in children, is for the patient to wake up with scrotal pain in the middle of the night or in the morning.

[3] Pain due to testicular torsion is usually constant and not relieved by rest. This is compared to pain from epididymo-orchitis that classically worsens with movements and is relieved by rest.

[4] Time is critically important in the diagnosis and management of testicular torsion. Most testicles remain viable when they are detorted within 6 hours. It is generally believed that the testis suffers irreversible damage after 8 hours of ischaemia, and few testicles remain viable when they are detorted after 24 hours after torsion. Infertility may result, even with a normal contralateral testis. This may be due to disruption of the immunologic 'blood–testis' barrier, and exposure of antigens from germ cells and sperm to the general circulation, with subsequent development of anti-sperm antibodies.

[5] Nearly 90% of patients may have associated nausea and vomiting.

[6] It is important to assess urinary symptoms that may suggest underlying UTI as a cause for epididymo-orchitis. This is, however, a less common cause in this age group.

[7] Sexually active patients need to be assessed for sexually transmitted infections (STIs). Common STIs such as chlamydia and gonorrhoea are frequent causes of epididymo-orchitis in males <35 years of age. For patients with a reasonable index of suspicion for STI, first-pass urine PCR should be performed, and appropriate empirical treatment initiated.

[8] Trauma can lead to scrotal haematoma and testicular rupture.

[9] Intermittent testicular torsion, characterised by the sudden onset of acute and intermittent sharp testicular pain and scrotal swelling, with rapid resolution (within seconds to a few minutes) and long intervals without symptoms, should be considered in patients with recurrent history of testicular pain without other identifiable causes.

Examination

- The patient appears in distress and **uncomfortable at rest** [1].
- Vital signs are unremarkable. Of note, temperature is **37.2°C** [2].
- Examination of the penis does not demonstrate any **meatal stenosis** [3].
- Testicular examination reveals an **exquisitely tender, high-riding left testicle in a horizontal lie** [4]. Right testicle is non-tender with normal vertical lie.

- **Cremasteric reflex** [5] is absent on the left side, and **Prehn's sign** [6] is negative.
- No **'blue-dot' sign** [7] is present.
- The abdomen does not appear distended, and there is no evidence of **surgical scars** [8].
- **Abdomen is not tender** [9] and no **inguinal hernia** [10] can be detected.

1 Patients with testicular torsion are often very uncomfortable, even when resting in bed. The pain is exacerbated with movements. The pain associated with epididymo-orchitis, however, can be relieved with rest.

2 Fevers in patients with an acute scrotum can suggest an infective cause such as epididymo-orchitis. Beware of concomitant viral illness in young patients which may complicate the clinical picture.

3 Meatal stenosis may cause chronic urinary retention and recurrent UTIs. This can lead to infective causes of acute scrotal pathology.

4 These are classic examination findings of acute testicular torsion. Twisting of the spermatic cord draws the testis high up in the scrotum and the ischaemic pain from lack of blood flow can be severe. Prolonged torsion can also induce oedema and the scrotum often appears swollen on examination.

5 The cremasteric reflex is the elevation of the testes in response to stroking of the upper inner thigh. This reflex is absent in testicular torsion.

6 According to Prehn's sign, the elevation of the scrotal contents relieves the pain in patients with epididymitis and aggravates or has no effect on the pain in patients with testicular torsion. Negative Prehn's sign indicates no pain relief with lifting the affected testicle, which points towards testicular torsion. However, this is not a reliable clinical feature.

7 Torsion of the appendix testis is a common cause of acute testicular pain in this age group. It typically demonstrates a non-tender testicle and a tender localised mass that is palpable, usually at the superior pole of the testis. The appendix may be ischaemic or gangrenous and appears through the scrotum as the 'blue-dot sign'.

8 Surgical scars can give hints about previous operations such as correction of undescended testis.

9 It is important to perform a thorough abdominal examination, as intra-abdominal pathology can cause referred pain to the testicles. Renal colic is an example.

10 Indirect inguinal hernias can cause acute scrotal tenderness. Patients would more often present with pain and prominent scrotal swelling.

Investigations

- FBE reports a **mildly elevated WCC** [1] . Other blood tests are within normal limits.
- A **urine dipstick is normal** [2] .

- An urgent scrotal ultrasound demonstrates **absent blood flow to the left testicle** [3] .

1 Infection and inflammation are common causes of an elevated WCC. In this patient, the presence of testicular torsion may explain these findings.

2 Urine dipstick is a good screening tool in patients with testicular pain, especially if epididymo-orchitis is suspected, as UTI is a common cause. In patients who are sexually active, a urine STI screen should also be performed. Dipstick is also useful if renal colic is a differential diagnosis, as it can detect microscopic haematuria.

3 When available, a Doppler ultrasound scan of the testicles done in a timely manner can assist in diagnosis of testicular torsion. Ultrasound can assess testicular and epididymal size, scrotal fluid, scrotal wall thickening, enlarged appendix testis, twisting of the spermatic cord, and arterial flow in the testis and epididymis. Demonstration of decreased testicular perfusion or twisting of the spermatic cord is consistent with testicular torsion. However, if there is a high index of suspicion for testicular torsion, surgical exploration of the scrotum should not be delayed by ultrasound.

Management

Immediate

Provide **analgesia** [1] and keep the patient **fasted** [2] . Seek **urgent Urology review** [3] .

Short-term

Perform emergency **scrotal exploration** [4] . Following the procedure, keep the patient in hospital overnight for **monitoring** [5] . Review the patient's surgical site to look for signs of **haematoma** [6] . The patient can be discharged if vital signs remain normal and **pain** [7] is controlled with oral analgesia.

Long-term

Follow the patient up in an **outpatient clinic** [8] if necessary for continuing wound management and monitoring for postoperative complications.

1 Ensure the patient is given adequate analgesia. This also helps to alleviate the anxiety in young patients undergoing surgery.

2 Keeping the patient fasted is crucial in the preoperative management of the patient. It reduces the risk of aspiration in the setting of general anaesthesia. Ideally, patients should be fasted off solid foods for 6 hours, and clear fluids for 2 hours prior to induction of anaesthesia.

3 Testicular torsion falls under the domain of Urology, and patients suspected of having torsion need to be assessed urgently. The viability of a torsed testicle is dependent upon the duration and completeness of torsion – 4–6 hours: ~100%; >12 hours: 20%; >24 hours: 0%.

4 The treatment for testicular torsion involves surgical exploration of the scrotum, as well as detorsion and fixation (orchidopexy) of both testes. Orchidectomy (removal of the testis) is performed if the testicle is non-viable.

5 Patients should be monitored postoperatively to ensure that they completely recover from anaesthesia, that they do not develop acute complications of surgery, and for pain control.

6 Review the surgical site to ensure proper closure, as well as the amount of bleeding or development of haematoma, and any signs of infection from the wound.

7 Pain from testicular torsion should be significantly improved postoperatively if managed appropriately. If ongoing severe pain is reported, look for signs of complication. Patients can be discharged if comfortable on simple oral analgesia.

8 The need for ongoing follow-up depends on the outcomes of the surgery. Most patients are well enough to be managed by their GP. Some will require follow-up visits to ensure adequate recovery and healing of wound, or to discuss future placement of testicular prosthesis in patients who required orchidectomy for non-viable testicle.

CASE 80: Urinary retention

History

- A **78-year-old male** [1] presents to the ED with a 12-hour history of **difficulty passing urine** [2].
- His past medical history includes **stroke, T2DM** [3], ischaemic heart disease and HTN.
- He reports worsening **suprapubic pain and only being able to pass dribbles of urine** [4].
- His premorbid lower urinary tract symptoms include **hesitancy, reduced flow, incomplete emptying and terminal dribble** [5].

- He also reports **daytime frequency, urgency and nocturia four times per night** [6], but no **dysuria or macroscopic haematuria** [7].
- He denies change in bowel habits and **last opened his bowels yesterday** [8].

[1] Lower urinary tract symptoms caused by benign prostatic hyperplasia (BPH) commonly affect men over the age of 60 years.

[2] This presentation suggests the patient may be in acute urinary retention as a complication of BPH.

[3] Stroke and diabetes can cause various bladder dysfunction and may contribute to worsening lower urinary tract symptoms.

[4] These are common presenting symptoms of acute urinary retention. The risk of BPH progression to worse symptoms, acute retention or surgical intervention is higher in men with larger prostate size, higher PSA, older age, low urine flow rates and more severe symptoms.

[5] This set of symptoms represents voiding or obstructive lower urinary tract symptoms. This results from progressive bladder outlet obstruction from BPH.

[6] This set of symptoms is indicative of irritative lower urinary tract symptoms. With progressive bladder outlet obstruction, the bladder may become overworked, leading to symptoms of overactive bladder. There are a number of other causes for irritative lower urinary tract symptoms.

[7] These are red-flag lower urinary tract symptoms which should prompt further investigation. When haematuria is present, underlying malignancy needs to be ruled out in the first instance.

[8] Constipation can be a common cause of acute urinary retention.

Examination

- The patient appears **uncomfortable** [1].
- The vital signs are unremarkable apart from a **borderline tachycardia** [2].
- **Mucous membranes are dry** [3].
- Examination of the **cardiorespiratory system is otherwise unremarkable** [4].
- The patient's **abdomen appears distended and tender to palpation over the suprapubic region** [5].

- The **bladder is percussible to the umbilicus** [6].
- There is no **flank tenderness** [7] on examination.
- **Digital rectal examination** [8] reveals a large prostate gland with benign features.
- **Post-void bladder scan** [9] demonstrates residual urine volume of 1.2L.

1 Acute urinary retention can be very distressing to patients and needs prompt relief.

2 The patient's tachycardia can be due to pain and discomfort from the retention. Otherwise, his vital signs suggest he is stable and not acutely septic or unwell.

3 The appearance of dry mucous membranes suggests the patient is dehydrated.

4 A systematic examination should include the cardiorespiratory system to ensure there are no coexisting abnormalities, given the patient's history.

5 Abdominal distension is consistent with urinary retention, and the bladder can be palpable in severe retention.

6 A full bladder is dull on percussion. If the patient's bladder is palpable up to the umbilicus, this means they are in retention with a large volume.

7 Examine the abdomen and flanks to ensure there is no coexisting pathology. This can include bowel pathology and renal colic.

8 It is important to perform a DRE to assess the prostate. Abnormalities such as size and signs of malignancy such as firmness, nodularity and irregularities can be detected.

9 A post-void bladder scan will confirm the diagnosis of urinary retention, defined as a residual volume of >400ml. It is a simple and rapid bedside test.

Investigations

- FBE reports a **mildly elevated WCC** [1] .
- UEC demonstrates **acute renal failure** [2] with a creatinine of 300μmol/L and an eGFR of 10ml/min/1.73m^2.
- **Electrolyte levels** [3] are normal. CRP level is normal.
- A **urine dipstick** [4] shows trace leucocytes, but no microscopic haematuria or nitrites are detected.
- **CT KUB demonstrates bilateral hydroureteronephrosis down to the vesicoureteric junction (VUJ)** [5] , but no obstructing lesions or stones are seen.
- Renal tract ultrasound shows an **enlarged prostate at 85cc** [6] , moderate bilateral hydronephroureterosis down to the bladder.

1 Infection and inflammation are common causes of an elevated WCC. Patients with acute urinary retention can cause this pattern.

2 When bladder outlet obstruction secondary to BPH is severe and prolonged, the bladder may decompensate. This results in absent or ineffective contractions that do not empty the bladder. Chronic hydronephrosis can lead to renal impairment. This is obstructive nephropathy.

3 It is important to ensure electrolyte levels are stable in acute renal failure as they can have significant implications. Electrolytes including sodium, potassium, magnesium and phosphate should be monitored at least daily.

4 Urine dipstick can be used to check for UTI, as that can contribute to urinary retention.

5 This is a typical imaging finding of obstructive nephropathy – chronic retention causing back pressure up to the kidneys appearing as enlarged kidneys and ureters, commonly associated with renal impairment.

6 Renal tract ultrasound is useful to assess prostate size and upper tract dilatation as well as post-void residuals. A prostate size on renal ultrasound of around 25cc is considered normal. In this instance, the patient's prostate is grossly enlarged and confirms bilateral hydronephrosis consistent with obstructive nephropathy.

Management

Immediate

Insert an **IDC** [1]. Monitor vital signs and urine output for **post-obstructive diuresis** [2]. Replace excessive urine output with **IV fluids** [3]. Seek advice from the **Urology team** [4].

Short-term

Monitor **urine output, renal function and electrolytes** [5]. Commence **combination therapy of an alpha blocker and 5-alpha-reductase inhibitor** [6]. Educate the patient about **catheter and leg bag management** [7]. Discharge the patient when **urine output normalises and UECs stabilise** [8]. Arrange for **elective transurethral resection of the prostate (TURP)** [9].

Long-term

Follow the patient up in clinic after TURP to **review histopathology** [10] and the patient's **lower urinary tract symptoms** [11].

---

[1] It is critical to insert an IDC promptly to relieve the patient's discomfort and bladder outlet obstruction. Do not use excessive force if resistance is encountered, to avoid creating false passages. Ensure the catheter is inserted to the hilt before inflating the balloon.

[2] Post-obstructive diuresis is the prominent polyuria that occurs after relieving complete obstruction of the urinary system. Post-obstructive diuresis is present when urine output is ≥200ml/hour for 2 consecutive hours. Most commonly, it is due to osmotic diuresis secondary to accumulation of non-absorbable solutes especially urea. Other contributing factors can include physiological diuresis, nephrogenic diabetes insipidus, impaired proximal tubular sodium reabsorption and circulating hormones.

[3] There are different protocols for fluid replacement during post-obstructive diuresis. It is reasonable to replace 50–100% of the urine output with IV fluids. Ensure not to perpetuate the diuresis by overzealous fluid replacement.

[4] Urinary retention and obstructive nephropathy are managed by the Urology team.

[5] Urine output should be monitored hourly, with UEC and CMP being monitored twice daily in the initial period. Renal function should improve significantly with relief of obstruction, even though it may never return to baseline.

[6] Alpha blockers cause relaxation of smooth muscle in the bladder neck and prostate. 5-alpha-reductase inhibitor blocks the conversion of testosterone to dihydrotestosterone. Combination therapy improves voiding symptoms, reduces prostate volume and vascularity.

[7] Obstructive nephropathy is an indication for TURP and the IDC needs to remain *in situ* until surgery. The patient needs to be taught how to manage catheter and urinary bags at home.

[8] When urine output normalises and there is adequate improvement in renal function, the patient can be discharged home with an IDC.

[9] Elective TURP can be performed under general or spinal anaesthesia. A resectoscope is used to shave away the prostate transurethrally. A 3-way IDC will be inserted postoperatively to ensure bleeding settles. The patient would normally stay in hospital for 2 nights following.

[10] Up to 10% of patients undergoing TURP are found to have incidental prostate cancer, thus a scheduled review of the histopathology is crucial to ensure nothing is missed.

[11] Finally, patients should be reviewed to ensure their lower urinary tract symptoms improve postoperatively. If symptoms persist, look for other causes by doing further investigations.

History

- A **69-year-old** [1] **male** [2] with **high blood pressure, elevated cholesterol** [3] and a **20 pack year smoking history** [4] presents with **constant mild lower back and flank pain** [5] worsening over the past few weeks [6].
- He also notes **nausea and vomiting and early satiety** [7].
- He does not have a history of other **artery aneurysms** [8] but has a cousin who had a **AAA repaired** [9].
- He states he has **not experienced these symptoms before** [10].
- He denies **pain in his limbs or fever and malaise** [11].
- He also denies feeling **light-headed** or having a **syncopal episode** [12].
- Further he does not have any **urinary symptoms, changes in bowel habit or rectal bleeding** [13].

[1] Patients at greatest risk for abdominal aortic aneurysms (AAA) are those who are older than 65 years.

[2] Estimated prevalence of abdominal aortic aneurysm in developed countries is 2–8% and is higher in men (4–8% in those >50 years) compared with women (1–1.3%). For men, diameter alone defines the presence of a AAA and predicts clinical events. However, for women, although the aorta is still considered aneurysmal when its diameter exceeds 3.0cm, the diameter is less predictive of clinical events. An aortic size index, calculated as diameter (cm)/body surface area (m^2), is more predictive of clinical events than absolute aortic diameter in women.

[3] Important risk factors for the development of AAA include older age, male gender, atherosclerosis and HTN. The most important negative risk factors include non-Caucasian ethnicity, female gender and diabetes. Other less frequent causes include Marfan and Ehlers–Danlos syndromes, collagen vascular diseases and mycotic aneurysm.

[4] The natural history of AAA is one of progressive expansion. On average, AAAs expand at around 0.3cm per year and tend to be more rapid in smokers, which is also a strong risk factor. The likelihood that an aneurysm will rupture is increased for those with aneurysm diameter >5.5cm, a faster rate of expansion (>0.5cm over a 6-month period), those who continue to smoke, and in females. Other factors include recent surgery and medical factors such as uncontrolled HTN which may increase aortic wall stress.

[5] Back pain can be caused by erosion of the AAA into adjacent vertebrae and flank pain can certainly be experienced by the patient, usually unimpressive some time before rupture. Other areas of pain include abdomen or groin. In patients with abdominal pain, rupture of the aneurysm

must be excluded. In some cases, isolated groin pain may occur with retroperitoneal expansion and pressure on the femoral nerves.

[6] The picture of gradually developing symptoms over a period of time is consistent with an expanding AAA that has begun to encroach on surrounding structures. A ruptured AAA on the other hand would result in immediate symptoms such as abdominal pain and syncope.

[7] AAAs are usually asymptomatic until they expand or rupture. The development of these symptoms may be a sign that the AAA is rapidly expanding and has become large enough to compress surrounding structures. It could also suggest the AAA is an inflammatory or infectious aneurysm.

[8] It is common that a patient will have multiple aneurysms of other large vessels (aorta, femoral, iliac, popliteal).

[9] First-degree relatives with a AAA are a strong risk factor for developing the disease.

[10] The majority of patients are asymptomatic which was likely our patient's case prior to coming in. It is common for previously unknown AAAs to become apparent incidentally or through imaging studies performed for other indications. Additionally, only 20–30% of patients who present to an ED with rupture have a known history of AAA.

[11] Patients with symptomatic AAA most commonly present with abdominal, back or flank pain, which may or may not be associated with AAA rupture. AAA can also present with other clinical manifestations, such as limb ischaemia (acute or chronic) or other systemic manifestations (fever, malaise).

[12] The classic presentation of AAA rupture is not present in this patient. Such symptoms include severe pain, hypotension

and a pulsatile abdominal mass. Patients with rupture into the retroperitoneum may attribute their symptoms to other causes and delay seeking medical attention.

13 Common misdiagnoses of AAA (especially ruptured) are renal colic, perforated viscus, diverticulitis, GI haemorrhage and ischaemic bowel.

Examination

- The patient appears in **slight discomfort** [1], but there are **no signs of respiratory distress** [2].
- The patient's capillary refill time is **less than 2 seconds** [3] and there is no pallor of the palmar creases.
- Pulse is **100bpm** [4] and regular.
- BP is **within normal limits** [5].
- Temperature is **37.5°C** [6].
- The conjunctivae are **not pale** [7].
- Heart sounds are dual with **no murmurs** [8].

- The abdomen does not appear **distended or rigid** [9], and **palpation of the aorta estimated a size around 5.5cm** [10].
- The mass palpated was **pulsatile** [11] and upon auscultation, **no bruits were present** [12].
- **Femoral, popliteal and pedal pulses were palpated** [13] and found and there were no signs of **bruising or bleeding on the flanks nor around the umbilicus** [14].

1 General inspection of the patient can guide the clinician's level of concern for the acuity of the patient's pathology. For example, if this patient looked visibly uncomfortable, pale and in severe pain, this may raise the suspicion that the patient has had a AAA rupture. Although from general inspection of the vitals they seem within the normal range, it is important to continually monitor for signs of decline. Further, patients may have normal vital signs in the presence of a ruptured AAA as a consequence of retroperitoneal containment of haematoma.

2 Respiratory distress would be another sign that the patient is acutely unwell and increase the clinician's level of concern.

3 A normal capillary refill time (<3 seconds) indicates that the patient is perfusing well and thus would likely have preserved end-organ perfusion, which is reassuring as it points away from a potential rupture. In addition, it suggests the patient is adequately hydrated. Other signs of adequate hydration are warm peripheries, normal skin turgor, moist mucous membranes and normal urine output.

4 The pulse rate is on the upper limit of normal. This is reassuring as in a potential ruptured AAA, the clinician would worry about a compensatory tachycardia as a response to loss of volume due to rupture.

5 Similarly, BP is currently within the normal range and stable. This along with other important vital signs must be monitored for a rapid drop that is indicative of blood loss.

6 Temperature is normal in this patient. However, if raised in a patient with suspicion of an expanding AAA, this could point to an inflammatory or infective process.

7 Conjunctival pallor is another sign of anaemia.

8 Heart murmurs may suggest valvular heart disease or structural heart defects. It is important to investigate these peri-operatively in the context of fitness for general

anaesthetic, and to quantify any increased risk of peri-operative complications.

9 A distended abdomen would be in keeping with a potential rupture of a AAA.

10 Most clinically significant AAAs are palpable upon routine physical examination; however, the sensitivity of palpation depends on the experience of the examiner, the size of the aneurysm, and the size of the patient. AAAs are palpated in the upper abdomen; the aorta bifurcates into the iliac arteries just above the umbilicus. The clinician need not be afraid of properly palpating the abdomen, because there is no evidence to indicate that aortic rupture can be precipitated by this manoeuvre. The average adult infra-renal aorta is approximately 2cm and usually >3cm is considered aneurysmal.
- Small aneurysms have a diameter <4.0cm
- Medium aneurysms have a diameter 4.0–5.5cm
- Large aneurysms have a diameter >5.5cm
- Very large aneurysms have a diameter ≥6.0cm.

11 A pulsatile mass is consistent with that of a AAA.

12 An abdominal bruit is non-specific for an unruptured aneurysm, but the presence of an abdominal bruit or the lateral propagation of the aortic pulse wave can offer subtle clues and may be more frequently found than a pulsatile mass.

13 Peripheral pulses are felt to determine if an associated aneurysm (femoral/popliteal) or occlusive disease exists. When assessing a patient for AAA, the physical exam should include a complete peripheral arterial vascular examination to assess for signs of thromboembolism or other peripheral aneurysms.

14 Given the aorta is in a retroperitoneal position, you will see Cullen's sign (peri-umbilical ecchymosis) and Grey Turner's sign (flank ecchymosis) with a ruptured AAA.

Investigations

- **FBE** [1] results are normal.
- **UEC** [2] results are normal.
- **LFT** [3] results are normal.
- **Blood typing** [4] was performed.
- **Urine analysis** [5] was normal.
- **ECG** [6] reveals no abnormalities.

- **Imaging tests** [7] were then ordered.
- While consideration was made for **abdominal ultrasound** [8], a **non-enhanced CT abdomen** [9] was performed instead given the patient's **stable condition** [10], which detected an unruptured stable AAA at **5.5cm** [11].

[1] An FBE with differential is used to assess transfusion requirements and the possibility of infection and inflammation, which are common causes of an elevated WCC.

[2] UECs are important in the setting of a surgical emergency. First, it identifies any electrolyte abnormalities that most often need correction prior to surgery. Secondly, it assesses renal function and fitness for IV contrast in the setting of imaging (such as a CT abdomen and pelvis), as well as serving as a prognosticator for postoperative recovery. Additionally, it provides valuable information in ruling in or out renal colic, which is the most common misdiagnosis for a ruptured AAA.

[3] In patients with abdominal pain, LFTs are useful to ensure that there are no confounding hepatobiliary illnesses. Additionally, it informs operative risk and guides postoperative management.

[4] Blood must be typed and cross-matched to prepare for the possibility of transfusion, including clotting factors and platelets. Laboratory studies are not routinely obtained as part of the evaluation of asymptomatic AAA. However, a WCC, blood cultures and ESR should be performed in patients with systemic symptoms (e.g. fever, weight loss) to evaluate for an infectious cause of AAA or inflammatory aneurysm.

[5] Urinalysis can help assess for haematuria from potential renal colic and rule out any sources of infection as synthetic materials are used in interventions for AAAs.

[6] ECG findings provide a baseline assessment of cardiac rhythm as a preoperative assessment should surgery be required.

[7] A diagnosis of AAA is established with imaging studies that demonstrate the aneurysm in the patient suspected of having AAA on the basis of risk factors or on physical examination. A definitive diagnosis requires abdominal imaging to show a focal aortic dilatation meeting aneurysm criterion (>1.5 x normal diameter, or >3.0cm in the infrarenal segment). Abdominal US and CT are both highly sensitive and specific for diagnosing AAA but are used under different circumstances. Plain radiography should not, however, be ordered for the sole purpose of evaluating suspected AAA due to low diagnostic yield. Its use can waste time, delay care, and place the patient at risk for aortic rupture and death.

[8] Ultrasound is the standard imaging tool for AAA. The aorta is measured from outside wall to outside wall in both longitudinal and transverse views. When performed by trained personnel, it has a sensitivity of nearly 100% and a specificity approaching 96% for the detection of infrarenal AAA. Ultrasound can also detect free peritoneal blood. This is usually the test of choice for asymptomatic AAAs but also for patients who are haemodynamically compromised. Obesity, abdominal tenderness and bowel gas may limit ultrasound images.

[9] CT is the imaging test of choice for symptomatic AAA that are also stable enough to have the imaging taken. Contrast-enhanced CT aortography is generally not needed to establish a diagnosis of ruptured AAA but may be essential for planning surgical repair. In patients with symptoms of more than one hour, findings of rupture on CT scan are usually obvious (e.g. retroperitoneal haematoma, extravasation of contrast). Other findings on abdominal CT may be associated with unstable aneurysms or 'impending rupture' (e.g. crescent sign, breaks in aortic wall calcification, aortic blebs).

[10] A disadvantage of CT is the need to send the patient out of the ED for an extended period of time. If the patient is unstable, or investigations are needed in a more time-critical manner, a bedside ultrasound should be performed. Further investigations such as angiography can be considered.

[11] Non-enhanced CT is used to size aneurysms. A CT can also clearly define the anatomy of the aneurysm and other intra-abdominal pathologic conditions. It also helps to identify anatomic relations that are relevant to surgical repair. These include the location of the renal arteries, the length of the aortic neck, the condition of the iliac arteries, and the presence of anatomic variants such as a retro-aortic left renal vein or a horseshoe kidney.

Management

Immediate

Monitor **vital signs** [1], obtain IV access and **administer fluid if necessary** [2]. **Seek advice** [3] from the vascular surgery team. Monitor for **sudden onset pain** [4] and ensure they have **access** [5] to surgery should that need arise.

Short-term

Manage the patient as a **symptomatic but unruptured** [6] AAA compared to cases that are **asymptomatic** [7] or **ruptured** [8]. Assess the patient as a surgical candidate for either an **open** [9] or **endovascular repair** [10] for his symptomatic AAA, with the approach ultimately decided by the **consultant surgeon** [11]. Watchful waiting includes **medical management of HTN** [12]. During the admission, monitor for rupture and **haemorrhagic shock** [13]. If a surgery has been performed, keep the patient in hospital for **monitoring** [14] and assess for postoperative complications by **auscultation of the lungs** [15] and **examination of the lower limbs** [16]. The patient may be discharged if **vital signs remain stable** [17] and they are **back to their premorbid level of function** [18].

Long-term

Follow the patient up in an outpatient clinic for continuing wound management and monitoring for postoperative complications or also for **monitoring the progress of the AAA** [19] if conservative management was chosen.

---

[1] Ensure the patient remains haemodynamically stable prior to operative treatment. In particular, BP and HR are important to stabilise as they are prognosticators for postoperative recovery. Oxygen may be provided and monitoring via ECG and vital signs is essential.

[2] Large-bore (14 or 16 gauge) IV lines should be inserted so that shock can be corrected with fluid and blood products.

[3] Ensure an expeditious referral is made to the vascular surgery team for early contact and advice.

[4] Patients >50 with sudden onset abdominal pain should be presumed to have a ruptured AAA and receive attentive management and resuscitation as necessary.

[5] If not already, the patient should be transported to a facility capable of operative treatment of a AAA.

[6] Aneurysm repair is indicated for patients with symptoms (abdominal/back/flank pain, thromboembolism) that cannot unequivocally be attributed to another aetiology, regardless of aneurysm diameter. For patients with symptomatic AAA such as in this case, the first priority is to determine whether there is any immediate concern that the aneurysm has ruptured or is at high risk for impending rupture, which may be suggested by clinical symptoms or signs, or certain radiologic features (e.g. broken calcification, asymmetry) that may indicate instability of the aneurysm. Patients should be admitted for further evaluation and if the patient is a candidate for repair, it should be performed during the same hospitalisation and whether to proceed with open surgical or endovascular approach is primarily based upon an anatomic assessment of aortoiliac anatomy.

[7] If the patient is asymptomatic, management depends on the patient's risk for rupture compared with the expected risk of peri-operative morbidity and mortality associated with repair. When the risk of rupture exceeds the risk of repair, repair is recommended. Conversely, if the risk of repair is greater than the risk of rupture, conservative management and surveillance is recommended. The assessment of rupture risk depends primarily upon the diameter of the aneurysm at diagnosis and the patient's medical comorbidities. The risk of rupture has been shown to be lower in small or medium-sized aneurysms (<5.5cm in diameter). This diameter threshold for AAA repair is not absolute and may depend on the patient's stature and location of the aneurysm. Other factors that need to be taken into account include the patient's age and gender, faster expansion rates, and the presence of other peripheral aneurysms. Patients who are not candidates for repair or refuse repair should create an advance directive detailing their wishes in the event of rupture. Family members should be made aware of these wishes, given that the patient may not be able to report these wishes at the time of aneurysm rupture.

[8] If the AAA is ruptured, the management should be guided by the haemodynamic status of the patient. The haemodynamically unstable patient (persistent in spite of resuscitation) with known AAA who presents with classic symptoms/signs of rupture (hypotension, flank/back pain, pulsatile mass) should be taken as an emergency to the operating room for immediate control of haemorrhage, resuscitation and repair of the aneurysm. While it is ideal to obtain imaging prior to intervention, it is not required. Volume resuscitation should be limited to the least amount

necessary to maintain mentation and stabilise BP and pulse rate. For patients with suspected ruptured AAA who are haemodynamically stable, abdominal imaging (preferably CT aortography) should be performed urgently to confirm the rupture prior to repair, rule out other potential aetiologies as a cause of abdominal pain and hypotension, and determine if an endovascular repair is feasible. Both open and endovascular techniques can be successfully employed in the treatment of ruptured AAA.

9 Open surgical repair involves replacing the diseased aortic segment with a tube or bifurcated prosthetic graft through a midline abdominal or retroperitoneal incision.

10 Endovascular aneurysm repair (EVAR) involves the placement of modular graft components delivered via the iliac or femoral arteries to line the aorta and exclude the aneurysm sac from the circulation. EVAR requires fulfilment of specific anatomic criteria. With contemporary techniques, including custom-made fenestrated and branched devices, most patients can be considered candidates for EVAR in experienced endovascular centres.

11 Guidelines from major medical and surgical societies recommend an individualised approach to the patient when choosing between open and endovascular repair, taking into account the patient's age, risk factors for peri-operative morbidity and mortality, anatomic factors, and experience of the surgeon. Given the need for lifelong surveillance with endovascular repair, younger patients with low operative risk may benefit more from open surgical repair, whereas older patients and those with high operative risk may benefit more from endovascular repair, provided their aortoiliac anatomy is appropriate.

12 Elevated AAA wall tension is a significant predictor of impending rupture. Accordingly, the clinician may wish to achieve acute BP control in patients with AAA and elevated BP. Agents commonly used include antihypertensive agents and analgesics.

13 Haemorrhagic shock is managed by means of fluid resuscitation, blood transfusion and immediate surgical consultation. The concept of permissive hypotension, whereby aggressive fluid resuscitation is avoided so as not to aggravate bleeding by raising the BP too much, should be taken into consideration. Treatment for coagulopathy may be initiated in the ED for patients who are receiving warfarin or heparin.

14 Patients must be monitored postoperatively for any immediate complications of surgery. These include signs of shock (septic or hypovolaemic), infection, reaction to anaesthesia, DVT and PE, urinary retention or renal failure.

15 Listen for any crepitations. The presence of crackles in the lung may indicate either an infective process (such as hospital-acquired pneumonia or aspiration pneumonia), or atelectasis.

16 Recent surgery and subsequent immobilisation in bed postoperatively are major risk factors for the development of DVT. Inspect the calves for unilateral swelling and erythema. Palpate the calves to ensure they are not tender. If clinically suspicious, order a Doppler ultrasound of the affected leg to diagnose, and then start the patient on anticoagulation.

17 If the patient remains afebrile, is haemodynamically stable and looks well, they are generally well enough to be discharged home.

18 The patient should ideally be able to function at the level that they were able to prior to becoming ill. If unsure, refer to the allied health team (primarily physiotherapy, occupational therapy and social work) for further assessment on fitness for discharge home at a functional level.

19 Regarding surveillance, ultrasounds are routinely performed on a schedule that depends primarily upon the diameter of the aneurysm. It is usually performed every year but may also occur on a more frequent interval (e.g. every 6 months) depending on the characteristics of the aneurysm or patient-related factors.

CASE 82: Acute limb ischaemia

History

- A 60-year-old man presents with an **acutely** [1] **painful left leg** [2] that started an hour ago and reports a **change in sensation** [3] in the toes.
- He has a history of **hypertension, hypercholesterolaemia, diabetes and a 10 pack year smoking history** [4].
- He was diagnosed with **peripheral vascular disease** [5] a year ago and has had improving intermittent claudication with medication and exercise. He reports this pain is unlike the usual cramping and burning pain he experiences on exercise and is now present at rest.

- He **denies paralysis** [6] of the leg, rather just slight weakness.
- He reports his **heart racing and at times feeling dizzy** [7] in the prior month.
- He denies having had a **heart attack in the past, having any vessel aneurysms or any back pain** [8].
- The doctor in the ED is concerned about the **sudden** [9] presentation and proceeds to urgent investigation as the patient is at risk of potentially **losing their limb** [10].
- At this point, the most likely **differential** [11] is that of an embolic obstruction, which is a vascular emergency.

[1] Acute limb ischaemia is defined as a sudden decrease in limb perfusion that threatens the viability of the limb. Complete or even partial occlusion of the arterial supply to a limb can lead to rapid ischaemia and poor functional outcomes within hours. It has an incidence of 1.5 cases per 10 000. The later the patient presents to a hospital, the more likely that irreversible damage to the neuromuscular structures will have occurred (more common if >6 hours post symptom onset), which will ultimately result in a lost limb.

[2] The vast majority of cases involve the lower limbs (>80%) and it is a vascular emergency as it can lead to extensive tissue necrosis which may ultimately result in limb amputation or death.

[3] The classical features of acute limb ischaemia include the six Ps. These are pain, pallor, pulselessness, perishingly cold (poikilothermia), paraesthesia and paralysis for the limb distal to the side of occlusion.

[4] Risk factors include atrial fibrillation, recent MI, aortic atherosclerosis, large vessel aneurysmal disease (e.g. aortic aneurysm, popliteal aneurysm) and prior lower extremity revascularisation (angioplasty/stent, bypass graft). Others are similar to risk factors for cardiovascular disease and peripheral arterial disease such as smoking, diabetes, obesity, HTN and hypercholesterolaemia.

[5] Arterial thrombosis and cardiac emboli are responsible for the majority of cases. Thrombosis occurs most commonly due to plaque rupture in an atherosclerotic segment in patients in peripheral arterial disease on which a thrombus forms. This is an acute on chronic presentation, presents

slower and the patient will usually have a past history of intermittent claudication or other symptoms. It is important to assess for patients with established peripheral arterial disease whether they are compliant with their medications (e.g. antiplatelets). A thrombus may also form in the context of hypotension, hypovolaemia, thrombophilia and malignancy. Embolisation occurs when a thrombus from a proximal source travels distally to occlude the artery. The original thrombus may arise in the left atrium in association with atrial fibrillation or as a post-MI mural thrombus. Other sources include prostheses (heart valves or bypass grafts) and aneurysms (particularly popliteal and abdominal aortic aneurysms). It is also possible that there is a traumatic cause which is usually the result of injury during interventional procedures, such as percutaneous coronary intervention. These have increased in prevalence over the last two decades.

[6] Usually, the affected limb will have pain at rest as well as altered sensation (paraesthesia). If paralysis is present in the affected limb, this is a late sign and urgent intervention needs to be administered. Both paraesthesia and paralysis require emergency surgical review, regardless of the cause.

[7] In the history, the causes of potential embolisation should be explored. The patient's symptoms suggest undiagnosed atrial fibrillation.

[8] The patient also has a history of chronic limb ischaemia which may thrombose. Other potential causes for the presentation are less likely as the patient has not had a recent MI (resulting in a mural thrombus) or a symptomatic AAA or peripheral aneurysms.

9 It is also important to differentiate between embolic and thrombotic causes. The major difference is that the sudden nature of embolic limb ischaemia means that the body does not have sufficient time to build up compensatory collateral circulation. As such it makes urgent intervention in embolic acute limb ischaemia a necessity, should the limb be able to be salvaged.

Clinical features	Thrombosis	Embolism
Onset	Gradual and vague	Sudden
Severity	Less severe	Severe
Peripheral arterial disease	History of peripheral arterial disease symptoms	Unlikely
Previous vascular surgery or endovascular interventions	Likely	Unlikely
Cardiac history	Unlikely	History of atrial fibrillation, recent MI

10 The Rutherford classification for clinical categories of acute limb ischaemia is detailed below. This highlights the variability in the presentation of acute limb ischaemia.

Rutherford category	Prognosis	Sensory loss	Motor deficit	Arterial Doppler	Venous Doppler
Viable (1)	No immediate threat	None	None	Audible	Audible
Marginally threatened (2A)	Salvageable if promptly treated	Minimal (toes or none)	None	Inaudible	Audible
Immediately threatened (2B)	Salvageable if immediately revascularised	More than toes, rest pain	Mild/moderate	Inaudible	Audible
Irreversible (3)	Major tissue loss, permanent nerve damage inevitable	Profound	Profound paralysis	Inaudible	Inaudible

11 The main differential diagnoses for acute limb ischaemia is critical limb ischaemia. Critical limb ischaemia has a longer onset over 2 weeks with gradually worsening rest pain. The pulses may be reduced or absent and rather than looking pale, the leg is usually pink and warm, and signs of peripheral arterial disease such as ulcers and gangrene are seen. There is less urgency to act with critical limb ischaemia than acute, which is an emergency. Other differential diagnoses include an acute DVT, peripheral neuropathy, compartment syndrome and thromboangiitis obliterans (Buerger's disease).

Examination

- The patient appears **uncomfortable** [1]; however, there are **no signs of respiratory distress** [2].
- The patient's capillary refill time in his hand is <2 seconds and there is no **pallor of the palmar creases** [3].
- Pulse is borderline tachycardic and **irregularly irregular** [4].
- The patient is normotensive. Temperature is **37.5°C** [5].
- Heart sounds are dual with **no murmurs** [6].
- On abdominal examination, palpation of the aorta was normal and **no bruits were auscultated** [7].
- On general inspection of the legs, the **left is paler** [8] and **cool to touch** [9].
- The capillary refill is **difficult to ascertain** [10] and the patient is **able to move** [11] the leg although it is **weaker** [12] compared to the normal leg.
- The **popliteal pulse, posterior tibial pulse and dorsalis pedis pulse** [13] could not be felt on the left leg, although present on the right.
- No **bruits** [14] over the vessels were heard and **Buerger's test** [15] was not performed as the clinician clinically believes there is an **embolic obstruction** [16].

1 General inspection of the patient can, at times, guide the clinician's level of concern for the acuity of the patient's pathology. The patient that looks visibly uncomfortable increases the suspicion of the seriousness of the presentation.

2 Respiratory distress may indicate hypoxia and should prompt the clinician to determine a cause and treat appropriately.

3 Inspect the upper limbs for signs of peripheral cyanosis, tar staining (indicating smoking) and xanthomata (high cholesterol). Temperature and capillary refill are also important telling signs of limb perfusion. Assess the relevant pulses (radial, radio-radial delay, brachial, carotid pulse) and measure BP.

4 The irregularly irregular pulse may indicate atrial fibrillation.

5 A concurrent fever could point towards a more infectious embolic cause of the acute limb ischaemia (e.g. septic emboli from infective endocarditis).

6 Heart murmurs may suggest valvular heart disease or structural heart defects. It is important to investigate these peri-operatively in the context of fitness for general anaesthetic, and to quantify any increased risk of peri-operative complications. Additionally, the murmurs may point to a source of embolism formation such as from valvular dysfunction.

7 On the abdomen, palpate the aorta for an aneurysm and auscultate the aorta and renal arteries for vascular bruits.

8 On general inspection look for marbled white skin appearance and signs of peripheral arterial disease such as gangrene and ulcers (arterial ulcers are typically small, well defined deep painful ulcers, most commonly in the most peripheral regions of a limb). Missing digits indicate previous amputation and scars may be indicative of previous surgical procedures such as bypass surgery or healed ulcers. Muscle wasting and hair loss are also signs present with peripheral arterial disease and xanthomata are indicative of hyperlipidaemia. Make sure to adequately expose the patient's limbs and abdomen for the examination.

9 The classical features of acute limb ischaemia include the six Ps as mentioned above. Assess whether the limb is cold to touch, assess for reduced or complete loss of light touch sensation in the distal limb.

10 Check the capillary refill time which when >2 seconds indicates poor peripheral perfusion.

11 Assess for paralysis by asking the patient to wiggle their toes and move their fingers.

12 Assess for muscle weakness by testing for power.

13 Check for pulses; the intensity of these can be graded from 0 to 4+ where 0 is no palpable pulse and 4+ a bounding pulse. A normal contralateral limb with palpable pulses is a sensitive sign for an embolic occlusion in the abnormal limb. The relevant pulses in the legs are the femoral pulse (also making sure to assess for radio-femoral delay), popliteal pulse, posterior tibial pulse and dorsalis pedis pulse.

14 Bruits (detected by auscultation over the large and medium-sized arteries, e.g. carotid, brachial, abdominal aorta, femoral, with the diaphragm of the stethoscope using light to moderate pressure) and the presence of a 'thrill' (palpable vibratory sensation over a vessel in which a loud bruit is audible, indicative of marked turbulence in local blood flow suggesting significant vascular pathology) should be noted.

15 Buerger's test may also be performed. With the patient supine, raise both of the patient's feet to 45° for 1–2 minutes. The development of pallor indicates that peripheral arterial pressure is unable to overcome the effects of gravity, resulting in loss of limb perfusion. If a limb develops pallor, note at what angle this occurs (e.g. 25°); this is known as Buerger's angle. A Buerger's angle of <20° indicates severe limb ischaemia. Sit the patient up and ask them to hang their legs down over the side of the bed. Gravity should now aid reperfusion of the leg, resulting in the return of colour to the patient's limb. The leg will initially turn a bluish colour due to the passage of deoxygenated blood through the ischaemic tissue. Then the leg will become red due to reactive hyperaemia secondary to post-hypoxic arteriolar dilatation (driven by anaerobic metabolic waste products).

16 The difference between embolism and thrombosis in the examination is:

Clinical examination	Thrombosis	Embolism
Appearance and feet	Less cold, cyanotic	Cold, mottled
Palpation of artery	Hard and calcified	Soft but tender
Contralateral leg pulses	Absent	Present

Investigations

- The ECG shows an **irregularly irregular rhythm** [1] .
- **FBE, UEC and coagulation studies** [2] are normal.
- A **lactate level** [3] is slightly elevated and a **group and hold was ordered** [4] .
- A **Doppler ultrasound** [5] was performed, confirming the obstruction and given the **time-critical** [6] nature of the presentation, the vascular surgery team was called for urgent surgery.
- An **echocardiogram** [7] is ordered as well, to be performed after initial management.

[1] A 12-lead ECG assesses for cardiac arrhythmia as an aetiology of embolism, most commonly atrial fibrillation.

[2] Send baseline bloods such as FBE, UEC, coagulation screen. A thrombophilia screen should be performed generally in a younger patient (<50 years) with no risk factors for acute limb ischaemia.

[3] A lactate is helpful in assessing and tracking the degree of tissue hypoperfusion and severity of ischaemia.

[4] A group and hold is important should the patient require imminent surgery.

[5] Duplex ultrasound/Doppler scan is useful to investigate and confirm the absence of pulses. Further imaging should be conducted in consultation with the vascular surgeon.

[6] Following this, CT/MR angiography is the gold standard to guide revascularisation of the limb. It is important, however, that this is performed when viable and delaying treatment is not threatening of limb viability. The imaging will provide more information regarding the anatomical location of the occlusion and can help decide the operative approach (such as femoral vs. popliteal incision). Digital subtraction angiography is also a potential choice here that provided detailed information.

[7] Other sources of imaging would include echocardiography if an embolus of cardiac origin is suspected. Consider performing a bubble study to assess for patent foramen ovale. In patients with a patent foramen ovale, paradoxical embolism can occur, where a thrombus of venous origin is carried to the arterial side (via a right-to-left shunt).

Management

Short-term

Monitor **vital signs** [1] and keep the patient **fasted** [2] . Obtain IV access. Start the patient on high flow oxygen and administer **heparin** [3] . Analgesia such as paracetamol and opioids should also be provided. Speak to the **vascular surgery team** [4] as soon as possible to assess **limb viability and treatment options** [5] . This patient is assessed to need **surgical** [6] rather than **conservative management** [7] . An embolectomy with a Fogarty catheter is assessed to be most suitable, given the **embolic nature** [8] of the acute limb ischaemia compared to **thrombotic** [9] . After the procedure, **monitor the patient for reperfusion injury** [10] , **auscultate the lungs, examine the lower limbs** [11] and check the **wound site** [12] . It is important to assess for **compartment syndrome** [13] and any **changes in sensation** [14] to the lower limbs. Additionally, an **echocardiogram** [15] should be performed and medications provided to rate and rhythm control the **atrial fibrillation** [16] along with anticoagulation in consultation with cardiology.

Long-term

Long-term management of this patient includes addressing **cardiovascular risk factors** [17] . **Follow-up** [18] with the GP and surgeon is important to prevent progression of the peripheral vascular disease this patient has.

[1] Ensure the patient remains haemodynamically stable prior to operative treatment. In particular, BP and HR are important to stabilise as they are prognosticators for postoperative recovery. Patients may deteriorate from the damage from an acutely ischaemic limb. Resuscitate if unstable.

[2] Keeping the patient fasted is crucial in the preoperative management of the patient. It will reduce the risk of aspiration in the setting of anaesthesia should a procedure be required.

3 A therapeutic dose of heparin or preferably a bolus dose then heparin infusion should be initiated as soon as is practical. This is to prevent further extension of embolism.

4 Acute limb ischaemia is a surgical emergency. Complete arterial occlusion will lead to irreversible tissue damage within 6 hours. Early senior surgical support is vital.

5 Further management depends on the severity of acute limb ischaemia. In viable limbs, patients will not have significant tissue loss, nerve damage, or significant sensory loss. Patients should have arterial anatomy defined and undergo revascularisation. A revascularisation procedure should be performed within 6–24 hours. In a threatened limb, urgent revascularisation procedure within 6 hours is warranted. In non-viable limbs, on the other hand, there will be signs of tissue loss, nerve damage and sensory loss, and amputation will be necessary. Irreversible limb ischaemia (mottled non-blanching appearance with hard woody muscles) requires urgent amputation or taking a palliative approach. Irreversible limb ischaemia will inevitably progress to gangrene and requires amputation of the non-viable parts of the limb. Furthermore, in acute limb ischaemia due to compartment syndrome, fasciotomies should be performed. In acute limb ischaemia due to a dissecting aneurysm, stenting and/or surgical repair is warranted.

6 Surgical (including endovascular) revascularisation is first line. The exact form of intervention depends on the type of occlusion (i.e. thrombus vs. embolus), duration of ischaemia, location, the viability of the limb and risks associated with treatment. Surgical intervention is mandatory for Rutherford 2b ischaemia.

7 Conservative management can often be considered for those with Rutherford 1 and 2a; a prolonged course of heparin may be the most effective non-operative management of acute limb ischaemia. Any patient started on conservative management via heparin will need regular assessment to determine its effectiveness through monitoring aPTT and clinical review. Surgical interventions may be warranted if no significant improvement is seen.

8 If the limb is viable and an embolic cause is suspected, the first-line approach is an embolectomy with a balloon (Fogarty) catheter. Angiographic studies may be carried out during the initial phase, provided that the mobility and sensation of the toes and ankle are normal, the ankle pressure is >30mmHg measured with a Doppler stethoscope, and no cyanosis or muscle tenderness is present. If the foot is cyanotic or the motor function impaired, circulation must be restored immediately with emergency surgery. Alternative options include percutaneous catheter-directed thrombolysis (with e.g. urokinase, alteplase, etc.) or bypass surgery.

9 If the limb is viable and a thrombotic cause is suspected, the first-line approach is percutaneous catheter-directed thrombolysis. Alternative options include surgical thrombectomy, percutaneous mechanical thrombus extraction or bypass surgery.

10 Acute limb ischaemia has a high mortality rate of 15–20% and a similarly high 30-day mortality rate of ~15% following surgical intervention. Around a third of deaths result from metabolic complications, in the form of reperfusion injury. Surgical revascularisation causes sudden reperfusion of ischaemic tissue in the affected limb, which can, in turn, lead to reperfusion injury. This can consist of massive oedema resulting in compartment syndrome and hypovolaemic shock. The sudden release of built-up substances can lead to various systemic complications. This includes hyperkalaemia due to the release of K^+ ions which can cause cardiac arrhythmias. Systemic acidosis can result from the release of H^+ ions and acute kidney injury can occur due to the release of myoglobin: patients may require emergency renal replacement therapy. Other severe complications include DIC and multi-organ dysfunction. Symptomatic treatment should be initiated and in severe cases, amputation of the affected extremity may be necessary. It is thus imperative that the patient is closely monitored and rapidly treated. Electrolyte imbalances may need potential haemofiltration.

11 Patients must be monitored postoperatively for any immediate complications of surgery. These include signs of shock (septic or hypovolaemic), infection, reaction to anaesthesia, DVT and PE, urinary retention or renal failure.

12 Review the surgical site to ensure proper closure, as well as the amount of ooze and any signs of infection from the wound. Examine the skin around the site for erythema. Check for warmth of the wound site. Determine if the patient's pain is in proportion to the surgical wound.

13 Compartment syndrome, due to oedema formation on reperfusion of the limb and confinement of the muscles in their tight fascia, can ultimately lead to muscle necrosis and is an emergency.

14 Peripheral nerve injury can lead to chronic severe neuropathic pain in the limb.

15 An echocardiogram should be performed to look for further clots in the heart.

16 It is important to correct for the cause of the embolic acute limb ischaemia. In our patient's case, it is imperative to control the atrial fibrillation to prevent further episodes. The patient should be start on an antiplatelet agent or anticoagulant based on his CHA_2DS_2-VASc score.

17 It is important for the patient to reduce their risk of cardiovascular disease. This involves creating a plan and speaking about smoking cessation. Alternatives such as nicotine patches may be provided as well as medication such as acamprosate. Careful attention to modifying diet and creating an exercise plan is important, especially as our patient has high cholesterol, high BP and diabetes. Medications such as statin therapy should be commenced as well as medications for managing diabetes and HTN. Long-term anticoagulation should be given in the setting of atrial fibrillation to prevent thrombus formation.

18 Since the patient does not have lifestyle-limiting claudication, exercise therapy will be beneficial, as will the antiplatelet therapy as a way to reduce risk of MI, stroke and vascular death. Follow-up visits annually are recommended (to monitor for development of coronary, cerebrovascular, or leg ischaemic symptoms). However, if there is no improvement, patients should be referred to a vascular specialist and have their anatomy defined and assessed for revascularisation.

CASE 83: Carotid artery disease

History

- A **70-year-old** [1] **male** [2] presents with **sudden onset left arm weakness and numbness that lasted 30 minutes** [3].
- He also reports **temporary vision loss** [4] in the left eye.
- **He has a background history** [5] **of HTN** [6], **hypercholesteraemia** [7] and diabetes.
- He has a **50 pack year smoking history** [8].
- Ten years ago, he underwent **coronary artery stenting for an MI** [9].

- He denies seizures or a history of **seizures** [10]. He does not recall a loss of consciousness.
- He does not have a **headache** [11] or any **vomiting** [12].
- He denies **recent trauma** [13] to the head.
- The patient has a history of **depression** [14].
- He is **retired, engages in minimal physical activity and has a poor diet** [15].

1 Age is the most important risk factor for stroke and increases the risk of having carotid artery stenosis. Stroke rate doubles every 10 years after 55 years of age. 15 million people suffer from stroke worldwide each year and of these, 5 million die within 1 year and 5 million have a permanent disability. Approximately 10–15% of ischaemic strokes are associated with carotid artery disease. Atherosclerotic carotid artery stenosis is the most common cause and can be the source of low flow or atheroembolism.

2 Carotid artery stenosis is considered asymptomatic if the patient has not experienced stroke or transient ischaemic attack (TIA) symptoms. Asymptomatic carotid artery stenosis affects around 7% of women and 12% of men aged >70 years. All patients with ischaemic stroke or TIA symptoms in the carotid circulation territory must be screened for carotid stenosis.

3 Symptomatic carotid disease is defined as focal neurologic symptoms (e.g. weakness, paraesthesia, dysarthria, aphasia, spatial neglect, homonymous visual loss, amaurosis fugax) in the distribution of a carotid artery with a significant stenosis. This does not include non-specific symptoms such as dizziness. A deficit lasting <60 minutes is often a TIA which is confirmed by a normal brain CT scan. Some TIAs may last up to 24 hours. In patients with high-grade stenosis, repeated TIAs may occur, all lasting <1 minute. A deficit lasting >24 hours is more likely to be a stroke. A CT scan can be normal or show signs of infarction. Watershed infarction (where perfusion pressure is lowest between the main arterial territories of the brain) can occur in carotid artery stenosis.

4 Atheroembolisation can cause amaurosis fugax which is a painless and temporary loss of vision due to obstruction of the retinal or ophthalmic artery. It is often described as a curtain falling over the eye. Other visual problems that

can occur in the setting of carotid artery disease include homonymous hemianopia (due to emboli lodging in the optic radiation) and complete blindness from ischaemic optic neuropathy (rare).

5 Past medical history is important in determining fitness for surgery as well as any risk factors for carotid stenosis. Many people with carotid artery disease are asymptomatic. It is common for carotid stenosis to be an incidental finding in patients with multiple cardiovascular risk factors (e.g. peripheral vascular disease, aged >65 years, coronary artery disease, HTN, hypercholesterolaemia or smoking history).

6 High systolic BP is a risk factor for carotid artery stenosis. Furthermore, patients with hypertension are 3 times more likely to have stroke compared to normotensive patients.

7 Hypercholesterolaemia is a risk factor for carotid artery stenosis in patients >65 years.

8 Smokers have a 50% increased risk for atheroembolic stroke compared to non-smokers. Hence, it is an independent predictor of carotid artery disease. This patient has a heavy smoking history which predisposes him to carotid artery stenosis.

9 A history of cardiovascular disease places patients at higher risk of having carotid artery stenosis. This includes peripheral vascular disease or coronary artery disease that has required intervention. Approximately 20% of patients with symptomatic cardiovascular disease have coronary artery disease.

10 Seizure is the most frequent mimic of cerebral ischaemia. Patients often report a past history of epilepsy. Ideally, witnesses should be asked whether a seizure was observed prior to the patient's onset of weakness. Tongue biting, muscle pain, incontinence and confusion after the event suggest a seizure rather than a TIA.

11 Those with a history of migraine headaches may experience a complex migraine that presents with symptoms similar to those of stroke. Patients can experience an aura prior to the onset of weakness. It may be associated with nausea and vomiting. This is a diagnosis of exclusion.

12 Vomiting may indicate raised ICP. This can be due to a migraine or a space-occupying lesion (e.g. intracranial haemorrhage or mass).

13 Recent trauma predisposes the patient to haemorrhage which can create a compressive mass-like effect on the brain, leading to initial symptoms of headache and vomiting. Compared to ischaemia, space-occupying lesions may have

a more gradual onset of symptoms. Furthermore, complete resolution of symptoms usually only occurs in a TIA.

14 Those with conversion disorder can present with sudden onset focal neurological deficits. The deficits often do not fit in a vascular territory and examination can demonstrate discrepancies. There may be a history of psychiatric illnesses and psychosocial stressors. This is again a diagnosis of exclusion. Given that this patient's symptoms appear to match a single territory and he has significant risk factors for carotid artery disease, he should be investigated for that first.

15 Overall health can be assessed by collecting a social history. This patient appears to be sedentary with a poor diet. These are risk factors for obesity and diabetes, which are implicated in the development of cardiovascular disease.

Examination

- The patient appears **comfortable** [1] .
- The patient's capillary refill time is **<2 seconds** [2] .
- Pulse is 90bpm and **regular** [3] .
- RR is 18 breaths per minute. BP is **125/80mmHg** [4] .
- He is **afebrile** [5] .
- Heart sounds are dual with **no murmurs** [6] .
- A **cervical bruit** [7] is heard over the right carotid artery.

- There are no **surgical scars or radiation** [8] over the neck.
- The **peripheral neurological examination** [9] performed is normal. He has intact normal sensation, no weakness, normal gait and intact coordination.
- A **cranial nerve exam** [10] is performed and is normal.

1 General inspection of the patient can, at times, guide the clinician's level of concern for the acuity of the patient's pathology. For example, a patient who looks uncomfortable and is not moving in bed may raise the suspicion of a severe stroke requiring immediate treatment.

2 An adequate capillary refill time indicates the patient is perfusing well and thus would likely have preserved end-organ perfusion. In addition, it suggests the patient is adequately hydrated. Other signs of adequate hydration are warm peripheries, normal skin turgor, moist mucous membranes and normal urine output.

3 An irregular pulse rate may indicate an underlying arrhythmia which could be a possible cause of thromboembolic stroke.

4 Monitoring vitals including BP is important in ensuring the patient is haemodynamically stable for further investigation. If the patient is not stable, then resuscitation should occur.

5 Fever may indicate infection. An abscess in the brain may act as a space-occupying lesion causing focal neurological deficits, as seen in this patient. However, this is unlikely as the patient has had resolution in his symptoms.

6 Heart murmurs may suggest valvular heart disease or structural heart defects. Cardiovascular disease is a risk factor

for carotid artery stenosis. It is important to investigate heart problems peri-operatively as well in the context of fitness for general anaesthetic, and to quantify any increased risk of peri-operative complications.

7 Carotid bruit is not a sensitive or specific sign for carotid artery disease. However, the presence of it prompts doctors to further investigate. High-grade stenosis is only found in <2% of individuals with a bruit. This is because more patients are asymptomatic and hence screening is required in those with significant risk factors.

8 Evidence of previous surgeries or radiation is important to note as adhesions, scarring, altered tissue planes or altered anatomy may be present in the area and complicate future surgeries in the same region. The surgeons will take this into consideration before deciding to operate on a patient.

9 A full peripheral neurological examination is extremely important in the assessment of a possible stroke or TIA. On general observation, symmetry and wasting should be noted. The patient should be examined for tone in both the upper and lower limbs. As stroke is an upper motor neurone defect, it is expected that the patient displays spastic paralysis and increased tone. Power in each muscle group (both lower and upper limbs) is measured via a grading system out of 5, where 0 is no muscle contraction at all and 5 is normal power against full resistance. Reflexes should be elicited and observed for hyper- or hyporeflexia. Coordination should be measured in the both the upper and lower limb bilaterally. Sensory testing for dull and sharp touch should be performed for every dermatome. If possible, the patient should be observed for gait and balance.

10 A full cranial nerve exam should be performed. This includes assessing for facial asymmetry, weakness, changes in sensation, dysarthria, hearing or balance problems and visual problems.

Investigations

- FBE reports a normal **WCC** [1].
- **UEC results are normal** [2].
- A **CT brain** [3] shows a right frontoparietal infarction.
- **Arterial duplex ultrasonography** [4] reveals a 70% stenosis of the right internal carotid artery.

- **CT angiography** [5] of the head, neck and chest reveals a significantly narrowed right carotid artery lumen (80%) which correlates with ultrasound findings.

1 Infection and inflammation are common causes of an elevated WCC. In this patient, a normal WCC alongside a normal body temperature means that infection is unlikely.

2 UECs are important in the setting of a surgical emergency. First, it identifies any electrolyte abnormalities that most often need correction prior to surgery. Secondly, it assesses renal function and fitness for IV contrast in the setting of imaging (such as a CT abdomen and pelvis), as well as serving as a prognosticator for postoperative recovery.

3 In symptomatic patients, a CT head is ordered immediately to assess ischaemic brain injury and rule out intracranial haemorrhage. Ischaemia on imaging presents as hypoattenuation (darkening) of the brain parenchyma, loss of grey–white matter differentiation and effacement of the sulci. MRI can be used as well to assess ischaemic brain injury; however, it is time-consuming and not appropriate in the emergency setting. However, it is interesting to note that MRI provides more accurate information about any stroke lesions compared with CT, it is more sensitive to recent ischaemia and it can also identify intracranial haemorrhage.

4 Duplex ultrasonography is the first test ordered when carotid stenosis is suspected in asymptomatic or symptomatic patients. Duplex ultrasonography has a sensitivity of 99% and

a specificity of 86% for high grade stenoses. Ultrasound will reveal elevated blood flow velocities and allow visualisation of the plaque in the carotid arteries.

5 Carotid stenosis is confirmed with a second imaging test. CT angiography (CTA) of the head, neck and chest should also be ordered if results of duplex ultrasonography are ambiguous or fall in the moderate stenosis range (50–69%) where revascularisation is considered. CTA provides important information on the anatomy or the arteries proximal and distal to the cervical carotid artery. It provides a view of the aortic arch before any stenting is performed. As CTA is the best modality to measure the degree of carotid artery stenosis, it is a necessary investigation when planning for carotid artery stenting or endarterectomy. It has a sensitivity of 85% and a specificity of 90% for diagnosing stenoses of >70%. As CTA requires iodinated contrast, caution should be taken with patients with renal insufficiency. Magnetic resonance angiography (MRA) is less commonly performed but has the benefit of not requiring ionising radiation. Both CTA and MRA are non-invasive. Cervical angiography is the definitive test for quantifying the severity of stenosis; however, it is rarely used due to its invasive nature and it carries a risk of causing atheroembolic stroke.

Management

Immediate

Given the **symptomatic** [1] **nature** [2] of the patient's stenosis, **refer** [3] to vascular surgery. Commence the patient on **aspirin** [4] as well as **statin** [5] therapy.

Short-term

The patient is **assessed to be appropriate** [6] for a **carotid endarterectomy** [7]. On the day of the

operation, monitor **vital signs** [8], obtain IV access and monitor for **signs of stroke** [9]. Following the procedure, keep the patient in hospital for **monitoring** [10]. Review the patient's **surgical site** [11], **auscultate the lungs** [12] and **examine the lower limbs** [13]. The patient may be discharged if **vital signs remain stable** [14].

Long-term

The patient was educated about the importance of addressing his **hypertension, hypercholesterolaemia and smoking** [15] and encouraged to have an **active lifestyle** [16]. The patient was told that as long as he adheres to medical advice, this **prognosis looks good** [17]. He has a regular follow-up **appointment booked** [18] and is advised to **present** [19] should he experience any similar symptoms.

[1] Symptomatic patients include those with TIA, stroke, and transient monocular blindness (amaurosis fugax) which is the case in our vignette. As the plaques within the carotid bulb enlarge and the overlying fibrin cap is eroded, ulcerations may appear over the surface. This becomes a source of atheroemboli to the retina and cerebral cortex. The majority of large ulcerations occur in association with high-grade stenoses and will warrant carotid endarterectomy on the basis of the degree of stenosis.

[2] In asymptomatic carotid artery stenosis, pharmacotherapy is generally considered the first-line therapy in patients with <70% stenosis. If medical management is selected, aspirin is the preferred antiplatelet agent due to its benefits in preventing MI in vascular patients. Clopidogrel and ticagrelor are reasonable alternatives should contraindications exist. Patients already on anticoagulation (e.g. warfarin) for an unrelated indication should not be given antiplatelet agents for carotid stenosis except in special circumstances (e.g. presence of a stent), and should continue on the anticoagulant with the additional goal of preventing atheroembolic stroke. It is imperative that risk factors such as cigarette smoking, hypercholesterolaemia and hypertension are managed with the appropriate guidelines. This also includes increased physical activity and exercise. All patients with asymptomatic stenosis at a high risk of a vascular event should be considered for statin therapy aiming for a target LDL cholesterol level of <1.8mmol/L. The benefit of endarterectomy is small in these patients and it comes with great risks. In patients with asymptomatic carotid artery stenosis, the annual risk of stroke is <1% if medical management of cardiovascular risk factors is adhered to. In cases where the asymptomatic carotid stenosis is >70%, carotid endarterectomy or stenting should be considered.

[3] Rapid referral to a specialist as soon as the neurological event occurs is recommended, and early revascularisation (i.e. within 2 weeks) in patients whose neurological symptoms have stabilised is important.

[4] Antiplatelet therapy should be started preoperatively to reduce the risk of complications such as stroke and MI. It should be initiated at diagnosis and continued indefinitely after the procedure. Aspirin alone, clopidogrel alone, or the combination of aspirin plus extended-release dipyridamole, are preferred antiplatelet agents in symptomatic patients.

[5] All patients should receive high-dose statin therapy, treating to a target LDL cholesterol level of <1.8mmol/L.

Patients should start or continue statin therapy prior to endarterectomy or stenting; statins should not be stopped during the peri-operative period and should be continued long-term if tolerated. Alternative cholesterol-lowering medications should be used for those patients who are intolerant to statins.

[6] It is important to assess for suitability for arterial surgery (e.g. very high lesion close to the base of the skull, radiation-induced stenosis, tracheostomy, or restenosis after a prior carotid endarterectomy). If there is not a high level of suitability, it is reasonable to perform carotid artery stenting. This is riskier in older patients but can be considered as an alternative to surgery in younger patients (aged ≤65 years) in centres where carotid stenting is regularly performed. Dual antiplatelet therapy (e.g. aspirin and clopidogrel) is preferred in stented patients and are used for the first 1–3 months followed by aspirin alone.

[7] If the patient has had a recent stroke or TIA with a high-grade carotid stenosis (at least 70%), they must be referred for urgent carotid endarterectomy. The surgery provides maximal benefit if performed within 2 weeks of the stroke or TIA as the risk of a recurrent stroke/TIA is greatest during this time period. For symptomatic patients with stenosis between 50% and 69%, the benefit is marginal. Similarly, there is little benefit if surgery is delayed after 3 months.

[8] Ensure the patient remains haemodynamically stable prior to operative treatment. In particular, BP and HR are important to stabilise as they are prognosticators for postoperative recovery.

[9] While carotid endarterectomy can reduce the rate of future stroke, the surgery itself comes with significant risks, including stroke itself.

[10] Patients must be monitored postoperatively for any immediate complications of surgery. These include signs of shock (septic or hypovolaemic), infection, reaction to anaesthesia, DVT and PE, and urinary retention.

[11] Review the surgical site to ensure proper closure, as well as the amount of ooze and any signs of infection from the wound. Examine the skin around the site for erythema. Check for warmth of the wound site.

[12] Listen for any crepitations. The presence of crackles in the lung may indicate either an infective process (such as hospital-acquired pneumonia or aspiration pneumonia) or atelectasis.

13 Recent surgery and subsequent immobilisation in bed postoperatively are major risk factors for the development of DVT. Inspect the calves for unilateral swelling and erythema. Palpate the calves to ensure they are not tender. If clinically suspicious, order a Doppler ultrasound of the affected leg to diagnose, and then start the patient on anticoagulation.

14 If the patient remains haemodynamically stable and looks well, they are generally well enough to be discharged home.

15 Risk factors such as cigarette smoking, hypercholesterolaemia and HTN must be managed according to appropriate guidelines. It is important to explain to the patient how these may lead to more atherosclerotic plaques forming. Blood thinning medications may be commenced, the statin started pre-operatively continued and resources to cease smoking provided. The GP is an important part of monitoring this behaviour and these conditions.

16 Lifestyle modifications include increased physical activity and exercise as appropriate. The patient can be provided information on these exercises and referred to an exercise physiologist to craft a personalised programme. This is an important component of secondary prevention.

17 Prognosis is related to the degree of carotid stenosis. Patients with asymptomatic carotid stenosis ≤70% managed with pharmacological therapy demonstrate progression to high-grade stenosis at a generally modest rate of no more than 5% per year. Carotid artery revascularisation is effective in preventing stroke, and <1% of patients per year have a stroke after carotid endarterectomy. Both carotid endarterectomy and stenting are anatomically durable procedures, and restenosis occurs in approximately 6% of patients over 2 years after either procedure.

18 Patients may be followed up annually after the postoperative visits associated with revascularisation. Clinical evaluation should include assessment for development of new TIA or stroke-like symptoms, which might require referral to a neurologist for confirmation of the diagnosis. Testing might include non-invasive duplex ultrasound examination to identify potential recurrent stenosis or the development of stenosis in the contralateral carotid artery. Patients placed on pharmacological management and who have not had revascularisation might also be followed annually for possible disease progression in the form of increasing degrees of stenosis.

19 Recurrent high-grade stenosis after a prior carotid endarterectomy or stenting occurs infrequently (approximately 6% over 2 years). Restenosis is generally a consequence of neointimal hyperplasia when it occurs within the first 2 years after surgery and commonly due to new atherosclerotic plaque when it occurs beyond 2 years after surgery. Residual stenosis is a stenosis found within 30 days of the carotid intervention. Regarding optimal treatment for the relatively rare occurrence, there is no consensus; some countries tend towards medical management while others suggest medical along with surgical. Hence it is imperative to address all the relevant risk factors.

CASE 84: Chronic limb ischaemia

History

- A **60-year-old** [1] male presents complaining of **right-sided calf** [2] **cramping while walking** [3], for **2 years** [4].
- He reports that in the last month, his pain has **not improved with rest** [5].
- He reports **pain at night and needing to hang his legs off the bed** [6] to feel comfortable.
- He has a 20 pack year **smoking history, diabetes, HTN and hyperlipidaemia** [7].

- He has a **family history** [8] of peripheral vascular disease.
- He regularly eats **greasy takeaways and rarely exercises** [9]. He works from home on a computer.
- He denies any **lesions on his feet** [10], **buttock pain or erectile dysfunction** [11].
- He denies his legs being **pale, cold or paralysed** [12].
- He does not experience **pain radiating down the lateral aspect of his leg and his pain is unrelieved by sitting/leaning forward** [13].

[1] The prevalence of peripheral arterial disease (PAD) increases with age, beginning at 40 years of age. 15–20% of individuals over 70 years of age have PAD.

[2] The lower limbs are more commonly affected, although upper limbs and gluteals can also be affected.

[3] An early symptom of the disease is intermittent claudication, which is a cramping/burning type pain in the calf, thigh or buttock after walking a fixed distance (claudication distance) that is then relieved by rest within minutes. The pathophysiology of peripheral vascular disease centres around damage, inflammation and structural defects of blood vessels. The inner wall of the arteries is lined by a thin layer of cells which ensures that the lining remains smooth and allows for unobstructed flow of blood. With ageing, plaque – which is made up of cholesterol, calcium or fibrous tissue – starts building up on the inner walls of the artery. The accumulation of these atherosclerotic plaques in the artery make it narrow and stiff. Eventually the blood flow is blocked due to atherosclerosis and this results in decreased supply of oxygen to organs and muscles.

[4] The long time frame of symptoms indicates chronic limb ischaemia. Those with acute limb ischaemia have a time-critical threat to limb viability that occurs within 2 weeks. Over a 5-year period, of those patients with intermittent claudication, 10–20% will develop worsening symptoms and 5–10% will develop critical limb ischaemia.

[5] Rest pain is when the patient experiences pain in the legs, especially the toes, at all times. These symptoms are a progression from intermittent claudication as the arterial disease advances and the blood supply to the legs is severely reduced. There are 4 stages of chronic limb ischaemia via the Fontaine classification. Stage 1 is asymptomatic. Stage 2 is when the patient experiences intermittent claudication. In

stage 3 the patient experiences ischaemic rest pain. In stage 4, the patient may develop ulceration/gangrene or both.

[6] Ischaemic rest pain is classically described as a burning pain in the ball of the foot and toes that is worse at night when the patient is in bed. The pain is exacerbated by the recumbent position because of the loss of gravity-assisted flow to the foot. Ischaemic rest pain is located in the foot, where tissue is furthest from the heart and distal to the arterial occlusions. Patients with ischaemic rest pain often need to dangle their legs over the side of the bed or sleep in a recliner to regain gravity-augmented blood flow and relieve the pain.

[7] Common risk factors include smoking, diabetes mellitus, HTN and hyperlipidaemia. Diabetes increases the risk of amputation associated with severely infected and non-healing wounds. Elevated homocysteine levels are also related to chronic limb ischaemia.

[8] A family history of peripheral artery diseases places the patient at greater risk of the disease.

[9] The patient's poor lifestyle contributes to his risk of atherosclerosis, which is the most common cause of peripheral vascular disease. Rarer causes of claudication are aortic coarctation, arterial fibrodysplasia, arterial tumour, arterial dissection, arterial embolism, thrombosis vasospasm and trauma. Other rare causes are Takayasu's arteritis, temporal arteritis, thoracic outlet obstruction and Buerger's disease.

[10] Minor knocks and bruises in the feet may struggle to heal due to the lack of adequate blood supply and nutrition. These then become ulcers and the tips of the toes may turn black (necrosis). Given the patient does not have this and the recency of his ischaemic rest pain, it is unlikely he

has critical limb ischaemia, which is the advanced form of chronic limb ischaemia. It is defined by a few criteria. First, having ischaemic rest pain for >2 weeks' duration requiring opiate analgesia. Secondly, there is the presence of ischaemic lesions or gangrene. Thirdly, the ankle–brachial index (ABI) is <0.5. Chronic limb ischaemia can result in sepsis secondary to infected gangrene, amputation and overall reduces the mobility and quality of life of the sufferer.

11 Buttock and thigh pain and erectile dysfunction indicates Leriche syndrome which is a form of PAD affecting the aortic bifurcation.

12 The patient is unlikely to have acute limb ischaemia, which is a sudden decrease in limb perfusion that threatens limb viability. It is associated with pain, paralysis, paraesthesia, pulselessness, pallor and perishingly cold temperature.

13 Another differential is spinal stenosis. Hence it is important to rule out pain radiating down the lateral aspect of the leg (tensor fascia lata) and having pain that occurs on standing alone and is relieved by position change, such as sitting or stooping forwards (lumbar spine flexion).

Examination

- The patient has a **BMI of 30** [1] and appears **uncomfortable** [2].
- There are no **signs of respiratory distress** [3].
- On inspection of the legs, **no wounds or ulcers** [4] were seen.
- The leg has slight **pitting oedema up to the shins** [5] and **capillary refill of the toes is sluggish** [6].
- The patient is not tachycardic. BP is elevated at **150/90mmHg** [7].

- Buerger's test revealed **pallor of the legs at 30 degrees** [8].
- **Popliteal and pedal pulses were palpated and were weaker on the right** [9].
- The leg was **not pale, pulseless, cool to touch and there were no changes in sensation** [10].
- Heart sounds are dual with **no murmurs** [11].

1 A BMI of 30 (obesity) is a risk factor for peripheral vascular disease.

2 General inspection demonstrates the ischaemic rest pain the patient is experiencing.

3 Respiratory distress would be another sign that the patient is acutely unwell and increase the clinician's level of concern.

4 Look for non-healing wounds that may be due to arterial insufficiency and gangrene.

5 Patients who keep their legs in a dependent position for comfort for night pain often present with considerable oedema of the feet and ankles.

6 The long capillary refill time indicates that there is likely to be an obstruction.

7 Hypertension may indicate that the patient has poor BP control. This is also a risk factor for PAD.

8 Buerger's test is used to assess the adequacy of the arterial supply to the leg. Both legs are examined simultaneously as the changes are most obvious when one leg has a normal circulation.

9 Diminished pulse indicates reduced blood flow due to obstruction.

10 The patient is unlikely to have acute limb ischaemia, which is a sudden decrease in limb perfusion that threatens limb viability. It is associated with pain, paralysis, paraesthesia, pulselessness, pallor and perishingly cold temperature.

11 Murmurs could indicate heart pathology that may have occurred in the past due to this patient's cardiovascular risk factors.

Investigations

- An **ankle–brachial index** [1] was performed which showed a value of **0.6** [2].
- A **UEC** [3] showed normal kidney function, **blood glucose** [4] was 8.0mmol/L and **lipid profile** [5] showed a high serum LDL cholesterol.
- **ECG** [6] showed sinus rhythm with no abnormalities.
- **Duplex ultrasound** [7] was performed which

showed severe stenosis of the right anterior tibial artery.
- **CT angiography** [8] was performed to accurately establish the location of the stenosis.
- Other blood tests such as a **thrombophilia screen** [9] were not performed.

1 The diagnosis of chronic limb ischaemia is clinical. The resting ABI is the initial diagnostic test for PAD. It is recommended in all patients with suspected lower limb disease with a history of exertional leg symptoms, non-healing wounds/foot ulcers, or abnormal lower extremity pulse examination. It can be used to quantify the severity of chronic limb ischaemia. ABI is performed by measuring the systolic pressure of the left and right brachial arteries and the left and right posterior tibial and dorsalis pedis artery pressures. The ABI is the highest of the dorsalis pedis and posterior tibial arteries' pressure divided by the higher of the left and right arm brachial artery pulse pressure.

2 Normal ABI is >0.9. Mild ABI is 0.8–0.9. Moderate ABI is 0.5–0.8. Severe ABI is <0.5. The patient's low ABI value indicates narrowing of the peripheral arteries. Rest pain, ulcers and necrosis combined with reduced pressures (ABI <0.5) in the legs is referred to as critical limb ischaemia. This is an indicator that the blood supply to the leg is severely depleted and here invasive intervention is warranted on an urgent basis to ensure that the leg does not deteriorate any further. It should be noted that any ABI value >1.2 should be interpreted with caution, as calcification and artery hardening may cause a falsely high ABI. Patients with either severely stenosed or completely occluded arteries may also have a normal ABI is there is an abundant collateral system present. If the patient is diabetic or has chronic kidney disease, the ABI test measured by standard procedure may not be accurate due to calcification (hardening) of the arteries. In such patients, measuring blood pressure of the toe (toe pressure) may provide more accurate results. An exercise ABI can also be performed, but it does not provide information about the location of the lesion. It is useful, however, in establishing the diagnosis of lower extremity PAD in symptomatic patients when resting ABIs are normal or borderline.

3 It is important to assess renal function when angiography is to be performed.

4 A higher than normal serum blood glucose demonstrates poor control.

5 The patient's lipids are also high, which is a risk factor for developing PAD.

6 An ECG may show changes associated with ischaemia and hypertrophy due to cardiovascular risk factors.

7 If the ABI/toe brachial index is abnormal, the next test to guide the therapeutic decision should be duplex ultrasonography of the lower-extremity arteries. The duplex ultrasound is both cost-effective and non-invasive and should be done first to verify stenoses. The location and degree of stenosis can also be assessed by duplex ultrasound. The accuracy is diminished in tortuous, calcified prosthetic bypass grafts, and in vessels with multiple stenoses. In the aortoiliac arterial segment, accuracy can also be diminished due to bowel gas and body habitus. If this is also abnormal (i.e. it shows stenoses or occlusions), an angiography is warranted.

8 CTA and MRA comprise the gold standard for establishing diagnosis, but require IV contrast.

9 Any patient presenting with chronic limb ischaemia aged <50 years without significant risk factors should have a thrombophilia screen and homocysteine levels checked. A lower homocysteine level has been associated with a reduced risk of cardiovascular events.

Management

Immediate

Leading up to the surgery, keep the patient **fasted** [1] and monitor **vital signs** [2] and **urine output** [3] . Refer the patient to **vascular surgery** [4] for intervention. Commence **aspirin** [5] a few days prior to surgery.

Short-term

An **angioplasty** [6] procedure is deemed most appropriate compared to **bypass surgery** [7] . Given the patient did not have critical limb ischaemia with gangrenous feet, **amputation** [8] is not considered. After the surgery, the catheter, guidewire and guide catheter are removed. Pressure will be applied to the puncture site until the bleeding has stopped. Continue to **monitor the patient, auscultate the lungs, examine the lower limbs** [9] and check the **wound site** [10] . The patient may be discharged if vital signs remain stable. Usually patients only stay for several hours and may be able to return home on the same day. Once the patient returns home (not driving themselves), they rest and continue to drink plenty of fluids. They should not lift **heavy objects, exercise strenuously or smoke for at least 24 hours** [11] . **Follow-up appointments** [12] are scheduled.

Long-term

The patient is encouraged to **cease smoking and take medications for his comorbidities including diabetes, HTN and hyperlipidaemia** [13] . A **regular exercise plan** [14] was implemented. A **statin** [15] , **aspirin** [16] and **regular follow-ups** [17] with the GP and surgeon are scheduled. The plan varies depending on the degree of symptoms from **asymptomatic** [18] to **critical limb ischaemia** [19] .

1 Keeping the patient fasted is crucial in their preoperative management. It allows the patient to have bowel rest, as well as reducing the risk of aspiration in the setting of anaesthesia. Ideally, patients should be fasted off solid foods for 6 hours, and clear fluids for 2 hours prior to induction of anaesthesia.

2 Ensure the patient remains haemodynamically stable prior to operative treatment. In particular, BP and HR are important to stabilise as they are prognosticators for postoperative recovery.

3 Urine output is an indicator of fluid balance. If urine output dwindles, this may be a sign of acute renal failure and early recognition is key to effective treatment. There are many causes of acute renal failure, some of which include IV contrast (in the setting of diagnostic imaging), some IV antibiotics (such as the cephalosporins) and some general anaesthetics and sedatives.

4 The vascular surgery team will decide which surgical intervention is best suited for the patient. They tend to perform interventions on patients if risk factor modification has already been discussed and supervised exercise has failed to improve symptoms. Any patients with critical limb ischaemia should be urgently referred for surgical intervention.

5 Aspirin is an antiplatelet agent that will help minimise the risk of blood clots during the procedure.

6 There are two main surgical options available. The first is angioplasty with or without stenting and the second is bypass grafting, which is typically used for diffuse disease or in younger patients. A combination such as surgery to clean a specific lesion allowing access for angioplasty to another region may also be implemented. Angioplasty is an endovascular procedure that opens up narrowed and blocked arteries by inflating a small balloon inserted via the groin. After an angioplasty, a stent (wire mesh tube) may be placed within the artery to hold the artery open. With X-ray guidance, the doctor will advance a thin wire through the catheter to the treatment site of the artery to penetrate the blockage and provide support for the therapy delivery system. A tiny deflated balloon will be advanced to the blockage along the wire that is already in place. Once the balloon is inside the blockage, the balloon will be inflated. Inflating the balloon squeezes the plaque against the wall of the artery, widening the artery opening. Next, if a stent is required, another tiny catheter with a stent mounted on it will be advanced to the blockage. Once the stent is inside the blockage and properly placed, it will be deployed into the artery. The stent locks in place against the artery wall, forming a scaffold to help keep the artery open. After the stent is fully expanded, additional X-rays will be taken to determine if the stent is fully open and how much blood flow has improved.

7 The surgeon may perform a bypass surgery, where a graft (healthy blood vessel removed from another part of the body) is attached to re-route blood away from the block.

Surgical bypass is a treatment option reserved for patients with advanced atherosclerosis where there is risk of losing the leg with no intervention. Often this is the only choice left to improve the blood supply to the leg when keyhole endovascular options have already failed. In addition to this, duplex ultrasound, MRA or CTA is used to determine the extent of arterial involvement for preoperative planning. Bypass surgery is performed under general or regional anaesthesia depending on the patient's overall fitness level and after discussion with the anaesthetists. In most instances the tube chosen for the bypass procedure is the patient's own vein which is harvested from the leg and in some cases an artificial tube made of medical grade PTFE (Teflon). The surgeon initially harvests the vein from the leg (usually the same leg undergoing bypass) by making an incision along the inside of the thigh. After this, the surgeon exposes the artery above and below the level at which the artery is blocked. Next a blood thinner (heparin) is administered to ensure that the blood remains thin and prevents clots from forming whilst the blood is temporarily blocked for the surgery. Clamps are placed at each end of the blocked section of artery to ensure that there is no blood loss during the bypass procedure. Next the graft is sutured in carefully using very fine sutures after tunnelling it under the skin and muscles of the thigh. The blood flow is then restored, and the suture lines are checked by the surgeon to ensure that it holds. An angiogram may be performed to confirm that the graft is working properly. Following this the surgeon closes the incision with stitches. After surgery, the patient will have to stay in hospital for 3–10 days for monitoring. Surgical bypass carries risks such as bleeding from the suture line, graft blocking, wound healing problems, infections and major amputation.

8 Amputations are considered for any patients who are unsuitable for revascularisation with ischaemia causing incurable symptoms or gangrene leading to sepsis. Two years following a below-knee amputation for chronic limb ischaemia, 15% require a further above-knee amputation, 30% have died, and only 40% have full mobility. The 5-year mortality rate in those diagnosed with chronic limb ischaemia is around 50%.

9 Patients must be monitored postoperatively for any immediate complications of surgery. These include signs of shock (septic or hypovolaemic), infection, reaction to anaesthesia, DVT and PE, urinary retention or renal failure.

10 Review the surgical site to ensure proper closure, as well as the amount of ooze and any signs of infection from the wound. Examine the skin around the site for erythema. Check for warmth of the wound site. Determine if the patient's pain is in proportion to the surgical wound.

11 Increased intra-abdominal pressure may cause damage to the wound as well as potentially compromise the stent/angioplasty procedure.

12 Long-term patency of lower extremity revascularisation should be monitored with a surveillance programme of serial reviews and Doppler ultrasounds.

13 All patients regardless of their symptoms should have aggressive risk factor modification. This includes controlling BP, lipid control, smoking cessation and diabetes control. This is because death from a cardiac cause has a relative risk of 3–6 in patients with peripheral vascular disease.

14 In terms of lifestyle advice, smoking cessation, regular exercise and weight reduction should be recommended.

15 High dose statin therapy such as atorvastatin should be commenced.

16 Antiplatelet therapy such as aspirin or clopidogrel should be commenced and is recommended for all patients.

17 This should be in close consultation with the GP and vascular surgeon. The course of chronic limb ischaemia is variable, and many patients' symptoms do improve on lifestyle changes and medical management alone.

18 Patients with claudication which does not limit their lifestyle should be advised to keep walking. Antiplatelet therapy (aspirin alone or clopidogrel alone) is recommended to reduce risk of MI, stroke and vascular death. First-line therapy for patients with lifestyle-limiting claudication is a supervised 12-week exercise programme and medication for symptom relief. A supervised exercise training programme consists of 30–45 minutes per session, 3 times a week for 12 weeks. If supervised exercise therapy is not feasible, community-based walking programmes have also shown some benefit. Symptom relief can be achieved with pentoxifylline, cilostazol or naftidrofuryl. If there is clinical improvement with an exercise programme and medication, follow-up visits annually are recommended (monitor development of coronary, cerebrovascular or leg ischaemic symptoms). However, if there is no improvement, patients should be referred to a vascular specialist and have their anatomy defined and assessed for revascularisation. Studies have shown that revascularisation in combination with exercise therapy is more effective than exercise therapy alone.

19 In patients with chronic severe limb ischaemia (critical limb ischaemia) who experience ischaemic rest pain, gangrene and non-healing wounds/foot and leg ulcers, ischaemic aetiology must be established urgently by physical examination and vascular studies. If patients have documented PAD, they should immediately be referred to a vascular specialist for revascularisation. Patients who were able to walk before the episode of critical limb ischaemia, have a life expectancy of >1 year, and are able to withstand surgery may be candidates for revascularisation. If the patient is not a candidate for revascularisation, they should be assessed for amputation where necessary and be on appropriate risk factor reduction medication.

CASE 85: Chronic venous insufficiency

History

- A **50-year-old** [1] male presents with a 5-month history of a **large ulcer on his right lower leg** [2].
- His legs have been chronically **swollen** [3] for over 5 years; the swelling **tends to get worse as the day progresses** [3].
- He reports **leg pain, heaviness, itching** [4] and **skin that feels tight** [5].

- He also reports some **dilated veins** [6] on both legs.
- His **brother and father** [7] both had similar problems in their legs.
- He has two documented episodes of **DVT** [8] in the affected leg 5 years earlier.
- He is obese with an **unhealthy lifestyle and has a 10 pack year smoking history** [9].

[1] A risk factor for developing chronic venous disease is advancing age. The disease affects about 7% of the population. Chronic venous insufficiency may be twice as common in women; however, estimates may be influenced by female life longevity. Chronic venous insufficiency refers to a wide spectrum of vein abnormalities that may be morphologic (e.g. venous dilatation) and/or functional (e.g. venous reflux) and are of long duration. The pathophysiology is due to inadequate muscle pump function, incompetent venous valves (reflux), venous thrombosis, or non-thrombotic venous stenosis. These cause elevated venous pressure (venous hypertension) which initiates a sequence of anatomic, physiologic and histologic changes leading to vein dilatation, skin changes or skin ulceration. The CEAP (Clinical, aEtiology, Anatomy, Pathophysiology) Comprehensive Classification System for Chronic Venous Disorders is used to grade chronic venous insufficiency. The factors responsible for a transition from mild to more severe clinical manifestations (increasing CEAP category), and whether there necessarily is a sequential progression, are not well known. Disease progression and increasing severity of symptoms appear to be related to the extent of venous valvular incompetence.

[2] Venous ulceration and bleeding are recognised complications. The prevalence of venous leg ulcers, the most extreme form of chronic venous insufficiency, is approximately 1–2%.

[3] Swelling of the legs is a common symptom of chronic venous insufficiency due to congestion. It tends to worsen towards the end of the day and on prolonged standing, and tends to improve with elevation. While periodic elevation may reduce the swelling, the more severe cases usually require additional compression.

[4] Other symptoms include pain, leg heaviness or aching, skin dryness, tightness, itching, and irritation and muscle

cramps. Burning and itching of the skin is mainly associated with venous stasis and eczema.

[5] More severe cases exhibit progressive skin changes, venous stasis dermatitis, lipodermatosclerosis and frank ulceration. Lipodermatosclerosis characteristically results from capillary proliferation, fat necrosis, and fibrosis of the skin and subcutaneous tissues.

[6] The clinical presentation of chronic venous insufficiency is also associated with dilated tortuous veins. Vein-related problems, when symptomatic, include a wide range of clinical signs that vary from minimal superficial venous dilation to chronic skin changes with ulceration. Chronic vein abnormalities are present in up to 50% of individuals. Patients may also present with superficial thrombophlebitis which presents as localised pain, tenderness and erythema in the involved area.

[7] Family history of venous disease is a strong risk factor for developing chronic venous insufficiency.

[8] Another risk factor is prior DVT. In spite of the well-known association, a history of DVT is obtained in fewer than one-third of patients with severe clinical manifestations of chronic venous disease (e.g. skin changes, ulcer).

[9] Increased BMI, smoking and sedentary lifestyle are all contributors to the severity of his condition. The proportion of the population suffering from obesity and chronic venous insufficiency is increasing, and obese patients are more likely to be symptomatic as a result of their venous disease. Other risk factors include prolonged standing, lower extremity trauma, some hereditary conditions (e.g. Klippel–Trénaunay syndrome), high oestrogen states and pregnancy.

Examination

- The patient appears **overweight** [1] and **all vitals are within normal limits** [2] .
- The capillary refill time on toes is **<2 seconds** [3] .
- On general inspection of the legs, there is **hyperpigmentation and dryness** [4] of the skin.
- Further, an **'upside-down champagne bottle'** [5] appearance is evident and there is a **large venous ulcer in the medial right ankle** [6] .
- There are **veins varying in size and appearance** [7] , some appearing **tortuous** [8] while others appearing thread-like over the calves bilaterally.
- There is **no pallor and all lower limb pulses are intact** [9] .
- **Swelling** [10] of the legs reaches the ankles.

[1] General inspection of the patient can provide clues to risk factors (e.g. obesity). It is important to examine the patient while they are standing.

[2] Assessing vitals for haemodynamic stability is important in all patients. Instability would require urgent medical attention and management.

[3] An adequate capillary refill time indicates the patient is perfusing well and thus would likely have preserved end-organ perfusion. In addition, it suggests the patient is adequately hydrated.

[4] Hyperpigmentation (usually a reddish-brown discolouration) of the ankle and lower leg is also known as brawny oedema. It results from extravasation of blood and deposition of haemosiderin in the tissues due to long-standing ambulatory venous hypertension. Dry, scaling, eczematous skin changes are typical of venous stasis dermatitis. Severe chronic venous insufficiency is associated with characteristic skin changes such as atrophie blanche, lipodermatosclerosis and hyperpigmentation. Atrophie blanche is characterised by localised, frequently round areas of white, shiny, atrophic skin surrounded by small dilated capillaries and sometimes areas of hyperpigmentation.

[5] Lipodermatosclerosis is a localised chronic inflammatory and fibrotic condition affecting the skin and subcutaneous tissues of the lower leg, especially in the supramalleolar region. When severe it may even lead to contracture of the Achilles tendon. This leads to the upside-down champagne bottle appearance.

[6] Venous ulcers are located in the gaiter area (between the malleolus and mid-calf) of the calf, proximal and posterior to the medial malleolus, and occasionally superior to the lateral malleolus. Ulceration may be healed or active.

[7] Signs of chronic venous insufficiency include telangiectasias (dilated intradermal venules <1mm in diameter), reticular veins (dilated, non-palpable subdermal veins ≤3mm in diameter), and corona phlebectatica (also known as malleolar flare or ankle flare). It consists of a fan-shaped pattern of small intradermal veins on the ankle or foot and is thought to be a common early physical sign of advanced venous disease.

[8] Palpation for bulges is consistent with varicose veins (dilated, palpable, subcutaneous veins >3mm in diameter). Primary varicose veins are not commonly associated with significant oedema or skin changes, but occasionally pure superficial venous system incompetence can be associated with oedema, skin changes and even frank ulceration. Varicose veins are generally thought to be more common in women than men. Varicose veins are present in 10–30% of the general population, with increasing rates in older individuals. Visible varicose veins typically are most concerning to patients as they are visually obvious. However, it is important to note that varicose veins are often associated with superficial axial venous reflux (e.g. great saphenous vein, small saphenous vein). Prior to treating patients with varicose veins, it is important to assess the superficial as well as deep veins for evidence of reflux.

[9] Arterial insufficiency must be ruled out, as it is a possible cause of some of the patient's symptoms. The affected limb usually appears pale due to obstructed blood flow, is cold to touch, has prolonged capillary refill time and may have reduced or absent lower limb pulses.

[10] Ankle swelling (usually unilateral but may be bilateral) due to oedema is also common. It characteristically indents with pressure and initially occurs in the ankle region but may extend to the leg and foot.

Investigations

- **Venous duplex ultrasonography** [1] showed **venous reflux** [2] bilaterally in deep and superficial veins.
- No other **investigations** [3] were required for this patient.

1 The diagnosis of chronic venous disease is suggested by the presence of typical symptoms (leg pain, fatigue, heaviness) and physical examination findings, and confirmed by the presence of venous reflux (superficial or deep). Hence the majority of symptomatic patients should undergo venous duplex ultrasonography to evaluate the nature and extent of venous reflux, which impacts the choice of treatment. Any combination of superficial, perforator or deep venous reflux can be present. It should be noted that duplex ultrasound is operator-dependent.

2 Venous reflux is defined as a duration of retrograde flow >500 milliseconds for superficial or perforator veins, or >1000 milliseconds for deep veins.

3 Other investigations to consider include ascending phlebography, CT venography, magnetic resonance venography and CT abdomen and pelvis. Ascending

phlebography identifies the site and level of obstruction, as well as the presence and location of collaterals, but it has been supplanted by duplex imaging, except when used by a specialist to evaluate treatment options for complex chronic venous insufficiency. CT and magnetic resonance venography provide excellent anatomical detail, so are useful in evaluating congenital and complex or advanced cases of chronic venous insufficiency. Patients with unilateral leg oedema suggesting iliac vein obstruction should be evaluated with a CT scan to rule out a pelvic or abdominal mass. If no evidence of extrinsic compression is found, the patient should be referred to a vascular specialist for further investigations, including an ascending phlebography. Intravascular ultrasound is also used in specialised centres as a secondary test to evaluate the significance of iliac vein obstruction in complex cases of chronic venous insufficiency. It is extremely useful in the diagnosis and therapy of iliac vein disease.

Management

Immediate

Refer the patient to the **vascular surgeons** [1] for consultation and consideration for **surgery** [2], given he is **symptomatic** [3] rather than **asymptomatic** [4]. **Clean and dress** [5] the patient's ulcer.

Short-term

Conservative measures should be trialled including **skin care, leg elevation, exercise** [6] and **compression therapy** [7]. These basic management

principles are important in treating the patient's **lipodermatosclerosis** [8]. As the patient has experienced **bleeding from the vessels** [9] in his legs, offer sclerotherapy. It is ultimately decided the patient's varicose veins are best managed with endovenous ablation.

Long-term

Follow the patient up to assess for complications following intervention. He is then regularly monitored for recurrence.

1 A referral should be made to the vascular surgeons, given this patient is experiencing late signs of chronic venous insufficiency. They will book an appointment with the patient, assess them and consent them for a procedure if deemed appropriate and necessary.

2 There are several minimally invasive chronic venous insufficiency treatments. The majority of patients are able to be managed via endovascular intervention; however, for <10% of patients who require surgical treatment, the options include vein ligation and stripping, microincision/ambulatory phlebectomy, and bypass surgery.

- Radiofrequency vein ablation (RVA): RVA uses a tiny catheter to deliver radiofrequency energy into the vein, closing it off. Once the vein is no longer supporting blood flow, it will shrink and be reabsorbed by the body.
- Endovenous laser therapy (EVLT): EVLT is a similar process to RVA. Instead of radiofrequency energy, EVLT uses laser energy to close the affected vein and seal off

blood flow. As with RVA, the vein will then shrink and disappear.
- Sclerotherapy involves the injection of a solution directly into spider veins or small varicose veins, which causes them to collapse and disappear. Several sclerotherapy treatments are usually required to achieve the desired results. Sclerotherapy is simple, relatively inexpensive, and can be performed in the doctor's office. Sclerotherapy can eliminate the pain and discomfort of these veins and helps prevent complications such as venous haemorrhage and ulceration. It is also frequently performed for cosmetic reasons. Sclerotherapy and surface laser therapy of telangiectasias and reticular veins are generally considered cosmetic treatments and are not typically available on the NHS in the UK, though occasionally sclerotherapy will be carried out on the NHS for treating veins that have bled. It is important to note that such treatment does not prevent the future

development of venous reflux and the occurrence of chronic venous disease.

- Angioplasty: if your symptoms are more severe, your vascular specialist may recommend angioplasty, which can help open a blocked vein using a balloon catheter.
- Ligation and stripping often are performed in combination. Vein ligation is a procedure in which a vascular surgeon cuts and ties off the problem veins. Most patients recover in a few days and can resume their normal activities. Stripping is the surgical removal of larger veins through two small incisions. Stripping is a more extensive procedure and may require up to 10 days for recovery. It usually causes bruising for several weeks after surgery.
- Microincision/ambulatory phlebectomy is a minimally invasive procedure in which small incisions or needle punctures are made over the veins, and a phlebectomy hook is used to remove the problem veins.
- Vein bypass in the leg is similar to heart bypass surgery, just in a different location. It involves using a portion of healthy vein transplanted from elsewhere in the body to reroute blood around the vein affected by the chronic venous insufficiency. Bypass is used for treatment of chronic venous insufficiency in the upper thigh and only in the most severe cases, when no other treatment is effective.

3 Patients with chronic venous disorders are managed according to clinical severity and the nature and level of underlying venous reflux. Initial conservative measures are recommended for most symptomatic patients and include skin care, leg elevation, exercise and compression therapy, as indicated. Patients who are refractory to conservative measures should undergo comprehensive review for further procedures. Whether then to offer additional treatment for symptomatic venous disease depends upon the response to conservative measures, ongoing symptoms, extent of disease, presence of reflux (superficial, deep, perforator), patient expectations, and likelihood that treatment would provide a durable benefit either with respect to appearance or improvement in symptoms. The majority of patients with chronic skin changes or venous ulcers will exhibit some degree of venous reflux (superficial, deep), and up to 20% with venous ulceration have isolated saphenous incompetence and may be candidates for superficial venous ablation.

4 Asymptomatic patients: some individuals with large dilated veins do not have significant complaints and may not find the appearance of their veins concerning. On the other hand, some people find even the smallest veins cosmetically troublesome, even in the absence of symptoms. In the absence of symptoms, telangiectasias, reticular veins and small varicose veins (<6mm) can generally be treated without further diagnostic studies as these patients are not as likely as patients with symptoms to have underlying venous reflux.

5 Performing a thorough clean of the wound allows optimal healing. Depending on the ulcer, preference and cost, different types of dressings can be used in the various stages of wound healing. Ulcers heal more effectively in a moist environment; hence occlusive dressings are well suited for such wounds. Non-absorbent, absorbent and debriding are a few of the many dressing types. Contaminated wounds usually require frequent dressing changes. Conversely, clean and dry ulcers should have their dressings changed weekly as frequent changes remove healthy cells. Apart from infection, other factors to consider in the healing of an ulcer include diabetes, thrombophilia and malnutrition. These conditions should be controlled before considering surgical management. In the case that the ulcer is infected, antibiotics should be promptly administered.

6 Although our patient is in the later stages of chronic venous insufficiency, conservative management strategies can help in the early stages and be beneficial overall. This includes avoiding long periods of standing or sitting. Patients should be encouraged to flex, extend their legs, feet and ankles around 10 times every 30 minutes in order to keep the blood flowing in the leg veins. Should a long period of standing be necessary, the patient should take frequent breaks and elevate their feet. Regular exercise and losing weight are important. Elevating legs while sitting or lying down is beneficial and compression stockings and good skin hygiene are essential. The patient should not use any skin creams or bath products without the doctor's approval as venous ulcers may become irritated and infected. It is also imperative that the patient adopts a healthy lifestyle and stops smoking. Regarding eczematous skin changes and stasis dermatitis, moisturising cream to combat skin dryness and flaking is beneficial.

7 Graded compression stockings are the cornerstone of chronic venous insufficiency treatment, supplemented by further specialised procedures, the choice of which depends on the specific associated clinical features. Graded compression knee-high stockings are the mainstay treatment for related oedema, stasis dermatitis and small venous leg ulcers. As therapy may be lifelong, patient compliance is of critical importance. An estimated 30–65% of patients are non-compliant with compression therapy. Recurrence of venous leg ulcers in patients compliant with stocking use is half that in those who are non-compliant. Non-compliance with prescribed stockings is the primary cause of compression therapy failure. Studies have concluded that compression stockings were more effective in healing venous ulcers compared to no compression therapy. For ulcer healing, multilayer dressings are more effective than single-layer dressings. Stockings must be put on first thing in the morning and should be removed only when the patient is recumbent (usually just before going to bed).

8 As our patient also has lipodermatosclerosis, it is important to address this problem. Physical activity (walking) should be encouraged to increase the functionality of the calf muscle pump. Weight reduction is effective if obesity is a factor. Mechanical compression therapy using compression stockings or socks is the mainstay of treatment, encouraging venous return and assisting with symptom control, but may be poorly tolerated in some individuals. Elevation of the legs can help reduce oedema and pain. Several medical options can also be offered.

9 Bleeding: telangiectasias, reticular veins or varicose veins that are superficial or located near bony prominences are prone to bleeding. Bleeding from dilated superficial veins can generally be managed with direct pressure and elevation of the limb. If bleeding continues, the bleeding point can be suture ligated. Patients with stigmata of recent venous bleeding or recurrent bleeding may be candidates for sclerotherapy of the site or vein excision, depending upon the location and size of the vein. Even in the presence of venous insufficiency, sclerotherapy reduces the risk of future bleeding at the treated site.

CASE 86: Deep venous thrombosis

History

- A 70-year-old male developed **pain in his right calf** [1] **three days after a right hip replacement** [2].
- He reports he noticed it this morning and that his leg appears **swollen and warm** [3].
- He did not report any **chest pain, haemoptysis** or **difficulty breathing** [4].
- He does not have any significant past medical history, nor does he have a **family history of DVT or clotting disorders** [5].

- He is concerned about having a clot in his leg which was **explained to him as a potential complication** [6], and asks if it is.
- He does not report any **trauma to the area or cuts/ wounds** [7].

[1] Leg pain in DVT occurs in 50% of patients, but this is entirely non-specific. Tenderness occurs in 75% of patients but is also found in 50% of patients without objectively confirmed DVT. When tenderness is present, it is usually confined to the calf muscles or along the course of the deep veins in the medial thigh. Pain and/or tenderness away from these areas is not consistent with venous thrombosis and usually indicates another diagnosis. The pain and tenderness associated with DVT do not usually correlate with the size, location or extent of the thrombus.

[2] The patient has some common risk factors for DVT including a history of immobilisation or prolonged hospitalisation, recent surgery and age >65 years.

[3] DVT should be suspected in patients presenting with symptoms including leg oedema (most specific), leg pain, warmth or erythema over the area of thrombosis. Symptoms are confined to the calf in patients with isolated distal DVT, while patients with proximal DVT may have calf or whole leg symptoms. A thrombus that does not cause a net venous outflow obstruction is often asymptomatic. Thrombi that involve the iliac bifurcation, the pelvic veins, or the vena cava produce leg oedema that is usually bilateral rather than unilateral. High partial obstruction often produces mild bilateral oedema that is mistaken for the dependent oedema of right-sided heart failure, fluid overload, or hepatic or renal insufficiency.

[4] Although most DVTs are occult and resolve spontaneously without complication, DVT-associated PE needs to be ruled out as it is associated with a 10% mortality rate. Therefore, symptoms such as dyspnoea, pleuritic chest pain and haemoptysis should be screened for.

[5] Other risk factors for DVT include family history of VTE, malignancy, hormone replacement therapy, oral contraceptives, pregnancy, stroke, heart failure, previous VTE and obesity. Less common risk factors include collagen-vascular and myeloproliferative disorders, nephrotic syndrome and heparin-induced thrombocytopenia.

[6] DVT simply cannot be diagnosed or excluded based on clinical findings, and diagnostic tests must be performed whenever the diagnosis of DVT is being considered. Even with patients with classic symptoms, as many as 46% have negative venograms. Furthermore, as many as 50% of those with image-documented venous thrombosis lack specific symptoms. Given the risks of untreated DVT (e.g. fatal pulmonary emboli) and the risk of anticoagulation (life-threatening bleeding), an accurate diagnosis of DVT is essential.

[7] Differentials include cellulitis and calf muscle tear/ haematoma. Another possibility is a large or ruptured Baker's cyst.

Examination

- The patient appears in **slight discomfort** [1] but there are no signs of respiratory distress.
- The patient's capillary refill time is <2 seconds. Pulse rate is **within normal limits** [2] and regular.

- BP is **unremarkable** [3].
- Heart sounds are dual with **no murmurs** [4].
- The abdomen is soft and non-tender. **No lymphadenopathy of masses** [5] were palpated.

- On examination of the legs, the right calf is **swollen with a circumference 4cm greater** [6] than the left and appears **erythematous** and **tender** [7].
- There is **slight pain** on **dorsiflexion of the right foot** [8].
- Pulses are palpable and there is no **widespread oedema or blanched appearance** [9] along the whole leg.

- There are **no varicose veins** or **signs of venous access** [10] seen.
- **Respiratory examination** [11] reveals equal air entry with vesical breath sounds.
- The surgical wound site **looks clean** [12] and in the process of healing.

1 General inspection of the patient can guide the clinician's level of concern for the acuity of the patient's pathology. For example, if this patient looked visibly uncomfortable with difficulty breathing, this may raise the suspicion that the patient has had a PE secondary to a DVT. Although from general inspection of the vitals they seem within the normal range, it is important to continually monitor for any changes.

2 The pulse is within the normal range. This is reassuring as tachycardia is a common finding of PE.

3 Similarly, BP is currently within the normal range and stable. This along with other important vital signs must be monitored.

4 Heart murmurs may suggest valvular heart disease or structural heart defects. It is important to investigate these peri-operatively in the context of fitness for general anaesthetic, and to quantify any increased risk of peri-operative complications.

5 Masses may indicate malignancy, which is a risk factor for clot development.

6 Oedema is the most specific symptom of DVT, leading to a difference in calf or thigh circumference. One meta-analysis reported that patients with a difference in calf circumference were twice as likely to have DVT.

7 While no single physical finding or combination of symptoms and signs is sufficiently accurate to establish the diagnosis of DVT, these findings greatly point us in the direction of DVT diagnosis. Patients with venous thrombosis may have variable discolouration of the lower extremity. The most common abnormal hue is reddish purple from venous engorgement and obstruction. Interestingly, the features of

DVT are often non-specific and patients are asymptomatic. Of patients evaluated for DVT of the lower extremity, only a quarter have the disease.

8 Pain can occur on dorsiflexion of the foot (Homans' sign) with a straight knee. However, Homans' sign is neither sensitive nor specific: it is present in fewer than one-third of patients with confirmed DVT and is found in >50% of patients without DVT.

9 In rare cases, the leg is cyanotic from massive iliofemoral venous obstruction. This ischaemic form of venous occlusion was originally described as phlegmasia cerulea dolens ('painful blue inflammation'). The leg is usually markedly oedematous, painful and cyanotic. Petechiae are often present.

10 A differential for DVT is superficial thrombophlebitis. This is characterised by the finding of a palpable, indurated, cord-like, tender, subcutaneous venous segment. 40% of patients with superficial thrombophlebitis without coexisting varicose veins and with no other obvious aetiology such as IV catheters, IV drug abuse and soft tissue injury have an associated DVT.

11 As many as 40% of patients have silent pulmonary embolism when symptomatic DVT is diagnosed. Approximately 4% of individuals treated for DVT develop symptomatic PE. Almost 1% of postoperative hospitalised patients develop PE. The 10–12% mortality rate for PE in hospitalised patients underscores the need for prevention of this complication.

12 It is important to evaluate the surgical site as a potential site of infection.

Investigations

- Assessment of the patient's **pre-test probability** [1] was conducted using the **Wells score** [2].
- As he has had **major surgery, localised tenderness and calf swelling** [3], he scored a total of **3 points** [4].
- He has not **previously** [5] had a DVT.

- Given his high probability of having a DVT, a **D-dimer did not need to be ordered** [6] and **compression ultrasonography with Doppler** [7] was performed.

- It showed **non-compressibility of the obstructed vein** and **abnormal flow** [8].
- Given his **high risk of pulmonary embolism** [9] he

underwent a **CTPA** [10] which was negative.
- **No routine bloods** [11] were performed, and an **ECG showed normal sinus rhythm** [12].

1 Clinically assessing the pre-test probability is useful when determining whether to do D-dimer testing in select patients, and also allows for the strategic use of ultrasonography for diagnosis. This guides diagnostic testing which aims to 'rule in' (>85% post-test probability of DVT) or 'rule out' DVT (<2% post-test probability of DVT in the next 3 months) with an acceptable level of certainty, thereby justifying instituting or withholding therapy, respectively.

2 Validated clinical prediction rules (Wells criteria) should be used to estimate the pre-test probability of DVT. This is extremely important as it will determine whether D-dimer levels and ultrasonography are performed.

3 The components of the Wells score include:
- paralysis, paresis or recent orthopaedic casting of a lower extremity (1 point)
- recently bedridden for >3 days or major surgery within the past 4 weeks (1 point)
- localised tenderness in the deep vein system (1 point)
- swelling of an entire leg (1 point)
- calf swelling 3cm greater than the other leg, measured 10cm below the tibial tuberosity (1 point)
- pitting oedema greater in the symptomatic leg (1 point)
- collateral non-varicose superficial veins (1 point)
- active cancer or cancer treated within last 6 months (1 point)
- alternative diagnosis more likely than DVT (e.g. Baker's cyst, cellulitis, muscle damage, post-thrombotic syndrome, inguinal lymphadenopathy, external venous compression) (minus 2 points).

4 The total score in an individual patient denotes the following risk of DVT:
- 0 or fewer points – low probability
- 1–2 points – moderate probability
- 3–8 points – high probability.

5 The modified Wells score contains all the components of the original Wells score, with one additional point given to those with a history of previously documented DVT. The modified score classifies patients according to whether or not DVT is likely (a score of ≥2) or unlikely (a score of ≤1).

6 In appropriately selected patients with low pre-test probability of DVT or PE, it is reasonable to obtain a high-sensitivity D-dimer. The D-dimer assay has a high sensitivity (up to 97%); however, it has a relatively poor specificity (as low as 35%) and therefore should only be used to rule out DVT, not to confirm the diagnosis of DVT.
- Normal D-dimer level (<500ng/ml) – patients with a low pre-test probability in whom the D-dimer level is normal do not need further testing.

- Positive D-dimer level (>500ng/ml) – in patients with a low pre-test probability in whom the D-dimer is positive, whole leg ultrasonography or proximal compression ultrasonography (CUS) should be performed.

7 In patients with intermediate to high pre-test probability of lower-extremity DVT, CUS with Doppler is recommended. This is a combination of ultrasonography to visualise the vein and Doppler to assess blood flow abnormalities, as the examiner applies gentle pressure to normally compressible veins using an ultrasound probe.

8 Positive findings include non-compressibility of the obstructed vein, visible hyperechoic mass and absent or abnormal flow in Doppler imaging. Although alternative imaging modalities are available (CT or MRI venography), they are rarely, if ever needed. If the whole leg ultrasonography is negative for DVT, no further testing is required. If the ultrasonography is positive, patients should be treated if a proximal or distal DVT is identified.

9 Patients should also be investigated for the pre-test probability of having a PE via the Wells criteria or PE rule-out criteria.

10 Patients at high risk of PE should be investigated with diagnostic imaging studies (e.g. ventilation-perfusion scan, multidetector helical CT and pulmonary angiography). PE is most often diagnosed by means of ventilation-perfusion lung scanning, which is reported as having a low, moderate or high probability of depicting PE. When the results of these studies are equivocal, the use of spiral CT scans may be able to demonstrate intravascular thrombosis. In many institutions, the criterion standard for diagnosing PE is CT pulmonary angiography.

11 Possible laboratory tests are coagulation studies (e.g. PT and aPTT) to evaluate for a hypercoagulable state due to conditions such as thrombophilia (younger patients with positive family history or unusual thrombus location). Similarly, protein S, protein C, ATIII, factor V Leiden, prothrombin 20210A mutation, antiphospholipid antibodies and homocysteine levels can be measured. Routine laboratory tests are not useful diagnostically, but may provide clues as to the underlying cause and may influence treatment decisions if DVT is confirmed. Additionally, for cases of idiopathic thrombosis, general tumour screening is necessary. This includes FBE, UECs, LFTs, urinalysis and CXR. It is also important to confirm the patient is up to date on all age-appropriate cancer screening

12 Electrocardiography may demonstrate ST-segment changes in patients with PE. The classically documented finding is the S1Q3T3 pattern, denoted by a deep S wave in lead I, Q wave and inverted T wave in lead III. However, this finding is neither sensitive nor specific for PE, and is only found in 20% of patients with PE.

Management

Immediate

To treat the **immediate risk** [1] of DVT, commence the patient on **anticoagulation** [2], such as LMWH. More **aggressive/invasive methods** [3] are not deemed appropriate. Monitor for **signs of bleeding** [4] and **platelet numbers** [5] as well as **renal function** [6]. Once safe, continue treatment from **home** [7] and encourage **mobility** [8]. If the patient **remains stable** [9] and is **not at high risk of bleeding** [10], consider transitioning to **long-term anticoagulation agents** [11]. **Continued** assessment for bleeding risk [12] should be conducted. After **3 months** [13], consider ceasing anticoagulation if not meeting **indications for lifetime therapy** [14]. Ensure no signs of **recurrent** [15] DVT.

Long-term

Long-term follow-up with specialists [16] is not necessary but **post-thrombotic syndrome** [17] should be monitored for.

1 The primary objectives for the treatment of DVT are to prevent PE, reduce morbidity, and prevent or minimise the risk of developing post-thrombotic syndrome (PTS). The mainstay of medical therapy has been anticoagulation as it is non-invasive and treats 90% of patients with no immediate demonstrable physical sequelae of DVT. There is also a low risk of complications, and studies have indicated an improvement in morbidity and mortality following this treatment.

2 The first phase of anticoagulation therapy for DVT is the initiation phase. Initiation (5–21 days following diagnosis) aims to arrest the active prothrombotic state and inhibit thrombus propagation and embolisation. Many different agents may be utilised.

3 Additional therapies include pharmacological thrombolysis. The goal of this is for faster resolution and it should be administered if there is a slow response to anticoagulation, or PE with haemodynamic instability; it can also be considered for acute proximal DVT of the leg. The agents used for this purpose include streptokinase, urokinase and tissue plasminogen activator. Another option is catheter-directed thrombolysis, where the thrombolytic agent is administered directly at the site of obstruction via a venous catheter. The indications for this procedure include an insufficient response to anticoagulation and thrombolysis, extensive thrombus (e.g. massive iliofemoral vein thrombosis associated with limb ischaemic or vascular compromise) and phlegmasia cerulea dolens. Low dose heparin is required to be administered prior to the procedure. Inferior vena cava filter insertion is indicated in patients with DVT at high risk of developing PE who have contraindications to anticoagulation, thrombolysis and thrombectomy (e.g. active bleeding, recent major surgery, recent intracranial haemorrhage).

4 Care should be taken to minimise the risk of major haemorrhage throughout the treatment period.

5 Monitor for the development of heparin-induced thrombocytopenia (HIT) if heparin or LMWH is used. This is achieved by measuring platelets. Heparin or LMWH should be discontinued if the platelet count falls to <100 x 10⁹/L. Fondaparinux is not associated with HIT.

6 For most patients treated with LMWH or fondaparinux, no therapeutic monitoring of anticoagulation is needed. Changes in patient weight may require adjustment of the dose. Renal function indices, such as serum creatinine and urea, should be obtained to determine initial and ongoing appropriateness of LMWH and fondaparinux, as both require discontinuation or dose adjustment in renal impairment. Frequent INR monitoring of patients who are treated with warfarin is required. This is preferably done by experts or specialised anticoagulation clinics, whenever possible. Anticoagulant therapy, although potentially life-saving, has inherent bleeding risks. Rivaroxaban, apixaban, edoxaban and dabigatran do not require laboratory monitoring for anticoagulant effect. It is recommended that attention be directed to any changes in renal or liver function testing as clinically indicated.

7 Home treatment is the option for most cases. Outcomes are at least as good as those achieved with hospitalisation, with lower cost and improved patient satisfaction. The criteria for hospitalisation include DVT that is best treated with IV unfractionated heparin (UFH), the presence or suspicion of PE, DVT that will undergo interventional therapy (catheter-directed thrombolysis), highly symptomatic DVT (pain and oedema needing analgesia), inability to educate the patient adequately in outpatient or ED setting, coexisting comorbidity requiring hospital management, or the presence of risk factors for bleeding that require close observation (e.g. chronic liver disease with varices, GI bleeding, bleeding disorder, malignancy).

8 It is important to encourage early mobilisation as early as tolerated and minimise bedrest.

9 The second phase on anticoagulation is long-term (up to 3 months) with the goal of preventing a new thrombus while the original clot is stabilised, and intrinsic thrombolysis is under way. Patients with proximal DVT of the leg and some patients with distal DVT of the leg should generally receive anticoagulation for at least 3 months. The choice of agent depends on patient factors such as hepatic function, renal function, pregnancy, presence of cancer, obesity, concomitant medications and the ability to monitor drug–drug interactions, and the risk of bleeding. Choice may also depend on individual physician or patient preference or recommendations in local guidelines.

10 For patients at increased risk of bleeding (e.g. recent surgery, peptic ulceration) treatment with intravenous UFH is preferred initially because it has a short half-life and its effect can be reversed quickly with protamine. Once it is clear anticoagulation is tolerated, selection of an appropriate anticoagulation regimen can take place.

11 In terms of direct oral anticoagulants (DOACs), rivaroxaban, apixaban, edoxaban and dabigatran are as effective as UFH, LMWH and warfarin for the treatment of DVT, and are generally recommended over warfarin, UFH and LMWH outside of special populations. All have a longer half-life than UFH or LMWH and a shorter half-life than warfarin, and all have a rapid onset of action. The patient will stay on this for a minimum of 3 months. During this time, follow-up and re-evaluation are based on the patient's level of risk for bleeding, comorbidities, and the anticoagulant agent selected.

12 Patients treated with warfarin continue to report for INR measurements. The frequency of measurements depends on the stability of INR values at each visit. Commonly INR is measured 1–2 times weekly after initial dose titration, with the time between measurements progressively extending if values remain in range. The target range of 2–3 is maintained. Patients taking dabigatran or edoxaban remain on the same dose started following the initiation with a parenteral agent, unless renal function substantially declines, warranting discontinuation. Apixaban and rivaroxaban doses are adjusted following the initiation phase (7 days for apixaban, 21 days for rivaroxaban). If extended LMWH is used, the dose depends on the agent and should be adjusted to the patient's weight.

13 The next phase of anticoagulation is set between 3 months to an indefinite time. Recommendations for continuation of anticoagulant therapy beyond 3 months vary by patient group. In patients who receive extended anticoagulation therapy, there is usually no need to change the choice of anticoagulant. Anticoagulation may also be discontinued after a course of at least 3 months. There is

consensus that patients who have an index DVT that occurs in the setting of a major transient provocation have a relatively low risk of developing recurrent VTE in the next 5 years, with estimates in the range of 15%.

14 Anticoagulant therapy is recommended for 3–12 months depending on site of thrombosis and on the ongoing presence of risk factors. If DVT recurs, if a chronic hypercoagulability is identified, or if PE is life-threatening, lifetime anticoagulation therapy may be recommended. This treatment protocol has a cumulative risk of bleeding complications of <12%.

15 Recurrent venous thrombosis refers to either clinical progression or worsening, documented objectively by venous duplex ultrasound, of the DVT, or the development of PE while on adequate anticoagulation. The early development of recurrent DVT may be caused by ongoing activation of clotting owing to an underlying cancer, antiphospholipid syndrome, or HIT, or simply because of inadequate or delayed initiation of treatment. If extension/worsening of DVT or PE occurs during an initial period of treatment with heparin, HIT should be considered, and a platelet count ordered immediately. If there is any suspicion of HIT, it is recommended that heparin is discontinued and treatment with a suitable alternative (e.g. argatroban) is initiated. For patients who have recurrent VTE while taking warfarin (with an INR in the therapeutic range) or dabigatran, rivaroxaban, apixaban or edoxaban, treatment should generally be changed to LMWH. DOAC interactions with medications reducing serum concentrations (e.g. P-glycoprotein inducers with dabigatran and edoxaban, P-glycoprotein and strong CYP3A4 inducers with rivaroxaban and apixaban) should be evaluated and modified where possible, to mitigate effects. However, recurrent VTE while on anticoagulants at therapeutic doses is unusual and should prompt evaluation of the recurrent VTE and of adherence to therapy. D-dimer testing in this situation may be helpful, as the initial D-dimer level is likely to be initially elevated, and it should fall if parenteral therapy is effective. The possibility of an underlying malignancy or antiphospholipid syndrome should also be considered. If progression or recurrence occurs in a patient already taking LMWH, the dose should be adjusted upwards by about 25% (as long as HIT has been excluded).

16 Consultations with the following specialists may be indicated: haematologist, vascular surgeon, radiologist/interventional radiologist.

17 Post-thrombotic syndrome (PTS) is a chronic complication of DVT that manifests months to many years after the initial event. Symptoms range from mild erythema and localised induration to massive extremity swelling and ulceration, usually exacerbated by standing and relieved by elevation of the extremity. After symptomatic DVT is treated with anticoagulation, the incidence of PTS at 2 years is 25–50% despite long-term anticoagulation for iliofemoral DVT, and after 7–10 years, the incidence is 70–90%. The only current treatment is use of compression hose and elevation.

CASE 87: Diabetic foot

History

- A **62-year-old male** [1] of **Bangladeshi descent** [2] with **T2DM** [3] presents with a 3-day history of **swelling, redness and pain** [4] of the **right foot** [5].
- It is **worse at night** [6] and he complains of **malaise** [7] over the last few weeks.
- A **blister from wearing new shoes** [8] has persisted on his forefoot for 3 months.
- Despite daily dressings, the area has **not healed** [9].
- The patient has had multiple **ulcers in his feet previously** [10].
- He reports chronic **numbness** [11] in his feet.

- The patient has missed his last few GP appointments and cannot recall his last **blood glucose level** [12].
- His **past medical history** [13] consists of **chronic kidney disease** [14] and **hypertension** [15].
- His **medications** [16] include **metformin** [17], **ramipril** [18] and rosuvastatin.
- He denies a history of **stroke, heart attack, peripheral vascular disease** [19] or **eye disease** [20].
- He is a **smoker** [21] with a 40 pack year history and drinks 5 units of **alcohol** [22] each day.
- He is a **retired taxi driver** [23].

[1] Diabetes mellitus is a very common chronic disease. Those aged >45 years are at greater risk of developing diabetes.

[2] Patients of South Asian descent are approximately three times more likely to develop diabetes than those of European descent. They are also more likely to suffer from complications of diabetes, such as macro- and microvascular disease.

[3] Type 2 diabetes mellitus (T2DM) is the most common type of diabetes in adults (>90%). It is due to insulin resistance and a progressive loss of insulin secretion from pancreatic beta cells, both of which lead to hyperglycaemia. It is detected either through screening or the presentation of hyperglycaemic symptoms. Type 1 diabetes mellitus (T1DM) is an autoimmune destruction of pancreatic beta cells which leads to insulin deficiency in the body. About 5–10% of diabetes in adults are type 1 and of these, 25% initially present with diabetic ketoacidosis.

[4] These signs of inflammation may indicate an underlying infection. Those with diabetes have some degree of immunosuppression and hence are at greater risk of developing infections compared to non-diabetics. Patients with sensory neuropathy may still be able to feel the onset of foot pain when an infection is present. Erythema of the foot may suggest cellulitis. The extent of the redness should be noted on examination.

[5] The location of the symptoms should be enquired about and noted. Often, symptoms arise in the feet and occasionally the calves. Foot deformity compromises balance and gait and hence predisposes patients to foot injuries and ulcers. These anatomic changes also impair microcirculation and skin integrity, which again increases the risk of ulcer development

and poor healing. A history of prior foot injuries should be ascertained from these patients.

[6] The time course of symptoms should be included in the history. Symptoms related to diabetic foot are often worse at night, may wake the patient up from sleep and are relieved with walking.

[7] Malaise can be a sign of infection.

[8] A small friction blister from new shoes may appear harmless; however, in diabetic patients with a poor ability to heal wounds, this can evolve into a diabetic ulcer.

[9] Poorly controlled glucose levels can reduce blood circulation that is required for skin repair. This means that diabetic patients have poor wound healing. Although cuts, scratches and blisters can occur on any site of the body, injury to the feet is most common. Hence, a small sore on the foot can develop into an ulcer which can result in infection (fungal, bacterial, gangrene) and limb amputation. Therefore, self-checks for ulcers, blisters, cracks, ingrown toenails and calluses should be performed regularly.

[10] A previous history of ulcer or amputation is the most important risk factor for diabetic foot. 30% of patients with foot ulcers have had a previous ulcer. Amputation of the leg increases the risk of ulceration on the contralateral foot due to increased pressure on the foot and abnormal gait.

[11] Neuropathy can present as burning, tingling or numbness. This compromises the patient's protective sensation and predisposes them to injury and the development of ulcers. Due to the lack of pain sensation or pressure perception, ulcers can go unnoticed by the patient. This gives rise to infections and anatomic deformities, e.g.

hammer toes, collapsed arch of the foot, and rocker bottom feet associated with Charcot foot. Other sensory changes may include fatigue, cramping or aching in the legs.

12 A thorough history of the patient's diabetes and glycaemic control is of utmost importance as it requires optimal management. The duration of diabetes, presence of micro- and macrovascular disease, recent BGLs or HbA1c and compliance with lifestyle measures (exercise, diet) and/ or medications should all be enquired about. A poorly controlled BGL increases the risk of developing microvascular and macrovascular complications. Those with a fasting plasma glucose ≥7.0mmol/L, 2-hour oral glucose tolerance test ≥11.1mmol/L, random plasma glucose ≥11.1mmol/L or HbA1c ≥6.5% are considered to have high blood glucose levels. HbA1c (also known as glycated haemoglobin) measures the last 3-month average BGL, as the lifespan of red blood cells is around 3–4 months.

13 Past medical history is important in determining risk factors for the development of diabetic foot and fitness for surgery if required. Recognising risk factors for diabetic foot is important because it allows early management which reduces morbidity related to foot ulceration.

14 Diabetes is the leading cause of kidney disease. High blood glucose damages blood vessels which contributes to diabetic nephropathy. CKD is an abnormality in kidney function or structure lasting for ≥3 months. Most patients are asymptomatic due to the ability of the kidneys to compensate for loss of function in nephrons. Only when a significant proportion of nephrons are damaged will symptoms appear. These symptoms include peripheral oedema and uraemia. If untreated, CKD can progress to end-stage renal disease, which requires dialysis or renal transplant.

15 Many diabetic patients develop HTN which is also a major risk factor in the development of CKD. Hence, BP control is crucial.

16 It is important to be aware of the medications a patient is on. They may be taking a drug that is worsening their condition; for example, some antipsychotics can cause metabolic syndrome and diabetes. They may be missing medications required for their conditions or the patient could be non-compliant with taking regular medications. All of these factors increase the risk of having poorly controlled BGLs.

17 Metformin is a common medication used in the treatment of diabetes. It belongs to the biguanide class. It works by activating AMP-dependent protein kinase to decrease gluconeogenesis, increase glucose uptake by cells and increase insulin sensitivity.

18 Ramipril is an antihypertensive within the group of ACE inhibitors. ACE inhibitors are known to be renal protective as they block the renin–angiotensin–aldosterone system (RAAS). This results in a reduction in systemic BP which protects glomeruli and reduces proteinuria.

19 Severe diabetes can lead to macrovascular complications. These include cerebrovascular accidents, cardiovascular disease (i.e. myocardial ischaemia, ischaemic heart disease) and peripheral vascular disease. All of these diseases contribute to the patient's morbidity and mortality. Peripheral vascular disease compromises blood flow to the extremities and this hinders the healing of any ulcers or infection.

20 Microvascular complications of diabetes include retinopathy, neuropathy and nephropathy. Retinopathy occurs when blood vessels of the retina are damaged due to high blood glucose. It is one of the leading causes of blindness in developed countries and affects up to 80% of patients who have diabetes for longer than 20 years. Visual impairment also hinders the ability for patients to inspect their feet for injuries. Neuropathy can present as sensory neuropathy (paraesthesia, numbness, pain) or autonomic neuropathy (postural hypotension, gastric paresis).

21 Smoking is a risk factor for diabetic complications.

22 Alcohol increases the risk of metabolic syndrome and hence can contribute to diabetic complications.

23 A thorough social history is important in order to understand the patient's risk factors for developing diabetic foot (e.g. occupation, physical activity, diet) and manage those with their GP.

Examination

- The patient appears **overweight** [1].
- He is **febrile and mildly tachycardic** [2].
- He does not use **mobility aids** [3] and is wearing **flip flops** [4].
- His **capillary refill time** [5] on the toes is 3 seconds.
- The foot appears **dry and cracked with calluses** [6] on the soles.
- On removal of the dressing, there is a **right foot ulcer** [7] located at the first metatarsophalangeal joint.
- There is **malodorous pus** [8] over the wound bed.
- Blanching **erythema** [9] extends 5cm from the ulcer border.
- There is **mild pitting oedema** [10] up to the ankle.
- There is no obvious **foot deformity** [11] or **gangrene** [12].

- The **dorsalis pedis pulse is weak** [13].
- **Sensation is absent** [14] over the soles of the feet bilaterally.

- **Cardiovascular exam** [15] is normal.
- There is no evidence of **previous surgeries** [16].

1 General inspection of the patient can illustrate the context of their condition to the doctor. A patient who appears overweight or obese is more likely to have poorly controlled diabetes. Waist circumference (abdominal or central obesity) is a stronger predictor of diabetes and cardiovascular disease than weight alone. BMI is useful but can be misleading in the elderly and in muscular individuals.

2 Vitals provide a clue to the acuity of the patient's condition. A patient who is febrile and tachycardic may indicate that they have an acute infection or possibly even sepsis. This requires urgent medical attention.

3 Diabetic complications, such as stroke or amputation, will require the patient to use some sort of mobility aid to move around.

4 Ill-fitting, unsupportive or non-protective footwear places patients at risk of foot injuries and the development of diabetic foot. Hence, observing the patient's footwear is important in assessing the cause of foot injuries (i.e. blister/ ulcer). An offloading shoe is designed to reduce weight-bearing pressure on the forefoot which promotes faster healing from wounds or post-surgery.

5 An adequate capillary refill time indicates the patient is perfusing well and thus would likely have preserved end-organ perfusion. In peripheral arterial disease, blood flow to the extremities may be hindered, which will present as delayed capillary refill.

6 A comprehensive examination of the foot should be performed. Inspection involves looking for ulcers, calluses, blisters, ingrown toenails and cracking of the skin. Calluses occur due to friction and high pressure associated with poor footwear. They need to be trimmed down in these patients as they can grow thick, break down and become ulcers. Similarly, ingrown toenails cause trauma to adjacent skin and tissue and can result in an open sore.

7 About 10% of people with diabetes will develop a diabetic foot ulcer at some point in their life. An ulcer is a full-thickness epithelial defect. Diabetic ulcers occur most often in areas of high pressure, such as the forefoot distal to the tarsometatarsal joint. In non-ambulatory patients, ulcers occur often at the heel. As an ulcer is an open wound, it is vulnerable to infection (e.g. localised infection, cellulitis, abscess, sepsis, osteomyelitis). Hyperglycaemia further hinders wound healing, which increases infection risk. The size, depth, site and bed of the ulcer should be noted.

8 Malodorous wounds and pus may indicate the presence of infection.

9 The location and extent of erythema should be noted as it may indicate cellulitis with or without deep soft tissue infection. The area should be palpated for fluctuance which would indicate an underlying abscess (deep soft tissue infection).

10 Oedema of the foot, ankle or calf may suggest infection.

11 Foot deformities contribute significantly to abnormal gait and balance due to improper distribution of pressure across the foot when walking. They also pose a challenge with footwear. Hence, deformities increase the risk of mechanical and pressure injuries which lead to the development of diabetic foot. On examination, the feet should be observed for hallux valgus (also known as bunions), hammer toes or mallet toes. Charcot's mid-foot deformity is uncommon and associated with mid-foot ulcers due to the inability to offload the area for healing.

12 Gangrene is tissue necrosis due to impaired blood circulation or infection. This presents as altered skin colour (black), coldness, numbness, swelling and pain. The feet and hands are usually affected. Dry gangrene occurs due to ischaemic tissue and is often secondary to peripheral artery disease. Wet gangrene (infected gangrene) is caused by bacterial infection which emits a foul odour. *Clostridium perfringens* is the most common aetiology. Due to stagnant blood bacteria rapidly proliferate, leading to sepsis. There is a high mortality associated with infected gangrene and thus emergency amputation is often needed to limit the systemic effects of the infection. As diabetes is a risk factor for peripheral vascular disease and infections, it can give rise to both wet and dry gangrene.

13 An absent or weak pedal pulse is concerning for peripheral artery disease. Other signs of poor perfusion include cold temperature and pale skin colour. These require immediate referral to the vascular team for investigation and management. Normal pulses indicate good arterial perfusion to the limb. Adequate perfusion is necessary for wound healing. Up to 30% of diabetic patients have peripheral arterial disease.

14 Peripheral sensory neuropathy significantly contributes to the development of foot ulcers and increases the risk of amputation. Between 40% and 60% of diabetics have sensory neuropathy. The type of sensory change (numbness, paraesthesia) and location should be noted.

15 Cardiovascular disease is macrovascular complication. Heart murmurs may suggest valvular heart disease or structural heart defects. It is important to investigate these peri-operatively in the context of fitness for general anaesthetic, and to quantify any increased risk of peri-operative complications.

16 Evidence of previous surgeries should be noted, including previous amputation.

Investigations

- FBE reports a significantly increased **WCC** [1] .
- **UEC results are normal** [2] .
- **CRP is elevated** [3] .
- **Blood glucose** [4] is raised at 15mmol/L.
- **Ulcer swabs and blood samples** [5] are sent for culture and sensitivity analysis.

- The patient has an **ABI of 1.3** [6] .
- An X-ray shows **no underlying bony erosion or fractures** [7] .
- **MRI** [8] does not show signs of osteomyelitis.
- **Angiography** [9] reveals severe stenosis of the right posterior tibial artery.

1 Infection and inflammation are common causes of an elevated WCC. In this patient, the presence of a malodorous ulcer in the setting of poorly controlled diabetes may explain these findings. In our patient, the combination of fever, tachycardia and raised WCC is concerning for a severe (limb- or life-threatening) infection.

2 UECs are important in the setting of a surgical emergency. First, they identify any electrolyte abnormalities that most often need correction prior to surgery. Secondly, they assess renal function and fitness for IV contrast in the setting of imaging (such as an angiography), as well as serving as a prognosticator for postoperative recovery.

3 C-reactive protein is one of many acute phase reactants that accompanies inflammatory states. During infection or inflammation, CRP is elevated. However, CRP has medium sensitivity and specificity for infection, hence it is used to monitor the patient's condition and response to treatment over time.

4 All diabetic patients with complications should have a blood glucose ordered. Blood glucose is often elevated in the presence of infection.

5 Microbiological cultures should be sent for analysis if infection is suspected. Samples should be taken from the base of the wound. Blood cultures should also be ordered as the patient may be septic. Once an organism is identified, the sensitivities are useful in guiding directed antibiotic treatment.

6 An ankle–brachial index (ABI) is the ratio of BP at the ankle to the BP in the upper arm. It is a popular test for quickly assessing peripheral vascular disease. A normal ratio is 0.9–1.2. Values <0.9 indicate arterial stenosis. ABI is unreliable on patients with arterial calcification as stiff arteries create falsely high ankle pressures. Hence, ratios of ≥1.3 should also be further investigated. Patients with diabetes, kidney failure or a heavy smoking history are more likely to have some sort of calcification in their arteries.

7 An X-ray of the foot is required in all patients to look for fractures, osteomyelitis and deformities. The films should ideally occur while the patient is weight-bearing in order to visualise foot deformities. Gout is a possible differential that can be investigated with X-ray. On imaging, gout may present as joint space narrowing, tophaceous arthritis and bony erosions. Osteomyelitis may appear as hypolucency or cortical destruction on X-ray; however, it requires an MRI to accurately diagnose.

8 If osteomyelitis is present, soft tissue fluid collections are visualised on MRI. T1 sequences would show hypointense areas of bone, while T2 sequences display hyperintense areas.

9 Angiography is the gold standard for diagnosing peripheral artery disease. Haemodynamically significant stenosis between the aorta and the feet requires urgent intervention.

Management

Immediate

Initiate sepsis protocol [1] . Monitor **vital signs** [2] and **urine output** [3] . Obtain IV access and **administer antibiotics** [4] and **fluid** [5] . **Seek advice** [6] from the vascular surgery team.

Short-term

Perform **basic wound care** [7] . Debride the wound and drain any collection found. Look closely for any areas of **gangrene** [8] . Perform **balloon angioplasty of the right posterior tibial artery** [9] . Following the procedure, keep the patient in hospital for **monitoring** [10]. Review the patient's **surgical site** [11] and **auscultate the lungs** [12] and **examine the lower limbs** [13]. Provide **offloading footwear** [14]. The patient may be discharged if **vital signs remain stable** [15] and they are **back to their premorbid level of function** [16].

Long-term

Follow the patient up in the **vascular outpatient clinic** [17] for monitoring of postoperative complications and diabetic foot progression. **Multidisciplinary care** [18] should be provided to the patient, as well as **dietary advice** [19].

[1] As the patient has signs of possible sepsis, a sepsis protocol should be initiated. This includes regular monitoring of vitals, taking blood cultures, measuring lactate (often through a VBG), administering oxygen if needed, and providing IV antibiotics and fluids.

[2] Ensure the patient remains haemodynamically stable. A BP that is dropping despite fluid therapy may require inotropes/vasopressors.

[3] Urine output is the best indicator of fluid balance. If urine output dwindles, this may be a sign of acute renal failure and early recognition is key to effective treatment. It is best monitored through an indwelling urinary catheter.

[4] IV broad-spectrum antibiotics are required immediately in the setting of suspected sepsis. The type of antibiotic used may depend on the hospital or community but usually IV gentamicin and flucloxacillin are used. Once cultures and sensitivities return, targeted therapy may commence.

[5] Intravenous fluid is integral in fluid resuscitation and stabilisation of circulation. In the setting of inflammation and infection, third spacing may occur, where too much fluid moves from the intravascular space into the interstitium. IV fluid management is based around four principles – resuscitation, maintenance, replacement (any fluid losses such as from the GI tract) and redistribution (e.g. third spacing). A 500ml bolus of a crystalloid solution (e.g. normal saline, Hartmann's solution) is adequate for resuscitation. Fluid overload should be avoided in patients with congestive heart failure. Following this, ensure the patient is on a fluid chart in order to monitor fluid input and output. Replace the losses based on this chart, and also ensure that adequate maintenance fluid is being given.

[6] Diabetic foot and associated peripheral vascular disease fall under the vascular surgeon's domain, and care should be directed by their advice. They will usually come to assess the patient themselves and consent the patient for a surgical intervention if necessary.

[7] After resuscitation, the wound should be cleaned and dressed with a non-adherent dressing covered with absorptive material. This type of dressing maintains a moist environment which is optimal for wound healing. If the wound has tunnelling or large amounts of exudate or necrotic tissue, it should be debrided beforehand. If there is an abscess or joint space infection, it should be drained.

In patients with a large skin defect but healthy granulation tissue, a split-thickness skin graft can assist with wound healing. However, the use of split-thickness skin graft is less effective for high pressure areas, such as the plantar forefoot.

[8] If there are areas of irreversible gangrene, then amputation may be performed. Diabetes is the most common non-traumatic cause of limb amputation.

[9] Once soft tissue infection has been controlled, surgical bypass or endovascular intervention (balloon intervention +/– stenting) may be required to establish normal perfusion to the limb extremity. Both methods have been shown to be equally effective in avoiding lower limb amputation. It is possible for stenosis to reoccur after endovascular intervention, hence repeat procedures may be required. If there is osteomyelitis, then the infected bone will need to be surgically removed. Foot deformities (e.g. bunions, hammer toes) should also be surgically corrected later.

[10] The patient must be monitored postoperatively for haemodynamic instability, reaction to anaesthesia, DVT and PE, urinary retention or renal failure. Monitoring for the resolution of infective symptoms is also important.

[11] Review the surgical site to ensure proper closure and that there are no signs of infection from the puncture site. Examine the skin around the site for erythema. Check for warmth of the surgical site.

[12] Listen for any crepitations. The presence of crackles in the lung may indicate either an infective process (such as HAP or aspiration pneumonia), or atelectasis. To prevent postoperative atelectasis, the patient should be given adequate analgesia and an incentive spirometer (both encourage deep breathing which prevents lung collapse).

[13] Look for any other wounds or ulcers that may have been initially missed. These can be continuing sources of infection for the patient. Any changes in skin colour or sensation should be noted. Recent surgery and subsequent immobilisation in bed postoperatively are major risk factors for the development of DVT. Inspect the calves for unilateral swelling and erythema. Palpate the calves to ensure they are not tender. If clinically suspicious, order a Doppler ultrasound of the affected leg to diagnose, and then start the patient on anticoagulation.

14 Repetitive trauma sustained during mobilisation is the most common cause of ulcers in diabetic patients. Preventing trauma allows ulcer healing. Offloading footwear protects the feet and helps distribute pressure more evenly across the foot bed.

15 If the patient remains afebrile, is haemodynamically stable and looks well, they are generally well enough to be discharged home.

16 The patient should ideally be able to function at the level that they were able to prior to becoming ill. If unsure, refer to the allied health team (primarily physiotherapy, occupational therapy and social work) for further assessment on fitness for discharge home at a functional level.

17 The need for ongoing follow-up depends on the severity of the illness, the complexity of the procedure and the patient's risk for postoperative complications. Some patients are fit and well enough to be managed by their GP, whilst some will require several follow-up visits with the vascular surgeons to ensure adequate recovery and resolution of any lingering symptoms.

18 Patients with poorly controlled diabetes often have several comorbidities, hence a multidisciplinary approach is most appropriate. This includes referring the patient on to any podiatry or orthotics service if available, a diabetes nurse educator, dietitian and exercise physiologist. These experts can provide the patient with advice on how to reduce the risk of developing a foot ulcer in the future.

19 Dietary advice and supplements (if appropriate) should be provided, as diabetic patients often have malnutrition and sarcopenia. Malnutrition impairs wound healing. Furthermore, having a well-balanced, healthy diet improves diabetes, which can reduce the risk and severity of many diabetic complications.

CASE 88: Lymphoedema

History

- A **65-year-old female** [1] presents with an 8-month history of progressive **left arm swelling** [2] .
- She was diagnosed with left **breast cancer** [3] 2 years ago for which she underwent a **partial mastectomy with axillary lymph node dissection** [4] and received **radiotherapy** [5] .
- She reports no other **past medical history** [6] , **past surgery** [7] and no significant **family history** [8] .
- Her hand feels **heavy and weak** [9] .

- She is concerned about the appearance of her **enlarged arm** [10] .
- She denies **fever, pain or any obvious skin changes** [11] .
- She reports **no swelling in the lower limbs** [12] .
- She also denies **recent overseas travel** [13] .
- She denies recent **trauma** [14] .
- She has a **healthy diet and is physically active** [15] . She does not smoke nor drink alcohol.

[1] Lymphoedema is a chronic, progressive collection of protein-rich fluid in tissue resulting from developmental (primary) or acquired (secondary) disruption of the lymphatic system. Approximately 140–250 million people worldwide have lymphoedema. Secondary lymphoedema occurs after injury to the lymphatic system. 90% of cases are caused by nematode infection, lymph node dissection, radiotherapy or neoplastic infiltration. More than 16 million cases are attributable to filariasis (nematode infection). Primary lymphoedema in children is rare (1.15 per 100 000), with both sexes being equally affected.

[2] Differentials for unilateral upper limb swelling include lymphoedema, DVT and superior vena cava (SVC) syndrome. Secondary lymphoedema is often unilateral compared to primary lymphoedema, which more frequently presents as bilateral swelling. Swelling begins distally due to gravity and progresses proximally.

[3] Most cases of secondary lymphoedema have a history of malignancy. Advanced TNM stage is associated with greater rates of lymphoedema. This may be due to lymph node metastasis. However, the effect of TNM staging is confounded by higher rates of surgery and radiation in these patients.

[4] 38% of women experience lymphoedema following mastectomy with axillary lymph node dissection and radiation for breast cancer. Removal of lymph nodes means that lymphatic fluid is more likely to accumulate within the tissue of distal limbs. Following breast cancer treatment, the risk of lymphoedema is proportional to the cancer stage and extent of treatment.

[5] Radiation near lymph nodes causes fibrosis of the lymphatic drainage system, leading to obstruction and lymphoedema. Women receiving axillary radiation for breast cancer are 6–7 times more likely to develop lymphoedema

than those not receiving radiation. Hence, a history of radiation is important and should cover the indication, location and frequency of radiation.

[6] Past medical history is important in determining differentials for unilateral limb swelling. It is also required to assess fitness for surgery.

[7] A history of previous surgery is important to assess patients who are candidates for surgery. Furthermore, certain surgical procedures predispose patients to developing lymphoedema, particularly lymph node dissections in treatment for malignancy. In addition to cancer surgeries, patients undergoing orthopaedic surgeries are at risk of developing chronic lymphoedema secondary to lymphatic system damage. Total hip and total knee arthroplasty are both associated with developing bilateral lower limb lymphoedema.

[8] Primary lymphoedema is usually idiopathic and sporadic. 10–15% of cases report a family history of disease. In hereditary lymphoedema, interstitial lymph accumulates due to obstruction, malformation or hypoplasia of various lymphatic vessels. Autosomal dominant inheritance is most common (e.g. Milroy disease, Meige disease); however, recessive forms have been described. Rarely, lymphoedema may occur as part of a genetic syndrome (e.g. Noonan syndrome, Turner syndrome, lymphoedema–distichiasis syndrome).

[9] The hands and feet are usually involved in lymphoedema. Swelling can occur in these regions alone or in combination with the arm and/or leg. Lymphatic channels, derived from outpouching of veins, drain proteinaceous fluid (lymph) into regional lymph nodes. The lymphatic system returns fluid from the interstitium into the circulatory system. Lymphatic stasis occurs when channels or nodes

are dysfunctional, and can lead to fat hypertrophy and immunological problems. Lymphoedema becomes clinically evident when approximately 80% of lymphatic drainage is dysfunctional. Enlargement of the extremities can create a feeling of heaviness and/or weakness leading to functional disability.

10 Changes to the shape and size of the affected limb as well as skin changes can occur due to chronic swelling associated with lymphoedema.

11 DVT may occur in the upper extremity and would present as unilateral erythema, warmth and pain. There may be an associated history of prior DVT, prolonged immobility of the limb or a hypercoagulable state. In lymphatic filariasis (elephantiasis), the skin and underlying tissues thicken. Elephantiasis mainly affects the lower extremities.

12 If bilateral swelling of the lower limbs was present, other differentials to consider include chronic venous insufficiency, lipoedema, obesity, congestive heart failure, hypoalbuminaemia (e.g. renal failure, protein-losing enteropathies, hepatic failure). Lymphoedema caused by insufficiency in both the lymphatic and venous system is known as phlebolymphoedema, which can arise from a congenital defect.

13 Lymphatic filariasis is caused by parasitic nematodes, also known as roundworms (e.g. *Wuchereria bancrofti*, *Brugia malayi*). These worms obstruct lymphatic channels directly and cause regional inflammation. Chronic cases may evolve into elephantiasis. Different species of filarial worms tend to affect different parts of the body (e.g. limbs, genitalia). The parasite is spread to humans via blood-feeding vector such as mosquitoes and is often found in tropical regions of Africa and Asia. Hence, a history of travel to endemic areas must be noted. Travellers must exercise caution when travelling to such areas.

14 Significant penetrating trauma can cause damage to the lymphatic system, giving rise to lymphoedema. Areas which are particularly susceptible to this include the axilla and groin. Blunt or minor trauma is unlikely to increase the risk of developing lymphoedema; however, it may do so in patients who already have a decreased number of functioning lymphatics (e.g. previously dissected lymph nodes).

15 Obesity may increase the risk of developing upper or lower extremity lymphoedema following treatment for cancer. Such patients should be encouraged to lose weight and may be considered for bariatric weight-loss surgery.

Examination

- The patient appears **comfortable** [1].
- There are **no signs of respiratory distress** [2].
- The patient's capillary refill time is **<2 seconds** [3].
- The patient does not appear to have **pallor** [4].
- Pulse is **80bpm** [5] and regular.
- RR is 18 breaths per minute. BP is **120/80mmHg** [6].
- Temperature is **37.3°C** [7].
- No **lymphadenopathy** [8] exists in the neck, axillae or groin.
- Heart sounds are dual with **no murmurs** [9].
- Auscultation reveals vesicular breathing sounds and **equal air entry** [10].
- There is evidence of **surgical scars** [11] across the right chest wall post breast surgery.
- No **abnormal masses** [12] are palpable in the axillae.
- Her left arm is diffusely swollen and **non-tender** [13] with **non-pitting oedema** [14] present up to the shoulder.

- Her **arm circumference** [15] on the left is 38cm compared to 33cm on the right.
- **Stemmer's sign** [16] is not elicited as there is no swelling or oedema in the lower limbs.
- **Skin** [17] over her left arm appears intact and not thickened or roughened.
- A **groin examination** [18] is not performed in this patient.
- There is no swelling or skin changes in the **lower limbs** [19].
- She does not appear **obese** [20].
- She has **full range of movement** [21] in her shoulder, elbow, wrist and fingers.

1 A general inspection assists in the initial assessment for the acuity of the patient's pathology. For example, a patient who appears comfortable and interactive is less concerning than one who appears visibly distressed or ill. Such patients are more likely to require urgent medical attention.

2 The presence of respiratory distress indicates some level of hypoxia or metabolic acidosis. The cause for respiratory distress should be sought by the treating clinician and treated appropriately. In the case of a DVT, shortness of breath and tachypnoea may indicate a PE. If there is swelling in the lower limbs, a differential would be congestive heart failure, which would also present as shortness of breath due to pulmonary oedema.

3 An adequate capillary refill time indicates the patient is perfusing well and thus would likely have preserved end-organ perfusion. In addition, it suggests the patient is adequately hydrated. Other signs of adequate hydration are warm peripheries, normal skin turgor, moist mucous membranes and normal urine output.

4 Pallor indicates anaemia. Anaemia can lead to reduced oxygen delivery, and most importantly reduced end-organ oxygen utilisation. Anaemia in itself may cause respiratory distress, but it is also a negative prognosticator for postoperative recovery. Those with heart disease may have anaemia of chronic disease.

5 If tachycardia is present, it may suggest infection, anxiety, anaemia or arrhythmia. This would require further investigation and management of the underlying problem.

6 In the setting of severe infection or dehydration, patients may present with hypotension. The most important thing to determine in a patient with hypotension is if the patient is in shock. If so, fluid resuscitation and identifying the cause of shock is imperative. Other features that are highly suspicious of shock include abnormal mental state, tachycardia, oliguria, tachypnoea, metabolic acidosis and hyperlactataemia.

7 Fever is a characteristic feature of most infections.

8 Infections can cause lymphadenopathy. As lymph nodes are where microorganisms are filtered, tender and mobile nodes are characteristic of infection/inflammation. Nematodes, in particular, occupy the lymphatic system including the lymph nodes in filariasis.

9 Heart murmurs may suggest valvular heart disease or structural heart defects. It is important to investigate these peri-operatively in the context of fitness for general anaesthetic, and to quantify any increased risk of peri-operative complications.

10 Bi-basal crackles on auscultation may indicate pulmonary oedema secondary to congestive heart failure or hypoalbuminaemia (e.g. renal failure, protein-losing enteropathies) which can be causes of lower limb oedema. Although this is not the case here, it is an important differential to consider if the patient's swelling was in the legs instead of the arm.

11 Evidence of previous surgeries may indicate removal of or injury to lymph nodes, thus leading to lymphoedema.

12 An onset of lymphoedema following cancer treatment years after the primary surgery may be indicative of a tumour. Further investigations should be performed to rule out recurrence of cancer leading to lymphatic obstruction or the development of lymphangiosarcoma.

13 Lymphoedema is usually painless. A DVT is more likely to present as pain in the limb.

14 Lymphoedema typically presents with unilateral limb swelling. However, it can also occur in other parts of the body (e.g. abdomen, genital region, face, neck). Pitting oedema is present early in the disease. Other causes of pitting oedema include heart failure, liver disease and renal disease. However, oedema in these cases is bilateral. Non-pitting oedema is a sensitive but non-specific feature in lymphoedema with advanced disease. This is due to the fact that lymphoedema stimulates adipose tissue deposition and thus pitting will not occur with later stages.

15 The circumference of extremities can be obtained to calculate limb volume. The measurement can be taken at any point along an arm or leg as long as anatomical landmarks are used. This is to ensure that the measurements are comparable across both sides. These measurements can be used during the initial evaluation to assess severity and during follow-ups to track response to treatment.

16 Stemmer's sign is the inability to pinch the skin on the dorsum of the second toe. This sign demonstrates lymphoedema due to fluid accumulation complicated by skin fibrosis. A negative sign, however, does not exclude lymphoedema. This phenomenon can be demonstrated on any other affected part of the body.

17 Advanced lymphoedema may present with skin changes secondary to fat deposition and skin tension over the affected region. Such changes include hyperkeratosis (thickening of skin), papillomatosis (roughened skin) and induration. Subcutaneous fibrosis, cobblestoning and wart-like skin changes may be seen. The skin may break down in severe cases with lymph exudate (lymphorrhoea). Lymphorrhoea impairs wound healing and increases infection risk.

18 A genital examination is not always indicated when examining for lymphoedema; however, it is interesting to note that different species of filarial worms tend to affect different parts of the body. For example, *Wuchereria bancrofti* can affect the limbs, vulva and scrotum in women and men, respectively. When the scrotum is affected, a hydrocele can form. *Brugia timori*, however, rarely affects the genitals.

19 Inspection of the lower limbs is an important part of a medical examination. Swelling or enlargement of the lower limbs may give rise to other differentials, such as congestive heart failure, hypoalbuminaemia (e.g. nephrotic syndrome, liver failure), lipoedema, lower limb DVT and chronic venous insufficiency. It is important to be aware that patients can have both lymphoedema and generalised oedema; for example, a cancer patient who has undergone lymph node dissection may have heart failure as a comorbidity. In DVT the patient may present with unilateral erythema, warmth and pain of the affected limb. Squeezing the calves may elicit pain if there is a thrombus present. Chronic venous insufficiency is often associated with pain, ulceration and skin pigment changes in both legs. Post-thrombotic syndrome presents similarly to chronic venous insufficiency; however, it is often unilateral and a prior history of DVT can distinguish this condition from lymphoedema. Lipoedema is an enlargement of the extremities (whilst sparing hands and feet) due to abnormal fat deposition. It often presents with limb tenderness and a negative Stemmer's sign.

20 Obesity is an independent risk factor for lymphoedema. A BMI of ≥50 may lead to lymphoedema arising without a past history of lymphatic injury or surgery. It is believed that the increased production and retention of fluid by adipose tissue contributes to the development of lymphoedema

in these individuals. Severely obese patients are at risk of developing massive localised lymphoedema (also known as a pseudotumour) which enlarges over years but is benign.

21 Functional status should be assessed during the examination. There may be a limited range of motion or an inability to perform certain tasks (e.g. tying knot, buttoning, writing). The patient may have an ambulation aid if there is lymphoedema in the lower extremities. Any functional limitation should be referred on to physical therapy for assessment and management.

Investigations

- FBE reports a normal **WCC** [1].
- **UEC results are normal** [2].
- **Duplex ultrasound** [3] of the left arm yields normal results.
- **Lymphoscintigraphy** [4] shows slow lymphatic flow, likely secondary to axillary lymph node dissection.

- **MRI** [5] shows thickened skin and accumulation of fluid above the muscle fascia.
- A **genetic test** [6] is not ordered due to the lack of family history.

1 A raised WCC may indicate infection. Filariasis as a cause of lymphoedema is an example of this. A normal WCC may lower suspicion of infection but does not rule it out. If there is additional history arousing suspicion of filariasis, a blood smear is indicated and will show the presence of microfilariae.

2 UECs are important in the setting of a surgical emergency. First, they identify any electrolyte abnormalities that most often need correction prior to surgery. Secondly, they assess renal function and fitness for IV contrast in the setting of imaging (such as a CT abdomen and pelvis), as well as serving as a prognosticator for postoperative recovery.

3 In patients with lymphoedema, a duplex ultrasound is used to evaluate the venous system for patency, competency and reflux. This in turn helps to rule out DVT as a differential. Ultrasound in itself, however, has poor diagnostic sensitivity and specificity for lymphoedema. Enlarged lymph nodes or other lesions causing lymphatic obstruction can be identified on CT or MR imaging.

4 Usually, a history and physical examination that is consistent with lymphoedema is sufficient to establish a diagnosis. Additional imaging is reserved for cases where the history and physical exam does not yield a definitive diagnosis or in cases where lymphatic obstruction (e.g. caused by a tumour) is suspected. The gold standard test to confirm lymphoedema is lymphoscintigraphy. Lymphoscintigraphy evaluates lymphatic function by

taking radiographical images after the injection of Tc99m-labelled substance into the dorsal web space of the affected extremity or genitalia. After contrast injection, the presence of dermal backflow, delayed or absent transport or lack of lymph node visualisation is consistent with lymphoedema. Lymphangiography, which involves injecting radio-opaque contrast into the lymphatic channels, is useful for mapping anatomical obstructions for preoperative planning rather than for diagnostic purposes. However, it is rarely used as it can cause lymphangitis and exacerbation of lymphoedema.

5 MRI is necessary to order if malignancy is suspected in a patient. As MRI is able to take detailed images, it can differentiate lymphoedema (cutaneous oedema) from various other diseases (e.g. lipoedema, venous disease, vascular anomaly). Both CT and MRI will reveal increased fat density, thickening skin and honeycombing of fluid and fibrous tissue above the muscle fascia in lymphoedema. However, CT is less useful than MRI as it has poorer resolution of soft tissue structures and also increases the patient's exposure to radiation. It is important to note that MRI and CT scans are non-specific and do not evaluate lymphatic function.

6 Genetic testing may be ordered for patients with primary lymphoedema. Although most cases are sporadic, some have a syndromic or familial basis.

Management

Immediate

It is likely that the patient has lymphoedema secondary to axillary lymph node dissection post partial mastectomy. Provide the patient with static **compression bandaging** [1] over the arm. Advise them to **elevate** [2] the arm when possible and provide education on **skin care** [3].

Short-term

Recommend **exercise** [4] and **weight control** [5] to reduce symptoms. **Intermittent pneumatic compression** [6] can be used later on if her oedema does not subside. Consider **psychosocial support** [7] if the patient appears anxious about the physical appearance of her arm. There are no **medications** [8] required for the cause of her lymphoedema.

Long-term

Follow the patient up in the lymphoedema **outpatient clinic** [9] as necessary to monitor the condition and its **complications** [10], and consider **surgery** [11] if it is unresolved.

[1] The first-line treatment for lymphoedema is compression using static garments, massage and/or pneumatic compression devices. Medical grade garments (at least 30mmHg) can assist in reducing swelling of the arm. Controlled compression therapy can also be used where the garment is progressively tightened to increase lymphatic flow. Multi-layered bandaging with joint padding has been shown to be more effective than single-layered garments. It is important to educate patients on the purpose of wearing compression garments as these can reduce range of motion and cause discomfort, both of which lead to poor compliance and worsening of oedema. Manual lymph drainage is an additional technique that may be performed by a trained therapist. However, this can be time-consuming and resource-intensive. Furthermore, evidence suggests that this may have minimal benefit.

[2] Patients are encouraged to elevate the affected extremity whenever they can, to reduce oedema. Elevating a limb allows gravity to assist in the drainage of lymphatic fluid.

[3] Skin care is extremely important in patients with lymphoedema. Trauma to the skin must be avoided. Cuts, even if minor, can lead to cellulitis and hence worsen lymphoedema through lymphatic injury. Protective clothing and shoes should be worn to avoid such injuries, especially when outdoors. Using a regular skin moisturiser and keeping the skin clean with frequent bathing also helps to minimise infection and skin breakdown. Poor skin care may lead to lymphorrhoea, fungal growth, hyperkeratosis, ulceration and papillomatosis.

[4] Exercise, such as weightlifting, may minimise symptoms, increase strength and reduce the incidence of lymphoedema exacerbations. Patients should be informed that exercise is not contraindicated with lymphoedema. An exercise therapist may be useful in educating patients on movements/activities to improve the condition.

[5] Obesity increases the risk of developing upper limb lymphoedema following breast cancer treatment. Hence, it is important for patients to be informed on the importance of maintaining a normal BMI. Obesity can also cause bilateral lower extremity lymphoedema. As obesity-induced lymphoedema is irreversible, those who are obese may be considered for bariatric weight-loss surgery before this condition develops.

[6] Intermittent pneumatic compression applies compression using a distal-to-proximal pressure gradient. It helps to reduce oedema alongside the use of static compression garments.

[7] Patients with chronic lymphoedema may struggle with frequent infections, poor skin, reduced limb function and an abnormal physical appearance. Providing psychosocial support and recommending support groups will assist such patients with their overall wellbeing.

[8] For patients with lymphoedema secondary to filariasis, anthelmintic agents are used to eradicate microfilariae. Examples include ivermectin and albendazole. The infectious disease team should be contacted to advise on drug and dosing recommendations.

[9] The need for ongoing follow-up depends on the severity of the illness and the patient's risk for postoperative complications. Some patients are fit and well enough to be managed by their GP, whilst some will require several follow-up visits to ensure adequate recovery and resolution of any lingering symptoms. If there is no definitive cure for the patient, a long-term approach between both the patient and doctor is required.

[10] Complications should be monitored and asked about on every follow-up. These include pain, limitations in limb function, skin changes and mental health. It would be ideal for the patient to function at the level that they were able

to prior to becoming ill. If needed, a referral to allied health would be most useful (e.g. physiotherapy, occupational therapy and social work) for further assessment on functional level as well as fitness for discharge.

11 Surgery is reserved for patients unresponsive to conservative measures or those with significant morbidity. Suction-assisted lipectomy is the first-line surgical treatment for extremity lymphoedema. This is an excisional technique used to remove diseased tissue. It is important to note that excisional procedures are not curative and will require the patient to use compression garments lifelong. Conversely, physiological procedures aim to re-establish lymphatic connections by creating new channels, anastomoses or transferring lymphatics to the affected area. The two most commonly performed procedures are vascularised lymph node transfer and lymphatic–venous anastomosis. Other procedures include free-tissue transfer, lymphangioplasty, lymphatic grafting and lymph node–venous anastomosis. Physiological procedures are less predictable than excisional ones, hence in moderate or severe disease, excision is required to remove excess fibrous and adipose tissue.

CASE 89: Type B aortic dissection

History

- A **60-year-old** [1] **male** [2] with a history of **untreated hypertension** [3] and **stable angina** [4] presents with **sudden and severe tearing pain** [5] **in the back radiating to both arms** [6].
- He denies **sensory changes, limb weakness** [7] and **syncope** [8].
- He is a **heavy smoker** [9], drinks alcohol socially and does not use **illicit drugs** [10].

- He denies any **shortness of breath** [11] or **chest pain** [12]; however, he does complain of associated **severe abdominal pain** [13].
- He denies recent **trauma** [14], **connective tissue disease** [15], **vasculitis** [16] or **known valvular or structural heart disease** [17].

[1] Aortic dissection is a tear in the inner layer of the aorta that leads to a progressively growing haematoma in the intima–media space. Incidence is highest at ages 40–80, with a peak between 50 and 65 years. It is estimated that 2–3.5 people per 100 000 are affected every year. In those aged <40, less than 40% of cases are due to HTN. Advanced age can pose as a contraindication to surgery.

[2] The incidence of aortic dissection is higher among men in a male-to-female ratio of 3:1. In females <40 years, half of all aortic dissections occur during pregnancy.

[3] HTN is the most common and important risk factor for aortic dissection. Approximately 70% of patients with dissection have elevated pressure which increases the risk of rupture. Past medical history is important in determining fitness for surgery as well as any contributing or causative factors for the patient's pain.

[4] Approximately 30% of patients with dissection have an history of atherosclerosis, hence it is important to assess cardiovascular risk factors.

[5] Pain from an aortic dissection is characterised by its abrupt and maximal severity at onset. It is often described as 'tearing' or 'ripping'. Painless dissection occurs in about 10% of patients, commonly in those with neurologic complications and Marfan syndrome. Delays in diagnosis often occur in patients presenting with atypical symptoms. Therefore, atypical symptoms of aortic dissection should always be considered.

[6] The location of pain may indicate where the dissection arises. Anterior chest pain may mimic acute MI and is usually associated with anterior arch or aortic root dissection. Any dissection involving the ascending aorta is classified as a Stanford type A dissection. These dissections generally require surgery due to their complications relating to aortic regurgitation and cardiac tamponade. Neck or jaw pain may

indicate aortic arch involvement extending into the great vessels. Tearing pain in the intrascapular area may indicate dissection in the descending aorta. Any dissection not involving the ascending aorta is a Stanford type B dissection. Type B dissections can often be managed with medical therapy, such as beta blockers and vasodilators. As the dissection evolves, the pain typically migrates.

[7] Dissection that involves the carotid arteries can compromise cerebral blood flow, leading to stroke. Symptoms include hemiparesis or paraesthesia. Paraplegia may arise from spinal cord ischaemia.

[8] Syncope and altered mental status are the most common neurologic findings. These may be caused by hypovolaemia, increased vagal tone, arrhythmia or stroke. Up to 20% of patients may present with syncope and no pain. Those presenting with syncope are more likely to have a type A dissection and cardiac tamponade.

[9] Tobacco use is associated with atherosclerotic and vascular disease and therefore dissections.

[10] Cocaine or amphetamine use can increase the risk of aortic dissection through acute HTN, vasoconstriction, increased stroke volume and vasospasm.

[11] Dyspnoea may indicate new-onset heart failure due to acute aortic insufficiency, cardiac tamponade or a haemothorax if the dissection ruptures into the pleura. PE is a differential which may also present as shortness of breath.

[12] Acute coronary syndrome (ACS) can be difficult to distinguish from an aortic dissection. It is an important differential and is typically described as central and crushing chest pain. However, note that dissection through the coronary ostia may in itself cause an acute MI. Pleuritic chest pain may indicate PE or pericarditis. Pericarditis may be a differential or a complication of slow extension of the dissection into the pericardium.

13 Abdominal aortic dissection can cause mesenteric ischaemia, presenting as abdominal pain. If the renal arteries are involved, renal ischaemia and infarction can arise, leading to oliguria or anuria. Similarly, dissection into the iliac arteries may present as claudication. If these conditions are suspected, immediate management should be instituted without delay.

14 Blunt chest trauma (e.g. motor vehicle accident) or iatrogenic injury (e.g. valve replacement, graft surgery, cardiac catheterisation) can lead to aortic dissection. Heavy lifting can also cause transient elevation in BP and thus dissection.

15 Vasculitis with aortic involvement have been associated with dissection. These include syphilis, Takayasu arteritis, giant cell arteritis, polyarteritis nodosa and Behçet's disease.

16 Connective tissue disorders, such as Marfan syndrome and Ehlers–Danlos syndrome, affect blood vessel wall strength and predispose patients to both aneurysms and aortic dissection. These patients are often young with a family history of dissection.

17 Bicuspid aortic valve predisposes to both aneurysms and dissections, presumably related to weakness of the aortic wall. Aortic coarctation is also a risk factor for dissection due to its association with long-standing HTN.

Examination

- The patient appears to be in significant pain but is otherwise **alert without signs of respiratory distress or pallor** [1].
- BP in his **right arm is 150/80mmHg** [2] which is **the same as his left arm** [3]. **Radial pulses are strong and regular bilaterally** [3].
- There is no sign of a **collapsing pulse** [4]. Pedal pulses are strong bilaterally.
- Pulse rate is regular at **110bpm** [5].
- Capillary refill time is **<2 seconds** [6]. RR is 18 breaths per minute. Temperature is 37°C.
- There is no **jugular venous distension** [7].

- Precordial examination reveals a **normal first and second heart sound** [8] and no **murmurs** [9].
- Auscultation of the lungs reveals vesicular breathing sounds and **equal air entry** [10].
- The abdomen is **soft but generally tender and mildly distended** [11].
- **Power is intact in all muscle groups** [12]. Strength is normal on the left side. Sensation and coordination are intact bilaterally.
- Cranial nerve examination is normal. His overall **aortic dissection detection risk score is 1** [13].

1 General inspection is important in assessing the patient's overall haemodynamic status, as it will determine whether immediate surgical management is required. As aortic dissection can result in fatal complications, fast and accurate diagnosis is crucial. Without intervention, the mortality rate increases by 1–2% per hour. Pallor may indicate anaemia due to cardiac tamponade or hypovolaemic shock. Altered mental status may be seen in shock, diminished carotid blood flow or direct extension of the dissection into the carotid arteries.

2 Hypertension is present in 70% of type B dissections. It may be due to a pre-existing hypertensive condition (the most important risk factor for dissection) or increased sympathetic drive secondary to pain. BP must be closely monitored, as a sudden change to hypotension may indicate cardiac tamponade, severe aortic regurgitation or acute MI secondary dissections involving the ascending aorta. Although rare, hypotension in type B dissections usually implies rupture of the aorta leading to hypovolaemic shock.

3 Depending on the dissection site, there may be discrepancies in pulse and BP due to an intimal flap or compression by haematoma. A BP differential >20mmHg between the two arms should increase the suspicion of aortic dissection. A pulse deficit may be unilateral or bilateral

depending on the level of the intimal flap. Hence, careful attention is needed when examining carotid, brachial and femoral pulses for asymmetry and bruits. Occlusion of the subclavian artery can result in reduced peripheral pulses in the left arm, while occlusion of the brachiocephalic trunk can result in reduced blood circulation in the right arm. Occlusion of a femoral artery leads to a decreased pedal pulse on one side.

4 Corrigan's sign (also known as water hammer or collapsing pulse) describes rapid visible arterial pulsations with a noticeable increase in amplitude of peripheral pulses seen in aortic regurgitation.

5 Tachycardia may be due to anxiety, pain-induced sympathetic stimulation or reflex from blood volume loss.

6 A capillary refill time <2 seconds is reassuring for adequate end-organ perfusion. Other signs to look for include warm peripheries, good skin turgor, moist mucus membranes and normal urine output.

7 Proximal aortic dissections may result in pericardial tamponade secondary to haemopericardium. It can present with raised JVP, muffled heart sounds and low blood pressure (Beck's triad). Similarly, proximal tears leading to aortic regurgitation may feature raised JVP. Pericardial friction rubs may suggest the presence of pericarditis as a result of dissection into the pericardium.

8 A loud second heart sound may be heard due to either systemic HTN where there is a dilated proximal aorta or pulmonary HTN due to severe aortic regurgitation.

9 A diastolic decrescendo murmur indicates aortic incompetence secondary to a dissection that propagates proximal to the initial tear. Other signs of aortic regurgitation include bounding pulses and wide pulse pressure. Severe regurgitation may result in signs suggestive of congestive heart failure: dyspnoea, orthopnoea, bi-basal crackles or elevated JVP.

10 Unilateral dullness to percussion and decreased breath sounds may indicate a pleural effusion or a haemothorax due to dissection rupture. Bi-basal crackles on the other hand may indicate pulmonary oedema secondary to aortic valve regurgitation.

11 Severe and persisting abdominal pain that is disproportionate to examination findings should raise suspicion of mesenteric or renal ischaemia.

12 Focal neurological deficits are due either to propagation of the dissection to involve branch arteries, or to mass effects compressing on surrounding structures. Diminished carotid blood flow can lead to stroke (e.g. hemiplegia, paraesthesia) or altered consciousness. Horner syndrome, characterised by miosis, anhidrosis and ptosis, arises from compression of the superior cervical sympathetic ganglion. Compression of the left recurrent laryngeal nerve may result in hoarseness of voice. The interruption of intercostal vessels can lead to spinal cord ischaemia and thus acute paraplegia.

13 Aortic dissection detection risk score (ADD-RS) is a highly sensitive bedside clinical tool used to assess the risk of acute aortic dissection. One score is given for the presence of a high risk condition (Marfan syndrome, family history, aortic valve disease, known aneurysm, recent aortic manipulation), characteristic pain (abrupt, severe or tearing pain in the chest, back or abdomen) and examination findings (perfusion deficit, new murmur, hypotension). A score of 2–3 indicates a high risk patient who requires definitive imaging.

Investigations

- An **ECG** [1] reveals signs of left ventricular hypertrophy without signs of ischaemia.
- FBE shows a **normal haemoglobin level** [2].
- **UEC results are normal** [3].
- **LFT results are normal** [4].
- **Lactate is elevated at 3.5mmol/L** [5].
- **Cardiac enzymes are within normal limits** [6].
- Blood is sent for **typing and cross-match** [7].
- **D-dimer assay is mildly elevated** [8].
- **CXR shows mild mediastinal widening** [9].
- **There is no lung pathology visible on CXR** [10].
- **CT angiography shows a type B aortic dissection** [11] originating distal to the left subclavian artery with its intimal flap extending past the coeliac trunk, just proximal to the right main renal artery.

1 An ECG is obtained in the initial evaluation of patients with chest or back pain. Aortic dissection that does not involve coronary ostia can be distinguished from ACS by the absence of ECG changes characteristic of ischaemia. However, if dissection involves the ostia and leads to coronary ischaemia, ECG is not helpful in differentiation. Furthermore, ECG findings can be variable in dissection. 30% of patients have normal ECGs, while 42% show non-specific ST and T wave changes. Ischaemic changes on ECG were present in 15% of patients. Due to the association between HTN and aortic dissection, signs of left ventricular strain may be present. Differentiating between ACS and dissection is of particular importance because thrombolytic therapy may be fatal in aortic dissection. Other findings on ECG may include pericarditis changes or electrical alternans in cardiac tamponade.

2 An FBE may reveal anaemia in the case of haemorrhage.

3 Renal function tests are required to identify any renal perfusion compromise. This would be shown as elevated creatinine and urea.

4 Liver function tests may reveal elevated ALT and AST if hepatic perfusion is compromised.

5 Elevated lactate levels obtained from a venous or arterial blood gas may be indicative of poor tissue perfusion or end-organ damage.

6 Cardiac enzymes, including serial troponins, are vital in identifying the presence of MI. It may be a differential or a complication of dissection. Cardiac-specific troponins I and T tend to be elevated within 3–5 hours after injury to the heart. Therefore, ECG and troponins must be repeated at 3 hours for high-sensitivity pathology tests or 6–8 hours for point-of-care tests.

7 A blood type and cross-match should be ordered in preparation for surgery, as some cases may require surgical intervention or transfusion.

8 D-dimer reflects activation of the extrinsic pathway of the coagulation cascade due to exposed tissue factor from an intimal tear. It carries a high sensitivity (90–95%) but a low specificity (56%). Hence, D-dimer may be a useful screening tool in low risk patients where clinical diagnostic uncertainty remains. As this tool has not been externally validated on its own, it should not be relied on in screening for aortic dissection. However, it is of value when considering the differential diagnosis of PE.

9 60–90% of aortic dissections present with mediastinal widening on imaging. Pleural effusion can be found in 20% of cases. Other less specific findings on CXR include displacement of calcification, aortic kinking and opacification of the aortopulmonary window. If the dissection extends through the adventitia into the pleural space, a haemothorax may be evident on imaging. Congestive heart failure as a complication of proximal dissections may result in pulmonary oedema, which is visible on imaging as Kerley B lines and upper lobar diversion.

10 Plain CXR is used to help differentiate various causes of pain in the thoracic region (e.g. pneumothorax, acute heart failure).

11 Definitive imaging with CTA of the chest, abdomen and pelvis is required in high risk patients, those with abnormal CXR, unexplained hypotension or in cases where there is no alternative diagnosis. Identification of a double (false) lumen is highly suggestive of aortic dissection. Other findings may include aortic dilatation and haematoma. Contrast leak indicates rupture. MRA is an alternative for stable patients with contraindications to CTA. Transthoracic or transoesophageal echocardiography may be used in unstable patients or those with renal insufficiency or contrast allergy. However, CTA remains the gold standard investigation in aortic dissection.

Management

Immediate

The patient's **vitals** [1] and **urine output** [2] are monitored. An **IV beta blocker is administered followed by a vasodilator** [3]. The patient is kept fasted [4]. **IV access is obtained and fluid** [5] is administered. The vascular surgery team is contacted for **advice and consultation** [6].

Short-term

Analgesics [7] are given. Given the suspicion of mesenteric ischaemia, the decision is made for **emergency aortic dissection repair surgery** [8]. **Continuous monitoring is performed intra-operatively** [9]. Following the procedure, the patient stays in hospital for **monitoring** [10] and **pain control** [11]. The patient may commence a graded **diet as tolerated** [12]. The patient's **surgical site** [13] is reviewed. A **cardiovascular** [14] and **respiratory** [15] examination is serially performed. The **lower limbs are examined** [16]. Once **stable** [17] with a return to **premorbid functioning level** [18], the patient may be discharged.

Long-term

The patient is followed up in the outpatient clinic to monitor for **postoperative complications** [19] and **manage cardiovascular risk factors** [20].

1 Vital signs must be monitored carefully. Haemodynamic instability calls for advanced life support. Control of BP and bleeding are urgent priorities. Supplemental oxygen, IV fluid resuscitation and inotropes (e.g. noradrenaline, dobutamine) should be given as appropriate in cases of renal failure and hypovolaemic shock. Coagulopathy should be corrected.

2 Urine output reflects fluid balance. Reduced urine output (<0.5ml/kg/hr) may indicate acute renal failure. Recognising this early allows treatment to be initiated quickly and effectively. The most likely cause for acute renal failure in this case is hypovolaemia which requires IV fluid resuscitation to maintain end-organ perfusion. Dissection extending to the renal arteries may cause obstruction of blood flow to the kidneys. This calls for immediate surgical management. Other causes of acute renal failure include IV contrast for imaging, general anaesthetics and sedatives.

3 BP control is essential in all patients to prevent further propagation of the dissection and reduce the risk of acute rupture. IV beta blockade (e.g. labetalol, esmolol) is used to achieve a heart rate <60bpm and a systolic BP of 100mmHg. IV vasodilator therapy, such as sodium nitroprusside or glyceryl trinitrate (GTN), should also be given if BP reduction is inadequate with a beta blockade. A beta blocker must be given prior to a vasodilator, as reflex tachycardia may increase aortic wall stress and hence worsen a dissection.

4 Keeping the patient nil by mouth is important in preparing them for potential surgery. It enables bowel rest and reduces the risk of aspiration during anaesthesia. Patients should be fasted off solid foods for 6 hours, and clear fluids for 2 hours prior to induction of anaesthesia.

5 IV fluid resuscitation is necessary in haemodynamic instability. Haemorrhage will cause hypovolaemia and thus compromise end-organ perfusion. Fluids are also important to maintain hydration in the patient who is fasting prior to surgery. A fluid bolus of 20ml/kg or 0.9% normal saline is often used for resuscitation. After the bolus, the patient's fluid status is reassessed, and maintenance fluids may be charted accordingly. Fluid charts are important in monitoring input and output as well as assessing overall hydration status. These charts are useful in identifying and replacing fluid losses.

6 As a type B aortic dissection falls under the vascular surgery team, advice should be sought from the relevant surgeon. They will come to assess the patient and consent them for open surgery or endovascular stent-graft repair.

7 Pain control is an important first-line therapy to reduce sympathetic tone and facilitate haemodynamic stability. Morphine is an analgesic which causes vasodilation and reduces heart rate through vagal tone stimulation.

8 Indications for surgery include persistent pain, branch occlusion, leak, continued extension despite optimal medical management and any type A dissection. Those with uncomplicated type B dissections are usually managed medically with BP and pain control. If complications occur (e.g. rupture, ischaemia, expansion), open surgery is performed to cover the tear and re-establish blood flow into the compromised branch vessels. Endovascular treatment with aortic stent implantation may be used instead in type B dissections if the open operative risk is too high.

9 Intra-operatively, all vitals and related parameters are monitored closely in order to identify complications early.

10 Postoperative monitoring is important to identify any complications of surgery. This includes shock due to bleeding, cardiac arrhythmias, infection, adverse anaesthetic reactions, acute renal failure and thromboembolism. FBC, UEC and LFTs should be monitored in case of dissection into other organs.

11 Postoperative pain control is important as it aims to minimise discomfort and facilitate early mobilisation and functional recovery, and prevents the development of chronic pain. It has also been shown to reduce length of stays and hospital costs.

12 Diet can be slowly introduced as tolerated following surgery. Following suspicion of mesenteric or small bowel ischaemia, patients are usually kept nil by mouth until bowel activity restarts (either as bowel sounds or passing flatus). A clear fluid diet is the first stage of oral intake after surgery. It keeps the patient hydrated and allows clinicians to stop administering IV fluids.

13 The surgical site should be reviewed to ensure that it is closed properly and able to heal well. Any exudates or signs of infection must be managed accordingly. The wound should be examined for erythema, warmth, swelling and pain. If pain is disproportionate to the surgical wound, then further investigations should be performed. Wound dehiscence is a complication that should be monitored and managed early, as it may increase risk of infection and scarring.

14 A cardiovascular examination should be performed to monitor for postoperative complications. Cardiac arrhythmia is a common risk which usually requires medical treatment. Less common risks include myocardial ischaemia and DVT.

15 A respiratory examination should be performed to monitor for postoperative complications. These include pneumothorax or haemothorax which will require a chest drain. Less common complications include atelectasis, pneumonia and PE.

16 Immobilisation in bed postoperatively is a major risk factor for the development of DVT. Look for unilateral swelling, tenderness and erythema in the calves by inspection and palpation. If clinically suspicious, order a Doppler ultrasound of the affected leg to diagnose, and then start the patient on anticoagulation.

17 If the patient remains afebrile, is haemodynamically stable and looks well, they are generally well enough to be discharged home.

18 The patient should ideally be able to function at the level that they were able to prior to becoming ill. If unsure, refer to the allied health team (primarily physiotherapy, occupational therapy and social work) for further assessment on fitness for discharge home at a functional level.

19 All patients with aortic dissection should be followed up with imaging. Those with uncomplicated dissections should have serial surveillance imaging with either CTA or MRA at 1, 3, 6 and 12 months after discharge, and then annually thereafter to monitor for any changes. Patients who have undergone thoracic endovascular aortic repair should undergo CTA at 1 and 12 months postoperatively, followed by CTA or MRA annually for 3 years.

20 No patient is considered cured on discharge. The aim of surgery is to improve the quality of life and longevity. Adequate BP control is vital in the long-term management of these patients. BP control should ideally be maintained at 90–120mmHg systolic. Beta blockers and ACE inhibitors are usually required. Additional antihypertensives, such as CCBs or diuretics, may be used if necessary. At least 40% of patients will require combination treatment to control BP. Other than HTN, cardiovascular risk factors, such as dyslipidaemia and diabetes mellitus, should be intensively managed. Smokers must be encouraged to cease smoking.

CASE 90: Varicose veins

History

- A **47-year-old** [1] **female** [2] presents with **fatigue and heaviness in her legs** [3].
- It is associated with **dilated veins over the calves which worsen later in the day** [4] and with prolonged standing. It is worst on the inner aspect of her calves.
- She reports the **skin colour** [5] around her veins appearing darker than before.
- Her legs feel **itchy and dry** [6].
- She has an **urge to move her legs** [7].
- There is **swelling in both ankles** [8] at the end of each day.
- There is a painful **ulcer** [9] above her right ankle present over the last 4 weeks.
- She has not noticed any **bleeding** [10] from the veins.

- These veins first appeared 25 years ago after her second **pregnancy** [11] and were asymptomatic. Over the last decade, the veins have enlarged and recently have become increasingly painful.
- She denies **pain in the calves** [12] and there is no **past history of DVT** [13].
- She recalls her **mother having similar veins** [14] in the legs.
- Other **past medical history** [15] includes T2DM and a cholecystectomy 20 years ago for cholecystitis.
- She works as an accountant and admits to **long periods of sitting** [16].
- She does **not smoke** [17], and drinks alcohol socially.
- She engages in minimal **physical activity** [18] outside of work but reports having a **healthy diet** [19].

[1] The prevalence of varicose veins increases with age. Hence, age is a risk factor for varicose veins. Furthermore, the prevalence of varicose veins in western countries is higher than in developing countries. Veins are blood vessels that normally return blood from the leg upwards, back to the heart. Blood flow in the veins should also always travel from the superficial veins to the deeper veins in the legs. Blood will not normally travel downwards in the reverse direction or outwards from deep to superficial veins as there are one-way valves inside the veins that prevent this occurring. In some people these valves can fail, and blood is thus permitted to not only travel towards the heart but can also travel backwards (reflux) down the leg, especially on standing. Veins that reflux are said to be incompetent or to have incompetent valves.

[2] Varicose veins are more common in women than men. Approximately 10–15% of men and 20–25% of women have visible varicose veins. Varicose veins are most often caused by incompetent venous valves. The dysfunction of such valves leads to blood pooling, increased pressure and thus distension of veins. This can take many years to develop.

[3] The feeling of heaviness in the legs can be caused by a number of diseases. Varicose veins and chronic venous insufficiency can cause heaviness in the legs due to the pooling of blood in the lower limbs. Overtraining can also cause fatigue in the legs; however, this is inconsistent with our patient's presentation as her issue appears chronic and she engages in minimal physical activity. Peripheral vascular

disease (PVD) can also cause heaviness and fatigue in the legs. It is associated with claudication (pain of the legs on walking/ standing).

[4] Varicose veins present as dilated tortuous veins. Dilated veins may cause pain, cramps, aching or fatigue in the legs after prolonged standing due to pooling of blood into the lower extremities. These symptoms often improve with elevation and are not present at the start of the day. Thrombophlebitis may be present with varicose veins. It is often described as causing severe pain, hyperpigmentation and erythema. Visible varicose veins typically are most concerning to patients as they are visually obvious. However, it is important to note that varicose veins are often associated with superficial axial venous reflux (e.g. great saphenous vein, small saphenous vein). Prior to treating patients with varicose veins, it is important to assess the superficial as well as deep veins for evidence of reflux.

[5] Skin colour changes (mottled orange-brown macular pigmentation) may indicate haemosiderin deposition due to chronic venous HTN. This is a feature of venous eczema. As haemosiderin can cause inflammation and injury to the surrounding soft tissues, patients are at risk of developing ulcers. Other than dysfunctional venous valves, morbid obesity can predispose patients to haemosiderin deposition due to reduced venous outflow.

[6] Venous eczema is caused by venous insufficiency. The causes include incompetent valves, obstruction of venous

outflow or dysfunctional calf muscle pump action. Fluid collection in tissue leads to an inflammatory response. It is characterised by red, itchy and blistered plaques, dry fissures and skin pigmentation. Some patients may complain of itching in the legs after physical activity or prolonged standing. Venous eczema can be complicated by secondary skin infection. This overlaps with lipodermatosclerosis (sclerosing panniculitis) which can similarly present as tender, itchy, indurated and erythematous skin. It is a chronic inflammatory condition characterised by fibrosis of the subcutaneous layer of the skin secondary to venous insufficiency and HTN.

7 Restless leg syndrome may be seen in patients with varicose veins. It describes a compulsive urge to move the legs. Other causes of restless legs include iron deficiency and kidney disease, Parkinson's disease and electrolyte disturbances.

8 Ankle swelling may be present with prolonged standing in patients with venous insufficiency and associated varicose veins. Chronic inflammation damages underlying lymphatic vessels, which can lead to lymphoedema. The accumulation of lymphatic fluid further increases the pressure in the lower limb.

9 The presence of varicose ulcers indicates chronic venous insufficiency. Increased venous pressure causes fibrin deposits around capillaries which hinder the delivery of oxygen to muscle and skin cells. The death of these cells leads to the formation of an ulcer (full-thickness skin loss). Venous ulcers are often characterised by location (often in the gaiter region) and are usually painless, unlike an arterial ulcer.

10 It is rare for varicose veins to bleed. If bleeding occurs, urgent referral is required.

11 Pregnancy and increasing numbers of births are risk factors for varicose veins. During pregnancy, total body fluid and intra-abdominal pressure are increased, both of which can cause venous distension. It has been suggested that progesterone can cause passive vein dilation leading to valvular dysfunction. Oestrogen triggers smooth muscle

relaxation and changes in collagen fibres, which similarly contributes to venous dilation.

12 Having varicose veins is a risk factor for DVT. Pain in the calves may indicate the presence of a DVT.

13 A past history of DVT is important as it can cause damage in the deep veins, leading to increased pressure, distension and varicose vein formation.

14 There may be a genetic link for varicose veins. Studies have shown that a history of varicose veins in an immediate family member increases the risk of developing varicose veins.

15 Past medical history is important in determining fitness for surgery, previous adverse reactions to general anaesthetics, allergies, current medications and any other contributing or causative factors for the patient's varicose veins. For example, diabetes mellitus is a risk factor for obesity, which can contribute to the development of varicose veins. Poor glycaemic control also has a negative impact on wound healing and affects preoperative medication management for diabetes.

16 Occupations that require prolonged standing or sitting may contribute to venous insufficiency and the development of varicose veins. Hence, a comprehensive social history which includes occupation and daily activities is required.

17 Smoking can increase one's risk of developing PVD. In PVD, lipids accumulate in the walls of arteries and hinder blood flow to the affected body part. Hence, it can similarly present as fatigue, heaviness and pain in the limb. Other risk factors to look for when assessing for PVD include HTN, cholesterol and diabetes. A smoking history is also important to ask about, as it is required in the assessment of peri-operative risk. Smoking is associated with an increased risk of peri-operative respiratory, cardiac and wound-related complications.

18 Lack of limb mobilisation worsens blood stasis in the lower extremities.

19 A poor diet and lack of physical activity may contribute to obesity, which can worsen venous insufficiency and the appearance of varicose veins.

Examination

- The patient appears **overweight** [1].
- Her **vitals are all within normal limits** [2].
- The patient's capillary refill time on both feet is **<2 seconds** [3].
- There are **veins varying in size and appearance** [4]; some appear tortuous while others appear thread-like over the calves bilaterally.
- There are many **small fine vein branches** [5].
- There is **hyperpigmentation and dryness** [6] to the skin.
- There is **no pallor and all lower limb pulses are intact** [7].
- The legs do not have an '**upside-down champagne bottle' appearance** [8].
- There is a small active **venous ulcer** [9] on the medial right ankle.
- There is evidence of **oedema up the ankle** [10].
- There is no **calf tenderness** [11].
- No **bleeding from the veins** [12] is observed.

1 General inspection of the patient can provide clues to risk factors (e.g. obesity).

2 Assessing vitals for haemodynamic stability is important in all patients. Instability would require urgent medical attention and management.

3 An adequate capillary refill time indicates the patient is perfusing well and thus would likely have preserved end-organ perfusion. In addition, it suggests the patient is adequately hydrated.

4 On examination of the skin, varicose veins appear as dilated and tortuous. These veins can be palpated for irregularities and bulges. The size can vary from 3–30mm. The size, severity and location of the varicose veins should be noted. In contrast to varicose veins, telangiectasias, also known as spider veins, appear very small (<1mm) and usually do not cause cosmetic concerns amongst patients. These sit much closer or within the overlying skin. Reticular veins sit in between telangiectasias and varicose veins. These veins are permanently dilated intradermal veins ranging between 1mm and 3 mm in diameter. They may be tortuous in appearance but are usually asymptomatic.

5 The presence of multiple fine vein branches visible on the skin suggests chronic venous HTN. This is known as corona phlebectatica.

6 The skin may appear brown and mottled due to the deposition of haemosiderin secondary to venous HTN. The legs should be examined carefully for ulcers, as haemosiderin can cause inflammation and destruction of local soft tissue. As haemosiderin leads to secondary changes in the microcirculatory system, capillaries become fibrotic and elongated. Itchy and dry skin demonstrates venous eczema.

Patients with such skin changes are regarded as having chronic venous insufficiency.

7 Arterial insufficiency must be ruled out, as it is a possible cause of some of the patient's symptoms. The affected limb usually appears pale due to obstructed blood flow, is cold to touch, has prolonged capillary refill time and may have reduced or absent lower limb pulses.

8 Lipodermatosclerosis usually affects the pretibial or medial aspect of the leg. The development of subcutaneous fibrosis leads to an 'upside-down champagne bottle' appearance in the legs due to narrowing of the distal lower limb. This is associated with poor wound healing due to chronic inflammation and fibrosis; thus, any coexisting venous ulcers may be difficult to treat.

9 The presence of varicose ulcers indicates chronic venous insufficiency. Venous ulcers are often located in the gaiter region and appear shallow and red-based with irregular borders. They are usually painless and can be either chronic or recurrent. Evidence of healed ulcers should be examined for as well. Venous ulcers should be differentiated from an arterial ulcer which is often punched-out in appearance and very painful.

10 Varicose veins reflect underlying venous HTN which can lead to bilateral oedema. Other causes of bilateral lower limb oedema include congestive cardiac failure and liver and renal failure.

11 Squeezing the calf may elicit pain if a DVT is present.

12 Any bleeding from varicose veins should be noted. Although rare, it can progress to haemorrhage, which requires urgent referral.

Investigations

Blood tests are not routinely indicated for initial work-up of varicose veins. The patient undergoes a **venous duplex ultrasound** [1] of the lower limbs which demonstrates the presence of reflux in the **great and small saphenous veins** [2].

1 Symptomatic patients should undergo venous duplex ultrasonography which assesses the nature of the reflux, which in turn affects the choice of treatment. According to the Clinical, aEtiological, Anatomical, and Pathophysiological (CEAP) criteria, varicose veins are ≥3mm in diameter and ultrasound demonstrated reverse flow. When using the ultrasound, the patient should be standing with their leg externally rotated. The superficial, deep and perforator veins can all be visualised. Reflux is defined as the closure of a valve only after 0.5 seconds in the superficial venous system and >1 second in the deep system. Reflux in the distal veins can be elicited by applying compression to the leg above the ultrasound. This acts to force blood back into the feet. For proximal veins, reflux can be identified through the use of Valsalva manoeuvre. Varicose veins can be differentiated from

reticular veins and telangiectasias by the absence of venous reflux on duplex ultrasound. Furthermore, not only is duplex useful to assess venous reflux, but DVT can also be ruled out with this investigation.

2 Veins are described in terms of anatomical location and direction. They can be axial (travelling caudal to cranial) or non-axial. They can be superficial or deep. They can also be communicating (between segments) or perforator (connecting superficial and deep veins). The anatomic classification of veins is important to be aware of, as findings from duplex ultrasonography will impact on treatment options. Examples of superficial veins are the great and small saphenous veins. Examples of deep veins include the popliteal and femoral veins.

Management

Immediate

Clean and dress [1] the ulcer. It is appropriate to trial conservative measures. This includes **skin care, leg elevation, exercise** [2] and **compression therapy** [3]. If the patient experiences recurrent ulcers and **ulcer infections** [4] following 12 months of conservative management, **refer to the vascular surgeons** [5] for consultation and consideration for surgery.

Short-term

Due to chronic symptoms affecting the patient's quality of life, a decision is made to consent and book her for endovenous ablation after discussing the **surgical options** [6]. Prior to surgery, **optimise the patient's overall health** [7]. Ensure **blood glucose levels** [8] are within normal range. After the operation, monitor for **procedure-specific complications** [9] and **general complications** [10]. Aim for **early mobility** [11] as tolerated, but avoid strenuous exercise or heavy lifting for 2 weeks. Give **IV fluids** [12] and **analgesia** [13] as required. Review the **surgical site and lower limbs** [14]. The patient can be discharged when **vital signs remain stable** [15] and they **can tolerate oral intake** [16].

Long-term

Follow the patient up in the **outpatient clinic** [17] for monitoring of symptoms and complications. If she has **recurrent symptoms, then further treatment** [18] may be required. Educate her on **lifestyle modifications** [19].

---

[1] Performing a thorough clean of the wound allows optimal healing. Depending on the ulcer, preference and cost, different types of dressings can be used in the various stages of wound healing. Ulcers heal more effectively in a moist environment; hence occlusive dressings are well-suited for such wounds. Non-absorbent, absorbent and debriding are a few of the many dressing types. Contaminated wounds usually require frequent dressing changes. Conversely, clean and dry ulcers should have their dressings changed weekly, as frequent changes remove healthy cells. Apart from infection, other factors to consider in the healing of an ulcer include diabetes, thrombophilia and malnutrition. These conditions should be controlled before considering surgical management. For clean chronic ulcers, skin grafts may be used to accelerate wound healing. However, the ulcer can recur.

[2] Varicose veins and venous ulcers are managed with exercise, limb elevation at rest and compression. Compression must not be used if arterial disease is also suspected. Cleansing of the skin wound is important in preventing infection and worsening of the ulcer. Debridement of dead tissue can be performed surgically or medically using wet and dry dressings and ointments. The purpose of debridement is to convert the wound from a chronic into an acute wound so that the normal stages of healing can be initiated.

[3] Compression bandages or stockings on the legs are used to improve quality of life, prevent progression of varicose veins and improve the healing rates of venous ulcers. It involves wrapping a stocking or bandage from the feet to just below the knee which creates an external pressure that aids the action of the calf muscle pump. If prolonged standing in one place cannot be avoided, compression stockings should be worn. In patients with evidence of continued reflux, compression stockings should be worn in the daytime (wearing at night is unnecessary). In 40–70% of patients, compression therapy results in the healing of chronic venous ulcers within 12 weeks.

[4] If the ulcer is infected with bacteria, antibiotics will be required. Signs of infection include increasing pain, erythema, heat and swelling around the wound (cellulitis). Long-standing ulcers are often colonised by microbes within a biofilm that is adherent to the underlying ulcer bed. Biofilms allow organisms to become more resistant to antibiotics and thus contribute to the poor healing of such ulcers.

[5] A referral should be made to the vascular surgeons if a patient is experiencing symptoms chronically with no response to conservative measures. They will book an appointment with the patient, assess them and consent them for a procedure if deemed appropriate and necessary.

[6] For symptomatic superficial tributary vein insufficiency with or without deep vein insufficiency, phlebectomy or foam sclerotherapy is the first-line treatment. Phlebectomy involves using a needle or small scalpel to remove portions of varicose vein. These stab incisions do not require closure. Foam sclerotherapy refers to the injection of a foamed sclerosant drug into small veins which causes shrinkage of the vessels. Recurrence is possible and requires repeat phlebectomies or sclerotherapy. For insufficiency of the truncal axial veins with or without deep vein insufficiency, endovenous thermal ablation using radiofrequency or laser is considered first line. Energy from radiofrequency causes closure of the vein, while laser results in thrombosis and vein destruction. It is usually performed on the great saphenous vein, anterior accessory saphenous vein or small saphenous vein. These veins can be visualised and accessed under ultrasound guidance.

7 Ensure the patient is systemically well prior to operative treatment in order to optimise postoperative recovery. This includes assessing whether the patient's comorbidities are managed or well controlled (e.g. COPD, cardiovascular disease, diabetes). If not well-controlled, the patient should be referred on to the relevant specialist for management prior to surgery. If the patient is sick (e.g. viral illness) then postponement of surgery should be considered unless it is required urgently.

8 Poorly controlled BGLs impact negatively on postoperative recovery and complicate the management of diabetic medications prior to surgery. Depending on the type of surgery and the patient's blood glucose control, the doctor may choose to continue their medications, cease their medications on the day of surgery or change their medication to insulin (if not already on insulin). The name of the diabetic medication that the patient is taking must be enquired about, as SGLT-2 inhibitors have been shown to cause euglycaemic ketoacidosis.

9 Complications to look out for in venous ablation include endothermal heat-induced thrombosis, phlebitis, skin injury secondary to heat, and paraesthesia. Complications to look out in those receiving foam sclerotherapy include haematoma, allergic reaction to sclerosant, VTE, thrombophlebitis, skin pigmentation and skin necrosis. Skin necrosis is rare and occurs when sclerosant is inadvertently injected outside the vein. It can cause extremely poor cosmetic outcomes. There have been a small number of cases reporting the occurrence of stroke after sclerotherapy treatment. As varicose vein stripping (phlebectomy) requires open surgery, the patient should be monitored for bleeding, infection and injury to the saphenous nerve (leading to paraesthesia).

10 Patients must be monitored postoperatively for any immediate complications of surgery. These include signs of shock (septic or hypovolaemic), infection, reaction to anaesthesia, DVT and PE, urinary retention or renal failure, and postoperative ileus.

11 The patient should mobilise early to keep blood in the legs flowing, which will minimise the risk of developing VTE. Recent surgery and subsequent immobilisation in bed postoperatively are major risk factors for this. Inspect the calves for unilateral swelling and erythema. Palpate the calves to ensure they are not tender. If clinically suspicious, order a Doppler ultrasound of the affected leg to diagnose, and then start the patient on anticoagulation.

12 As the patient is required to fast prior to and during surgery, IV fluids are important in maintaining the patient's fluid balance. Fluid balance can be assessed through history, examination and reading fluid charts. If the patient is hypovolaemic, they may have dry mucous membranes, poor skin turgor, thirst, low BP or tachycardia. The best indicator of fluid balance, however, is urine output so if a patient has an indwelling urinary catheter then that can be used.

13 Analgesia will be given during the patient's hospital stay and upon discharge. Adequate pain management reduces the risk of developing chronic pain symptoms.

14 Review the surgical site to ensure proper closure and that there are no signs of skin infection from the wound.

15 If the patient remains afebrile, is haemodynamically stable and looks well, they are generally well enough to be discharged home. The patient should be advised that if they notice any increased pain, swelling, discharge or fever, they should return to the hospital for assessment and management.

16 The patient must be able to tolerate oral intake prior to discharging home. This is to ensure they continue to stay hydrated, as they are unable to receive IV fluid whilst at home.

17 Ongoing follow-up is important in terms of assessing postoperative and general complications of varicose veins. Some patients are fit and well enough to be managed by their GP, whilst some will require follow-up visits with the vascular surgeons to ensure adequate recovery and resolution of any lingering symptoms. Most patients report a noticeable improvement in their symptoms within the first few weeks after the procedure. Repeat duplex ultrasound is required if symptoms recur. It may take up to 6 months for the full outcome of the intervention to become evident. Patients with varicose veins are at risk of developing long-term chronic venous insufficiency which is predominantly managed through lifestyle factors. Feet and legs should be checked regularly for cracks, sores and changes in colour.

18 In patients with significant recurrence rates leading to deep vein obstruction, specialist referral for stenting or reconstruction of the vein may be considered. The decision for this treatment to occur depends on the patient's symptoms, clinical severity and whether the patient is appropriate for long-term anticoagulation.

19 Patients should be counselled on the modification of lifestyle factors, including increasing physical activity and weight loss. Patients should avoid prolonged periods of standing or sitting. Intermittent leg elevation may be helpful. It is important to educate patients on compliance with wearing compression stockings if they have evidence of deep venous system insufficiency.

INDEX OF CONDITIONS